Intermittent Hypoxia and Human Diseases

Lei Xi • Tatiana V. Serebrovskaya
Editors

Intermittent Hypoxia and Human Diseases

Springer

Editors
Lei Xi, M.D.
Department of Internal Medicine
Virginia Commonwealth University
Richmond
Virginia
USA

Tatiana V. Serebrovskaya, Ph.D., D.Sc.
Bogomoletz Institute of Physiology
National Academy of Sciences
Kiev
Ukraine

ISBN 978-1-4471-2905-9 ISBN 978-1-4471-2906-6 (eBook)
DOI 10.1007/978-1-4471-2906-6
Springer Dordrecht Heidelberg New York London

Library of Congress Control Number: 2012937844

British Library Cataloguing in Publication Data
A catalogue record for this book is available from the British Library

Printed on acid-free paper

Springer is part of Springer Science+Business Media (www.springer.com)

Foreword

What is "intermittent hypoxia"? Does it play pathogenic roles in disease states, such as sleep-disordered breathing (sleep apnea), chronic pulmonary disease, cardiovascular disease, and cancer? Or, quite to the contrary, does exposure to intermittent hypoxia induce protective responses? As the 25 chapters of this excellent collection attest, "intermittent hypoxia" means different things to different investigators. Depending upon what is meant by this phrase, and in what context it occurs, the effect may be detrimental or beneficial.

In some cases, "intermittent hypoxia" refers to periods (up to several hours) of hypoxia that are followed by periods (again lasting hours) of normoxia. During these hypoxic episodes, the degradation of hypoxia-inducible factor 1α (HIF-1α) is inhibited, and the protein accumulates, dimerizes with HIF-1β, binds to hypoxia response elements, and activates the transcription of several hundred genes in each cell. Upon reoxygenation, HIF-1α is rapidly degraded, but the mRNAs and their translation products will persist for variable periods of time ranging from hours to days, depending upon their individual half-lives. The important point is that in these contexts, HIFs accumulate only during the periods of hypoxia.

In contrast, the intermittent hypoxia associated with sleep-disordered breathing consists of short periods of hypoxia lasting 15–30 s, followed by periods of reoxygenation lasting several minutes, with many cycles of hypoxia and reoxygenation occurring throughout the night. In this context, it is hypoxia and reoxygenation, rather than hypoxia *per se*, that is the stimulus for HIF-1 activation. Whereas continuous hypoxia increases HIF-1α protein levels by inhibition of prolyl hydroxylases leading to decreased ubiquitination-dependent degradation, intermittent hypoxia not only inhibits the hydroxylases but also induces increased HIF-1α synthesis by activating the mammalian target of rapamycin (mTOR). As a result, HIF-1α levels remain persistently elevated in between episodes of intermittent hypoxia and for several hours afterwards.

At the moment, the field of intermittent hypoxia research is at risk of collapsing under the weight of imprecise terminology. To distinguish between these various contexts, I suggest that the first context described, in which HIFs accumulate strictly during the periods of hypoxia, be known as "cyclic hypoxia" to distinguish it from the second context, which will retain the title "intermittent hypoxia." Both of these contexts should be distinguished from "continuous hypoxia," in which a single episode of hypoxia lasting minutes, hours, or days induces a response. As the reader tackles each chapter of this superb volume, it may be useful to ask the following questions: How do the authors define "intermittent hypoxia"? What cells are being exposed to this stimulus? What molecular pathways are mediating the observed pathological (maladaptive) or physiological (adaptive) response?

Baltimore, USA — Gregg L. Semenza, M.D., Ph.D.

Preface

> The beginning, middle, and end of the birth, growth, and perfection of whatever we behold is from contraries, by contraries, and to contraries; and whatever contrariety is, there is action and reaction, there is motion, diversity, multitude, and order, there are degrees, succession, and vicissitude.
>
> Giordano Bruno
> (Italian philosopher and astronomer, 1548–1600)

It might be hard to find a better example for the duality in life science than the effects of intermittent hypoxia on living organisms including human bodies. As the above-quoted wisdom of the controversial philosopher and astronomer Giordano Bruno (1548–1600), this universe and its miniature form – our life – are full of contraries and complexity. For these very reasons, we should not be surprised by the divergent or even controversial findings and notions surrounding the scientific field of intermittent hypoxia.

Dealing with these long-standing controversies and new concepts, this book provides an open forum for the most updated scientific understanding of both adaptive (beneficial) and maladaptive (detrimental) responses to intermittent hypoxia and their potential pathogenic and prophylactic roles in the development and progression of major human diseases. A total of 68 prominent experts from 9 countries (i.e., Austria, China, Germany, Israel, Russia, Spain, Turkey, Ukraine, and USA) have contributed their most updated research data and perspectives in both basic and translational aspects of intermittent hypoxia. This is our continued effort in promoting the translational research on intermittent hypoxia and its clinical applications in disease prevention and treatment around the globe. In this book, we paid special attention to several important topics related to intermittent hypoxia that have not been covered by our previous book – *Intermittent Hypoxia: From Molecular Mechanisms to Clinical Applications* (Nova Science Publishers, 2009; ISBN 9781608761272). For instance, from the 25 chapters of the present book, readers can find a number of new topics concerning the effects of intermittent hypoxia on cardiac arrhythmias, atherosclerosis, chronic obstructive pulmonary diseases, reproductive and occupational disorders, as well as cancer. This monograph is highly disease-oriented where all the fundamental research findings are selectively presented as mechanistic explanations of a particular human disease. Therefore, our present book is especially prepared for the interests of clinicians, allied healthcare professionals, athletic trainers, and translational medical researchers.

We like to take this opportunity to express our sincerest appreciation to each of the contributing authors for answering our calls and devoting their best effort to write their outstanding chapters for this book. We are truly honored by having a foreword written by Prof. Gregg Semenza (The Johns Hopkins Medical Institutions, USA), one of the world-renowned authorities in hypoxia biology and medicine. Our special thanks to Mr. Grant Weston (senior editor) of Springer-London for his constant encouragement, support, and extraordinary patience throughout the planning, editorial, and publication phases of this book.

Finally, we are indebted to our beloved families for their understanding and tolerance during the countless long hours we had spent at home for writing and editing this monograph in the past year. Without their sacrifice and moral support, the completion of this seemingly endless and overwhelming task would not be possible.

Richmond, Virginia, USA Lei Xi, M.D.
Kiev, Ukraine Tatiana V. Serebrovskaya, Ph.D., D.Sc.

Contents

Part I

Intermittent Hypoxia and Cardiovascular Disorders

1 Sleep-Disordered Breathing and Cardiac Arrhythmias: Role of Intermittent Hypoxia

Thomas Bitter

Abstract
Focusing on the role of intermittent hypoxia, this chapter intends to describe the association between sleep-disordered breathing and cardiac arrhythmias in specific. By showing pathophysiologies of different types of sleep-disordered breathing, we try to give an understanding of why sleep apnea is a common phenomenon among cardiac patients. Moreover, this chapter is intended to point out cardiovascular consequences and mechanisms, which are involved in an enhanced myocardial irritability and predispose patients with evident sleep-disordered breathing to suffer from cardiac arrhythmias. We thereby especially focus on intermittent hypoxia and its major role in the proarrhythmia pathological process. Finally, translating evidences from bench to bedside, we present clinical data that elucidate associations between sleep-disordered breathing and ventricular arrhythmias, atrial fibrillation, or conduction disturbances.

Abbreviations

Afib	Atrial fibrillation
AHI	Apnea-hypopnea index
BMI	Body mass index
CI	Cardiac index
CPAP	Continuous positive airway pressure
CRP	C-reactive protein
CSA	Central sleep apnea
CSR	Cheyne-Stokes respiration
LAD	Left atrial diameter
LVEDD	Left ventricular end-diastolic diameter
NO	Nitric oxide
NREM	Non-rapid eye movement
NT-proBNP	N-terminal pro–brain natriuretic peptide
NYHA	New York Heart Association
OSA	Obstructive sleep apnea
PAP	Pulmonary artery pressure
pCO_2	Partial pressure of carbon dioxide
PCWP	Pulmonary capillary wedge pressure
PG	Cardiorespiratory polygraphy
pO_2	Partial pressure of oxygen
PSG	Cardiorespiratory polysomnography
PV	Pulmonary vein
PVI	Pulmonary vein isolation
RAAS	Renin-angiotensin-aldosterone system
REM	Rapid eye movement
RFCA	Radiofrequency catheter ablation
ROS	Reactive oxygen species
SCD	Sudden cardiac death
SDB	Sleep-disordered breathing
SR	Sinus rhythm
TNF	Tumor necrosis factor

T. Bitter
Department of Cardiology, Heart and Diabetes Center North Rhine-Westphalia, Ruhr University Bochum, Georgstraße 11, D-32545 Bad Oeynhausen, Germany
e-mail: akleemeyer@hdz-nrw.de

L. Xi, T.V. Serebrovskaya (eds.), *Intermittent Hypoxia and Human Diseases*,
DOI 10.1007/978-1-4471-2906-6_1, © Springer-Verlag London 2012

1.1 Introduction

Cardiac arrhythmias, either evolving from the atrium or the ventricle, are of major socioeconomic impact. Atrial arrhythmias, most commonly presenting as atrial fibrillation (Afib), have shown an increasing prevalence and hospitalization rate over the past decades which is expected to grow even further [1]. For the individual, existence of atrial fibrillation is not only accompanied by symptoms leading to subjective and objective exercise capacity impairment, but also means a fivefold increase in stroke risk as well as an increased mortality risk [2, 3]. Conduction disturbances and moreover ventricular tachyarrhythmias on the other hand leading to sudden cardiac death (SCD) are a major contributor to mortality in the industrialized nations [4].

1.2 Pathophysiology of Cardiac Arrhythmias

1.2.1 Supraventricular Arrhythmias

The pathophysiology of cardiac arrhythmias involves the interaction of a triggering event and an arrhythmogenic substrate that induces electrical instability. In atrial fibrillation, profibrillatory changes of the atrial myocardium including atrial size enlargement, scarring, and fibroses are associated with conduction slowing and refractory periods lengthening, thus serving as a substrate [5]. In addition, rapid atrial rates such as those during periods of fibrillation increase myocyte calcium load. This induces adaptive mechanisms, for instance, a reduction in activity or downregulation of calcium channels which shorten atrial refractory period and thereby perpetuates atrial fibrillation as well [6, 7]. The most important initial trigger source for intermittent Afib was identified to be the muscular sleeve of the pulmonary veins. Compared to the neighboring left atrial muscle or the muscular sleeve of the pulmonary veins in patients without atrial fibrillation, this area presents with different electrophysiologic properties (e.g., shorter refractory periods) [8]. With ongoing remodeling, multiple reentrant wavelets occur, propagating in different directions, hence further promoting structural changes.

1.2.2 Ventricular Arrhythmias

Ventricular tachycardia often degenerates into ventricular fibrillation followed by asystole or pulseless electrical activity, resulting in sudden cardiac death. Two conditions seem to be of major importance in this respect: scar or fibrosis of different etiologies (cardiomyopathies, myocarditis, myocardial infarction, etc.) can act as an anatomic substrate initiating ventricular tachycardia, without active or clinically obvious myocardial ischemia [9]. Scar or fibrosis may contain regions with vital myocytes with slow conduction that can give rise to reentry circuits and cause sustained ventricular tachycardia [10]. Reentry is considered to be a major mechanism responsible for ventricular arrhythmias, though regional changes in automaticity, as well as triggered activity due to afterdepolarizations, are important as well [11].

In patients without myocardial scars or fibrosis, arrhythmias can be triggered by acute or chronic myocardial ischemia. Alternatively, during acute myocardial ischemia, cessation of blood flow results in redistribution of a number of ions across the cardiomyocyte membrane, including the net cellular K^+ loss and subsequent extracellular K^+ accumulation that result in intracellular Na^+ and Ca^{++} gain. This complex interplay between myocardial ischemia resulting in ionic imbalances, reduction in tissue pH, and neurohumoral changes contributes to electrophysiological changes that result in slowed conduction, reduced excitability and prolonged refractoriness, cell-to-cell uncoupling, and the generation of spontaneous electrical activity [12]. This process of arrhythmogenesis is probably further facilitated by metabolic changes including accumulation of free fatty acids and their metabolites, formation of lysophosphoglycerides, and impaired myocardial glycolysis [13].

1.3 Sleep-Disordered Breathing and Arrhythmias

1.3.1 Consequences of Sleep-Disordered Breathing

Since in 1973, Lown and coworkers investigated day-night cycles with respect to the occurrence of premature ventricular beats and proposed a protective effect of sleep on ventricular irritability; enormous efforts have been spent on explaining this phenomenon [14]. There is yet conceiving evidence that predominance of parasympathetic influence is one of the main factors [15]. Normal sleep consists of two main categories. With a 75% proportion of sleep duration, non-rapid eye movement (NREM) sleep forms the prevailing entity and is associated with an increase in parasympathetic nerve system activity and a decrease in

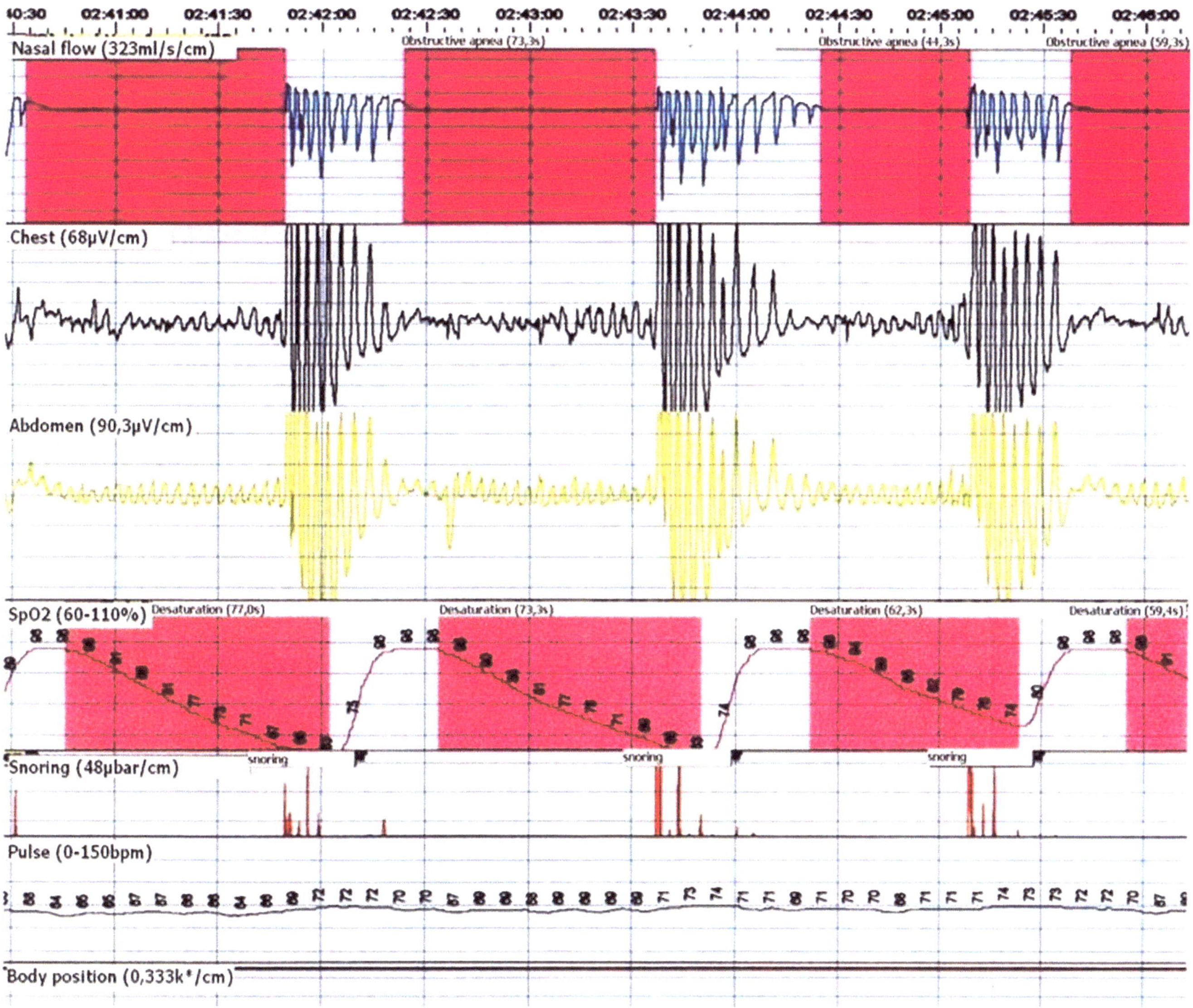

Fig. 1.1 Example of obstructive sleep apnea, diagnosed by cardiorespiratory polygraphy

sympathetic nerve tone activity. This in turn leads to a lowering of heart rate, catecholamine serum levels, vascular tone, blood pressure levels, and systemic vascular resistance [16]. Rapid eye movement sleep (REM) on the other hand is dominated by sympathetic tone, which means that with transition from NREM to REM sleep, all factors mentioned above increase.

Sleep-disordered breathing (SDB), most commonly presenting as either obstructive sleep apnea (OSA) or central sleep apnea (CSA) with Cheyne-Stokes respiration (CSR), has been recognized as comorbidity with potential interaction and impact on progression and outcome of patients with cardiovascular disease, probably by interrupting normal sleep pattern due to intermittent hypoxemias and consequent sympathetic activation. Obstructive sleep apnea affects 2–4% of the general population [17]. OSA can be summarized as a syndrome of elevated airway resistance due to nocturnal obstruction of upper airways, leading to hypopneas and/or apneas (Fig. 1.1). Apnea is defined as a ≥90% reduction of airflow lasting for ≥10 s. Hypopnea is defined as a ≥10 s lasting, ≥30% reduction of airflow accompanied by a ≥4% oxygen desaturation/arousal or a ≥10 s lasting, ≥50% reduction of airflow with a ≥3% desaturation or an arousal [18]. "Arousal" describes a transition from sleep to a state of wakefulness for at least 3 s and is usually blamed upon an increase in sympathetic drive as a result of intermittent hypoxemia in apneic or hypopneic phases of sleep-disordered breathing.

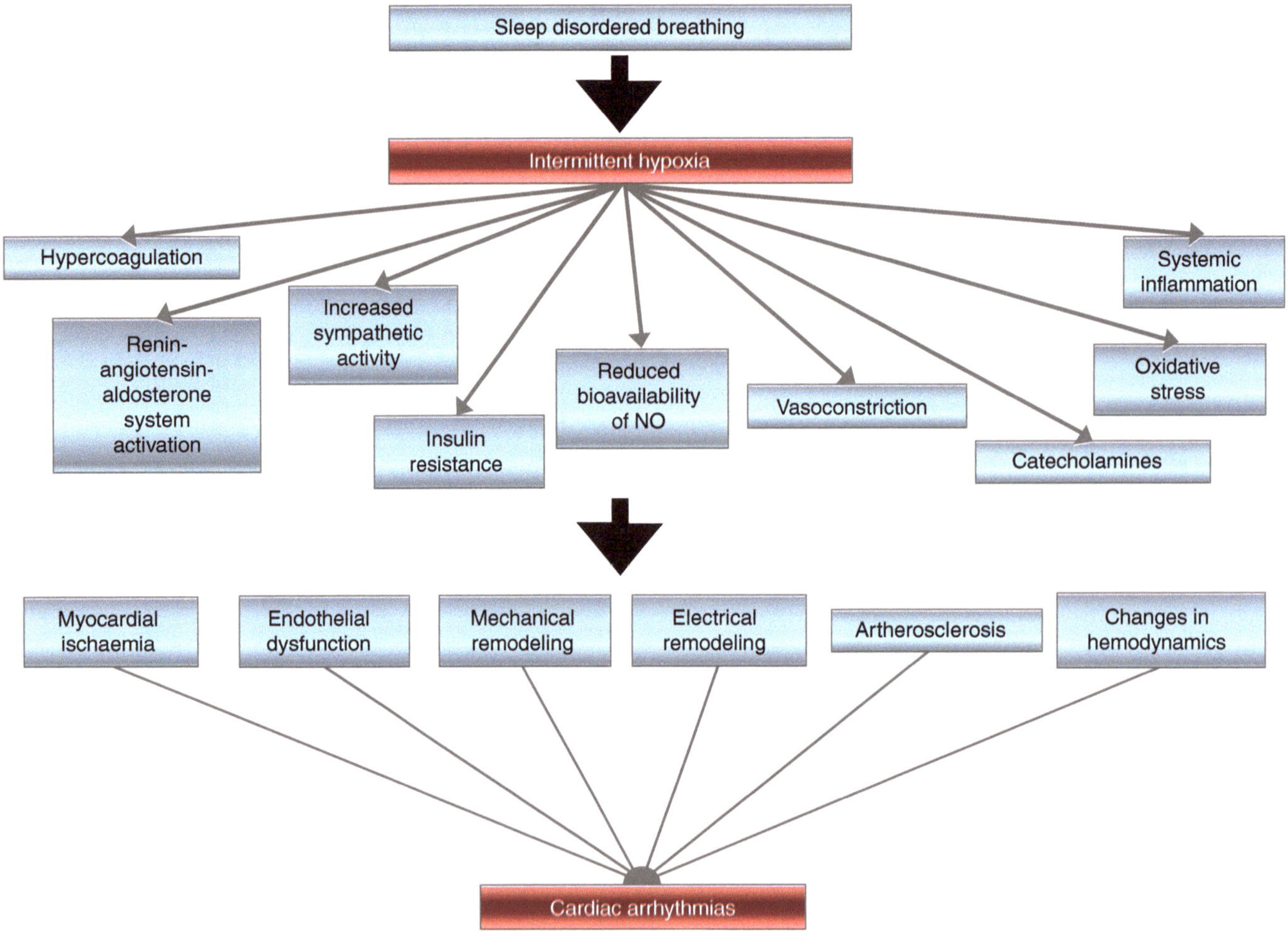

Fig. 1.2 Pathophysiological mechanisms linking obstructive sleep apnea to cardiac arrhythmias

1.3.2 Vasoconstriction

Intermittent hypoxemias per se as well as consequential increase in sympathetic nerve system activity or arousals have major impact on the cardiovascular system (Fig. 1.2). Even though severe hypoxemias are known to have a local vasodilatative effect via endothelial vasoactive substances such as nitric oxide (NO), adenosine, and eicosanoid, cycles of hypoxemias as well as carbon-dioxide retention in obstructive sleep apnea patients are rather associated with systemic vasoconstriction, potentially leading to ischemia as an underlying mechanism for the occurrence of arrhythmias [19, 20]. Activation of the sympathetic nerve system appears to be a key factor in this setting, thus leading to increased plasma levels of catecholamines and a reduced α- and β_2-adrenergic vascular response [21–23]. In addition, levels of angiotensin II and aldosterone are elevated in OSA patients as well [24, 25]. As angiotensin II induces vasoconstriction via AT_1 receptor, enhanced vasoconstrictor sensitivity to angiotensin II, as seen in OSA patients, additionally augments vasoconstriction [26].

1.3.3 Renin-Angiotensin-Aldosterone System

The renin-angiotensin-aldosterone system (RAAS) is also involved in electrical and mechanical remodeling. Likely due to an increase of intracellular calcium concentration, due to an augmented calcium influx via L-type calcium channels, and an increased availability of calcium contained in the sarcoplasmic reticulum, angiotensin II was shown to shorten the refractory period [27, 28]. In vitro, angiotensin II increases protein synthesis in myocardial fibroblasts and myocytes. Together with an increase in coronary artery permeability, allowing diffusion of growth factors into the myocardial interstitium, it promotes proliferation and growth [29–31]. On the other hand, angiotensin II causes oxidative stress with subsequent induction of apoptosis at both the endothelial and myocyte levels, and it is known to cause necrosis and fibrosis through its cytotoxic effect on cardiac myocytes [32]. In addition, increased aldosterone serum levels stimulate collagen synthesis by myocardial fibroblasts and may also play a role in myocyte death through their effect on electrolyte balance [33, 34].

1.3.4 Endothelin, Oxidative Stress

Endothelin-1, a potent vasoconstrictive neuropeptide, produced by endothelin-converting enzyme from big endothelin-1 as precursor peptide may also initiate ischemia via vasoconstriction. Studies suggest increased serum level of either endothelin-1 or big endothelin-1 to be found in OSA patients [35, 36]. Upregulation of endothelin-1 production may be mediated by a reduced NO bioavailability that was shown to inhibit conversion from big endothelin-1 to endothelin-1.

As briefly mentioned, NO has been recognized as an important mediator of endothelium-dependent vasodilatation. Several studies observed an altered vasodilatation in OSA patients as well as reduced plasma levels of NO as the possible underlying mechanism [37–39]. On intermittent hypoxemic periods, formations of free radicals or reactive oxygen species (ROS) emerge and react with NO to produce peroxynitrite, thereby diminishing bioavailability of NO [40, 41].

1.3.5 Inflammation

Another possible link between sleep apnea-derived hypoxemias and an enhanced myocardial irritability leading to arrhythmias is inflammation. An association with parameters of cell adhesion (CD15, CD11c), increased intracellular ROS, and increased adherence to human endothelial cells on monocytes has been demonstrated for OSA patients. Following the thesis that initiation of leukocyte-endothelial cell adherence can contribute to a critical impairment of endothelial function as well as atherosclerosis with consecutive hemodynamic impairment and ischemia [42], in addition, OSA patients face an increased expression of C-reactive protein, interleukin 6, interleukin 8, as well as functional and phenotypic changes of CD4 and CD8 T cells, followed by an increase in tumor necrosis factor (TNF) α and interleukin 4 as well as a decrease of interleukin 10 expression [43, 44]. Among these parameters, TNF-α, CRP, fibrinogen, as well as parameters of blood viscosity and platelet coagulation that were also found elevated in OSA patients seem to have particular importance as predictors for cardiovascular events [45–48].

1.3.6 Metabolic Dysregulation

Finally, OSA-related factors contribute to the development of metabolic dysregulation, for instance, insulin and leptin resistance [49, 50]. Increased sympathetic activity due to sleep fragmentation and intermittent hypoxemias alters hypothalamic-pituitary-adrenocortical axis function that in addition to the aforementioned changes in oxidative and inflammatory pathways is involved in insulin resistance and impaired pancreatic beta-cell function [50, 51]. Diabetes and metabolic syndrome are not only known major risk factors for coronary artery disease and atherosclerosis but also are independently associated with sudden cardiac death [52].

1.3.7 Intrathoracic Pressure Alterations

Inefficient respiratory excursions, a regular occurrence in the apneic or hypopneic phases of OSA, alter the transmural pressure and volume relations. This does not only lead to increased sheer stress with subsequent mechanical remodeling but also triggers extension-sensitive ion channels and hence promotes enhanced myocardial irritability [53].

1.3.8 Cheyne-Stokes Respiration

Cheyne-Stokes respiration as a specific entity of central sleep apnea has recently been demonstrated a highly prevalent comorbidity in patients with either systolic or diastolic heart failure [54–56]. Impaired hemodynamics (reduced cardiac index (CI), increased pulmonary capillary wedge pressure (PCWP), and enhanced pulmonary artery pressure (PAP)) that stimulate pulmonary vagal irritant receptors (J-receptors), circulatory delay, and/or increased sympathetic activity as typical consequences following congestive heart failure lead to a chemoreceptor sensitization and promote respiratory instability (Fig. 1.3) [57–59]. This in turn is associated with subsequent hyperventilation that, due to prevailing cortical control, does not become evident under stable conditions during daytime, but can be evoked with exercise testing or during sleep [57, 58, 60, 61]. As hyperventilation is accompanied by a loss in partial pressure of

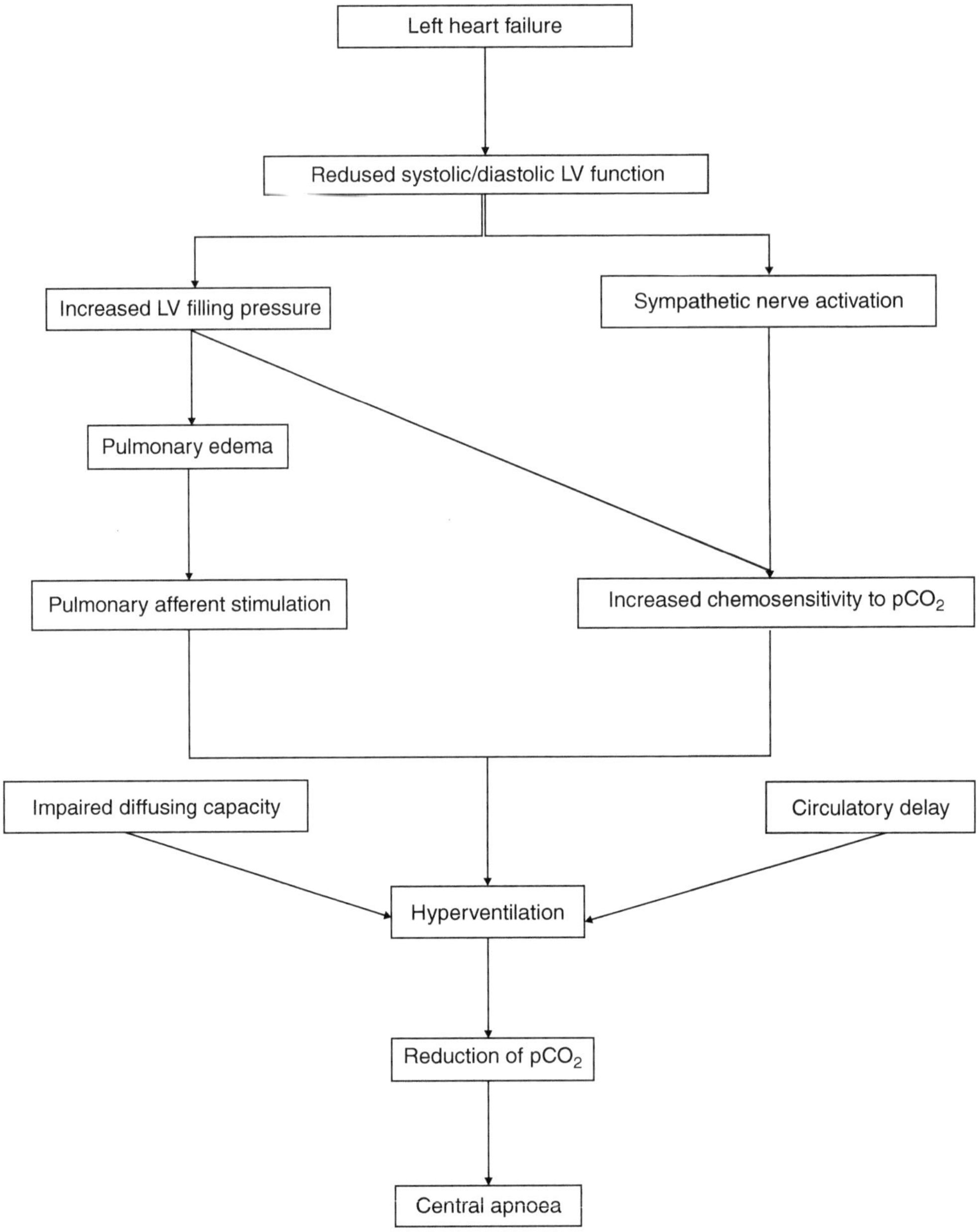

Fig. 1.3 Pathophysiological model of Cheyne-Stokes respiration in congestive heart failure

CO_2, hyperventilation periods are interrupted by intermittent hypopneas or apneas (Fig. 1.4). Therefore, Cheyne-Stokes respiration has been defined as at least 10 min of continuous cycles of waxing and waning tidal volumes with periods of hyperventilation separated by at least five central apneas or hypopneas per hour [18].

Unlike OSA, CSR has often been regarded as a marker of heart failure severity only [55]. Hence, pathophysiological consequences have not been investigated that thoroughly during past decades. This attitude has changed since CSR was identified as an independent prognostic predictor in patients with CHF [62]. Now there is conceiving evidence that marked sympathetic activations do occur with CSR as well, thus promoting adverse cardiovascular effects ending up in a vicious circle with progression of CSR with further impairment of cardiac function [63–65]. For hypoxemic periods are less extensive in CSR patients, recent investigations revealed sympathetic activation mainly associated with hyperventilation periods [64, 66]. Therefore, similar consequences for the cardiovascular system in patients with CSR compared to those with OSA can be assumed, even though this is not proven, yet.

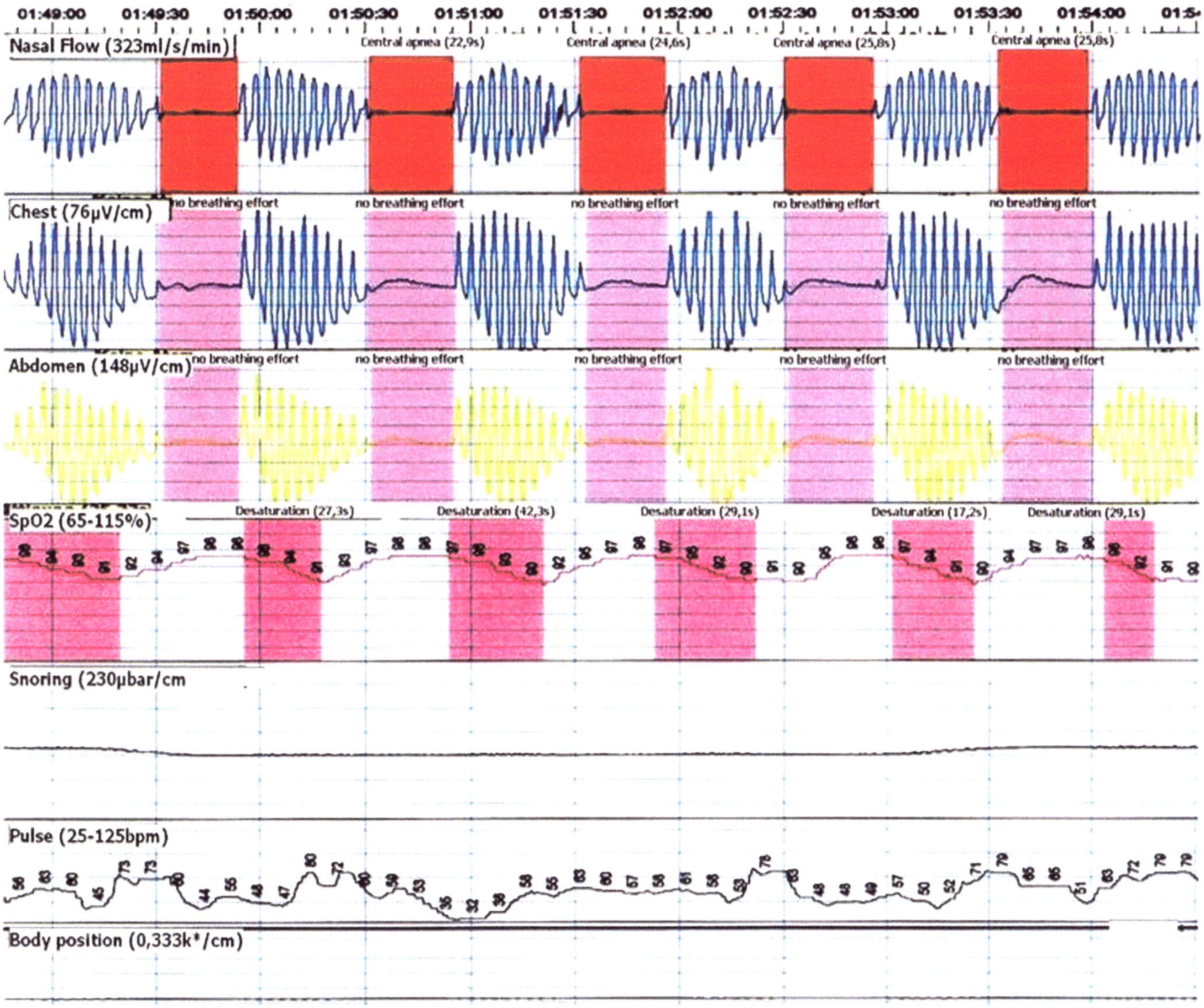

Fig. 1.4 Example of Cheyne-Stokes respiration, diagnosed by cardiorespiratory polygraphy

1.4 Clinical Evidence

1.4.1 Ventricular Tachycardia

Translating pathophysiological considerations to clinical results, several investigators found obstructive sleep apnea associated with a higher frequency of ventricular ectopia [67–69]. Among 228 subjects with sleep-disordered breathing compared to 338 patients without SDB, the odds ratio for complex ventricular ectopy (OR 1.74) as well as nonsustained ventricular tachycardia (OR 3.40) was markedly increased [69]. A recent study in 2,911 elder men also found Cheyne-Stokes respiration as an independent risk factor for complex ventricular ectopias (OR 1.55) [70]. Lanfranchi investigated 47 heart failure patients and found a higher incidence of nonsustained ventricular arrhythmias among patients with CSR [71]. In addition, a high prevalence of SDB (60%) was demonstrated in patients with known ventricular tachycardias or frequent premature ventricular beats who had a preserved systolic left ventricular function, supporting the hypothesis that SDB is an independent risk factor for the occurrence of malignant ventricular arrhythmias [72].

All studies investigated small numbers of patients and nevertheless presented unique results, outlining OSA and CSA being independently associated with ventricular tachycardias. We recently conducted a study in which 255 patients with congestive heart failure 6 months after implantation of a cardiac resynchronization device with cardioverter-defibrillator were included. After a follow-up period of 48 months, the event-free survival period from the first detected malignant arrhythmia (nonsustained ventricular tachycardia, sustained ventricular tachycardia, ventricular fibrillation) was found shorter in patients with either obstructive or central sleep apnea with Cheyne-Stokes respiration compared to patients without sleep-disordered breathing, and an independent association with both OSA (OR 1.69) and CSA (OR 2.06) was found [73]. However, ventricular ectopias and nonsustained ventricular tachycardias are of little predictive value with respect to life-threatening arrhythmias [74]. Thus, an exacerbated ventricular irritability per se will be of little impact with respect to an impaired prognosis.

Anyway, a known peak in sudden cardiac death during the night for obstructive sleep apnea patients has been previously recognized. Reviewing polysomnograms of 112 patients that died suddenly from cardiac cause, OSA patients presented with an increased risk for sudden cardiac death during sleeping hours (midnight to 5:59 a.m.), in contrast to the nadir of sudden cardiac death between 6 a.m. and 11:59 a.m. in the general population [75]. Because life-threatening arrhythmias are of significant interest in this respect, a short-term study investigated the effect of sleep-disordered breathing in 75 patients with heart failure and implanted cardioverter-defibrillator for 180 days postimplant. SDB was identified as independent predictor for life-threatening arrhythmias; however, no distinction was made between OSA and CSA [76]. Staniforth demonstrated an increased hazard for life-threatening arrhythmias in 101 heart failure patients with suspected CSA after an average follow-up of 6 months [77]. Unfortunately, diagnosis was based on pulse oximetry only, and multivariate analyses were not performed, so the impact of this study remains unclear. Our data from 255 patients, investigated by cardiorespiratory polygraphy initially and followed for 48 months, provided similar results. Again OSA (OR 2.10) and CSA (OR 3.41) were found independently associated with a shorter event-free survival period to first malignant ventricular arrhythmias requiring appropriate cardioverter-defibrillator therapy (antitachycardia pacing and/or shock) [73].

1.4.2 Atrial Fibrillation

Another important field of cardiac arrhythmias, in which sleep-disordered breathing is of major importance, is atrial fibrillation. A study published in 2004 reported a 49% prevalence of OSA in 152 patients with atrial fibrillation prior to cardioversion [78]. A major limitation was that diagnosis of OSA was based upon a questionnaire investigation only. Nevertheless, we found a similar prevalence of OSA in a study of 150 patients with persistent atrial fibrillation undergoing cardiorespiratory polygraphy [79]. In a younger cohort (mean age 55 years), Stevenson and colleagues also demonstrated a higher prevalence of SDB in patients with either persistent or paroxysmal atrial fibrillation compared to age- and sex-matched controls as well as an association of higher atrial fibrillation burden in patients with paroxysmal atrial fibrillation and evident sleep-disordered breathing compared to those without [80]. A link to aforementioned pathophysiological concepts was conducted recently by demonstrating that hypercapnia is associated with a 152% lengthening of effective refractory period promoting an increased vulnerability to AF [81]. Consequently, the incidence of atrial fibrillation among 3,542 patients followed for 16 years was higher in those with OSA and independently associated with the magnitude of nocturnal hypoxemias [78]. In secondary prophylaxis, obstructive sleep apnea was shown to be an independent risk factor for the recurrence of atrial fibrillation in patients with either persistent or paroxysmal atrial fibrillation undergoing cardioversion or invasive ablation therapy [82–84].

Cheyne-Stokes respiration in patients with atrial fibrillation again is less well investigated. In a group of 60 patients with CSA, a proportion of 27% patients presenting with Afib was demonstrated, thus suggesting an association of Afib with CSA [85]. In parallel, we found a 31% prevalence of CSA in patients with persistent Afib despite normal systolic LV function [79]. Data on prognostic implications of CSA in atrial fibrillation are not yet available.

1.4.3 Bradyarrhythmias and Conduction Disturbances

Due to the fact that final evidence for an association between sleep-disordered breathing and bradyarrhythmias is lacking, this paragraph briefly describes possible mechanisms involved and clinical data. Even though sympathetic activation in response to ongoing hypoxic phases is the most commonly addressed consequence of sleep apnea, hypoxic stimulation of the carotid body also results in vagotonia with subsequent bradycardia [86]. However, individual heart rate response to hypoxia was shown to depend upon intrinsic hypoxic chemosensitivity and the relative influence of hypoxia on vagal and sympathetic influence on the sinoatrial node [87]. Therefore, clinical investigations on the prevalence of bradyarrhythmias and conduction disturbances revealed nonuniform results. A recent study in 2,911 participants in the Outcome of Sleep Disorders in Older Men Study as well as results from the Sleep Heart Health Study did not display a statistical significance in occurrence of heart blocks or sinus pauses >3 s among patients with or without sleep-disordered breathing [69, 70]. These findings are different from those of several other investigations that found severe bradyarrhythmias more frequently among patients with sleep-disordered breathing compared to those without [67, 88, 89].

1.5 Treatment Effects

1.5.1 Obstructive Sleep Apnea

In obstructive sleep apnea, continuous positive airway pressure (CPAP) has proven as the therapy of choice [90]. As described before, OSA occurs when the upper airway becomes narrow as the muscles relax naturally during sleep. The CPAP machine stops this phenomenon by delivering a stream of compressed air via a hose to a nose mask or full-face mask, splinting the airway (keeping it open under air pressure) so that unobstructed breathing becomes possible, thus preventing apneas and hypopneas. In patients with OSA and cardiovascular disease, CPAP was shown, for instance, to improve arterial hypertension, outcome after coronary intervention, as well as overall prognosis in heart failure patients [91–93]. With respect to cardiac arrhythmias, Ryan et al. found a significant reduction of ventricular premature beats in ten heart failure patients receiving CPAP versus eight controls. In contrast, Craig and coworkers did not report a significant decrease in dysrhythmia frequency among 40 treated versus 43 subtherapeutic controls with moderate to severe OSA, but no CHF [94, 95]. Several uncontrolled studies revealed sinus bradycardia, and pauses were significantly reduced with CPAP therapy [88, 96, 97]. With respect to atrial fibrillation, it was shown that CPAP is able to restore the risk of recurrence after atrial fibrillation from 82% in 27 untreated to 42% in 12 treated patients [82].

1.5.2 Cheyne-Stokes Respiration

Focusing on CSR, neither data on therapeutic approaches to reduce life-threatening arrhythmias nor on effectively improving prognosis are available. The CANPAP trial investigated 258 heart failure patients with reduced left ventricular ejection fraction and CSR. One hundred and twenty-eight were randomized to receive CPAP therapy, whereas the remaining 130 did not. The authors could not find a reduced mortality of the treatment group 24 months after [98]. However, a prognostic benefit could be demonstrated for those patients with an AHI <15/h during therapy, a goal which is difficult to achieve with CPAP [99, 100]. Therefore, irrespective of previously published positive results that demonstrated a reduced ventricular irritability in CHF patients with CSR undergoing CPAP therapy, novel ventilator devices have recently been introduced [101]. Adaptive servoventilation (ASV) represents a bi-level ventilation system with automatic, anticyclic adaption of pressure support, which appears favorable in improving the apnea and hypopnea index compared to other therapy modalities in patients with Cheyne-Stokes respiration [100]. Recent investigations revealed positive effects on cardiovascular function in patients with heart failure and either reduced or preserved left-ventricular ejection fraction [102–104]. However, data on cardiac arrhythmias in patients with CSR undergoing ASV are rare so far. We therefore performed a large-scale study investigating a total number of 403 patients with congestive heart failure and either untreated moderate to severe CSR, treated CSR, or mild or no CSR. After 48 months, event-free survival period to detected cardiac arrhythmias as well as appropriate cardioverter-defibrillator therapies, adjusted for all significant covariates, was significantly shorter in patients with untreated CSR, but not in patients with treated CSR compared to those with mild or moderate CSR [73].

1.6 Summary

In summary, Cheyne-Stokes respiration and especially obstructive sleep apnea with subsequent intermittent hypoxemias and sympathetic activation can be regarded as a significant risk factor for cardiac arrhythmias. Different acute mechanisms following apneic phases, such as oxidative stress, inflammation, vasoconstriction, intrathoracic pressure changes, and metabolic changes, may serve as potential triggers for arrhythmias. Likewise, they promote electrical and mechanical remodeling of the heart and cardiovascular system as potential arrhythmogenic substrates.

References

1. Nieuwlaat R, Capucci A, Camm JA, et al. Atrial fibrillation management: a prospective survey in ESC member countries. The Euro Heart Survey on Atrial Fibrillation. Eur Heart J. 2005;26:2422–34.
2. Kannel WB, Wolf PA, Benjamin EJ, et al. Prevalence, incidence, prognosis and predisposing conditions for atrial fibrillation: population-based estimates. Am J Cardiol. 1998;82:2N–9.
3. Wolf PA, Dawber TR, Thomas HR, et al. Epidemiologic assessment of chronic atrial fibrillation and the risk of stroke: the Framingham study. Neurology. 1978;28:973–7.
4. Zheng ZJ, Croft JB, Giles WH, et al. Sudden cardiac death in the United States, 1989 to 1998. Circulation. 2001;104:2158–63.
5. Sanders P, Morton JB, Davidson NC, et al. Electrical remodelling of the atria in congestive heart failure: electrophysiologic and electroanatomic mapping in humans. Circulation. 2003;108:1461–8.
6. Courtemanche M, Ramirez RJ, Nattel S. Ionic mechanisms underlying human atrial action potential properties: insights from a mathematical model. Am J Physiol. 1998;275:301–21.
7. Lai LP, Su MJ, Lin JL, et al. Down-regulation of L-type calcium channel and sarcoplasmic reticular Ca^{2+}-ATPase mRNA in human atrial fibrillation without significant change in the mRNA of ryanodine receptor, calsequestrin and phospholamban: an insight into the mechanism of atrial electrical remodelling. J Am Coll Cardiol. 1999;33:1231–7.
8. Haissaguerre M, Jais P, Shah DC, et al. Spontaneous initiation of atrial fibrillation by ectopic beats originating in the pulmonary veins. N Engl J Med. 1998;339:659–66.
9. Ashikaga H, Sasano T, Dong J, et al. Magnetic resonance-based anatomical analysis of scar-related ventricular tachycardia: implications for catheter ablation. Circ Res. 2007;101:939–47.

10. van Dessel PF, de Bakker JM, van Hemel NM, et al. Pace mapping of postinfarction scar to detect ventricular tachycardia exit sites and zones of slow conduction. J Cardiovasc Electrophysiol. 2001;12: 662–70.
11. Vermeulen JT, McGuire MA, Opthof T, et al. Triggered activity and automaticity in ventricular trabeculae of the failing human and rabbit hearts. Cardiovasc Res. 1994;28:125–8.
12. Owens LM, Fralix TA, Murphy E, et al. Correlation of ischemia-induced extracellular ion changes to cell-to-cell electrical uncoupling in isolated blood-perfused rabbit hearts. Experimental Working Group. Circulation. 1996;94:10–3.
13. Pogwizd SM, Corr PB. Mechanisms underlying the development of ventricular fibrillation during early myocardial ischemia. Circ Res. 1990;66:672–95.
14. Lown B, Tykocinski M, Garfein A, et al. Sleep and ventricular premature beats. Circulation. 1973;48:691–701.
15. Crasset V, Mezzetti S, Antoine M, et al. Effects of aging and cardiac denervation on heart rate variability during sleep. Circulation. 2001; 103:84–8.
16. Hobson JA. Current concepts. Sleep: biochemical aspects. N Engl J Med. 1969;281:1468–70.
17. Young T, Palta M, Dempsey J, et al. The occurrence of sleep-disordered breathing among middle-aged adults. N Engl J Med. 1993;328: 1230–5.
18. Iber C, Ancoli-Israel S, Chesson Jr AL, et al. The AASM manual for the scoring of sleep and associated events: rules, terminology and technical specifications. AASM manual for scoring sleep. Westchester, Illinois: American Academy of Sleep Medicine; 2007.
19. Fletcher FC. Effect of hypoxia on sympathetic activity and blood pressure. Respir Physiol. 2000;119:189–97.
20. Brooks D, Horner LJ, Kozar LF, et al. Obstructive sleep apnea as a cause of systemic hypertension. Evidences from a canine model. J Clin Invest. 1997;99:106–9.
21. Imadojemu VA, Mawji Z, Kunselman A, et al. Sympathetic chemoreflex responses in obstructive sleep apnea and effects of continuous positive airway pressure therapy. Chest. 2007;131:1406–13.
22. Dimsdale JE, Ziegler MG, Ancoli-Israel S, et al. The effect of sleep apnea on plasma and urinary catecholamines. Sleep. 1995;18:377–81.
23. Mills PJ, Kennedy BP, Loredo JS, et al. Effects of nasal continuous positive airway pressure and oxygen supplementation on norepinephrine kinetics and cardiovascular responses in obstructive sleep apnea. J Appl Physiol. 2006;100:343–8.
24. Calhoun DA, Nishizaka MK, Zaman MA, et al. Aldosterone excretion among subjects with resistant hypertension and symptoms of sleep apnea. Chest. 2004;125:112–7.
25. Moller DS, Lind P, Strunge B, et al. Abnormal vasoactive hormones and 24-hour blood pressure in obstructive sleep apnea. Am J Hypertens. 2003;16:274–80.
26. Kraiczi H, Hedner J, Peker Y, et al. Increased vasoconstrictor sensitivity in obstructive sleep apnea. J Appl Physiol. 2000;89:493–8.
27. Shinagawa K, Mitamura H, Ogawa S, et al. Effect of inhibiting Na^+/H^+–exchange or angiotensin converting enzyme on atrial tachycardia-induced remodelling. Cardiovasc Res. 2002;52:438–46.
28. Nakashima H, Kumagai K, Urata H, et al. Angiotensin II antagonist prevents electrical remodelling in atrial fibrillation. Circulation. 2000;101:2612–7.
29. Sadoshima J, Izumo S. Molecular characterization of angiotensin II induced hypertrophy of cardiac myocytes and hyperplasia of cardiac fibroblasts: critical role of the AT1 receptor subtype. Circ Res. 1993;73:413–23.
30. Sadoshima J, Xu Y, Slayter HS, et al. Autocrine release of angiotensin II mediates stretch-induced hypertrophy of cardiac myocytes in vivo. Cell. 1993;75:977–85.
31. Weber KT, Brilla CG. Pathological hypertrophy and the cardiac interstitium: fibrosis and the renin-angiotensin-aldosterone system. Circulation. 1991;83:1849–65.
32. Ollivier JP, Bouchet VA. Prospects for cardioreparation. Am J Cardiol. 1992;70:27C–36.
33. Brilla CG, Zhou G, Matsubara L, et al. Collagen metabolism in cultured adult rat cardiac fibroblasts: response to angiotensin II and aldosterone. J Mol Cell Immunol. 1994;26:809–20.
34. Sheehan JP, Seelig MS. Interactions of magnesium and potassium in the pathogenesis of cardiovascular disease. Magnesium. 1984;3: 301–14.
35. Phillips BG, Narkiewicz K, Pesek CA, et al. Effects of obstructive sleep apnea on endothelin-1 and blood pressure. J Hypertens. 1999; 17:61–6.
36. Grimpen F, Kanne P, Schulz E, et al. Endothelin-1 plasma levels are not elevated in patients with obstructive sleep apnea. Eur Respir J. 2000;15:320–5.
37. Kato M, Roberts-Thomson P, Phillips BG, et al. Impairment of endothelium-dependent vasodilatation of resistance vessels in patients with obstructive sleep apnea. Circulation. 2000;102: 2607–10.
38. Carlson J, Rangemark C, Hedner J. Attenuated endothelium-dependent vascular relaxation in patients with sleep apnoea. J Hypertens. 1996;14:577–84.
39. Ip MS, Lam B, Chan LY, et al. Circulating nitric oxide is suppressed in obstructive sleep apnea and is reversed by nasal continuous positive airway pressure. Am J Respir Crit Care Med. 2000;162:2166–71.
40. Lavie L, Lavie P. Molecular mechanisms of cardiovascular disease OSAHS: the oxidative stress link. Eur Respir J. 2009;33:1467–84.
41. Christou K, Kostikas K, Pastaka C, et al. Nasal continuous positive airway pressure treatment reduces systemic oxidative stress in patients with severe obstructive sleep apnea syndrome. Sleep Med. 2009;10:87–94.
42. Dyugovskaya L, Lavie P, Lavie L. Increased adhesion molecule expression and production of reactive oxygen species in leucocytes of sleep apnea patients. Am J Respir Crit Care Med. 2002;165:934–9.
43. Yokoe T, Minoguchi K, Matsuo H, et al. Elevated levels of C-reactive protein and interleukin-6 in patients with obstructive sleep apnea syndrome are decreased by nasal continuous positive airway pressure. Circulation. 2003;107:1129–34.
44. Dyugovskaya L, Lavie P, Lavie L. Lymphocyte activation as a possible measure of atherosclerotic risk in patients with sleep apnea. Ann N Y Acad Sci. 2005;1051:340–50.
45. Ridker PM, Hennekens CH, Buring JE, et al. C-reactive protein and other markers of inflammation in the prediction of cardiovascular disease in women. N Engl J Med. 2000;342:836–43.
46. Ridker PM, Rifai N, Pfeffer M, et al. Elevation of tumor necrosis factor-alpha and increased risk of recurrent coronary events after myocardial infarction. Circulation. 2000;101:2149–53.
47. Wessendorf TE, Thielmann AF, Wang YM, et al. Fibrinogen levels and obstructive sleep apnea in ischemic stroke. Am J Respir Crit Care Med. 2000;162:2039–42.
48. Saletu M, Nosiska D, Kapfhammer G, et al. Structural and serum surrogate markers of cerebrovascular disease in obstructive sleep apnea (OSA): association of mild OSA with early atherosclerosis. J Neurol. 2006;253:746–52.
49. Al Lawati N, Mulgrew A, Cheema R, et al. Pro-atherogenic cytokine profile of patients with suspected obstructive sleep apnea. Sleep Breath. 2009;13:277–83.
50. Ronksley PE, Hemmelgarn BR, Heitman SJ, et al. Obstructive sleep apnoea is associated with diabetes in sleepy subjects. Thorax. 2009;64:834–9.
51. Shaw JE, Punjabi NM, Wilding JP, et al. Sleep disordered breathing and type 2 diabetes. A report from the International Diabetes Federation Taskforce on Epidemiology and Prevention. Diabetes Res Clin Pract. 2008;81:2–12.
52. Empana JP, Duciemetiere P, Balkau B, et al. Contribution of the metabolic syndrome to sudden death in asymptomatic men: the Paris Prospective Study I. Eur Heart J. 2007;28:1149–54.

53. Franz MF, Bode R. Mechano-electrical feedback underlying arrhythmias: the atrial fibrillation case. Prog Biophys Mol Biol. 2003;82:163–74.
54. Sin DD, Fitzgerald F, Parker JD, et al. Risk factors for central and obstructive sleep apnoea in 450 men and women with congestive heart failure. Am J Respir Crit Care Med. 1999;160:1101–6.
55. Oldenburg O, Lamp B, Faber L, et al. Sleep-disordered breathing in patients with symptomatic heart failure: a contemporary study of prevalence in and characteristics of 700 patients. Eur J Heart Fail. 2007;9:251–7.
56. Bitter T, Prinz C, Faber L, et al. Sleep-disordered breathing in heart failure with normal left ventricular ejection fraction. Eur J Heart Fail. 2009;11:602–8.
57. Solin P, Bergin P, Richardson M, et al. Influence of pulmonary capillary wedge pressure on central apnea in heart failure. Circulation. 1999;99:1574–9.
58. Javaheri S. A mechanism of central sleep apnoea in patients with heart failure. N Engl J Med. 1999;341:949–54.
59. Solin P, Roebuck T, Johns DP, et al. Peripheral and central ventilatory responses in central sleep apnea with and without congestive heart failure. Am J Respir Crit Care Med. 2000;162:2194–200.
60. Oldenburg O, Bitter T, Wiemer M, et al. Pulmonary capillary wedge pressure and pulmonary arterial pressure in heart failure patients with sleep-disordered breathing. Sleep Med. 2009;10:726–30.
61. Arzt M, Harth M, Luchner A, et al. Enhanced ventilatory response to exercise in patients with chronic heart failure and central sleep apnea. Circulation. 2003;107:1998–2003.
62. Javaheri S, Shukla R, Zeigler H, et al. Central sleep apnoea, right ventricular dysfunction, and low diastolic blood pressure are predictors of mortality in systolic heart failure. J Am Coll Cardiol. 2007;49:2028–34.
63. Van De Borne P, Mezzetti S, Montano N, et al. Hyperventilation alters arterial baroreflex control of heart rate and muscle sympathetic nerve activity. Am J Physiol Heart Circ Physiol. 2000;279: 536–41.
64. Trinder J, Merson R, Rosenberg JI, et al. Pathophysiological interactions of ventilation, arousals, and blood pressure oscillations during Cheyne-Stokes respiration in patients with heart failure. Am J Respir Crit Care Med. 2000;162:808–13.
65. Wedewardt J, Bitter T, Prinz C, et al. Cheyne-Stokes respiration in heart failure: cycle length is dependent on left ventricular ejection fraction. Sleep Med. 2010;11:137–42.
66. Leung RS, Floras JS, Bradley TD. Respiratory modulation of the autonomic nervous system during Cheyne-Stokes respiration. Can J Physiol Pharmacol. 2006;84:61–6.
67. Guilleminault C, Connolly SJ, Winkle RA. Cardiac arrhythmia and conduction disturbances during sleep in 400 patients with sleep apnoea syndrome. Am J Cardiol. 1983;52:490–4.
68. Shepard Jr JW, Garrison MW, Grither DA, et al. Relationship of ventricular ectopy to oxyhemoglobin desaturation in patients with obstructive sleep apnoea. Chest. 1985;88:335–40.
69. Mehra R, Stone KL, Varosy PD, et al. Nocturnal arrhythmias across a spectrum of obstructive and central sleep disordered breathing in older men: outcomes of sleep disorders in older men (MrOS sleep) study. Arch Intern Med. 2009;169:1147–55.
70. Mehra R, Benjamin EJ, Shahar E, et al. Association of nocturnal arrhythmias with sleep-disordered breathing: the Sleep Heart Health Study. Am J Respir Crit Care Med. 2006;173:910–6.
71. Lanfranchi PA, Somers VK, Braghiroli A, et al. Central sleep apnoea in left ventricular dysfunction: prevalence and implications for arrhythmic risk. Circulation. 2003;107:727–32.
72. Koshino Y, Satoh M, Katayose Y, et al. Association of sleep-disordered breathing and ventricular arrhythmias in patients without heart failure. Am J Cardiol. 2008;101:882–6.
73. Bitter T, Westerheide N, Prinz C, et al. Cheyne-Stokes respiration and obstructive sleep apnoea are independent risk factors for malignant ventricular arrhythmias requiring appropriate cardioverter-defibrillator therapies in patients with congestive heart failure. Eur Heart J. 2011;32:61–74.
74. Teerlink JR, Jalaluddin M, Anderson S, et al. Ambulatory ventricular arrhythmias in patients with heart failure do not specifically predict an increased risk of sudden death. PROMISE (Prospective Randomized Milrinone Survival Evaluation) Investigators. Circulation. 2000;101:40–6.
75. Gami AS, Howard DE, Olson EJ, et al. Day-night pattern of sudden death in obstructive sleep apnoea. N Engl J Med. 2005;352: 1206–14.
76. Serizawa N, Yumino D, Kajimoto K, et al. Impact of sleep-disordered breathing on life-threatening ventricular arrhythmia in heart failure patients with implantable cardioverter-defibrillator. Am J Cardiol. 2008;102:1064–8.
77. Staniforth AD, Sporton SC, Early MJ, et al. Ventricular arrhythmia, Cheyne-Stokes respiration, and death: observations from patients with defibrillators. Heart. 2005;91:1418–22.
78. Gami AS, Pressman G, Caples SM, et al. Association of atrial fibrillation and obstructive sleep apnea. Circulation. 2004;110: 364–7.
79. Bitter T, Langer C, Vogt J, et al. Sleep-disordered breathing in patients with atrial fibrillation and normal systolic left ventricular function. Dtsch Arztebl Int. 2009;106:164–70.
80. Stevenson IH, Teichtahl H, Cunnington D, et al. Prevalence of sleep disordered breathing in paroxysmal and persistent atrial fibrillation patients with normal left ventricular function. Eur Heart J. 2008; 29:1662–9.
81. Stevenson IH, Roberts-Thomson KC, Kistler PM, et al. Atrial electrophysiology is altered by acute hypercapnia but not hypoxemia: implications for promotion of atrial fibrillation in pulmonary disease and sleep apnea. Heart Rhythm. 2010;7:1263–70.
82. Kanagala R, Murali NS, Friedman PA, et al. Obstructive sleep apnea and the recurrence of atrial fibrillation. Circulation. 2003;107: 2589–94.
83. Tang RB, Dong JZ, Liu XP, et al. Obstructive sleep apnoea risk profile and the risk of recurrence of atrial fibrillation after catheter ablation. Europace. 2008;11:100–5.
84. Chilukuri K, Dalal D, Marine JE, et al. Predictive value of obstructive sleep apnoea assessed by the Berlin Questionnaire for outcomes after the catheter ablation of atrial fibrillation. Europace. 2009;11: 896–901.
85. Leung RS, Huber MA, Rogge T, et al. Association between atrial fibrillation and central sleep apnea. Sleep. 2005;28:1543–6.
86. Guilleminault C, Connolly S, Winkle R, et al. Cyclical variation of the heart rate in sleep apnoea syndrome. Mechanisms, and usefulness of 24 h electrocardiography as a screening technique. Lancet. 1984;1:126–31.
87. Sato F, Nishimura M, Shinano H, et al. Heart rate during obstructive sleep apnea depends on individual hypoxic chemosensitivity of the carotid body. Circulation. 1997;96:274–81.
88. Abe H, Takahashi M, Yaegashi H, et al. Efficacy of continuous positive airway pressure on arrhythmias in obstructive sleep apnea patients. Heart Vessels. 2010;25:63–9.
89. Grimm W, Becker HF. Obesity, sleep apnea syndrome, and arrhythmogenic risk. Herz. 2006;31:213–8.
90. Epstein LJ, Kristo D, Strollo PJ, et al. Clinical guideline for the evaluation, management and long-term care of obstructive sleep apnea in adults. J Clin Sleep Med. 2009;5:263–76.
91. Cassar A, Morgenthaler TI, Lennon RJ, et al. Treatment of obstructive sleep apnea is associated with decreased cardiac death after percutaneous coronary intervention. J Am Coll Cardiol. 2007;50: 1310–4.
92. Kasai T, Narui K, Dohi T, et al. Prognosis of patients with heart failure and obstructive sleep apnea treated with continuous positive airway pressure. Chest. 2008;133:690–6.

93. Barbe F, Duran-Cantolla J, Capote F, et al. Long-term effect of continuous positive airway pressure in hypertensive patients with sleep apnea. Am J Respir Crit Care Med. 2010;181:718–26.
94. Ryan CM, Usui K, Floras JS, et al. Effect of continuous positive airway pressure on ventricular ectopy in heart failure patients with obstructive sleep apnoea. Thorax. 2005;60:781–5.
95. Craig S, Pepperell JC, Kohler M, et al. Continuous positive airway pressure treatment for obstructive sleep apnoea reduces resting heart rate but does not affect dysrhythmias: a randomised controlled trial. J Sleep Res. 2009;18:329–36.
96. Kurlynka NV, Pevzner AV, Litvin A, et al. Treatment of patients with long nocturnal asystoles and obstructive sleep apnea syndrome by creating continuous positive air pressure in the upper respiratory tract. Kardiologiia. 2009;49:36–42.
97. Roche F, Xuong AN, Court-Fortune I, et al. Relationship among the severity of sleep apnea syndrome, cardiac arrhythmias, and autonomic imbalance. Pacing Clin Electrophysiol. 2003;26:669–77.
98. Bradley TD, Logan AG, Kimoff RJ, et al. Continuous positive airway pressure for central sleep apnea and heart failure. N Engl J Med. 2005;353:2025–33.
99. Arzt M, Floras JS, Logan AG, et al. Suppression of central sleep apnea by continuous positive airway pressure and transplant-free survival in heart failure: a post hoc analysis of the Canadian Continuous Positive Airway Pressure for Patients with Central Sleep Apnea and Heart Failure Trial (CANPAP). Circulation. 2007;115:3173–80.
100. Teschler H, Döhring J, Wang YM, et al. Adaptive pressure support servo-ventilation: a novel treatment for Cheyne-Stokes respiration in heart failure. Am J Respir Crit Care Med. 2001;164:614–9.
101. Javaheri S. Effects of continuous positive airway pressure on sleep apnoea and ventricular irritability in patients with heart failure. Circulation. 2000;101:392–7.
102. Philippe C, Stoica-Herman M, Drouot X, et al. Compliance with and effectiveness of adaptive servoventilation versus continuous positive airway pressure in the treatment of Cheyne-Stokes respiration in heart failure over a six month period. Heart. 2006;92:337–42.
103. Oldenburg O, Bitter T, Lehman R, et al. Adaptive servoventilation improves cardiac function and respiratory stability. Clin Res Cardiol. 2011;100:107–15.
104. Bitter T, Westerheide N, Faber L, et al. Adaptive servoventilation in diastolic heart failure and Cheyne-Stokes respiration. Eur Respir J. 2010;36:385–92.

Effects of Chronic Intermittent Hypoxia on Cardiac Rhythm Transcriptomic Networks

2

Sanda Iacobas and Dumitru Andrei Iacobas

Abstract

This chapter completes a series of four studies analyzing in a mouse model the genomic consequences of chronic obstructive sleep apnea during development from neonatal to puberty. Groups of two male and two female 1-day-old sibling mice each were subjected for 1, 2, or 4 weeks to normal atmospheric conditions or to chronic intermittent hypoxia, and the transcriptomes of their hearts profiled and compared. Our previous papers reported alterations of individual genes, gene ontology categories, translation regulators and responses to stress, and analyzed and quantified the topological changes of the heart rhythm determinant (HRD) genomic fabric, including the ranking of the HRD genes. HRD fabric was defined as the most stably expressed and interconnected gene web that might be responsible for the generation, maintenance, and modulation of the heart rhythm in each condition. Here, we introduce the new analysis of the network landscape to determine the ways by which Ca^{2+} and Wnt signaling pathways, translation initiation, and elongation factors, and SOX (i.e., sex-determining region Y-box) genes control the HRD fabric. We also analyze the changes in the networks by which connexin 43, the main protein that couples the cardiomyocytes by forming intercellular gap junction channels, modulates the HRD fabric during development under normoxic and hypoxic conditions. Remarkably, the amplitude of the transcriptomic alterations diminished from 1 to 4 weeks of hypoxia, indicating activation of certain acclimatization or accommodation mechanisms. In addition to regulation of expression level, our analyses revealed changes in the stability control and interlinking of functional gene networks as well as switch of dominant gene pairs. Thus, we found that *Hif1a-Jup*, *Lmna-Pcdh7*, and *Eef1a2-Gnao1* are the most important pairs at 1, 2, and 4 weeks normoxia, respectively, while *Jup-Slc25a20*, *Cdh16-Vezt*, and *Eif2ak4-Pcdh12* are the controlling pairs at 1, 2, and 4 weeks hypoxia, respectively. The analysis has shown that changes in expression control and coordination had substantial contributions to the overall transcriptomic differences. Moreover, with respect to magnitude, hypoxia transcriptomic effects are comparable to those associated to development. Altogether, these results indicate the profound remodeling of the HRD fabric and regulatory pathways in response to intermittent oxygen deprivation that may explain the cardiac arrhythmias experienced by teenagers suffering by chronic obstructive sleep apnea.

S. Iacobas • D.A. Iacobas (✉)
D.P. Purpura Department of Neuroscience,
Albert Einstein College of Medicine,
Bronx, NY, USA
e-mail: dumitru.iacobas@einstein.yu.edu

L. Xi, T.V. Serebrovskaya (eds.), *Intermittent Hypoxia and Human Diseases*,
DOI 10.1007/978-1-4471-2906-6_2, © Springer-Verlag London 2012

Abbreviations

CIH Chronic intermittent hypoxia
HRD Heart rhythm determinant
NOR Normoxia (normal atmospheric conditions)
PGA Prominent Gene Analysis
SIG Signaling genes
SOX Sex-determining region Y-box
TRA Transcription and translation regulators
WNT Wingless-related MMTV integration site

2.1 Introduction

Snoring is not only unpleasant to those living around you, but it is also bad for your heart. So bad that when chronic it may change the fate of genes responsible for the heart rhythm, generating lifelong arrhythmias. Chronic intermittent hypoxia, such as in obstructive sleep apnea, causes numerous heart problems, including hypertension, coronary artery disease, congestive heart failure, pulmonary hypertension, stroke, and cardiac arrhythmias [1–6]. Lethal cardiac arrhythmias are often associated with altered expression or mutation of key genes [7]. Variants in genes that encode cardiac ion channel α- and β-subunits lead to congenital syndromes such as abnormally long or short QT, Brugada, and catecholaminergic polymorphic ventricular tachycardia [8]. Moreover, inherited mutations in genes related to regulatory pathways of ion channels may also cause cardiac arrhythmias [8–12]. The multitude of arrhythmia forms suggests that normal cardiac rhythm requires appropriate co-expression of numerous and diverse molecular components.

Interestingly, there are substantial differences between effects of chronic intermittent and chronic constant hypoxia (such as in pulmonary disease or living at high altitude) [13–17]. These differences suggest that in addition to oxygen deprivation, the frequency of alternating normal and hypoxic atmospheric conditions may be of importance in developing adaptation mechanisms. Whether caused by constant or intermittent hypoxia, the wide diversity of clinical manifestation indicates high complexity of underlying molecular mechanisms that remain largely unresolved in spite of numerous models that have been proposed (e.g., [18–25]). In the following paragraphs, we focus on the heart rhythm determinant (HRD) gene fabric and signaling networks that modulate it. We have developed methods to select the most relevant genes and quantify the networks responsible for the cardiac function.

In a previous study [13], we have profiled the heart transcriptomes of 36 mice subjected for 1, 2, or 4 weeks of their early life to normal atmospheric conditions or to chronic constant or intermittent hypoxia, with two males and two females profiled in each condition. However, for the unity of the book, in this chapter, we discuss only the genomic consequences of the chronic intermittent hypoxia. We here introduce new analyses by which to reveal additional possible transcriptomic mechanisms that make chronic intermittent hypoxia an arrhythmogenic condition. They complete the analyses of individual genes and gene ontology (GO) categories that have been regulated [13], alteration of translation regulators and response to stress [16], alteration of HRD gene hierarchy and remodeling of the topology of HRD genomic fabric [17].

2.2 Materials and Methods

Results of this chapter were obtained by analyzing from new perspectives part of the data obtained in a previously described gene expression experiment [13] performed in the laboratory of Dr. Haddad (UCSF). Expression of 4,862 completely annotated unigenes was adequately quantified in all RNA samples (publically available in http://www.ncbi.nlm.nih.gov/geo/query/acc.cgi?acc=GSE2271). Of these genes, 54 were assigned to the heart rhythm determinant (HRD) fabric while other 44 genes were included in transcription and translation regulators (TRA) and 35 to signaling (SIG) gene cohorts owing to their influence on the HRD fabric. HRD genes were selected from the quantified genes in this experiment though our prominent gene analysis (PGA) as reported in a previous paper [17]. The selection includes the adrenergic receptor kinase beta 1 (*Adrbk1*), ankyrins (*Ank2*, *Ank3*), ion channels and transporters (*Atp1a1*, *Atp1a2*, *Atp2a2*, *Kcnh2*, *Slc25a20*, *Slc8a1*), regulators of heart rhythm (*Lamp2*, *Lmna*, *Sema3a*, *Ttr*), contraction (*Dmpk*, *Gnao1*), inotropy (*Csrp3*, *Gaa*), and development (*Id2*, *Nfatc3*, *Tbx5*). Direct and indirect epigenetic modulators (*Hand2*, *Hdac5*, *Mef2a*, *Mef2b*, *Mef2c*, *Mef2d*, *Smyd1*) were added because of their relation with various miRNA, short noncoding RNAs involved in posttranscriptional regulation whose altered expression was recently linked to arrhythmias [26–28]. Moreover, since generation of synchronized rhythmic heart contractions requires integration of electrical and mechanical properties, we have also incorporated in this study genes encoding components of the intercalated discs (specialized regions of the plasma membrane that link neighboring cardiac myocytes). Thus, we have profiled several adherens (*Jup*, *Vcl*, *Vezt*), members of the cadherin superfamily (*Cdh13*, *Cdh16*, *Cdh2*, *Cdh22*, *Cdh5*, *Dsc2*, *Dsg2*, *Pcdh12*, *Pcdh7*, *Pcdhgc3*) and cadherin-associated proteins (*Ctnna1*, *Ctnnal1*, *Ctnb1*, *Ctnd1*), plakophilins (*Pkp2*, *Pkp3*, *Pkp4*), and tight (*Cxadr*, *Tjp1*, *Tjp2*,) and gap junction proteins (*Gja1*). However, 6 HRD genes (*Gja1* = gap junction membrane channel protein alpha 1; *Itpr1/2* = inositol 1,4,5-triphosphate receptor 1/2; *Ryr1* = ryanodine receptor 1;

Slc8a1;*Ttr*=transthyretin) were included also in SIG cohort. In the TRA cohort, we have considered the effects on HRD fabric of hypoxia inducible factor 1 alpha subunit (*Hif1a*), 5 (eukaryotic) translation elongation (*Eef*), and 38 translation initiation (*Eif*) factors. SIG cohort includes SOX genes and genes involved in Ca^{2+} and Wnt signaling because their reciprocal interactions and interactions with Cx43 and other intercalated disc proteins control cardiomyogenesis [29–35].

2.2.1 Hypoxia Treatment

As described in Fan et al. [13], CD1 mice (Charles River) were placed in a hypoxia chamber (BioSpherix) with their mother starting on the second day after birth (P2) for 1, 2, or 4 weeks. O_2 concentration was switched between 21% and 11% every 4 min, continuously for 24 h/day for the entire period. At the end of each period, mice were anesthetized by inhalation of isoflurane (Baxter Pharmaceutical Products), the hearts removed, and quickly frozen in liquid nitrogen. The surgical procedures and protocols were approved by the Albert Einstein College of Medicine (AECOM) Animal Care and Use Committee.

2.2.2 Microarray Hybridization

Briefly, 60-μg total RNA extracted with TRIzol (Invitrogen) was used to synthesize a fluorescently labeled cDNA probe by direct incorporation of either Cy3 or Cy5 fluorescent dye (Amersham Biosciences). Fluorescent cDNA probes were treated with blocking solution for 1 h before being applied to pretreated and prehybridized microarray slides. Hybridization with 27 k cDNA mouse AECOM microarrays were performed in GeneMachines HybChamber overnight at 50°C. After incubation, each slide was washed to remove unbound cDNAs and SDS, dried, and scanned with a GenePix 4100A scanner (Axon Instruments) at 600 V (635 nm) and 550 V (532 nm). We adopted the "multiple-yellow" hybridization strategy in which each slide was hybridized with Cy5-labeled cDNA obtained from a male heart and Cy3-labeled cDNA from a female heart, both mice being from the same litter and subjected to the same treatment. The multiple-yellow strategy improves intrachip normalization since the mRNA content of the starting total RNA is affected only by the biological variability among animals, matched by gender, age, and condition. It improves also the interchip normalization and the green and red fluorescence signals obtained with the same scanner setting for all slides being compared separately, thus avoiding the inherent nonuniform bias toward one tag. This allowed all possible comparisons among conditions, time points, and sexes.

2.2.3 Scanning, Acquisition, and Normalization

Images were acquired and primarily analyzed with GenePix Pro 4.1 software. A gene was considered as quantifiable if its foreground fluorescence signal was more than twice the background. Any spot that was not quantifiable in all samples was removed from the analysis. The background-subtracted signals were normalized with an in-house-developed iterative algorithm described in [36], alternating intra-array and inter-array normalization until the average-corrected ratio differed by <5% from the previous one.

2.2.4 Analysis of Expression Regulation

Detection of significantly regulated genes relied on a composite criterion of $>|1.5\times|$ absolute fold change and p value <0.05 with a Bonferroni-type correction for the redundancy groups (set of spots probing the same gene) [37]. GenMAPP and MAPPFinder software (www.genmap.org, Gladstone Institute) were used for the first categorization of the altered genes [13].

2.2.5 Analysis of Expression Variability and Transcript Abundance Control

We have determined the relative expression variability (REV) of each gene as the chi-square statistical estimate of the coefficient of variability (CV) of transcript abundance in the set of biological replicas. This statistical measure was necessary to limit the effect of the nonuniform size of the redundancy group of spots on the gene's CV. By ordering the genes according to their REVs, we have determined the gene expression stability (GES) as a percentile of transcription control, with GES = 100 indicating the most controlled gene and GES < 1 indicating the least controlled one [16]. We have also studied whether the strength of the transcription control is age dependent and changes in hypoxia. The transcription control limits the so-called genomic noise (responsible for the expression variability within biological replicas) that we view as a transcriptomic tuning to the variability of local conditions.

2.2.6 Analysis of Expression Coordination and Gene Networking

Transcription variability allows calculation of Pearson correlation coefficient ρ between the expression levels of gene pairs in biological replicas and identification of synergistically (SYN, $\rho>0.90$), antagonistically (ANT, $\rho<-0.90$), and independently

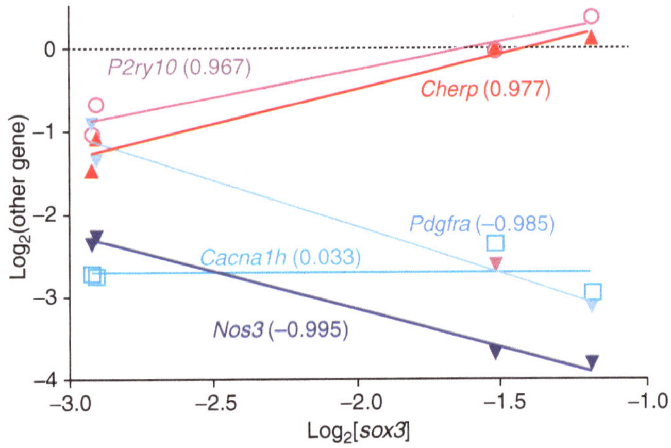

Fig. 2.1 Examples of synergistically (*Cherp*, *P2ry10*), antagonistically (*Nos3*, *Pdgfra*), and independently (*Cacna1h*) expressed partners of *Sox3* in hearts of 1-week-old mice grown under normal atmospheric conditions. Genes: *Cacna1h*=calcium channel, voltage-dependent, T-type, alpha 1 H subunit; *Cherp*=calcium homeostasis endoplasmic reticulum protein, *Nos3*=nitric oxide synthase 3; endothelial cell, *P2ry10*=purinergic receptor P2Y; G-protein coupled 10, *Pdgfra*=platelet-derived growth factor receptor; alpha polypeptide. Note that for synergistically expressed partners, the expression levels go in the same direction among biological replicas; for antagonistically expressed, they go in opposite directions, while no correlation can be established for independently expressed genes

(IND, $|\rho|<0.05$) expressed partners (examples in Fig. 2.1). Expression of each gene is expected to be tied to that of other genes so that amounts of encoded proteins respect the "stoichiometry" of the biological processes [38]. Expression coordination may occur between genes from the same GO category (examples in [17]) or between genes from different GO categories (as illustrated in Fig. 2.1 where the transcription factor *Sox3* is coordinately expressed with certain Ca^{2+}-signaling genes). This expression coordination between genes involved in different functional categories suggests that the functional pathways can modulate each other.

2.2.7 Prominence Gene Analysis

The most relevant HRD genes were selected from the adequately quantified genes in all conditions through our Prominence Gene Analysis (PGA), a variant of the principal component analysis (PCA). The essential difference between PGA and PCA is that genes with the largest variance among distinct conditions are no longer considered as "centroids." Instead, PGA selects the genes that can form the most interconnected and stably expressed network with respect to a particular biological process, molecular function, or cellular location. Thus, the interest is shifted from the most alterable genes in a series of (not necessarily causally related) conditions to the most influential ones in each condition. A gene is considered as prominent if it is (1) coordinated with that of numerous other genes (to control the fabric) and (2) resistant to the variation of the local conditions (to protect the fabric) [17, 39, 40].

2.2.8 "Gene Network Landscape"

In order to "visualize" and compare the topology of gene networking in different conditions, we here introduce a new measure in which each gene pair (γ,ε) is represented by a "mountain" whose height is proportional to the contribution of that gene pair to the coordination and stability of the gene network in condition *c* (e.g., CIH-2=2 weeks hypoxia). The "mountain height" *H* increases with the expression coordination of the two genes and decreases with their relative expression variability within the cohort(s) they belong to:

$$H_{\gamma,\omega}^{(\alpha)} = \frac{\langle X\rangle_{\Gamma}^{(\alpha)} \left|\rho_{\gamma,\omega}^{(\alpha)}\right| \langle X\rangle_{\Omega}^{(\alpha)}}{X_{\gamma}^{(\alpha)} X_{\omega}^{(\alpha)}}$$

$$\gamma \in \Gamma, \omega \in \Omega; \quad \Gamma,\Omega = HRD, SIG, TRA$$

$$\alpha = NOR-1/2/4\,,\; CIH-1/2/4$$

where $X_{\gamma/\omega}^{(c)}$ is the chi-square estimate of the individual gene expression variability and $\langle X\rangle_{\Gamma/\Omega}^{(c)}$ the average expression variability of gene cohorts Γ and Ω in condition α.

2.2.8.1 Overall Transcriptomic Differences

In our opinion, it is not enough to present a list of differently expressed genes to know how much the compared conditions differ from each other from transcriptomic point of view. Therefore, we have developed a comprehensive computational procedure by which to evaluate the *overall transcriptomic differences* $\Delta_{\text{tot}}^{(\alpha,\beta)}$ between conditions α and β (= NOR-1, NOR-2, NOR-4, CIH-1, CIH-2, CIH-4):

$$\mathrm{Card}_{\Gamma}\Delta_{\text{tot}}^{(\alpha,\beta)} = \underbrace{\sqrt{\sum_{\gamma\in\Gamma}\left[\left(1-p_{\gamma}^{(\alpha,\beta)}\right)\left(\left|x_{\gamma}^{(\alpha,\beta)}\right|-1\right)\right]^{2}}}_{\text{Change of expression level}} + \underbrace{\sqrt{\sum_{\gamma\in\Gamma}\left(\frac{X_{\gamma}^{(\beta)}}{\langle X\rangle_{\Gamma}^{(\beta)}}-\frac{X_{\gamma}^{(\alpha)}}{\langle X\rangle_{\Gamma}^{(\alpha)}}\right)^{2}}}_{\text{Change of transcription control}} + \underbrace{\sqrt{\sum_{\gamma\in\Gamma}\left(\frac{\mathrm{Card}_{\Gamma}}{\mathrm{Card}_{\Gamma}-1}\sum_{\varepsilon\in\Gamma,\varepsilon\neq\gamma}\left(\rho_{\gamma,\varepsilon}^{(\beta)}-\rho_{\gamma,\varepsilon}^{(\alpha)}\right)^{2}\right)}}_{\text{Change of networking}}$$

where $x_{\gamma}^{(\alpha,\beta)}$ = *expression ratio* (negative for downregulation) and $p_{\gamma}^{(\alpha,\beta)} = \mathrm{p}$ value of the significant regulation. In addition to quantifying the magnitude and statistical significance of expression regulation (expression ratio *x*, negative for downregulation), it considers also the changes in the transcription control and networking. This new measure that is not affected by the arbitrary cutoffs in expression regulation and significant coordination was used to quantify the global alterations induced by hypoxia as well as transformations during the development.

2.3 Results

2.3.1 Expression Regulation

Table 2.1 presents the genes (from the 127 analyzed in this chapter) that were significantly regulated by chronic intermittent hypoxia. Overall, hypoxia regulated expression of

Table 2.1 Significantly regulated genes in hearts of mice subjected for 1, 2, or 4 weeks of their early life to chronic intermittent hypoxia with respect to their normoxic counterparts

Gene	Symbol	CAT	CHR	1 week	2 weeks	4 weeks
Eukaryotic translation elongation factor 1 alpha 1	*Eef1a1*	TRA	9	2.21		
Eukaryotic translation elongation factor 1 alpha 2	*Eef1a2*	TRA	2		2.60	
Eukaryotic translation elongation factor 1 beta 2	*Eef1b2*	TRA	1		−2.11	1.66
Eukaryotic translation initiation factor 1A, Y-linked	*Eif1ay*	TRA	X	−1.62		
Eukaryotic translation initiation factor 1B	*Eif1b*	TRA	9	−1.87		
Eukaryotic translation initiation factor 2 alpha kinase 4	*Eif2ak4*	TRA	2		−1.60	
Eukaryotic translation initiation factor 2, subunit 1 (alpha)	*Eif2s1*	TRA	12	−2.34		
Eukaryotic translation initiation factor 2, subunit 2 (beta)	*Eif2s2*	TRA	2	−2.49		
Eukaryotic translation factor 3, subunit 12	*Eif3s12*	TRA	7	−3.93	1.89	
Eukaryotic translation factor 3, subunit 2 (beta)	*Eif3s2*	TRA	4		−1.93	
Eukaryotic translation factor 3, subunit 3 (gamma)	*Eif3s3*	TRA	15		2.36	
Eukaryotic translation factor 3, subunit 6 interacting protein	*Eif3s6ip*	TRA	15	−3.03		
Eukaryotic translation factor 3, subunit 9 (eta)	*Eif3s9*	TRA	5		−1.86	
Eukaryotic translation initiation factor 4E	*Eif4e*	TRA	3	−1.86	−4.07	
Eukaryotic translation initiation factor 5	*Eif5*	TRA	12		2.24	
Eukaryotic translation initiation factor 5A	*Eif5a*	TRA	11	−1.55	−2.23	−1.51
Wingless-related MMTV integration site 3A	*Wnt3a*	SIG	11	−1.94		
Wingless-related MMTV integration site 5B	Wnt5b	SIG	6	1.58		
SRY-box containing gene 11	*Sox11*	SIG	12		−2.35	
SRY-box containing gene 3	*Sox3*	SIG	X	2.39		
Calcium binding protein 39	*Cab39*	SIG	1	−1.89		
Calcium channel, voltage-dependent, alpha2/delta subunit 1	*Cacna2d1*	SIG	5		−1.72	
Erbb2 interacting protein	*Erbb2ip*	SIG	13	−1.69		
Yamaguchi sarcoma viral (v-yes-1) oncogene homolog	*Lyn*	SIG	4	2.15		
Nitric oxide synthase 3, endothelial cell	*Nos3*	SIG	5		1.65	
Neurogranin	*Nrgn*	SIG	9	−1.90		
Protein tyrosine phosphatase, non-receptor type 6	*Ptpn6*	SIG	6		−2.53	
RAS-related C3 botulinum substrate 1	*Rac1*	SIG	5		−3.11	
Inositol 1,4,5-triphosphate receptor 1	*ltpr1*	HRD	6	−2.21		
Ankyrin 2, brain	*Ank2*	HRD	3	1.55		
Cadherin 22	*Cdh22*	HRD	2		1.76	
Guanine nucleotide binding protein, alpha o	*Gnao1*	HRD	8		−2.88	
Inhibitor of DNA binding 2	*ld2*	HRD	12	−1.85		
Junction plakoglobin	*Jup*	HRD	11	1.97		
Potassium voltage-gated channel, subfamily H (eag-related), member 2	*Kcnh2*	HRD	5	1.93		
Protocadherin gamma subfamily C, 3	*Pcdhgc3*	HRD	18	1.90		
Sema domain, immunoglobulin domain (lg), short basic domain, secreted, (semaphorin) 3A	*Sema3a*	HRD	5		2.40	
Solute carrier family 25 (mitochondrial carnitine/acylcarnitine translocase), member 20	*Slc25a20*	HRD	9	−2.32	−2.41	
Vezatin, adherens junctions transmembrane protein	*Vezt*	HRD	10	−1.62	−1.56	2.28

Missing values indicate that no significant regulation was detected for that gene
CAT category, *CHR* chromosomal location
Negative numbers (grey background) indicate down-regulation

Fig. 2.2 Expression variability of some SIG genes in the heart of 1-week-old mice raised in normal atmospheric conditions (*NOR*-1) or chronic intermittent hypoxia (*CIH*-1). The *rectangles* represent the 95% confidence intervals of the binary logarithms of the relative (to the average gene) expression level within four biological replicas. Numbers above the rectangles are the GES scores. Note the nonuniform variability among the genes and the change in expression control induced by hypoxic conditions. Genes: *Egfr* = epidermal growth factor receptor, *Erbb3* = v-erb-b2 erythroblastic leukemia viral oncogene homolog 3 (avian), *Gnaq* = guanine nucleotide-binding protein, alpha q polypeptide, *Gnas* = (guanine nucleotide-binding protein, alpha stimulating) complex locus, *Il4* = interleukin-4, *Pax6* = paired box gene 6, *Pdgfrb* = platelet-derived growth factor receptor, beta polypeptide; protein phosphatase 3, *Ppp3ca* = catalytic subunit, alpha isoform, *Prkaca* = protein kinase, cAMP-dependent, catalytic, alpha

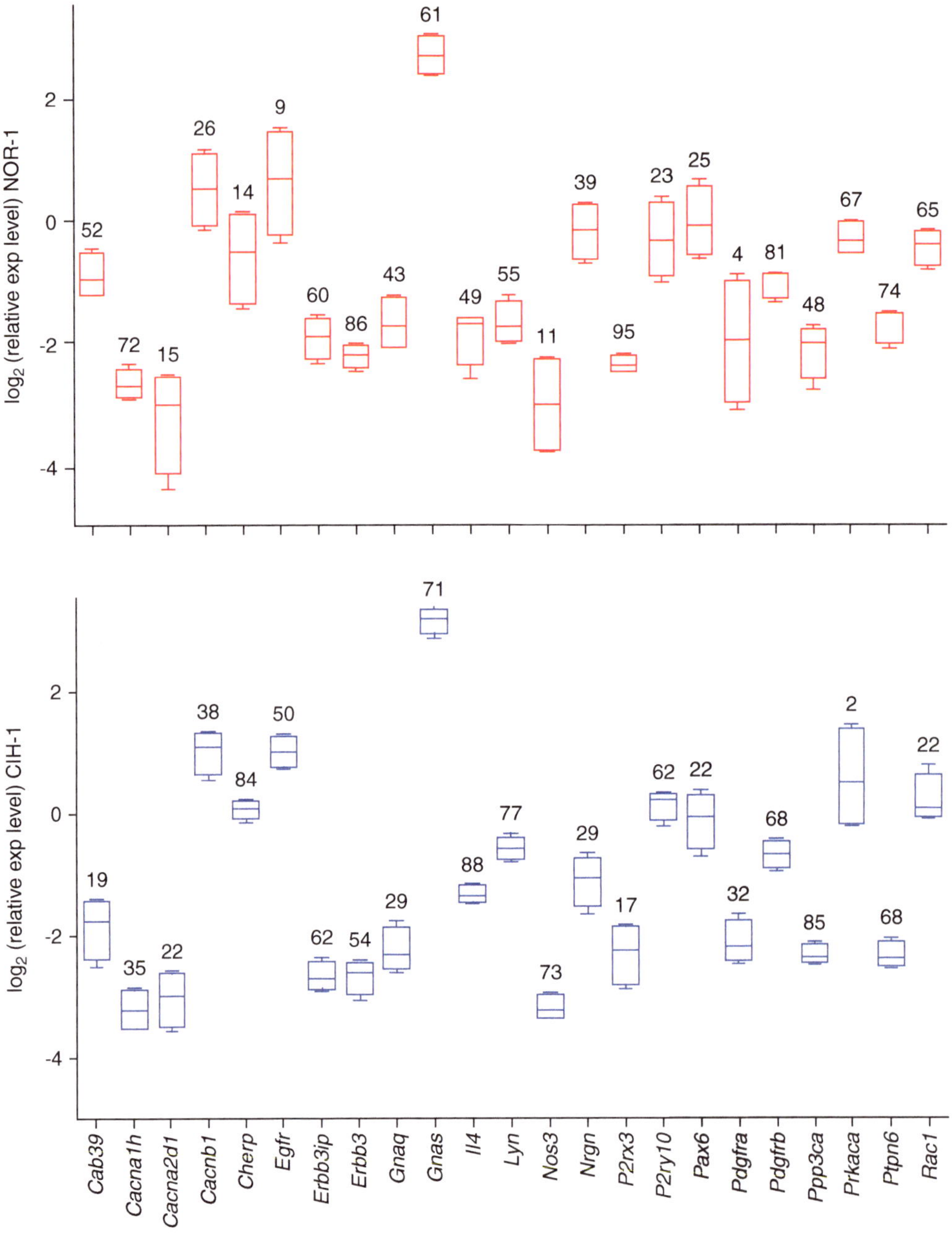

16.2% TRA, 11.6% SIG, and 8.6% HRD genes, the percentages decreasing from 1 to 4 weeks of oxygen deprivation. The reduction in number of regulated genes indicates activation of adapting mechanisms. Interestingly, after 1 week hypoxia, expression of *Wnt5b* (which promotes adipogenesis) was increased (as also reported in arrhythmogenic right ventricular cardiomyopathy [41]), while that of *Wnt3a* (required for cardiac differentiation in (human) embryonic stem cells [42]) was decreased.

2.3.2 Change in Transcription Control

Figure 2.2 illustrates the expression variability of certain SIG genes in hearts of 1-week-old mice subjected to normal atmospheric conditions or to chronic intermittent hypoxia and their GES scores in each condition. Note how hypoxia switched the controlling priorities of the cardiomyocytes. For instance, the tight control of *P2rx3* (= purinergic receptor P2X, ligand-gated ion channel, 3) in normoxia (GES = 95) was relaxed in

Table 2.2 The most stably expressed gene within the selection in each condition

Gene	Symbol	NOR-1	CIH-1	NOR-2	CIH-2	NOR-4	CIH-4
Most stable expressed							
Eukaryotic translation initiation factor 4, gamma 2	*Eif4g2*	**99.20**	41.24	24.68	26.10	76.92	51.65
Myocyte enhancer factor 2D	*Mef2d*	28.73	**99.75**	95.66	22.32	23.14	69.42
Protocadherin 7	*Pcdh7*	48.95	83.98	**99.94**	26.86	97.96	85.68
Vezatin, adherens junctions transmembrane protein	*Vezt*	47.10	93.29	81.00	**98.64**	26.53	32.25
Eukaryotic translation elongation factor 1 alpha 2	*Ef1a2*	3.85	87.66	67.44	57.84	**98.91**	31.16
Purinergic receptor P 2Y, G-protein coupled 10	*P2ry10*	22.79	61.50	44.01	73.49	69.05	**98.91**
Most unstably expressed							
SET and MYND domain containing 1	*Smyd1*	**0.80**	86.24	7.51	20.65	41.73	4.42
Eukaryotic translation elongation factor 2	*Eef2*	88.63	**1.09**	3.19	51.21	83.34	1.69
Gap junction membrane channel protein alpha 1	*Gja1*	17.89	8.17	**0.93**	15.08	34.97	**7.01**
Catenin (cadherin associated protein), alpha 1	*Ctnna1*	1.28	34.04	28.42	**0.14**	33.81	47.39
Solute carrier family 25 (mitochondrial carnitine/acylcarnitine translocase), member 20	*Slc25a20*	61.46	98.64	23.78	90.11	**2.34**	40.39
Yamaguchi sarcoma viral (v-yes-1) oncogene homolog	*Lyn*	55.16	76.94	37.76	27.05	75.95	**0.41**

The numbers are the GES scores (bold numbers on gray background for the most stably/unstably expressed genes). Note the differences among conditions and that chronic hypoxia switched genes such as *Smyd1*, *Eef2*, and *Lyn* between stably (GES > 75) and very unstably (GES < 5) expressed (compare normoxic and hypoxic values for the same duration)

hypoxia (GES = 17), while the loose control of *Cherp* (GES = 14) was significantly tightened in hypoxia (GES = 84).

The most stably and unstably expressed genes in each condition are presented in Table 2.2 together with their GES scores in all conditions. One may note that expression variability is highly influenced by both development (compare values at 1, 2, and 4 weeks) and oxygen deprivation (compare normoxic with hypoxic values). Although the analysis was limited to only 127 genes profiled in six conditions, Table 2.2 shows how large is the interval of expression control from <1 in the case of *Gja1* (at 2 weeks normoxia), *Ctnna1* (2 weeks CIH), and *Lyn* (4 weeks CIH) to >99 for *Eif4g2* (1 week normoxia), *Mef2d* (1 week CIH) and *Pcdh7* (2 weeks normoxia).

2.3.3 Alteration of Gene Networking

Figure 2.3 presents hypoxic alteration of part of the *Gja1*-dependent network that controls the HRD fabric by direct expression coordination or through coordination with its Ca^{2+}-signaling partners at 1, 2, and 4 weeks. We found a substantially lower number of significant coordinations in hypoxia. When all SIG and HRD genes are considered, the percent of the coordinately expressed genes in hypoxia decreases by 59% at 1 week, by 40% at 2 weeks, and only by 11% at 4 weeks with respect to the normoxic counterparts. The dynamics of the coordination differences suggests again activation of certain acclimatization or accommodation mechanisms. Although cardiomyocytes proliferate rapidly during fetal life, the heart growth shifts from hyperplasia to hypertrophy after birth, with most cardiac cells gradually ceasing to undergo DNA replication [43]. Interestingly, as Fig. 2.3 shows, the expression coordination increases also between the first and the second week of life both in normoxic and hypoxic conditions but decreases between the second and the fourth week.

2.3.4 Remodeling of the Network Landscape

Figure 2.4 presents the landscapes of HRD fabric and of SIG-HRD and TRA-HRD networks in hearts of 1-week-old mice regrown in normoxic or chronic intermittent hypoxic conditions. One may observe the profound remodeling of these "landscapes" as well as the change of dominant gene pairs for each network. Thus, the dominant pairs from normoxia (*Cdh16-Id2*, *P2rx3-Cdh16*, *Hif1a-Jup*) are replaced by: *Jup-Slc25a20*, *Wnt5b-Jup*, and *Eif5a-Mef2d* in hypoxia. Moreover, while the "mountains" of both HRD fabric and CAS-HRD networks are taller in 1 week hypoxia, those of TRA-HRD networks are taller in 1 week normoxia.

Table 2.3 lists the dominant pairs in all conditions. Note the change of dominant pairs both due to development and hypoxia and that the network has the largest scores at 2 weeks normoxia. We found that *Hif1a-Jup*, *Lmna-Pcdh7*, and *Gnao1-Pcdh7* are the most influential at 1, 2, and 4 weeks normoxia, respectively, while *Jup-Slc25a20*, *Cdh16-Vezt*, and *Eif2ak4-Pcdh12* are the leading pairs at 1, 2, and 4 weeks hypoxia.

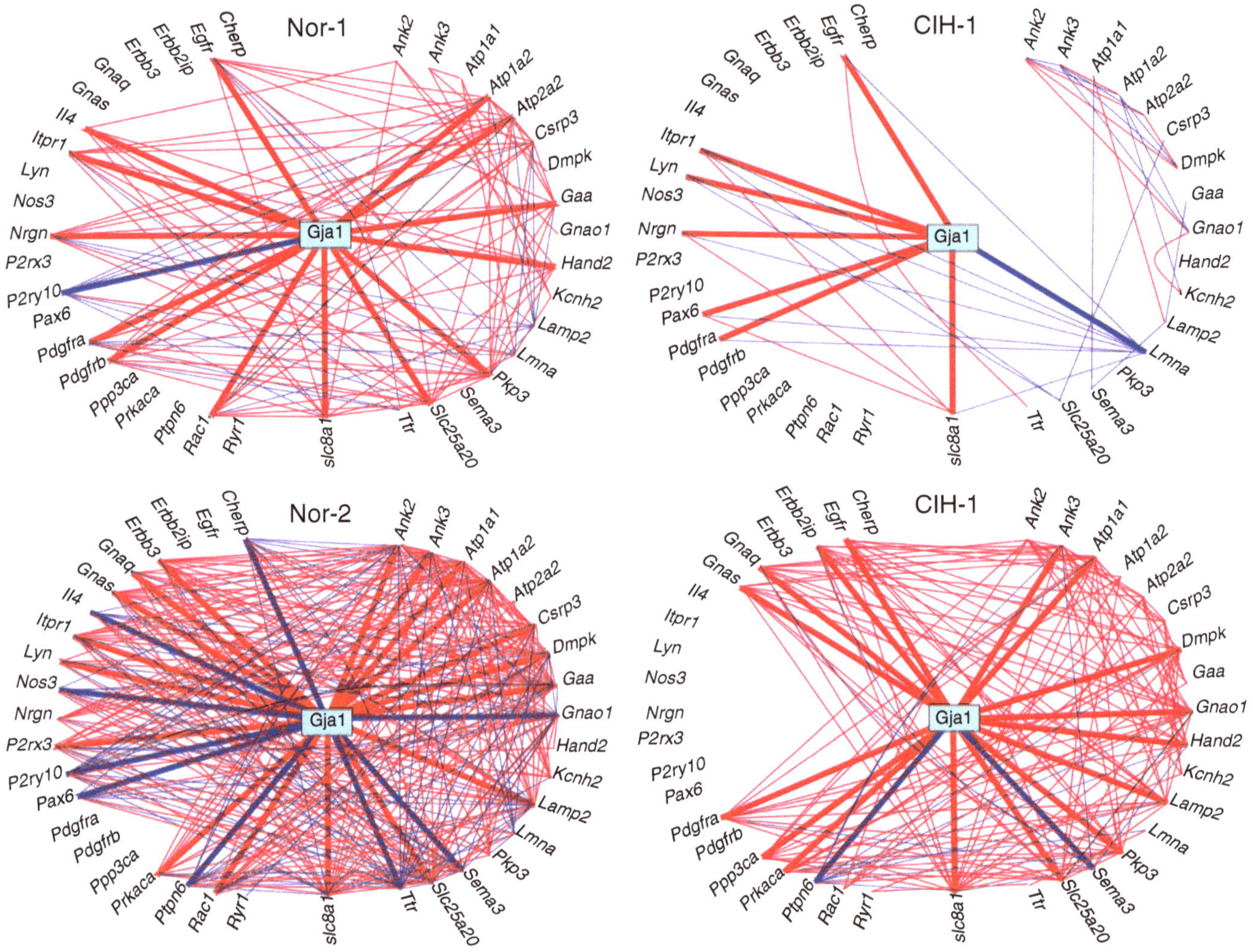

Fig. 2.3 Part of the *Gja1*-dependent network in controlling the heart rhythm determinant and its change during development in normoxic and hypoxic conditions. *Red/blue lines* (thicker for *Gja1* interlinks) indicate synergistic/antagonistic expression coordination of the linked genes. Note that Cx43 encoded by *Gja1* controls expression of HRD genes both by direct expression coordination and through coordination with its Ca^{2+}-signaling gene partners. Genes: *Atp1a1/2* ATPase, Na^+/K^+–transporting, alpha 1/2 polypeptide, *Atp2a2* ATPase, Ca^{2+}-transporting, cardiac muscle, slow twitch 2, *Csrp3* cysteine and glycine-rich protein 3, *Dmpk* dystrophia myotonica-protein kinase, *Gaa* glucosidase, alpha, acid, *Hand2* heart and neural crest derivatives expressed transcript 2, *Lamp2* lysosomal membrane glycoprotein 2, *Lmna* lamin A

2.3.5 Overall Transcriptomic Changes

Figure 2.5 presents the average transcriptomic alterations induced by chronic hypoxia in expression level, control, and coordination of the selected 127 genes as well as the differences between successive time points in the same treatment. Interestingly, coordination alteration is the largest at each treatment duration, pointing out that network remodeling is the most important arrhythmogenic transcriptomic factor and not the regulation of the expression levels of HRD genes. An important observation is that the overall alteration diminishes continuously from 1 to 4 weeks hypoxia indicating activation of transcriptomic adaptation mechanisms to the hypoxia stress. Although chronic hypoxia is a major stress, the developmental changes appear of similar magnitude if not even larger than those induced by hypoxia (compare values of different treatments for the same duration with different durations for the same treatment).

2.4 Discussion

2.4.1 Advantages and Limitations of the Transcriptomic Studies on Ischemic Animal Models

Numerous microarray studies have compared the heart transcriptomes of arrhythmic and non-arrhythmic humans and animal models (e.g., [44–48]), identifying significantly

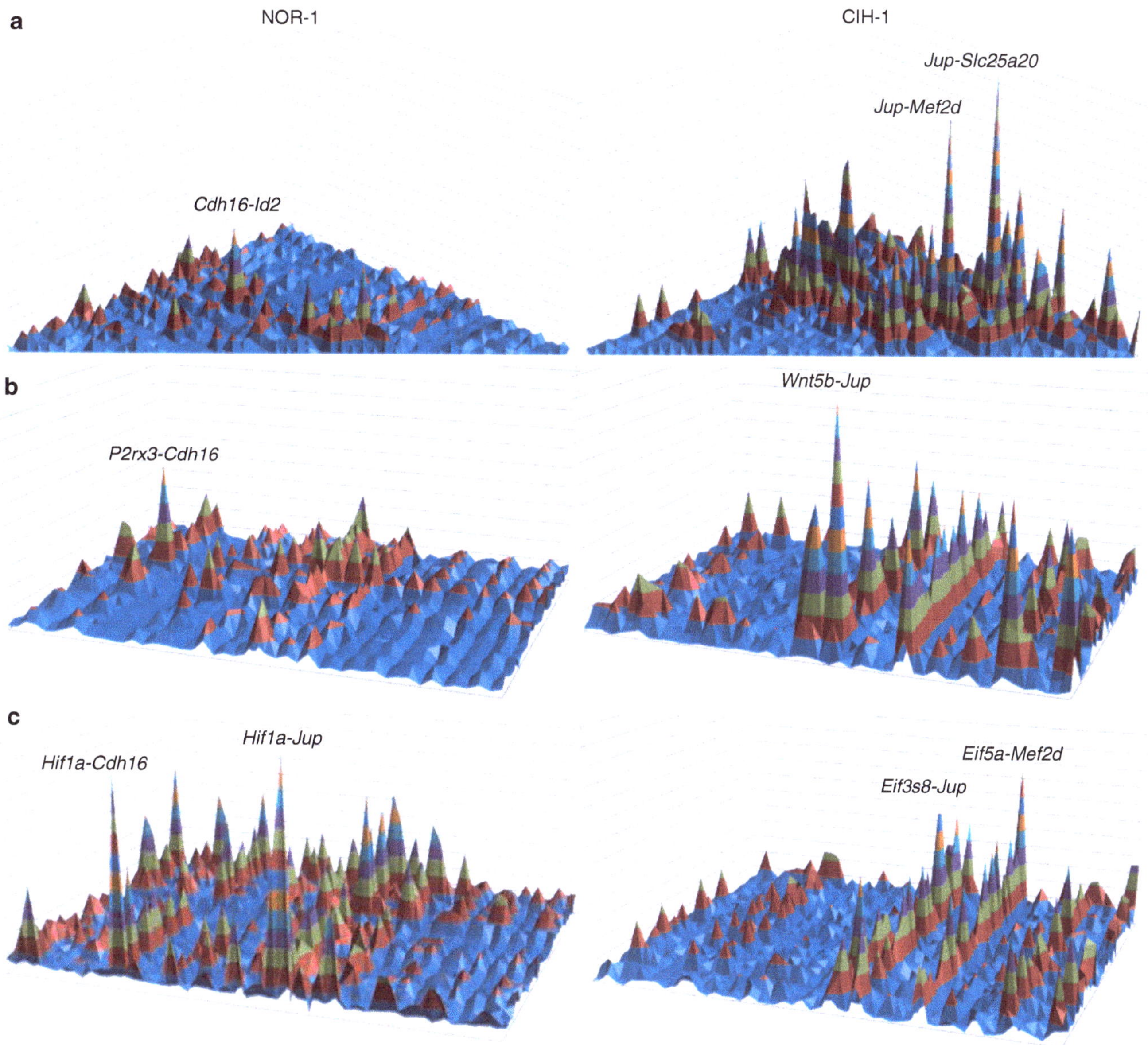

Fig. 2.4 Gene network landscapes at 1 week. (**a**) HRD fabric. Since the same set of HRD genes was considered on both horizontal axes, the landscape is mirrored with respect to the diagonal and therefore only half of it was represented. (**b**) SIG-HRD network. (**c**) TRA-HRD network. Note the profound remodeling of the landscapes, the differences in "mountain heights," and the change of dominant gene pairs. Genes: *Cdh16* cadherin 16, *Eif3s8* eukaryotic translation initiation factor 3, subunit 8

Table 2.3 The dominant gene pairs of each network in each condition

	HRD–HRD	SIG–HRD	TRA–HRD
NOR-1	*Cdh16–Id2* (12.38)	*P2rx3–Cdh16* (12.08)	*Hif1a–Jup* (25.56)
CIH-1	*Slc25a20–Jup* (34.71)	*Wnt5b–Jup* (23.68)	*Eif5a–Mef2d* (17.62)
NOR-2	*Lmna–Pcdh7* (61.56)	*Cacnb1–Pcdh7* (48.82)	*Eif1b–Pcdh7* (50.16)
CIH-2	*Cdh16–Vezt* (20.27)	*Pax–Vezt* (17.46)	*Eif3s12–Pcdh12* (11.12)
NOR-4	*Gnao1–Pcdh7* (20.35)	*Cacnb1–Pcdh7* (11.20)	*Eef1a2–Gnao1* (14.88)
CIH-4	*Pcdh 12–Sema3a* (9.21)	*P2ry10–Pcdh12* (14.94)	*Eif2ak4–Pcdh12* (16.56)

The numbers are the "heights" of the pairs. Note that the "tallest" pairs are at 2 weeks normoxia
Genes: *Cacnb1* calcium channel, voltage-dependent, beta 1 subunit, *Pcdh12* protocadherin 12

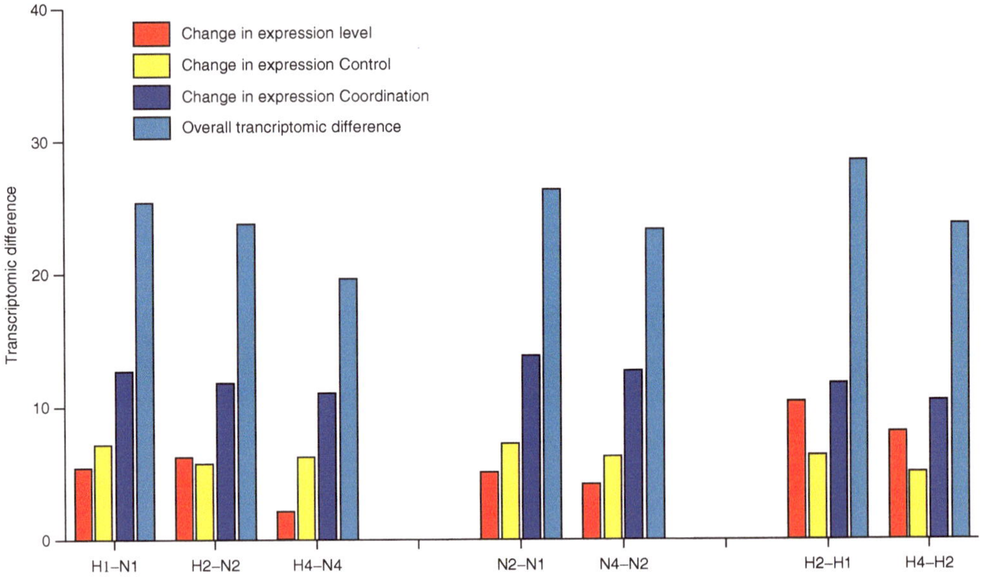

Fig. 2.5 Transcriptomic changes induced by hypoxia (H1-N1, H2-N2, H4-N4) or by development under normoxic (N2-N1, N4-N2) or hypoxic (H2-H1, H4-H2) conditions. Letters *N* and *H* indicate normoxia and hypoxia, while numbers indicate the duration of the treatment (in weeks). Note that change in expression coordination has the largest contribution in each comparison and that changes induced by hypoxia are of similar magnitude as those caused by development either in normoxic or hypoxic conditions

regulated genes and clustering them according to gene ontology (GO) terms and fold expression changes. These studies have had a high impact in delineating essential genomic alterations induced by or predisposing to the disease and in describing transcriptomic differences between normal and pathological conditions. However, although use of lab animals offers unlimited possibilities to investigate consequences of oxygen deprivation, no animal model reproduces exactly what happens in the human body. Even so, animal experiments are critical for narrowing the spectrum of possibilities since the hard cores of a great number of functional pathways were preserved during evolution.

2.4.2 The Endless Story of Gene Expression Analysis

For now, the most powerful and cost-effective tool to investigate complex molecular phenomena is the gene expression array. By quantifying thousands of genes at a time, practically the whole genome, gene expression studies allow endless possibilities to analyze data. The unlimited number of perspectives comes from the fact that genes are not lonely but team players, forming partially overlapping webs whose composition and topology adapt continuously to the variable local conditions. If only gene composition is considered, the complex gene network can be formally deconvoluted into 20,000 or so individual genes, ~200 millions distinct gene pairs, >1.3 trillion distinct triplets, $>6.6\times10^{15}$ quadruplets, and so on. This means as many distinct pathways in which genes may be involved as individuals, doublets, triplets, quadruplets, etc. Moreover, the same pathway may perform differently when conditions change. Because of this, interpretation of microarray data is a never-ending story.

This is our fourth paper analyzing from new perspectives the transcriptomic alterations in hearts of mice subjected in their early life to chronic intermittent hypoxia based on a gene expression experiment. In the first paper [13], we have identified the genes that were up- or downregulated in hypoxia when compared to normoxic counterparts and grouped them according to their GO categories as biological process, molecular function, or cellular localization. Expression regulation of selected genes was confirmed by qRT-PCR, Western blotting, and morphological and physiological observations. Although this was a huge amount of information by itself, it represents only the very tip of what we could learn from such studies.

Table 2.1 shows that in the first and second week of hypoxia, numerous translation regulators and signaling genes were downregulated, while after 4 weeks, only *Eif5a* was downregulated, *Eef1b2* and *Vezt* being upregulated. Interestingly, *Eif5a* was downregulated at all 3 time points that explain why apoptosis was enhanced in chronic constant hypoxia (where it was upregulated at 4 weeks) but not in CIH [13], confirming the role of *Eif5a* in the apoptosis induction [49].

2.4.3 Expression Variability

An important addition was to determine whether the new condition changed the strength of the control of transcript abundance by determining the change of the relative expression variability (REV score) and gene expression stability (GES percentile) [16]. Although the transcriptomic machinery is similar in (here) hearts of mice from the same litter, subjected to the same treatment, the local conditions in which genes are transcribed are never identical, making the genome a noisy system. Therefore, genes exhibit different expression levels in biological replicas, expression variability resulting from the transcriptomic tuning to the local conditions. Moreover, as illustrated in Fig. 2.1b, the variability is not uniform among the genes, our study revealing from very stably expressed (standard deviation negligible when compared to the average expression level) to very unstably expressed (standard deviation exceeding the average value). Since gene expression is regulated by numerous controlling mechanisms, a lower variability indicates a stricter control of the transcript abundance. Expression variability is expected to increase with relaxation of the control of transcript abundance by the homeostatic mechanisms. Very stably expressed genes are likely to be essential for cell survival, phenotype expression, and/or integration in superior, multicellular structures. Correspondingly, certain very unstably expressed genes may be involved in the adaptation to environmental changes. Thus, the analysis of expression variability may provide valuable indication with regard to the role of various genes in maintaining the function or ensuring adaptation of the system to the environment changes. Remarkably, genes such as *Smyd1*, *Eef2*, and *Lyn* were switched between stably and very unstably expressed, indicating profound reconfiguration of transcription control priorities. The relaxed control of *Eef2* at 1 and 4 weeks hypoxia may help its control by *Ampk* whose α_1 and α_2 subunits of AMPK are activated during myocardial ischemia [50].

2.4.4 Remodeling of the HRD Fabric

Figure 2.3 illustrates the plasticity of the HRD fabric whose topology was profoundly remodeled during development and altered by oxygen deprivation. However, when a particular relationship is fundamental for the cardiac function, it tends to be preserved, as the antagonistic expression of *Gja1* and *Sema3* at 2 weeks. Sema3a is important in maintaining normal heart rhythm through sympathetic innervation patterning, both disruption and overexpression of *Sema3a* being associated with reduced sympathetic innervations and attenuation of the epicardial-to-endocardial innervation gradient [51]. On the other hand, Cx43 encoded by *Gja1* influences the heart rhythm by modulating the innervation of the cardiac tissue as we have shown by both transcriptomic and immunostaining comparisons of the left ventricles of wild-type and Cx43 null neonatal mice [52].

2.4.5 Why Have We Focused on Functional Genomic Fabric?

All of our transcriptomic studies indicate that genes are not independently but rather coordinately expressed in transcellular transcription networks (e.g., [36–38]). Therefore, manipulation of a single gene has ripple effects on numerous others, located on all chromosomes and whose protein products are involved in a wide diversity of processes [52]. Because of expression coordination, practically, all genes are directly or indirectly involved in every functional pathway. However, genes are not of equal importance in controlling the pathway and an arbitrary cutoff (either as influence of a gene or as number of genes considered) should be established. Therefore, we have developed and tested the prominent gene analysis (PGA) [17, 39, 40] to identify the genes forming the most interconnected and stably expressed functional web. Expression coordination of web genes forces their expression levels to oscillate in synchrony. PGA is an alternative to the principal component analysis (PCA), both methods aiming to reduce the huge number of variables to the most informative ones. The difference is that while PCA considers "centroids" as the most alterable genes in a set of distinct conditions, PGA selects the most interconnected and stably expressed ones in the same condition. Genomic fabrics exhibit characteristic gene composition and topology depending on region, sex [39], and age [14, 16, 17]; responds by transcriptomic tuning to variable local conditions and environmental constraints [14, 16, 17]; and remodels in disease.

2.4.6 Network Landscape

The novel analysis of network landscape quantifies the role of each gene pair in interconnecting and stabilizing the web. Remarkably, genes encoding the protocadherins *Pcdh7* and *Pcdh12* and cadherin *Cdh16* are components of the most influential pairs within HRD fabric, underlying the role of the intercalated discs in synchronizing contraction of cardiomyocytes. The cadherins are a superfamily of calcium-dependent adhesion molecules with auxiliary functions in embryogenesis, stem cell fate and maintenance, cell polarity, and signal transduction [53]. However, genes encoding signaling proteins such as the purinergic receptors *P2rx3* and *P2ry10* and *Wnt5b*, as well as the translation regulators *Eef1a2*, *Eif1b*, *Eif2ak4*, *Eif3s12, and Eif5a* are forming also very influential pairs with HRD genes.

2.4.7 Overall Transcriptomic Changes

This new measure provides the most comprehensive way to evaluate the transcriptomic differences between two conditions. It includes the "transcriptomic recovery" that we have recently used to determine the reversion of gene expression alterations in hearts of mice with chronic chagasic cardiomyopathy after transplantation of bone marrow cells [54]. The analysis revealed two very interesting aspects: (1) that remodeling of the coordination network has the major contribution when comparing any two conditions and (2) that development and chronic hypoxia induce similar overall transcriptomic changes. The first aspect tells us that analysis of expression regulation is not enough to characterize the transcriptomic alterations induced by pathological conditions/development. Therefore, the list of biomarkers should be extended to include also the genes exhibiting large changes in expression control and coordination.

In summary, from this study, we have learned that chronic intermittent hypoxia is a major stress that profoundly remodels the heart rhythm genomic fabric and signaling pathways controlling this fabric, the overall transcriptomic alterations being comparable to the substantial changes during the development.

Acknowledgment The research was supported by award number HL092001 (DAI) from the National Heart, Lung, and Blood Institute (NHLBI). The content is solely the responsibility of the authors and does not necessarily represent the NHLBI official views.

References

1. Dursunoglu D, Dursunoglu N. Cardiovascular diseases in obstructive sleep apnea. Tuberk Toraks. 2006;54:382–96.
2. Jain V. Clinical perspective of obstructive sleep apnea-induced cardiovascular complications. Antioxid Redox Signal. 2007;9:701–10.
3. Park AM, Nagase H, Kumar SV, et al. Effects of intermittent hypoxia on the heart. Antioxid Redox Signal. 2007;9:723–9.
4. Schweitzer P. Cardiac arrhythmias in obstructive sleep apnea. Vnitr Lek. 2008;54:1006–9.
5. Serebrovskaya TV, Manukhina EB, Smith ML, et al. Intermittent hypoxia: cause of or therapy for systemic hypertension? Exp Biol Med. 2008;233:627–50.
6. Brisco MA, Goldberg LR. Sleep apnea in congestive heart failure. Curr Heart Fail Rep. 2010;7:175–84.
7. Nattel S, Maguy A, Le Bouter S, et al. Arrhythmogenic ion-channel remodeling in the heart: heart failure, myocardial infarction, and atrial fibrillation. Physiol Rev. 2007;87:425–56.
8. Mohler PJ, Wehrens XH. Mechanisms of human arrhythmia syndromes: abnormal cardiac macromolecular interactions. Physiology (Bethesda). 2007;22:342–50.
9. Dostanic I, Schultz Jel J, Lorenz JN, et al. The alpha 1 isoform of Na, K-ATPase regulates cardiac contractility and functionally interacts and co-localizes with the Na/Ca exchanger in heart. J Biol Chem. 2004;279:54053–61.
10. Lee RS, Lam CW, Lai CK, et al. Carnitine-acylcarnitine translocase deficiency in three neonates presenting with rapid deterioration and cardiac arrest. Hong Kong Med J. 2007;13:66–8.
11. Killeen MJ, Thomas G, Sabir IN, et al. Mouse models of human arrhythmia syndromes. Acta Physiol (Oxy). 2008;192:455–69.
12. Teng GQ, Zhao X, Lees-Miller JP, et al. Homozygous missense N629D hERG (KCNH2) potassium channel mutation causes developmental defects in the right ventricle and its outflow tract and embryonic lethality. Circ Res. 2008;103:1483–91.
13. Fan C, Iacobas DA, Zhou D, et al. Gene expression and phenotypic characterization of mouse heart after chronic constant and intermittent hypoxia. Physiol Genomics. 2005;22:292–307.
14. Iacobas DA, Fan C, Iacobas S, et al. Transcriptomic changes in developing kidney exposed to chronic hypoxia. Biochem Biophys Res Commun. 2006;349:329–38.
15. Douglas RM, Miyasaka N, Takahashi K, Hetherington HP, et al. Chronic intermittent but not constant hypoxia decreases NAA/Cr ratios in neonatal mouse hippocampus and thalamus. Am J Physiol Regul Integr Comp Physiol. 2007;292:R1254–9.
16. Iacobas DA, Fan C, Iacobas S, et al. Integrated transcriptomic response to cardiac chronic hypoxia: translation regulators and response to stress in cell survival. Funct Integr Genomics. 2008;8:265–75.
17. Iacobas DA, Iacobas S, Haddad GG. Heart rhythm genomic fabric in hypoxia. Biochem Biophys Res Commun. 2010;391:1769–74.
18. Ai J, Wurster RD, Harden SW, et al. Vagal afferent innervation and remodeling in the aortic arch of young adult Fischer 344 rats following chronic intermittent hypoxia. Neuroscience. 2009;164:658–66.
19. Naghshin J, McGaffin KR, Witham WG, et al. Chronic intermittent hypoxia increases left ventricular contractility in C57BL/6J mice. J Appl Physiol. 2009;107:787–93.
20. Chen L, Zhang J, Hu X, et al. The Na^+/Ca^{2+} exchanger-1 mediates left ventricular dysfunction in mice with chronic intermittent hypoxia. J Appl Physiol. 2010;109:1675–85.
21. Guan Y, Gao L, Ma HJ, et al. Chronic intermittent hypobaric hypoxia decreases beta-adrenoceptor activity in right ventricular papillary muscle. Am J Physiol Heart Circ Physiol. 2010;298:H1267–72.
22. Kc P, Balan KV, Tjoe SS, et al. Increased vasopressin transmission from the paraventricular nucleus to the rostral medulla augments cardiorespiratory outflow in chronic intermittent hypoxia-conditioned rats. J Physiol. 2010;588:725–40.
23. Liu JN, Zhang JX, Lu G, et al. The effect of oxidative stress in myocardial cell injury in mice exposed to chronic intermittent hypoxia. Chin Med J. 2010;123:74–8.
24. Tekin D, Dursun AD, Xi L. Hypoxia inducible factor 1 (HIF-1) and cardioprotection. Acta Pharmacol Sin. 2010;31:1085–94.
25. Zhang Y, Zhong N, Zhou ZN. Effects of chronic intermittent hypobaric hypoxia on the L-type calcium current in rat ventricular myocytes. High Alt Med Biol. 2010;11:61–7.
26. van Rooij E, Olson EN. MicroRNAs: powerful new regulators of heart disease and provocative therapeutic targets. J Clin Invest. 2007;117:2369–76.
27. Cai B, Pan Z, Lu Y. The roles of microRNAs in heart diseases: a novel important regulator. Curr Med Chem. 2010;17:407–11.
28. Girmatsion Z, Biliczki P, Bonauer A, et al. Changes in microRNA-1 expression and IK1 up-regulation in human atrial fibrillation. Heart Rhythm. 2009;6:1802–9.
29. Kormish JD, Sinner D, Zorn AM. Interactions between SOX factors and Wnt/beta-catenin signaling in development and disease. Dev Dyn. 2010;239:56–68.
30. Ai Z, Fischer A, Spray DC, et al. Wnt-1 regulation of connexin43 in cardiac myocytes. J Clin Invest. 2000;105:161–71.
31. Gessert S, Kühl M. The multiple phases and faces of Wnt signaling during cardiac differentiation and development. Circ Res. 2010; 107:186–99.
32. Nagy II, Railo A, Rapila R, et al. Wnt-11 signalling controls ventricular myocardium development by patterning N-cadherin and beta-catenin expression. Cardiovasc Res. 2010;85:100–9.
33. Garcia-Gras E, Lombardi R, Giocondo MJ, et al. Suppression of canonical Wnt/beta-catenin signaling by nuclear plakoglobin recapitulates phenotype of arrhythmogenic right ventricular cardiomyopathy. J Clin Invest. 2006;116:2012–21.
34. Malekar P, Hagenmueller M, Anyanwu A, et al. Wnt signaling is critical for maladaptive cardiac hypertrophy and accelerates myocardial remodeling. Hypertension. 2010;55:939–45.
35. Martin J, Afouda BA, Hoppler S. Wnt/beta-catenin signalling regulates cardiomyogenesis via GATA transcription factors. J Anat. 2010;216:92–107.
36. Iacobas DA, Iacobas S, Urban-Maldonado M, et al. Similar transcriptomic alterations in Cx43 knock-down and knock-out astrocytes. Cell Commun Adhes. 2008;15:195–206.

37. Spray DC, Iacobas DA. Organizational principles of the connexin-related brain transcriptome. J Membr Biol. 2007;218:39–47.
38. Iacobas DA, Iacobas S, Spray DC. Connexin-dependent transcellular transcriptomic networks in mouse brain. Prog Biophys Mol Biol. 2007;94:168–84.
39. Iacobas DA, Iacobas S, Thomas N, et al. Sex-dependent gene regulatory networks of the heart rhythm. Funct Integr Genomics. 2010;10:73–86.
40. Iacobas S, Iacobas DA. Astrocyte proximity modulates the myelination gene fabric of oligodendrocytes. Neuron Glia Biol. 2010;6:157–169.
41. Lombardi R, Dong J, Rodriguez G, et al. Genetic fate mapping identifies second heart field progenitor cells as a source of adipocytes in arrhythmogenic right ventricular cardiomyopathy. Circ Res. 2009;104:1076–84.
42. Paige SL, Osugi T, Afanasiev OK, et al. Endogenous Wnt/beta-catenin signaling is required for cardiac differentiation in human embryonic stem cells. PLoS One. 2010;5:e11134.
43. Chen HW, Yu SL, Chen WJ, et al. Dynamic changes of gene expression profiles during postnatal development of the heart in mice. Heart. 2004;90:927–34.
44. Liew CC, Dzau VJ. Molecular genetics and genomics of heart failure. Nat Rev Genet. 2004;5:811–25.
45. Gao Z, Xu H, DiSilvestre D, et al. Transcriptomic profiling of the canine tachycardia-induced heart failure model: global comparison to human and murine heart failure. J Mol Cell Cardiol. 2006;40:76–86.
46. Roberts R. Genomics and cardiac arrhythmias. J Am Coll Cardiol. 2006;47:9–21.
47. Jickling GC, Xu H, Stamova B, et al. Signatures of cardioembolic and large-vessel ischemic stroke. Ann Neurol. 2010;68:681–92.
48. Du CY, El Harchi A, McPate MJ, et al. Enhanced inhibitory effect of acidosis on hERG potassium channels that incorporate the hERG1b isoform. Biochem Biophys Res Commun. 2011;405:222–7.
49. Sun Z, Cheng Z, Taylor CA, et al. Apoptosis induction by eIF5A1 involves activation of the intrinsic mitochondrial pathway. J Cell Physiol. 2010;223:798–809.
50. Wong AK, Howie J, Petrie JR, et al. AMP-activated protein kinase pathway: a potential therapeutic target in cardiometabolic disease. Clin Sci. 2009;116:607–20.
51. Ieda M, Kanazawa H, Kimura K, et al. Sema3a maintains normal heart rhythm through sympathetic innervation patterning. Nat Med. 2007;13:604–12.
52. Iacobas DA, Iacobas S, Li WE, et al. Genes controlling multiple functional pathways are transcriptionally regulated in connexin43 null mouse heart. Physiol Genomics. 2005;20:211–23.
53. Delmar M, McKenna WJ. The cardiac desmosome and arrhythmogenic cardiomyopathies: from gene to disease. Circ Res. 2010;107:700–14.
54. Soares MBP, Lima RS, Souza BSF, et al. Reversion of gene expression alterations in hearts of mice with chronic chagasic cardiomyopathy after transplantation of bone marrow cells. Cell Cycle. 2011;10:1448–55.

Intermittent Hypoxia and Atherosclerosis

3

Demet Tekin, Elisa Chong, and Lei Xi

Abstract

Atherosclerosis is a common pathologic condition that is affecting millions of people in their large and small arteries, including the aorta, coronary, and cerebral arteries. Atherosclerotic lesions are characterized by focal thickening of the vascular tunica intima, through the accumulation of fatty deposits, platelets, and leukocytes in the endothelial cell layer, which eventually form the fatty streaks and plaques inside vascular walls. The subsequent ulceration and rupture of plaques could trigger the formation of thrombi that may partially or completely obstruct blood circulation and cause devastating consequences impairing the function and survival of vital organs. Therefore, atherosclerosis represents a distinguished basis of cardiac, cerebral, and peripheral vascular diseases. This chapter is aimed at providing a comprehensive and non-biased overview on the updated evidence of both detrimental and beneficial effects of intermittent hypoxia in the pathological process of atherosclerosis. Collectively, there is a remarkably abundant body of evidence for an atherogenic role played by chronic and severe intermittent hypoxia. On the other hand, a number of studies originated predominantly by Russian/Ukrainian scientists also demonstrated paradoxical anti-atherosclerosis prophylactic and therapeutic effects, which could be elicited by some well-controlled training/conditioning regimens with often mild or moderate levels of intermittent hypoxia. Considering these most updated evidence and divergent points of view, we have further discussed the possible molecular signaling pathways for both detrimental and protective mechanisms of IH. Nevertheless, many seemingly controversial areas require further investigations, which will undoubtedly bring new insights into the fundamental issue of prevention and treatment of atherosclerosis-associated cardiovascular diseases.

D. Tekin (✉)
Department of Physiology, School of Medicine,
Ankara University, Ankara, Turkey
e-mail: dtekin@medicine.ankara.edu.tr

E. Chong
Division of Cardiology, School of Medicine,
Virginia Commonwealth University,
Richmond, VA, USA

L. Xi
Division of Cardiology, School of Medicine,
Virginia Commonwealth University,
Richmond, VA, USA
e-mail: lxi@vcu.edu

L. Xi, T.V. Serebrovskaya (eds.), *Intermittent Hypoxia and Human Diseases*,
DOI 10.1007/978-1-4471-2906-6_3, © Springer-Verlag London 2012

Abbreviations

APOE	Apolipoprotein E
COX-2	Cyclooxygenase-2
CPAP	Continuous positive airway pressure
ELAM	Endothelial-leukocyte adhesion molecule
eNOS	Endothelial nitric oxide synthase
EPCs	Endothelial progenitor cells
EPO	Erythropoietin
FFA	Free fatty acid
FGF	Fibroblast growth factor
FMD	Flow-mediated dilation
HDL	High-density lipoprotein
HIF-1	Hypoxia inducible factor 1
ICAM	Intercellular adhesion molecule
IGF-1	Insulin-like growth factor
IH	Intermittent hypoxia
IHT	Intermittent hypoxia training
IL-6	Interleukin 6
IMT	Intima–media thickness
iNOS	Inducible nitric oxide synthase
LDL	Low-density lipoprotein
LTB4	Leukotriene B4
MCP-1	Monocyte chemotactic protein 1
NADPH	Nicotinamide adenine dinucleotide phosphate
NF-κB	Nuclear factor kappa B
NO	Nitric oxide
NOS	Nitric oxide synthase
OSA	Obstructive sleep apnea
PAI-1	Plasminogen activator inhibitor 1
PDGF	Platelet-derived growth factor
PMNs	Polymorphonuclear leukocytes
RDI	Respiratory disturbance index
ROS	Reactive oxygen species
SCD-1	Stearoyl coenzyme A desaturase 1
SMCs	Smooth muscle cells
SREBP	Sterol regulatory element-binding protein
TF	Tissue factor
TLR	Toll-like receptor
TNF-α	Tumor necrosis factor-alpha
TRLP	Triglyceride-rich lipoprotein
VCAM	Vascular cell adhesion molecule
VEGF	Vascular endothelial growth factor
VLDL	Very-low-density lipoprotein

3.1 Introduction

Human health is essentially dependent upon normal vascular function to maintain blood circulation, which supplies the critically important oxygen and nutrients to all vital organs in the human body. Blood vessels contain three basic structural components: (1) *tunica intima*, (2) *tunica media*, and (3) *tunica adventitia*. The *tunica intima* is composed of endothelial cell layer and a thin subendothelial layer with connective tissue and occasional smooth muscle cells. Endothelium is a special type of epithelium that acts as a semipermeable barrier between the blood plasma and the interstitial tissue fluid that controls the exchange of nutrients and fluid between plasma and artery wall. Endothelial cells perform several other functions, including production of (1) vasoactive factors that affect the vascular tone, such as vasodilatory nitric oxide and prostacyclin, and vasoconstrictive endothelin and angiotensin-II; (2) inflammatory mediators; and (3) growth factors such as vascular endothelial growth factor (VEGF) to help maintain the vasculature and regulate vasculogenesis and angiogenesis under normal and pathologic conditions. The endothelium also regulates blood coagulation. When endothelial cells are damaged by atherosclerotic lesions, the contact of subendothelial connective tissue with blood induces the aggregation of blood platelets and following coagulation pathways.

The *tunica media* consists of concentric layers of smooth muscle cells and variable amounts of elastic fibers and lamellae, reticular fibers of collagen type III, proteoglycans, and glycoproteins interposed among the smooth muscle cells, all of which is produced by these cells. Smooth muscle cells or fibers occur in the walls of all vessels larger than capillaries. By maintaining their attachments to neighbor cells and surrounding connective tissue matrix, smooth muscle cells provide the tonus of the artery.

The *tunica adventitia* consists principally of type I collagen and elastic fibers. This adventitial layer is gradually continuous with the stromal connective tissue of the organ through which the blood vessel runs. Collagen fibers are found throughout the wall: in the subendothelial layer, between muscle layers, and in the outer layers. Elastic material provides the resiliency for the vascular wall expanded under pressure. Elastin predominates in large arteries where it forms parallel lamellae regularly distributed between the muscle layers [89, 111].

3.2 Atherosclerosis

Atherosclerosis is a common pathologic condition that is affecting millions of people in their large and small arteries, including the aorta, coronary, and cerebral arteries. Atherosclerotic lesions are characterized by focal thickening of the vascular tunica intima, through the accumulation of fatty deposits, platelets, and leukocytes in the endothelial cell layer. As the lesions progress, proliferation of smooth muscle cells and connective tissue elements and the deposition of cholesterol in smooth muscle cells and macrophages occur throughout the

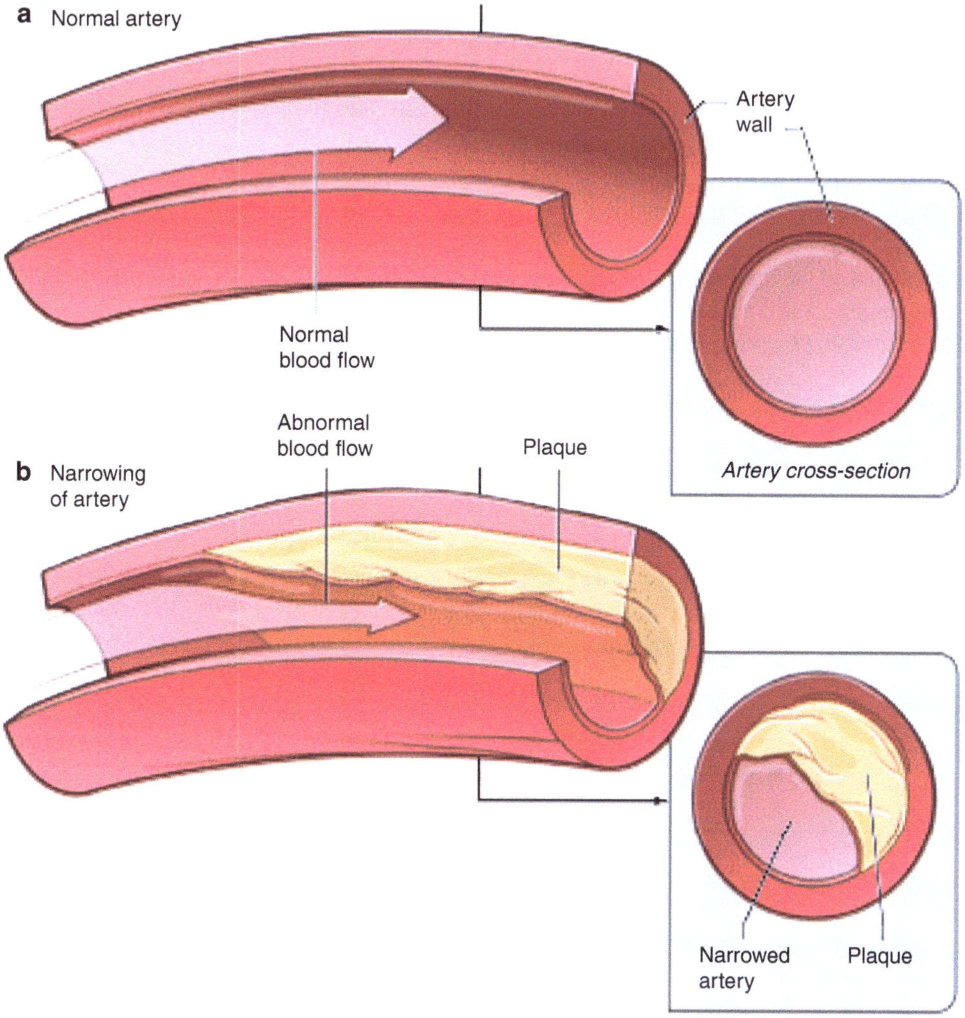

Fig. 3.1 Illustrative description of atherosclerosis. (**a**) Shows a normal artery with normal blood flow. (**b**) Shows an artery with plaque buildup (Adapted from the public health information posted by the National Heart Lung and Blood Institute, US Department of Health, and Human Services; (http://www.nhlbi.nih.gov/health/health-topics/topics/atherosclerosis/)

vascular tunica media. When heavily loaded with lipids, these cells are referred to as foam cells and form the fatty streaks and plaques that characterize atherosclerosis (Fig. 3.1). These changes may extend to the inner part of the tunica media, and the thickening may become so great as to occlude the vessel [23, 89]. Localized fibrous thickenings of the arterial wall are associated with lipid-infiltrated plaques that may eventually calcify. Old plaques are also prone to ulceration and rupture, triggering the formation of thrombi that obstruct blood flow. Therefore, atherosclerosis leads to vascular insufficiency in the limbs, abnormalities of the renal circulation, dilations (aneurysms), and even rupture of the aorta or other large arteries. It also leads to common severe and life-threatening diseases of the heart and brain because of the formation of intravascular clots at the site of the plaques [92]. High serum cholesterol, high blood pressure, infection, high blood iron or homocysteine levels, smoking, and hereditary factors are among the proposed etiological factors for atherosclerosis [23].

The pathogenetic events of atherosclerosis, which follow each other but sometimes appear parallel, are summarized below [11, 51, 52, 78, 92, 111].

3.2.1 Increased Permeability of the Endothelium to Macromolecules Such as Low-Density Lipoproteins

Shear stress and various vasoactive agents that induce endothelial cell constriction with the opening of endothelial junctions can increase the endothelial cell permeability especially at points where the arteries branch. This is followed by the infiltration of low-density lipoprotein (LDL) into subendothelial region. Genetic and environmental factors can also change the properties of endothelial adhesion factors without endothelial injury and initiate atherosclerosis in some individuals.

3.2.2 Subsequent Oxidation of LDL Cholesterol Particles and Endothelial Injury

Steep oxygen gradients within the arterial wall create local conditions for free radical generation. Peroxidative injury increases the atherogenic potential of both cholesteryl ester-rich (low-density) and triglyceride-rich (very-low-density and intermediate-density) lipoproteins. Oxidized LDLs initiate endothelial injury by activating the expression and release of proinflammatory molecules, such as natural antibodies; innate effector proteins, such as C-reactive proteins and the complement system; cytokines; chemokines; and adhesion molecules, such as intercellular adhesion molecule (ICAM), endothelial-leukocyte adhesion molecule (ELAM), and vascular cell adhesion molecule (VCAM), from endothelial cells, macrophages, or T cells. Oxidized LDLs inhibit NO production causing defective vasodilation. Modified LDLs activate Toll-like receptors (TLRs), particularly TLR4, which in turn induce proinflammatory gene expression and lead to macrophage infiltration by monocyte chemotactic protein-1 (MCP-1).

3.2.3 Leukocyte and Platelet Adherence to the Areas of Endothelial Injury

Proinflammatory cytokines draw white blood cells and platelets to the areas of endothelial injury, which in turn stimulate clotting, activate T and B cells, and release chemicals that act as chemoattractants to perpetuate the cycle of inflammation, clotting, and fibrosis.

3.2.4 Entrance of Leukocytes into the Subintimal Space

The endothelium becomes sticky to white blood cells by the activation of endothelial adhesion factors. Rolling and adherence are the first steps of leukocyte recruitment controlled by chemokines, cytokines, and adhesion molecules released into the media. Once attached to the endothelial layer, the monocytes and neutrophils begin to emigrate between the endothelial cells and into the interstitial space. In the interstitium, the monocytes mature into macrophages and, along with the neutrophils, continue to release cytokines, which further induce the inflammatory cycle.

3.2.5 Secretion of Growth Factors by Platelets, Injured Endothelium, and Macrophages

Proliferation has been attributed to growth factors, such as platelet-derived growth factor (PDGF), fibroblast growth factor (FGF), and insulin-like growth factor (IGF-1). Because these growth factors can be produced by the endothelium in vitro, it is likely that the dysfunctional endothelium in atherosclerosis also produces growth factors while shifting from a growth-inhibitory to a growth-promoting mode.

3.2.6 Recruitment of Smooth Muscle Cells from the Media to the Subintima Where They Proliferate

The release of cytokines, chemokines, and growth factors by inflammatory cells, including platelets, causes the migration and proliferation of smooth muscle cells (SMCs). Proliferating SMCs can internalize lipids and lipoproteins to form foam cells. Lipids accumulate both intracellularly and extracellularly. Subintimal SMCs can synthesize collagen, elastin, glycosaminoglycans, and other connective tissue elements that trap lipoproteins, therefore, ensuring plaque stability. SMCs can also synthesize PDGF and other growth factors that cause self-stimulation of SMC proliferation, tissue factor (TF), and plasminogen activator inhibitor-1 (PAI-1) that act locally to produce thrombin or inhibit fibrinolysis of the fibrin network used to facilitate cell migration and MCP-1, which increases monocyte chemoattraction into the lesion, thereby leading to lesion development.

3.2.7 Formation of Macrophage Foam Cells sand Fatty Streaks

Oxidized LDLs are recognized by a family of scavenger receptors expressed on macrophages. These scavenger receptors mediate the uptake of oxidized LDL into macrophages and the formation of foam cells. The foam cells form fatty streaks and the ones in the overlying endothelium can express MCP-1, resulting in further enhanced monocyte chemoattraction and adhesion. The streaks usually appear in the aorta during the first decade of human life, in the coronary arteries during the second decade, and in the cerebral arteries during the third and fourth decades.

3.2.8 Thrombus Formation, Plaque Rupture and Ulceration

Endothelial injury leads to platelet deposition, tissue factor-mediated activation of extrinsic coagulation to generate thrombin, cleavage of fibrinogen to fibrin, and formation of thrombus. Thrombin gives rise to endothelial expression of adhesion molecules and consequent monocyte attachment, together with secretion of platelet granular constituents. With continued injury and inflammation, platelet aggregation increases and a thrombus begins to form. Fibrous scar tissue replaces some of the vascular wall, changing the structure of the wall. This results in the formation of cholesterol and fat buildup, fibrous scar tissue deposits, platelet-derived clots, and smooth muscle cell proliferation. As plaques mature, a fibrous cap can form over them; the plaques with defective or broken caps are most prone to rupture. Furthermore, matrix metalloproteinases are secreted and activated by inflammatory cells that degrade extracellular matrix components and increase the vulnerability of atherosclerotic plaque to rupture. The lesions alone may distort vessels to the point that they are occluded, but it is usually rupture or ulceration of plaques that trigger thrombosis – the formation of blood clots that eventually block blood flow.

3.3 Obstructive Sleep Apnea and Cardiovascular System Diseases

Obstructive sleep apnea (OSA) is a chronic medical condition characterized by repeated episodes of apnea due to upper airway obstruction during sleep [138]. These episodes result in hypoventilation, hypoxemia, reoxygenation, recurrent arousals from sleep, and activation of the sympathetic nervous system. OSA occurs in 2–4% of middle-aged women and 4–9% of middle-aged men in the general population [1, 137]. The increased risk of cardiovascular diseases is among the other adverse consequences of OSA [87, 135]. An 18-year follow-up of the Wisconsin sleep cohort has shown that the untreated severe OSA patients are five times more likely to die from cardiovascular causes [139]. However, confounding variables, such as obesity, hypertension, smoking, alcohol intake, age, and level of exercise make this independent relationship difficult to prove [112]. On the other hand, continuous positive airway pressure (CPAP) therapy decreases cardiovascular morbidity and mortality in OSA patients. This proves OSA as an independent risk factor for its cardiovascular consequences. In a large cardiovascular outcome study, severe untreated OSA significantly increased the risk of fatal and nonfatal cardiovascular events [87].

In a prospective study from the Sleep Heart Health cohort, the investigators found that OSA, independent of several confounding variables, causes significant increases in all-cause and coronary artery disease-related cardiovascular mortality, particularly in men aged 40–70 years with severe form of OSA [106]. Recently, Shah et al. conducted a large observational cohort study showing that patients with OSA had an increased risk for the development of myocardial infarction, coronary revascularization events, and cardiovascular death, independent of other cardiovascular risk factors [121]. Furthermore, OSA has been implicated as an independent risk factor for the development of hypertension [97], stroke [135], coronary artery disease [100], congestive heart failure [131], cardiac arrhythmias [46], pulmonary hypertension [116], and aortic dissection [95]. The cardiovascular morbidities resulting from OSA have also been studied broadly in animal models to further elucidate the underlying molecular mechanisms. These studies were reviewed in details by Farré and colleagues [37].

It is notable that each cycle of apnea and following recovery of ventilation is accompanied by arterial oxyhemoglobin desaturation and resaturation into the normal levels. This situation creates a typical case of intermittent hypoxia in the OSA patients that could last throughout the night. Thus, the chronic exposure to intermittent hypoxia has been traditionally considered as one of the main causes of cardiovascular diseases in patients with OSA.

3.4 Detrimental Role of Intermittent Hypoxia in Initiation and Progression of Atherosclerosis

Intermittent hypoxia (IH) and its clinical version – OSA – are associated with atherosclerosis and conditions predisposing to atherosclerosis, including endothelial dysfunction, dyslipidemia, oxidative stress, endothelial and systemic inflammation, and hypercoagulation [4, 11, 28, 31, 43, 77, 78, 94, 125].

Savransky et al. investigated the induction of atherosclerosis in a murine model of OSA based on chronic IH combined with the preexisting hyperlipidemia. They found that 12 weeks of chronic IH led to the development of atherosclerotic lesions in the aortic origin and descending aorta in the mice on a high-cholesterol diet, whereas the mice on a regular diet were free of the disease. These results suggest that preexisting dyslipidemia, due to either genetic or environmental factors, is necessary for the expression of atherogenic properties of IH [117]. On the contrary, rabbits fed a normal diet and exposed to IH for 3 weeks developed arteriosclerotic changes in the aorta [54]. In another animal study, exposure to 12-h daily intermittent repetitive hypoxia for 3 weeks was found to strongly promote vascular disease indicated by intimal thickening both in normal and previously damaged arteries [72].

One of the characteristics of atherosclerosis is increased intima–media thickness (IMT) of the artery. Carotid IMT is evaluated by ultrasound, correlates well with anatomical measurements, and is an early marker of preclinical atheroma [78]. According to the results of several studies, intermittent nocturnal hypoxemia is associated with early signs of atherosclerosis represented by increased carotid IMT with correlated systemic inflammatory markers in OSA patients. This is also correlated to the severity, frequency, and duration of the hypoxemia [28, 90, 125]. The CPAP treatment significantly improves validated markers of atherosclerosis including carotid IMT and inflammatory responses in patients with OSA. These results provided evidence suggesting OSA is an independent risk factor for atherosclerosis [29]. Nevertheless, the demonstration of an independent association between OSA and atherosclerosis is difficult because the majority of the patients with OSA share several risk factors for atherosclerosis, including hypertension, diabetes, and obesity [133].

Recently, Drager and colleagues reported that the coexistence of OSA and hypertension has additive effects on the markers of atherosclerosis such as carotid IMT and diameter of the artery [30]. In addition to IMT, tomographic coronary calcium scoring is used for risk stratification of asymptomatic patients under the risk of coronary events. Coronary artery calcification is an active event and can be seen at all stages of atherosclerotic plaque formation and progression. The direct effects of OSA on the presence and extent of coronary atherosclerosis quantified by the tomographic coronary calcification scoring have been investigated in a cross-sectional observational study on 97 patients with OSA, who were asymptomatic for coronary artery disease. The results of the study revealed that OSA contributes to coronary artery disease risk with association to the severity of hypoxemia [67].

In the following sections, we further provide an in-depth analysis on the potential mechanisms related to the IH-induced detrimental effects on atherosclerosis, based on the evidence from both animal studies and clinical investigations in the OSA patients – a most commonly used model for studying the pathological consequences of chronic IH in humans.

3.4.1 IH and Endothelial Injury and Dysfunction

Vascular endothelium is a multifunctional, dynamic cell layer, which controls vascular functions through accepting or releasing several vasoactive mediators and inflammatory and growth factors. In addition to its physiological barrier function between blood and tissue, endothelium regulates hemostasis, vascular tone, and angiogenesis. The balance between vasoconstrictor and vasodilator factors has a crucial role in the maintenance of vascular homeostasis. On the other hand, oxidative stress, inflammatory mediators, hypercholesterolemia, and sympathetic activation are among the factors that initiate endothelial injury following a cascade of events leading to atherosclerosis. Endothelial injury is an important component in the initiation of the atherosclerotic process. Injured endothelium becomes proinflammatory and prothrombotic. Therefore, vasoconstriction, vascular smooth muscle proliferation, hypercoagulability, and thrombosis are among the potential consequences.

Endothelial dysfunction denotes impairment in endothelium-dependent vasodilation mediated by nitric oxide (NO). Flow-mediated dilation (FMD) is NO-dependent vasodilation that results from shear stress-mediated activation of endothelial NO synthesis in response to acute increases in blood flow [63]. Ultrasound assessment of FMD can be utilized for the evaluation of endothelial function and cardiovascular risk [22]. It was suggested that IH causes endothelial dysfunction, possibly due to decreased bioavailability of NO. In addition to vasodilation, other protective effects of NO are important for the prevention of atherosclerosis. These effects include the limitation of leukocyte recruitment and leukocyte expression of adhesion molecules and the prevention of vascular smooth muscle cell proliferation and platelet aggregation and adhesion [73]. Various evidences indicate that vascular endothelium is functionally impaired in patients with OSA. For instance, circulating markers of endothelial injury such as cell adhesion molecules, fibrinogen, and nitric oxide have been shown to be affected by OSA [33, 57, 58]. Endothelial NO availability deceases possibly via a direct effect of IH on the endothelial NO synthase (eNOS)-mediated NO production (reviewed in [39, 68]). As a result, NO-dependent FMD is impaired, as being a prognostic marker of atherosclerosis [98]. An impaired endothelium-dependent vasodilation in resistance arteries is also evident in OSA patients, and the severity of this impairment is correlated with the degree of nocturnal hypoxemia [58, 65, 71]. Another reason for decreased NO production could be the promotion of endothelial cell apoptosis by IH [25]. Indeed, patients with OSA have an increased number of circulating apoptotic endothelial cells, which are correlated with the abnormal endothelium-mediated vasodilation, thereby the process of atherosclerosis, and are reversible by CPAP therapy [36].

While hypoxia has several deleterious effects, cellular and systemic responses to hypoxia attempt to compensate for these effects. Endothelial progenitor cells (EPCs) are circulating bone-marrow-derived cells, which protect endothelium by increasing endothelial repair capacity. EPCs have important roles in vascular regeneration, neovascularization, and improving blood perfusion and, therefore, the recovery of ischemic tissues [7]. Hypoxia inducible factor-1alpha (HIF-1α), a major transcription factor in response to hypoxia, activates angiogenic VEGF [42, 120]. VEGF leads to mobilization of EPCs from the bone marrow and induces the angiogenic properties of these cells [7]. There are inconsistent findings in regard to EPC levels in patients with OSA suggesting that not all patients are exposed to hypoxia–reoxygenation to the same extent. However, recent evidence suggests that EPCs are decreased particularly in OSA patients with endothelial dysfunction and related cardiovascular morbidities [7, 60].

Endothelial injury that is related to oxidative stress and inflammation has also been reported in some in vitro studies. The expression of eNOS as a source of endothelial NO, cyclooxygenase-2 (COX-2), and inducible NO synthase (iNOS) as markers of vascular endothelial inflammation and endothelial nitrotyrosine as an indicator of nitrosative stress were evaluated in venous endothelial cells collected from OSA patients [60]. While the expression of eNOS was found to be decreased, implicating the reduced NO availability, the expressions of COX-2, iNOS, and nitrotyrosine were found to be increased. In addition to findings of vascular inflammation and oxidative stress, circulating endothelial progenitor cells were found to be increased, compromising the impaired endothelial repair mechanism. FMD is an indirect marker of arterial endothelial NO-mediated reactivity and was also reduced in these patients. The reversal of the above findings by CPAP verifies the independent effects of OSA on endothelial dysfunction [60].

3.4.2 IH and Dyslipidemia

Accumulated evidence suggests that IH induces dyslipidemia in either experimental IH or in patients with OSA. For example, the mice with exposure to IH for 5 days had increased serum cholesterol uptake and triglyceride levels in the liver [79]. Total cholesterol, high-density lipoprotein (HDL) cholesterol, phospholipids, and triglyceride levels were also upregulated in their serum, whereas an increase in low-density lipoprotein (LDL) cholesterol became evident after 4 weeks of IH [79]. In another animal experiment, chronic IH for 21 days increased triglyceride and very-low-density lipoprotein (VLDL) levels, while 4 days of IH did not affect plasma levels of total cholesterol, LDL, and triglycerides, suggesting a time-dependent effect of hypoxia on lipids [101]. Hypoxic stimulus to human macrophages in vitro causes an accumulation of triglyceride-containing cytosolic lipid droplets, which then convert to foam cells [12]. This proposed hyperlipidemia scheme, when combined with increased lipid peroxidation following macrophage foaming, would possibly lead to a progression of atherosclerosis in IH.

In addition, stearoyl coenzyme A desaturase (SCD-1), a hepatic enzyme of lipoprotein secretion, has been found to play a critical role in intermittent hypoxia-induced dyslipidemia and atherosclerosis [118]. Another factor related to hyperlipidemia is the sterol regulatory element-binding protein (SREBP), a transcription factor of lipid biosynthesis in the liver. It was demonstrated in a mouse model of IH that SREBP pathway mediates the IH-induced dyslipidemia. These authors suggested that the elements of SREBP pathway can be considered as potential therapeutic targets [80].

Another recent study on the mice fed with a high-cholesterol diet and exposed to 4 weeks of chronic IH demonstrated that hypoxia inactivated adipose lipoprotein lipase activity and, thus, inhibited the clearance of triglyceride-rich lipoproteins (TRLP) [32]. Interestingly, the same group also showed that increased levels of TRLP by IH were associated with atherosclerosis [117]. In the atherosclerosis-prone apolipoprotein E (APOE) knockout mice, IH accelerated the growth of advanced atherosclerotic plaques together with elevated levels of serum lipids [62].

Clinically, hyperlipidemia and lipid peroxidation in non-obese patients with OSA were found to be dependent on the severity of chronic IH [81]. In a large cross-sectional study (Sleep Heart Health Study), where 6,440 healthy subjects were screened for OSA, a significant correlation between the severity of hypoxia and the total serum cholesterol, HDL, and triglyceride levels, was observed [96]. In addition, Robinson et al. found a significant decrease in total cholesterol of OSA patients after CPAP therapy in their clinical trial [108].

It was reported that inflammatory cytokines (such as IL-2 and IL-6) upregulate serum amyloid alpha production in OSA patients [124]. Serum amyloid alpha is an apolipoprotein and an acute-phase reactant, which changes the high-density lipoprotein composition during inflammatory response. There is a strong relationship between serum amyloid alpha and atherogenesis as well as the future cardiovascular events [61].

Finally, Drager et al. proposed a putative mechanism for chronic IH-induced dyslipidemia. According to this mechanism, IH induces SREBP-1c and SCD-1through HIF-1 activation in the liver. The following increase of fatty acids and triglycerides leads to hepatic steatosis and an increase in lipoprotein secretion. IH also increases adipose tissue lipolysis resulting in an increased free fatty acid (FFA) flux to the liver, heart, and skeletal muscle. In addition, IH inhibits lipoprotein lipase clearance. All these effects would cause dyslipidemia with a rise in VLDL. Other potential factors, such as sympathetic activation, insulin resistance, and oxidative stress, may also involve in the IH-induced dyslipidemia in OSA patients [31].

3.4.3 IH and Oxidative Stress and Inflammation

Normal cellular energy metabolism produces reactive oxygen species (ROS) such as superoxide anion, hydrogen peroxide, and hydroxyl radicals. ROS can potentially originate from the mitochondrial respiratory chain, nicotinamide adenine dinucleotide phosphate (NADPH) oxidases, nitric oxide synthases (NOS), especially eNOS, cytochrome P450 enzymes, arachidonic acid pathway enzymes, lipoxygenases, and xanthine oxidoreductase in the endothelial cells. Antioxidant defense systems balance the detrimental effects of increased oxidants. An imbalance between oxidants and antioxidants caused by increased ROS production and/or decreased antioxidants results in enhanced oxidative stress, which may lead to DNA, protein and lipid peroxidation, depletion of intracellular adenosine triphosphate, alteration in calcium homeostasis, and cellular apoptosis. Considerable data indicated that ROS and oxidative stress are important features of cardiovascular diseases including atherosclerosis, hypertension, and congestive heart failure (reviewed in [123]).

IH is proposed to be a major mediator of cardiovascular alterations caused by OSA. Each episode of apnea, hypopnea, or both is usually followed by a marked decrease in arterial oxygen saturation, which rapidly normalizes after ventilation resumes. This hypoxia–reoxygenation might be analogous to recurrent episodes of ischemia–reperfusion injury, which refers to the damage that occurs after the restoration of blood flow to ischemic or hypoxic tissues. This reoxygenation–reperfusion phase is thought to result in the overproduction of ROS [136]. Therefore, IH may upregulate lipid peroxidation and reduces NO bioavailability by breaking this oxidant/antioxidant balance through the increase of ROS production. Indeed, lipid peroxidation is a putative mechanism of atherogenesis in chronic IH [117]. Furthermore, increased free radicals impair eNOS-mediated NO synthesis, promote NO breakdown, and increase peroxynitrite production. The endothelial expression of nitrotyrosine, an indicator of NO oxidation, increases in OSA, suggesting enhanced endothelial oxidative stress in these patients [60]. Therefore, OSA can be considered as an oxidative stress disorder. The hypoxia–reoxygenation process during sessions of OSA has been shown to promote atherosclerosis by generating ROS and by increasing ROS-mediated lipid peroxidation, systemic inflammation, adhesion molecule expression, and leukocyte activation [73, 74]. For instance, leukocyte activation, which increases leukocyte adhesion and ROS production, is apparent during the episodes of OSA [33]. Superoxide production of polymorphonuclear leukocytes (PMNs) in patients with OSA was also found to be increased, and CPAP treatment was able to reverse it back to the normal levels [119]. Superoxide radicals cause endothelial dysfunction by impairing endothelium-dependent vasodilation during IH through the limitation of NO production [65]. Oxidative stress and decreased NO bioavailability in OSA have been demonstrated in other studies. The plasma concentrations of 8-isoprostane (a specific biomarker of lipid peroxidation) and total nitrate and nitrite (the stable metabolites of NO reflecting overall NO production) were evaluated in men with OSA and without cardiovascular complications. The results revealed higher lipid peroxidation and lower NO production, which were normalized by CPAP therapy [3]. Another study showed that 2 weeks of IH attenuated endothelium-dependent vasodilation in skeletal muscle resistance arteries [102]. This impairment was accompanied by new collagen deposition in the *tunica media* and a decrease in maximal diameter of the artery. Urinary excretion of 8-isoprostane PGF2α was also elevated, suggesting increased oxidant stress at the systemic level. These findings indicate that exposure to chronic IH produces structural as well as functional deficits in skeletal muscle resistance arteries, accompanied by systemic evidence of oxidant stress [102]. When xanthine oxidase, an enzyme-mediating superoxide production, was inhibited by allopurinol, the impaired vasodilation recovers. The results indicate that xanthine oxidase and its resultant superoxide radical may play an important role in IH-induced vascular dysfunction [27]. Additional evidence proving the involvement of oxidative stress with atherosclerosis in human OSA were reported by Monneret et al., who showed a relationship between lipid peroxidation, carotid IMT, and the severity of IH in the patients with OSA [93]. Urinary 15-F_{2T}-isoprostane levels were examined as an indicator of lipid peroxidation in this study.

On the other hand, reduced effectiveness of the antioxidant system worsens the harmful effects of oxidant stress on vascular injury. Plasma levels of antioxidants such as glutathione peroxidase; vitamins A, E, and B_{12}; and homocysteine have been found to be lower in OSA patients than in age-matched controls, and the decreased antioxidant capacity was partially reversed by CPAP treatment [5]. Impairment of the antioxidant properties of albumin related only to OSA severity has also been demonstrated [38]. In addition, the application of antioxidants [14, 50, 60] along with CPAP therapy improved endothelial function in OSA patients [14, 60].

Since all of the above-mentioned effects of oxidative stress due to IH lead to endothelial dysfunction and subsequent vascular injury, which are related to multiple cardiovascular pathologies (such as atherosclerosis, hypertension, and ischemia reperfusion), it is difficult to draw clear-cut boundaries between the IH-induced oxidative stress, inflammation, and endothelial injury on its progression to atherosclerosis. These factors are likely interconnected with each other. We have therefore attempted to depict a summarized explanation for this complex relationship in Fig. 3.2.

Accumulating evidence supports a central role for inflammation in all phases of atherosclerosis, from the initiation of the fatty streak to the culmination of plaque rupture, which is represented as acute coronary syndrome [113]. IH is thought to cause vascular inflammation that leads to the progression of atherosclerosis. The initial insult comes from increased ROS production, which aggravates endothelial dysfunction. The T cell activation, ICAM-1 expression and leukocyte rolling associated with early inflammatory vascular remodeling were demonstrated in a mouse model of IH [4]. In addition, increased levels of inflammatory mediators and the expression of adhesion molecules in the vascular endothelium have been shown in patients with OSA [33]. Moreover, inflammatory responses are also exaggerated in OSA patients as well as in animal models of IH because of the activation of the inflammatory transcription factor, nuclear factor kappa B (NF-κB) pathway, and downstream gene products including inflammatory cytokines such as tumor necrosis factor-alpha (TNF-α) and interleukin-6 (IL-6), chemokines such as IL-8, adhesion molecules such as ICAM-1, and cell receptors. These mediators have also been linked to the pathogenesis of atherosclerosis [40, 112]. The cross talk between NF-κB and HIF-1 pathways potentiates the inflammatory response [66], even though HIF-1 is known for its adaptive responses to hypoxia [126]. Besides the upregulation of COX-2 and iNOS in vascular endothelial cells, NF-κB provides direct evidence of vascular endothelial inflammation in OSA. COX-2 increases superoxide production and vasoconstrictor and inflammatory prostanoid production, leading to platelet activation and endothelial dysfunction [39]. A recent study showed that leukotriene B4 (LTB4) receptors play a role in IH-induced atherogenesis [82]. LTB4 is a proinflammatory mediator that activates leukocyte cell recruitment, ROS production, and induction of gene expression. Accordingly, it was suggested that the LTB4 pathway can be a therapeutic target for IH-induced cardiovascular outcomes [82].

Endothelial inflammation is followed by or together with systemic inflammation in IH [114]. Patients with sleep apnea have increased circulating levels of inflammatory markers of vascular dysfunction such as IL-6, TNF-α, CRP, VEGF, and

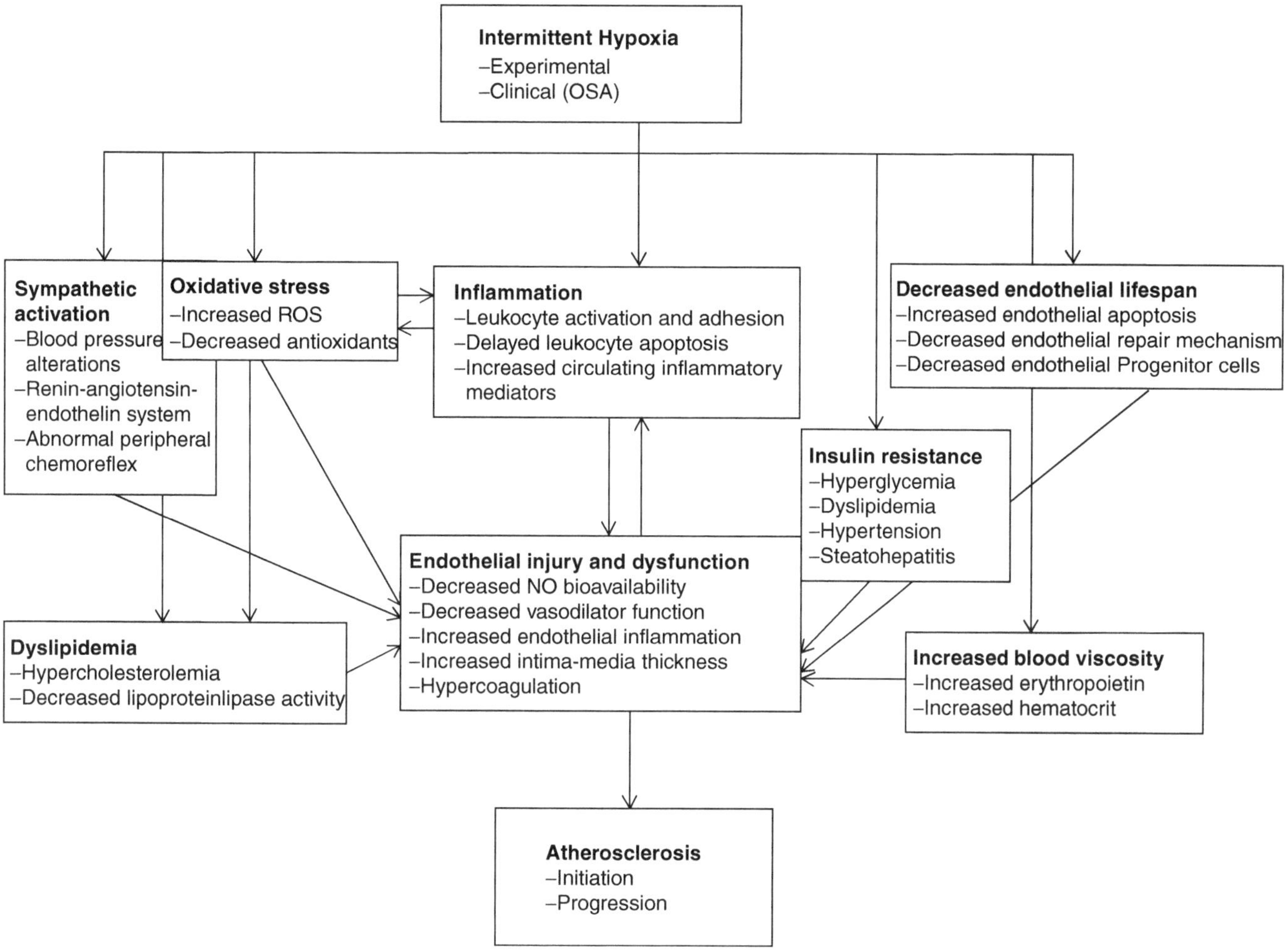

Fig. 3.2 The cross talk between pathophysiological variables plays potential role in intermittent hypoxia-induced atherosclerosis. The complex interactions between the consequences of intermittent hypoxia such as sympathetic activation, dyslipidemia, oxidative stress, inflammation, insulin resistance, increased blood viscosity, and decreased endothelial life span lead to endothelial injury and dysfunction, which is the main step for the initiation of atherosclerosis. It should be noted that oxidative stress has additional effects on dyslipidemia and inflammation, which are important in the progression of the atherosclerotic lesion

adhesion molecules [34, 49, 76, 113, 122]. The circulating adhesion molecules, ICAM-1, VCAM-1, and E-selectin, have been shown to be elevated in patients with OSA [39]. Another inflammatory marker, VEGF, is a heparin-binding glycoprotein, which induces angiogenesis by regulating endothelial cell functions such as vascular permeability, mitogenesis, activation, proliferation, and migration. VEGF involvement in inflammatory reactions may influence the atherosclerotic process. For example, the progression of coronary atherosclerosis in humans was found to be related to VEGF [56]. We and others have demonstrated that IH upregulates the cardiac expression of VEGF in animal experiments [10, 17, 127]. Plasma VEGF concentrations were higher in patients with sleep apnea syndrome [49, 76], and a yearlong treatment of nasal CPAP decreased the circulating high VEGF levels in these patients [76]. Similarly, plasma VEGF levels in mice subjected to chronic IH were found to be elevated [20]. Nevertheless, the exact role played by such an IH-induced upregulation of VEGF in the etiology of atherosclerosis remains to be further elucidated.

The adhesion of circulating leukocytes to the endothelial cells, which is mediated by adhesion molecules, is an important step for atherogenesis. Specifically, a decrease in apoptosis contributes to the activation of PMNs by adhesion molecules, which leads to a prolonged life span. Under normal conditions, PMNs are removed by apoptosis to limit their activation. The delayed PMN apoptosis was observed in patients with OSA, which returned to normal after the treatment, showing its relation to IH [35]. Because delayed apoptosis results in functional longevity of PMNs, it can also facilitate increased procoagulant activity, leukocyte plugging in the capillaries, and the release of proinflammatory cytokines and ROS, all of which promote endothelial cell damage and dysfunction and could possibly exacerbate systemic and myocardial damage [18]. A more detailed discussion of the inflammatory events in OSA can be found in Chap. 8 of this book by Dyugovskaya and Polyakov.

3.4.4 IH and Hypercoagulation

The ability of vascular endothelium to prevent platelet adhesion, thrombosis, and coagulant activity is critical because it can form both anticoagulant and procoagulant substances. Vascular damage, oxidative stress, and/or endothelial dysfunction may activate platelets. Platelet activation is followed by the secretion of inflammatory mediators from platelets, platelet–leukocyte interactions, increased platelet adhesion and aggregation to the vessel wall, and the involvement of platelets together with the thrombotic state of the vessel in atherogenesis.

Platelet activation has been shown to increase in patients with OSA, which returned to normal after CPAP treatment. The increased aggregability in OSA patients could be secondary to elevated nocturnal levels of catecholamines. In addition, increased hematocrit, fibrinogen, and blood viscosity could contribute to hypercoagulability and, therefore, the atherosclerotic process [122]. Likewise, repetitive arousal from sleep during OSA was found to be associated with prothrombotic factors [130]. Increased blood viscosity contributes to the hypercoagulability state of IH. Enhanced erythropoietin [16] and hematocrit levels [55] have been shown in patients with OSA. The rats subjected to chronic IH also exhibited higher hematocrit levels [88].

3.5 Prophylactic and Therapeutic Effects of Intermittent Hypoxia Training or Conditioning on Atherosclerosis

3.5.1 Original Concept of Using IH for Reduction of Atherosclerosis and Its Risk Factors

Until recent years, a number of Russian/Ukrainian studies related to IH and atherosclerosis have been largely unrecognized in the biomedical literature of Western countries. This chapter appears to be the first attempt to summarize the previously ignored evidence for a beneficial role of IH training or conditioning in prevention and treatment of atherosclerosis. The first PUBMED-retrievable article on such a topic was published in Russian language in 1993 by the research group of Dr. Felix Z. Meerson (1926–2010) – an internationally renowned pioneer in the field of adaptive medicine [2]. These investigators exposed the patients with essential hypertension to an IH regimen in a hypobaric pressure chamber. The adaptation to IH results in improvement of general condition of patients, decline in blood pressure and serum sodium concentrations, better microcirculation, and tissue oxygenation. Reduced total serum cholesterol and atherogenic index were also achieved in the hypercholesterolemia patients. These positive results on IH-induced attenuation of two major risk factors of atherosclerosis – hypertension and hypercholesterolemia – introduced a new concept regarding the usefulness of hypobaric IH regimen in treating atherosclerosis-related cardiovascular disorders.

This groundbreaking concept of therapeutic effects of IH on atherosclerosis and its pathogenic risk factors has been subsequently confirmed and expanded by a numbers of independent research laboratories in Russia [69, 84, 91, 128], Ukraine [105], Taiwan [21], and Russia/USA [86].

3.5.2 Therapeutic Effects of IH Training on Hypertension

The original observation of antihypertensive effect following adaptation to a well-controlled IH regimen [2] has been reinforced by the recent studies of Manukhina and colleagues in both hypertensive patients [84] and rats [86]. These researchers exposed the patients with stage 1 arterial hypertension to a 20-day normobaric IH-conditioning program, which consisted of 4–10 cycles of alternating 3-min hypoxia (10% inspired O_2) and 3-min room air breathing. Blood pressure was monitored for 24 h before and after IH, and NO synthesis was evaluated by 24-h urinary excretion of nitrate and nitrite – the stable metabolites of NO. They found that IH conditioning increased NO synthesis and decreased blood pressure in the hypertensive patients as compared with those of normotensive individuals. Significant inverse correlations were found between NO production and the disease duration, systolic, and diastolic blood pressure, respectively. The IH conditioning-induced enhancement of NO synthesis was especially robust in the patients with arterial hypertension for more than 5 years duration. The reduction in blood pressure persisted for at least 3 months. Accordingly, these authors suggested that IH conditioning exerted a robust, persistent therapeutic effect and can be considered as an alternative, nonpharmacological treatment for patients with stage 1 arterial hypertension [84].

These investigators also demonstrated in a rat model of spontaneous hypertension that IH conditioning prevented endothelial dysfunction and improved vascular NO storage [86]. The animal experiments were conducted in young (aged 4–8 weeks) spontaneously hypertensive rats, which were subjected to either IH (9.5–10% inspired O_2, 5–10 min, 5–8 times/day, for 20 days) or sham treatment. Endothelium-dependent relaxation to acetylcholine was measured in norepinephrine-precontracted, isolated aortic rings, and the NO stores were evaluated by percentage relaxation to *N*-acetylcysteine, which releases stored NO. It was shown that IH conditioning significantly suppressed the development of hypertension in these rats. Endothelial function declined from 54.7±4.6% to 28.1±6.4% relaxation to acetylcholine, the sham group, whereas it was sustained at 60.3±6.0% relaxation in the IH-conditioned rats. IH conditioning also induced formation of available NO stores and enhanced the capacity of aortic rings for NO storage [86]. These new data clearly demonstrated the antihypertensive effect of IH conditioning apparently via prevention of endothelial dysfunction and enhancement of NO stores in vascular walls.

3.5.3 Therapeutic Effects of IH Training on Hyperlipidemia

Following the original report on lipid-lowering effect of IH training in hypercholesterolemia patients [2], the effects of hypobaric IH on blood lipid concentrations were independently reevaluated in 46 male coronary heart disease patients who underwent acclimation to IH in a hypobaric chamber [128]. It was reported that total cholesterol decreased by 7% on completion of IH protocol and by 9% at 3 and 6 months after the IH training. HDL levels increased by 12% at 3-month post-IH follow-ups and remained significantly higher than baseline until 6 months. Conversely, LDL levels declined on completion of IH and were lower at 3-month (13%) and 6-month (11%) post-IH period. Similar changes were found in VLDL and triglycerides. The beneficial effects were more pronounced in the patients with higher baseline levels of serum lipids. The authors concluded that application of hypobaric IH training in coronary heart disease patients with abnormal lipid metabolism can lead to favorable changes of plasma lipid profile, which persist up to 6 months after the IH treatment.

More recently, Minvaleev examined antiatherogenic changes of serum lipid profile following: (1) the mountain and climatic treatment on Caucasian resorts, (2) hypobaric IH therapy, and (3) trekking in mountains with regular cold tests (the Tibetan Yoga gtum-mo) [91]. The investigator found that the maximal rate of antiatherogenic changes of serum lipid profile (decrease in the total cholesterol and in LDL, increase in HDL) is characteristic for a combination of three conditions: (1) moderate IH, (2) moderate physical activities, and (3) special exercises for increase of cold tolerance (the Tibetan Yoga gtum-mo) [91].

3.5.4 Inhibitory Effects of IH Training on Glucose Tolerance and Endothelial Dysfunction in Diabetic Animals

The use of IH conditioning for reducing risk factors in diabetic animals represents another recent advance in this research field. A Ukrainian laboratory first reported a restoring effect of IH training on endothelial function in experimental diabetes mellitus [105]. The authors reported apparent beneficial effects after IH training, such as a decrease of hyperglycemia and normalization of endothelium-dependent vascular reaction. The IH training led to an increase in constitutive NO synthase activity and a decrease in iNOS activity in the diabetic rat heart and aorta, whereas nitrite level (an indicator of NO synthesis) increased in both heart and aorta. IH training also diminished the levels of oxidative stress markers such as a hydrogen peroxide [105].

More recently, Chen and colleagues investigated the long-term effect of daily 8-h mild IH (14–15% inspired O_2) on glucose tolerance and muscle morphology in rats [21]. After 8 weeks of mild IH treatment, plasma glucose and insulin levels in the oral glucose tolerance test, epididymal fat mass, and body weight were significantly lower as compared to the normoxia control group. Capillary and fiber densities of soleus muscle were 33% and 35% higher in the IH group than those of the control group. These data indicate that long-term mild IH decreases the diffusion distance of glucose and insulin across muscle fibers and decreases adiposity in rats, which could account for the observed improvement in glucose tolerance and provide a clear rationale for further investigating the use of mild IH in the treatment of obesity and type 2 diabetes.

3.5.5 Direct Inhibition of IH Training on Experimentally Induced Atherosclerosis

The most compelling evidence of the direct effect of IH training on development of atherosclerosis was provided by Russian investigators in a model of high-cholesterol-fed rabbits [69]. During a 3-month period, 12 rabbits were fed with cholesterol (200 mg/kg) and exposed at the altitude of 6,000 m for 6 h/day (i.e., hypobaric IH). The controls ($n=10$) received high-cholesterol diet only. The IH-treated rabbits had less severe hypercholesterolemia (total cholesterol 20.6±2.3 mmol) than the normoxic controls (33.1±1.9 mmol/L, $P<0.05$). Similar results were also obtained in the levels of LDL cholesterol ($P<0.05$, IH versus control). Morphologic examination revealed that there were no atherosclerotic plaques in the aorta of IH-treated animals, in contrast to the controls. Whereas in the control group, the massive diffuse lipid deposits (features of atherosclerosis) were found and there were just tiny dot-like and small strip-like lipid patches in the IH group. The affected aortic areas were much smaller in the IH group (13.5%) than those in the control group (65%). Furthermore, IH exposure also reduced number of lipid inclusions in monocytes (303±13% vs. 370±5% in control, $P<0.05$). These data strongly suggest that hypobaric IH exerts antiatherogenic effect on experimental atherosclerosis.

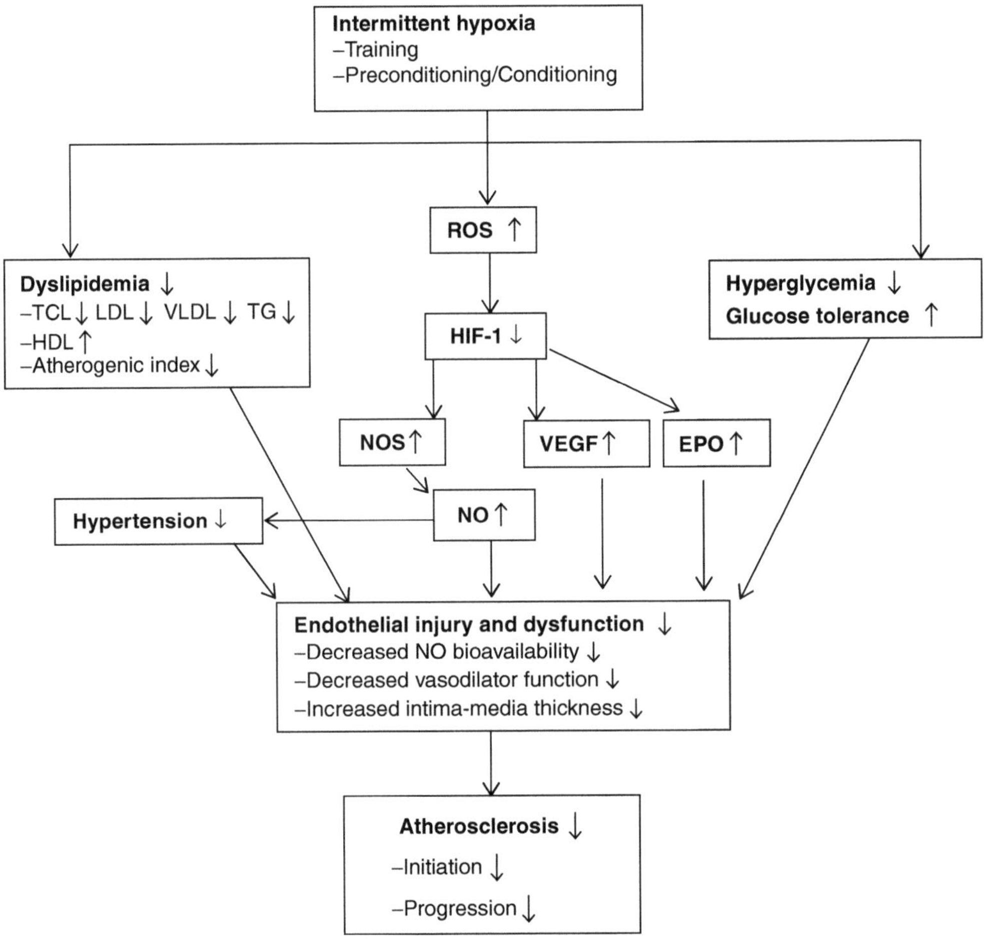

Fig. 3.3 Mechanistic explanation of prophylactic and therapeutic effects of intermittent hypoxia in limiting the pathological factors for atherosclerosis

3.5.6 Paradoxical Low Mortality in Elderly Men with Moderate Sleep Apnea

Interestingly, French researchers recently reported an unexpected survival advantage in elderly people with moderate sleep apnea [75]. They investigated retrospectively the rates of all-cause mortality in elderly people (≥65 years) diagnosed with sleep apnea and compared their mortality rates with that of age-, gender-, and ethnicity-matched national mortality data. Survival of 611 elderly people was ascertained after a follow-up of 5.2 ± 1.1 years. Their age was 70.4 ± 4.8 years, body mass index was 30.4 ± 5.9 kg/m^2, and respiratory disturbance index (RDI) was 28.9 ± 20.1 events/h. Seventy-five (12.27%) patients died during the follow-up period. In comparison with the demographically matched cohort from the general population, the standardized mortality rate of these patients was 0.67 [95% confidence interval: 0.53–0.80, $P<0.0006$]. In particular, there was a significant survival advantage for the moderate sleep apnea group (RDI 20–40 events/h) with a standardized mortality rate of 0.42 ($P<0.0002$) [75]. These authors related the paradoxical survival advantage of elderly people with moderate sleep apnea to a potential cardioprotective adaptive pathway activated by the chronic IH during sleep apnea in the elderly. However, whether or not this lower rate of all-cause mortality is mainly resulted from the antiatherogenic and cardiovascular protective effects of mild IH remains to be clarified.

3.5.7 Possible Mechanisms for the Beneficial Effects of IH on Atherosclerosis

In order to explain the largely unclear molecular mechanisms of the paradoxical beneficial effects afforded often by mild or moderate IH, we would propose a HIF-1–NO-dependent signaling cascade, as illustrated in Fig. 3.3. As previously mentioned, there is a good consensus that IH can activate HIF-1 and its down targets such as iNOS [6, 26, 104, 134], erythropoietin (EPO) [8, 13, 16, 47, 48, 53, 59, 70, 107, 109], and VEGF [10, 17, 47, 49, 76, 126, 127] in various organs and tissues in several mammalian species, including human, dog, rat, and mouse.

NO appears to play a central role in both pathogenesis and protection of the atherosclerosis-related pathologies. Several studies in humans and animals reported IH-caused reduction of NO production or bioavailability in various organ systems. For example, 14 days of chronic IH (10% inspired O_2 for 1 min at 4-min intervals, 12 h/day) impairs endothelium-dependent dilation in rat cerebral and skeletal muscle resistance arteries [103]. It was suggested that exposure to chronic IH reduces the bioavailability of NO in the cerebral and skeletal muscle circulations and severely blunts vasodilator responsiveness to acute hypoxia. This concept was confirmed in the subsequent human studies. The level of alveolar-derived exhaled NO was found to be lower in the OSA patients as compared to the healthy control subjects, and this impairment was associated with an increased risk of hypertension [41]. The alveolar NO concentration significantly improved after nasal CPAP therapy in the OSA patients (i.e., from 2.67 ± 0.41 to 4.69 ± 0.74 nL/L, $P=0.01$). Similarly, a recent report showed that exhaled NO was reduced upon chronic IH exposure at high altitude (3,800–4,000 m) in 81 well-acclimatized mine workers (age of 31.8 ± 6.7 years) [129]. Compared to the first day at altitude, the exhaled NO was reduced by 17.2% on day 3 ($P=0.001$) and 29.6% by the end of the 2–3-week shift ($P<0.001$). Furthermore, in a well-controlled laboratory study, ten healthy male subjects exposed to IH (2 min of hypoxia 45 mmHg alternating with 2 min of normoxia 88 mmHg for 6 h daily, for 4 consecutive days) had a increase in mean arterial pressure by 4 mmHg ($P<0.01$) and a decrease in NO derivatives by 55% ($P<0.05$) [44]. Chronic IH also had suppressive effects on both baseline and post-ischemic NOS activity/protein expression and NO release in dogs [115].

To the contrary, some well-controlled training/conditioning programs with the same stimulus – IH – were also reported to enhance NO production in cardiovascular system. More than a decade ago, it was shown that the rats adapted to hypobaric IH had a better NO reserve to be used in vascular NO deficiency found in the stroke-prone spontaneously hypertensive rats [85]. Also, in rodent models, IH upregulates cardiac iNOS mRNA and/or protein expression in mice [134] and rats [6, 26, 104]. The rats pretreated with chronic IH had significantly higher baseline levels of nitrate + nitrite content (the indicator of NO production) in myocardial tissues [26]. In hamsters exposed to IH consisted of 6 min of 8% O_2 breathing followed by 6 min of 21% O_2 for every 8 h for 21 days, there was an increase in plasma NO (nitrite/nitrate) levels [9]. The authors concluded that preconditioning with IH greatly reduces oxidative stress and stimulates NO-induced vasodilation during I/R injury, thus maintaining capillary perfusion. Furthermore, in 30 healthy sedentary men, exposure to the IH regimen of 12%, 15%, or 21% inspired O_2 for 1 h/day and 5 days/week for 4 weeks in a normobaric hypoxia chamber led to an increased plasma NO metabolite levels [132]. Whereas antihypertensive [85] and anti-ischemia effects of the IH-enhanced NO production have now been well established [6, 26, 134], the direct evidence in supporting the NOS-derived NO to block or retard development of atherosclerosis under IH remains unavailable.

In addition, another HIF-1-regulated hormone protein – EPO – has been shown to be effectively upregulated by IH [8, 13, 47, 48, 53, 59, 70, 107, 109]. With few exception [24], EPO has been shown to lead direct vascular protection in patients [45, 99] and laboratory animals [15, 83], apart from its hematopoietic effect. EPO is also well known to enhance myocardial resistance to ischemia–reperfusion injury [126]. The most relevant evidence was shown by multiple groups of investigators that systemic administration of exogenous EPO protects against various components of atherosclerosis [15, 45, 83, 99]. The first piece of evidence was reported in Watanabe heritable hyperlipemic rabbits [15]. EPO administration reduced lesion in vascular walls and impeded the progression of atherosclerosis in the rabbits. Long-term EPO therapy (12 months) in the hemodialyzed patients also decreased their vascular IMT and plasma levels of CC-chemokine, which recruits leukocytes from the blood compartment into tissues and participate in the progression of atherosclerosis [99]. In a mouse model of severe atherosclerosis, EPO suppressed the formation of macrophage foam cells of the lesions via the liver X receptor alpha-dependent upregulation of ATP-binding cassette transporters A1 and G1 [83]. It was shown that EPO markedly attenuated lipid accumulation in oxidized LDL-treated macrophages through an increase in cholesterol efflux. These phenotypes were also demonstrated in the EPO-overexpressed macrophages [83]. Another recent study was carried out in 15 chronic kidney disease patients (9 males and 6 females, mean age 63 years) with anemia; they were treated subcutaneously with recombinant human EPO (12,000 U once every 2 weeks for 6 months) [45]. The carotid IMT, a marker of atherosclerosis and several indicators of ROS production were significantly decreased ($P<0.001$) at the end of EPO treatment period. Taken together, future studies are warranted to demonstrate if the enhanced level of *endogenous* EPO following IH plays an essential role in the possible inhibitory effect of IH training/conditioning on atherosclerosis.

Furthermore, the role of IH-induced VEGF in various stages of atherosclerosis remains elusive and often contradictory. It is notable that recent studies demonstrated vascular adverse effects of anticancer agents that target VEGF [19, 64, 110]. For instance, patients treated with anti-VEGF agents are at increased risk for arterial thromboembolic events [19]. The rupture of atherosclerotic plaque was reported in a renal cancer patient treated with an anti-VEGF agent – sunitinib [110]. The observed adverse effects in clinics may be related to the downstream consequences of suppression of VEGF cellular signaling pathways that are important in the regulation and maintenance of microvasculature. Downregulation of VEGF can lead to vascular disturbances and even regression of blood vessels, which may be intensified by concurrent pathological conditions [64]. Based on these emerging views, we would cautiously hypothesize a mainly protective role played by the IH-induced VEGF in maintaining vascular homeostasis and stabilizing atherosclerotic plaques (Fig. 3.3). However, such a hypothesis needs to be verified in future experiments.

Conclusion

The IH associated with OSA can lead to atherosclerosis by creating endothelial dysfunction, endothelial injury, oxidative stress, vascular inflammation, hyperlipidemia, hypercoagulation, and sympathetic activation. These pathologies have interconnections by affecting each other in a circuit. Overall, endothelial dysfunction is the main initial step for atherosclerosis. The above-mentioned consequences of IH also contribute to both the initiation and progression of atherosclerosis along with endothelial dysfunction. Patients with OSA have been shown to develop cardiovascular system diseases such as atherosclerosis, hypertension, coronary artery disease, cerebrovascular disease, and cardiac failure. The causal relationship between IH and atherosclerosis and finally cardiovascular morbidities in the patients with OSA can be proven by the effects of CPAP therapy, which improves most of the adverse effects of IH and decreases the cardiovascular morbidity rate. Therefore, to a large extent, OSA can be considered as an independent risk factor for cardiovascular diseases.

Conversely, a number of studies originated predominantly by Russian/Ukrainian scientists also demonstrated paradoxical anti-atherosclerosis prophylactic and therapeutic effects, which could be elicited by some well-controlled training/conditioning regimens often with mild or moderate IH. Considering these most updated evidence and divergent points of view, we have proposed in this chapter the potential molecular signaling pathways for both detrimental and protective mechanisms of IH. Nevertheless, many seemingly controversial areas in IH research require further investigations, which will undoubtedly bring new insights into the fundamental issue of prevention and treatment of atherosclerosis-associated cardiovascular diseases.

Acknowledgments We like to thank Prof. Tatiana V. Serebrovskaya for sharing her vast knowledge of the relevant studies published in Russian and Ukrainian languages, which enabled us to provide a more balanced presentation of the less known and insufficiently recognized evidence for the beneficial role of intermittent hypoxia in limiting the atherogenic factors.

References

1. Al Lawati NM, Patel SR, Ayas NT. Epidemiology, risk factors, and consequences of obstructive sleep apnea and short sleep duration. Prog Cardiovasc Dis. 2009;51:285–93.
2. Aleshin IA, Kots IaI, Tverdokhlib VP, et al. The nondrug treatment of hypertension patients by their adaptation to periodic hypoxia in a barochamber. Ter Arkh. 1993;65:23–9 [In Russian].
3. Alonso-Fernández A, García-Río F, Arias MA, et al. Effects of CPAP on oxidative stress and nitrate efficiency in sleep apnoea: a randomised trial. Thorax. 2009;64:581–6.
4. Arnaud C, Dematteis M, Pepin JL, et al. Obstructive sleep apnea, immuno-inflammation, and atherosclerosis. Semin Immunopathol. 2009;31:113–25.
5. Barceló A, Barbé F, de la Peña M, et al. Antioxidant status in patients with sleep apnoea and impact of continuous positive airway pressure treatment. Eur Respir J. 2006;27:756–60.
6. Belaidi E, Beguin PC, Levy P, et al. Prevention of HIF-1 activation and iNOS gene targeting by low-dose cadmium results in loss of myocardial hypoxic preconditioning in the rat. Am J Physiol Heart Circ Physiol. 2008;294:H901–8.
7. Berger S, Lavie L. Endothelial progenitor cells in cardiovascular disease and hypoxia-potential implications to obstructive sleep apnea. Transl Res. 2011;158:1–13.
8. Berglund B, Aulin KP, Wide L. Effect of short-term and intermittent normobaric hypoxia on endogenous erythropoietin isoforms. Scand J Med Sci Sports. 2003;13:124–7.
9. Bertuglia S. Intermittent hypoxia modulates nitric oxide-dependent vasodilation and capillary perfusion during ischemia-reperfusion-induced damage. Am J Physiol Heart Circ Physiol. 2008;294: H1914–22.
10. Birot OJ, Peinnequin A, Simler N, et al. Vascular endothelial growth factor expression in heart of rats exposed to hypobaric hypoxia: differential response between mRNA and protein. J Cell Physiol. 2004;200:107–15.
11. Borissoff JI, Spronk HM, ten Cate H. The hemostatic system as a modulator of atherosclerosis. N Engl J Med. 2011;364:1746–60.
12. Boström P, Magnusson B, Svensson PA, et al. Hypoxia converts human macrophages into triglyceride-loaded foam cells. Arterioscler Thromb Vasc Biol. 2006;26:1871–6.
13. Brugniaux JV, Pialoux V, Foster GE, et al. Effects of intermittent hypoxia on erythropoietin, soluble erythropoietin receptor and ventilation in humans. Eur Respir J. 2011;37:880–7.
14. Buchner NJ, Quack I, Stegbauer J, et al. Treatment of obstructive sleep apnea reduces arterial stiffness. Sleep Breath. 2012;16(1): 123–33.
15. Buemi M, Allegra A, Corica F, et al. Does erythropoietin administration affect progression of atherosclerosis in Watanabe heritable hyperlipaemic rabbits? Nephrol Dial Transplant. 1998;13:2706–8.
16. Cahan C, Decker MJ, Arnold JL, et al. Erythropoietin levels with treatment of obstructive sleep apnea. J Appl Physiol. 1995;79:1278–85.
17. Cataldi A, Bianchi G, Rapino C, et al. Molecular and morphological modifications occurring in rat heart exposed to intermittent hypoxia: role for protein kinase C α. Exp Gerontol. 2004;39: 395–405.
18. Chello M, Anselmi A, Spadaccio C, et al. Simvastatin increases neutrophil apoptosis and reduces inflammatory reaction after coronary surgery. Ann Thorac Surg. 2007;83:1374–80.
19. Chen HX, Cleck JN. Adverse effects of anticancer agents that target the VEGF pathway. Nat Rev Clin Oncol. 2009;6:465–77.
20. Chen XY, Zeng YM, Huang ZY, et al. Effect of chronic intermittent hypoxia on hypoxia inducible factor-1 alpha in mice. Zhonghua Jie He He Hu Xi Za Zhi. 2005;28:93–6 [In Chinese].
21. Chen CY, Tsai YL, Kao CL, et al. Effect of mild intermittent hypoxia on glucose tolerance, muscle morphology and AMPK-PGC-1alpha signaling. Chin J Physiol. 2010;53:62–71.
22. Corretti MC, Anderson TJ, Benjamin EJ, et al. International brachial artery reactivity task force. Guidelines for the ultrasound assessment of endothelial-dependent flow-mediated vasodilation of the brachial artery: a report of the International Brachial Artery Reactivity Task Force. J Am Coll Cardiol. 2002;39:257–65.

23. Corwin EJ, Cannon JG. Cardiovascular system: conditions of disease or injury: atherosclerosis. In: Corwin EJ, editor. Handbook of pathophysiology. 3rd ed. Philadelphia: Wolters Kluwer Health/Lippincott Williams & Wilkin; 2008.
24. Desai A, Zhao Y, Lankford HA, et al. Nitric oxide suppresses EPO-induced monocyte chemoattractant protein-1 in endothelial cells: implications for atherogenesis in chronic renal disease. Lab Invest. 2006;86:369–79.
25. Dhar-Mascareño M, Cárcamo JM, Golde DW. Hypoxia-reoxygenation-induced mitochondrial damage and apoptosis in human endothelial cells are inhibited by vitamin C. Free Radic Biol Med. 2005;38:1311–22.
26. Ding HL, Zhu HF, Dong JW, et al. Inducible nitric oxide synthase contributes to intermittent hypoxia against ischemia/reperfusion injury. Acta Pharmacol Sin. 2005;26:315–22.
27. Dopp JM, Philippi NR, Marcus NJ, et al. Xanthine oxidase inhibition attenuates endothelial dysfunction caused by chronic intermittent hypoxia in rats. Respiration. 2011;82:458–67.
28. Drager LF, Bortolotto LA, Lorenzi MC, et al. Early signs of atherosclerosis in obstructive sleep apnea. Am J Respir Crit Care Med. 2005;172:613–8.
29. Drager LF, Bortolotto LA, Figueiredo AC, et al. Effects of continuous positive airway pressure on early signs of atherosclerosis in obstructive sleep apnea. Am J Respir Crit Care Med. 2007;176:706–12.
30. Drager LF, Bortolotto LA, Krieger EM, et al. Additive effects of obstructive sleep apnea and hypertension on early markers of carotid atherosclerosis. Hypertension. 2009;53:64–9.
31. Drager LF, Jun J, Polotsky VY. Metabolic consequences of intermittent hypoxia: relevance to obstructive sleep apnea. Best Pract Res Clin Endocrinol Metab. 2010;24:843–51.
32. Drager LF, Li J, Shin MK et al. Intermittent hypoxia inhibits clearance of triglyceride-rich lipoproteins and inactivates adipose lipoprotein lipase in a mouse model of sleep apnoea. Eur Heart J 2012;33:783–90.
33. Dyugovskaya L, Lavie P, Lavie L. Increased adhesion molecules expression and production of reactive oxygen species in leukocytes of sleep apnea patients. Am J Respir Crit Care Med. 2002;165:934–9.
34. Dyugovskaya L, Lavie P, Lavie L. Lymphocyte activation as a possible measure of atherosclerotic risk in patients with sleep apnea. Ann N Y Acad Sci. 2005;1051:340–50.
35. Dyugovskaya L, Polyakov A, Lavie P, et al. Delayed neutrophil apoptosis in patients with sleep apnea. Am J Respir Crit Care Med. 2008;177:544–54.
36. El Solh AA, Akinnusi ME, Baddoura FH, et al. Endothelial cell apoptosis in obstructive sleep apnea: a link to endothelial dysfunction. Am J Respir Crit Care Med. 2007;175:1186–91.
37. Farré R, Montserrat JM, Navajas D. Morbidity due to obstructive sleep apnea: insights from animal models. Curr Opin Pulm Med. 2008;14:530–6.
38. Faure P, Tamisier R, Baguet JP, et al. Impairment of serum albumin antioxidant properties in obstructive sleep apnoea syndrome. Eur Respir J. 2008;31:1046–53.
39. Feng J, Zhang D, Chen B. Endothelial mechanisms of endothelial dysfunction in patients with obstructive sleep apnea. Sleep Breath 2012;16:283–94.
40. Fitzpatrick SF, Tambuwala MM, Bruning U, et al. An intact canonical NF-κB pathway is required for inflammatory gene expression in response to hypoxia. J Immunol. 2011;186:1091–6.
41. Foresi A, Leone C, Olivieri D, et al. Alveolar-derived exhaled nitric oxide is reduced in obstructive sleep apnea syndrome. Chest. 2007;132:860–7.
42. Forsythe JA, Jiang B-H, Iyer NV, et al. Activation of vascular endothelial growth factor gene transcription by hypoxia-inducible factor 1. Mol Cell Biol. 1996;16:4604–13.
43. Foster GE, Poulin MJ, Hanly PJ. Intermittent hypoxia and vascular function: implications for obstructive sleep apnoea. Exp Physiol. 2007;92:51–65.
44. Foster GE, Brugniaux JV, Pialoux V, et al. Cardiovascular and cerebrovascular responses to acute hypoxia following exposure to intermittent hypoxia in healthy humans. J Physiol. 2009;587:3287–99.
45. Fujiwara N, Nakamura T, Sato E, et al. Renovascular protective effects of erythropoietin in patients with chronic kidney disease. Intern Med. 2011;50:1929–34.
46. Gami AS, Pressman G, Caples SM, et al. Association of atrial fibrillation and obstructive sleep apnea. Circulation. 2004;110:364–7.
47. Glaus TM, Grenacher B, Koch D, et al. High altitude training of dogs results in elevated erythropoietin and endothelin-1 serum levels. Comp Biochem Physiol A Mol Integr Physiol. 2004;138:355–61.
48. Gore CJ, Rodríguez FA, Truijens MJ, et al. Increased serum erythropoietin but not red cell production after 4 wk of intermittent hypobaric hypoxia (4,000–5,500 m). J Appl Physiol. 2006;101:1386–93.
49. Gozal D, Lipton AJ, Jones KL. Circulating vascular endothelial growth factor levels in patients with obstructive sleep apnea. Sleep. 2002;25:59–65.
50. Grebe M, Eisele HJ, Weissmann N, et al. Antioxidant vitamin C improves endothelial function in obstructive sleep apnea. Am J Respir Crit Care Med. 2006;173:897–901.
51. Griendling KK, Harrison DG, Alexander RW. Biology of the vessel wall: endothelial dysfunction and vascular smooth muscle abnormalities. In: Hurst JW, Fuster V, Walsh RA, editors. Hurst's the heart. 13th ed. New York: McGraw-Hill Medical; 2011.
52. Hansson GK. Inflammation, atherosclerosis, and coronary artery disease. N Engl J Med. 2005;352:1685–95.
53. Heinicke K, Prommer N, Cajigal J, et al. Long-term exposure to intermittent hypoxia results in increased hemoglobin mass, reduced plasma volume, and elevated erythropoietin plasma levels in man. Eur J Appl Physiol. 2003;88:535–43.
54. Helin P, Lorenzen I, Garbarsch C, et al. Arteriosclerosis and hypoxia. 2. Biochemical changes in mucopolysaccharides and collagen of rabbit aorta induced by systemic hypoxia. J Atheroscler Res. 1969;9:295–304.
55. Hoffstein V, Herridge M, Mateika S, et al. Hematocrit levels in sleep apnea. Chest. 1994;106:787–91.
56. Inoue M, Itoh H, Ueda M, et al. Vascular endothelial growth factor (VEGF) expression in human coronary atherosclerotic lesions: possible pathophysiological significance of VEGF in progression of atherosclerosis. Circulation. 1998;98:2108–16.
57. Ip MS, Lam B, Chan LY, et al. Circulating nitric oxide is suppressed in obstructive sleep apnea and is reversed by nasal continuous positive airway pressure. Am J Respir Crit Care Med. 2000;162:2166–71.
58. Ip MS, Tse HF, Lam B, et al. Endothelial function in obstructive sleep apnea and response to treatment. Am J Respir Crit Care Med. 2004;169:348–53.
59. Ishii M, Iwamoto T, Nagai A, et al. Polycythemia and changes in erythropoietin concentration in rats exposed to intermittent hypoxia. Adv Exp Med Biol. 2010;662:121–6.
60. Jelic S, Padeletti M, Kawut SM, et al. Inflammation, oxidative stress, and repair capacity of the vascular endothelium in obstructive sleep apnea. Circulation. 2008;117:2270–8.
61. Johnson BD, Kip KE, Marroquin OC, et al. Serum amyloid A as a predictor of coronary artery disease and cardiovascular outcome in women: the National Heart, Lung, and Blood Institute-Sponsored Women's Ischemia Syndrome Evaluation (WISE). Circulation. 2004;109:726–32.
62. Jun J, Reinke C, Bedja D, et al. Effect of intermittent hypoxia on atherosclerosis in apolipoprotein E-deficient mice. Atherosclerosis. 2010;209:381–6.

63. Juonala M, Viikari JS, Alfthan G, et al. Brachial artery flow-mediated dilation and asymmetrical dimethylarginine in the cardiovascular risk in young Finns study. Circulation. 2007;116:1367–73.
64. Kamba T, McDonald DM. Mechanisms of adverse effects of anti-VEGF therapy for cancer. Br J Cancer. 2007;96:1788–95.
65. Kato M, Roberts-Thomson P, Phillips BG, et al. Impairment of endothelium-dependent vasodilation of resistance vessels in patients with obstructive sleep apnea. Circulation. 2000;102:2607–10.
66. Kent BD, Ryan S, McNicholas WT. Obstructive sleep apnea and inflammation: relationship to cardiovascular co-morbidity. Respir Physiol Neurobiol. 2011;178:475–81.
67. Kepez A, Niksarlıoğlu EY, Hazırolan T, et al. Evaluation of association between obstructive sleep apnea and coronary risk scores predicted by tomographic coronary calcium scoring in asymptomatic patients. Anadolu Kardiyol Derg. 2011;11:428–35.
68. Khayat R, Patt B, Hayes Jr D. Obstructive sleep apnea: the new cardiovascular disease. Part I: obstructive sleep apnea and the pathogenesis of vascular disease. Heart Fail Rev. 2009;14:143–53.
69. Kitaev MI, Aĭtbaev KA, Liamtsev VT. Effect of hypoxic hypoxia on development of atherosclerosis in rabbits. Aviakosm Ekolog Med. 1999;33(5):54–7 [In Russian].
70. Knaupp W, Khilnani S, Sherwood J, et al. Erythropoietin response to acute normobaric hypoxia in humans. J Appl Physiol. 1992;73: 837–40.
71. Kraiczi H, Caidahl K, Samuelsson A, et al. Impairment of vascular endothelial function and left ventricular filling: association with the severity of apnea-induced hypoxemia during sleep. Chest. 2001; 119:1085–91.
72. Lau AK, Chaufour X, McLachlan C, et al. Intimal thickening after arterial balloon injury is increased by intermittent repetitive hypoxia, but intermittent repetitive hyperoxia is not protective. Atherosclerosis. 2006;185:254–63.
73. Lavie L. Intermittent hypoxia: the culprit of oxidative stress, vascular inflammation and dyslipidemia in obstructive sleep apnea. Expert Rev Respir Med. 2008;2:75–84.
74. Lavie L. Oxidative stress - a unifying paradigm in obstructive sleep apnea and comorbidities. Prog Cardiovasc Dis. 2009;51:303–12.
75. Lavie P, Lavie L. Unexpected survival advantage in elderly people with moderate sleep apnoea. J Sleep Res. 2009;18:397–403.
76. Lavie L, Kraiczi H, Hefetz A, et al. Plasma vascular endothelial growth factor in sleep apnea syndrome: effects of nasal continuous positive air pressure treatment. Am J Respir Crit Care Med. 2002; 165:1624–8.
77. Lavie L, Dyugovskaya L, Lavie P. Sleep-apnea-related intermittent hypoxia and atherogenesis: adhesion molecules and monocytes/endothelial cells interactions. Atherosclerosis. 2005;183:183–4.
78. Lévy P, Pépin JL, Arnaud C, et al. Obstructive sleep apnea and atherosclerosis. Prog Cardiovasc Dis. 2009;51:400–10.
79. Li J, Thorne LN, Punjabi NM, et al. Intermittent hypoxia induces hyperlipidemia in lean mice. Circ Res. 2005;97:698–706.
80. Li J, Nanayakkara A, Jun J, et al. Effect of deficiency in SREBP cleavage-activating protein on lipid metabolism during intermittent hypoxia. Physiol Genomics. 2007;31:273–80.
81. Li J, Savransky V, Nanayakkara A, et al. Hyperlipidemia and lipid peroxidation are dependent on the severity of chronic intermittent hypoxia. J Appl Physiol. 2007;102:557–63.
82. Li RC, Haribabu B, Mathis SP, et al. Leukotriene B4 receptor-1 mediates intermittent hypoxia-Induced atherogenesis. Am J Respir Crit Care Med. 2011;184:124–31.
83. Lu KY, Ching LC, Su KH, et al. Erythropoietin suppresses the formation of macrophage foam cells: role of liver X receptor alpha. Circulation. 2010;121:1828–37.
84. Lyamina NP, Lyamina SV, Senchiknin VN, et al. Normobaric hypoxia conditioning reduces blood pressure and normalizes nitric oxide synthesis in patients with arterial hypertension. J Hypertens. 2011;29:2265–72.
85. Manukhina EB, Mashina SYu, Smirin BV, et al. Role of nitric oxide in adaptation to hypoxia and adaptive defense. Physiol Res. 2000;49:89–97.
86. Manukhina EB, Jasti D, Vanin AF, et al. Intermittent hypoxia conditioning prevents endothelial dysfunction and improves nitric oxide storage in spontaneously hypertensive rats. Exp Biol Med. 2011;236:867–73.
87. Marin JM, Carrizo SJ, Vicente E, et al. Long-term cardiovascular outcomes in men with obstructive sleep apnoea-hypopnoea with or without treatment with continuous positive airway pressure: an observational study. Lancet. 2005;365:1046–53.
88. McGuire M, Bradford A. Chronic intermittent hypoxia increases haematocrit and causes right ventricular hypertrophy in the rat. Respir Physiol. 1999;117:53–8.
89. Mescher AL. The circulatory system: tissues of the vascular wall and structural plan of blood vessels. In: Junqueira LCU, Mescher AL, editors. Junqueira's basic histology: text & atlas. 12th ed. New York: McGraw-Hill Medical; 2010.
90. Minoguchi K, Yokoe T, Tazaki T, et al. Increased carotid intima-media thickness and serum inflammatory markers in obstructive sleep apnea. Am J Respir Crit Care Med. 2005;172:625–30.
91. Minvaleev RS. A comparison of rate of human lipid profile changes at moderate altitude. Fiziol Cheloveka. 2011;37:103–8 [In Russian].
92. Mitrovic I. Cardiovascular disorders: vascular disease. In: McPhee SJ, Hammer GD, editors. Pathophysiology of disease: an introduction to clinical medicine. 6th ed. New York: McGraw-Hill Medical; 2010.
93. Monneret D, Pepin JL, Godin-Ribuot D, et al. Association of urinary 15-F2t-isoprostane level with oxygen desaturation and carotid intima-media thickness in nonobese sleep apnea patients. Free Radic Biol Med. 2010;48:619–25.
94. Morgan BJ. Vascular consequences of intermittent hypoxia. Adv Exp Med Biol. 2007;618:69–84.
95. Naito R, Sakakura K, Kasai T et al. Aortic dissection is associated with intermittent hypoxia and re-oxygenation. Heart Vessels 2011 May 15. [Epub ahead of print]
96. Newman AB, Nieto FJ, Guidry U, et al. Sleep Heart Health Study Research Group. Relation of sleep-disordered breathing to cardiovascular disease risk factors: the Sleep Heart Health Study. Am J Epidemiol. 2001;154:50–9.
97. Nieto FJ, Young TB, Lind BK, et al. Association of sleep-disordered breathing, sleep apnea, and hypertension in a large community-based study. Sleep Heart Health Study. JAMA. 2000;283:1829–36.
98. Nieto FJ, Herrington DM, Redline S, et al. Sleep apnea and markers of vascular endothelial function in a large community sample of older adults. Am J Respir Crit Care Med. 2004;169:354–60.
99. Pawlak K, Pawlak D, Mysliwiec M. Long-term erythropoietin therapy decreases CC-chemokine levels and intima-media thickness in hemodialyzed patients. Am J Nephrol. 2006;26:497–502.
100. Peker Y, Kraiczi H, Hedner J, et al. An independent association between obstructive sleep apnoea and coronary artery disease. Eur Respir J. 1999;14:179–84.
101. Perry JC, D'Almeida V, Souza FG, et al. Consequences of subchronic and chronic exposure to intermittent hypoxia and sleep deprivation on cardiovascular risk factors in rats. Respir Physiol Neurobiol. 2007;156:250–8.
102. Philippi NR, Bird CE, Marcus NJ, et al. Time course of intermittent hypoxia-induced impairments in resistance artery structure and function. Respir Physiol Neurobiol. 2010;170:157–63.
103. Phillips SA, Olson EB, Morgan BJ, et al. Chronic intermittent hypoxia impairs endothelium-dependent dilation in rat cerebral and skeletal muscle resistance arteries. Am J Physiol Heart Circ Physiol. 2004;286:H388–93.
104. Portnychenko AH, Rozova KV, Vasylenko MI, et al. Age-dependent differences of the ultrastructural changes in the myocardium after hypoxical preconditioning and ischemia-reperfusion of the isolated heart in rats. Fiziol Zh. 2007;53:27–34 [In Ukrainian].

105. Prysiazhna OD, Kotsiuruba AV, Talanov SO, et al. Normalizing effect of intermittent hypoxic training on the function of endothelium in experimental diabetes mellitus. Fiziol Zh. 2007;53(2):3–7 [In Ukrainian].
106. Punjabi NM, Caffo BS, Goodwin JL, et al. Sleep-disordered breathing and mortality: a prospective cohort study. PLoS Med. 2009;6:e1000132.
107. Qin L, Xiang Y, Song Z, et al. Erythropoietin as a possible mechanism for the effects of intermittent hypoxia on bodyweight, serum glucose and leptin in mice. Regul Pept. 2010;165:168–73.
108. Robinson GV, Pepperell JC, Segal HC, et al. Circulating cardiovascular risk factors in obstructive sleep apnoea: data from randomized controlled trials. Thorax. 2004;59:777–82.
109. Rodríguez FA, Ventura JL, Casas M. Erythropoietin acute reaction and haematological adaptations to short, intermittent hypobaric hypoxia. Eur J Appl Physiol. 2000;82:170–7.
110. Ropert S, Vignaux O, Mir O, et al. VEGF pathway inhibition by anticancer agent sunitinib and susceptibility to atherosclerosis plaque disruption. Invest New Drugs. 2011;29:1497–9.
111. Ross R. Cell biology of atherosclerosis. Annu Rev Physiol. 1995;57:791–804.
112. Ryan S, McNicholas WT. Intermittent hypoxia and activation of inflammatory molecular pathways in OSAS. Arch Physiol Biochem. 2008;114:261–6.
113. Ryan S, McNicholas WT. Inflammatory cardiovascular risk markers in obstructive sleep apnoea syndrome. Cardiovasc Hematol Agents Med Chem. 2009;7:76–81.
114. Ryan S, Taylor CT, McNicholas WT. Systemic inflammation: a key factor in the pathogenesis of cardiovascular complications in obstructive sleep apnoea syndrome? Thorax. 2009;64:631–6.
115. Ryou MG, Sun J, Oguayo KN, et al. Hypoxic conditioning suppresses nitric oxide production upon myocardial reperfusion. Exp Biol Med. 2008;233:766–74.
116. Sajkov D, Cowie RJ, Thornton AT, et al. Pulmonary hypertension and hypoxemia in obstructive sleep apnea syndrome. Am J Respir Crit Care Med. 1994;149:416–22.
117. Savransky V, Nanayakkara A, Li J, et al. Chronic intermittent hypoxia induces atherosclerosis. Am J Respir Crit Care Med. 2007;175:1290–7.
118. Savransky V, Jun J, Li J, et al. Dyslipidemia and atherosclerosis induced by chronic intermittent hypoxia are attenuated by deficiency of stearoyl coenzyme A desaturase. Circ Res. 2008;103:1173–80.
119. Schulz R, Mahmoudi S, Hattar K, et al. Enhanced release of superoxide from polymorphonuclear neutrophils in obstructive sleep apnea: impact of continuous positive airway pressure therapy. Am J Respir Crit Care Med. 2000;162:566–70.
120. Semenza GL. O_2-regulated gene expression: transcriptional control of cardiorespiratory physiology by HIF-1. J Appl Physiol. 2004;96:1173–7.
121. Shah NA, Yaggi HK, Concato J, et al. Obstructive sleep apnea as a risk factor for coronary events or cardiovascular death. Sleep Breath. 2010;14:131–6.
122. Shamsuzzaman ASM, Gersh BJ, Somers VK. Obstructive sleep apnea: implications for cardiac and vascular disease. JAMA. 2003;290:1906–14.
123. Sugamura K, Keaney Jr JF. Reactive oxygen species in cardiovascular disease. Free Radic Biol Med. 2011;51:978–92.
124. Svatikova A, Wolk R, Shamsuzzaman AS, et al. Serum amyloid a in obstructive sleep apnea. Circulation. 2003;108:1451–4.
125. Szabóová E, Tomori Z, Donic V, et al. Sleep apnoea inducing hypoxemia is associated with early signs of carotid atherosclerosis in males. Respir Physiol Neurobiol. 2007;155:121–7.
126. Tekin D, Dursun AD, Xi L. Hypoxia inducible factor 1 (HIF-1) and cardioprotection. Acta Pharmacol Sin. 2010;31:1085–94.
127. Tekin D, Dursun AD, Baştuğ M, et al. The effects of acute and intermittent hypoxia on the expressions of HIF-1α and VEGF in the left and right ventricles of the rabbit heart. Anadolu Kardiyol Derg. 2011;11:379–85.
128. Tin'kov AN, Aksenov VA. Effects of intermittent hypobaric hypoxia on blood lipid concentrations in male coronary heart disease patients. High Alt Med Biol. 2002;3:277–82.
129. Vinnikov D, Brimkulov N, Redding-Jones R, et al. Exhaled nitric oxide is reduced upon chronic intermittent hypoxia exposure in well-acclimatized mine workers. Respir Physiol Neurobiol. 2011;175:261–4.
130. von Känel R, Loredo JS, Ancoli-Israel S, et al. Association between polysomnographic measures of disrupted sleep and prothrombotic factors. Chest. 2007;131:733–9.
131. Wang H, Parker JD, Newton GE, et al. Influence of obstructive sleep apnea on mortality in patients with heart failure. J Am Coll Cardiol. 2007;49:1625–31.
132. Wang JS, Chen LY, Fu LL, et al. Effects of moderate and severe intermittent hypoxia on vascular endothelial function and haemodynamic control in sedentary men. Eur J Appl Physiol. 2007;100:127–35.
133. Wolk R, Kara T, Somers VK. Sleep-disordered breathing and cardiovascular disease. Circulation. 2003;108:9–12.
134. Xi L, Tekin D, Gursoy E, et al. Evidence that NOS2 acts as a trigger and mediator of late preconditioning induced by acute systemic hypoxia. Am J Physiol Heart Circ Physiol. 2002;283:H5–12.
135. Yaggi HK, Concato J, Kernan WN, et al. Obstructive sleep apnea as a risk factor for stroke and death. N Engl J Med. 2005;353:2034–41.
136. Yamauchi M, Kimura H. Oxidative stress in obstructive sleep apnea: putative pathways to the cardiovascular complications. Antioxid Redox Signal. 2008;10:755–68.
137. Young T, Palta M, Dempsey J, et al. The occurrence of sleep-disordered breathing among middle-aged adults. N Engl J Med. 1993;328:1230–5.
138. Young T, Peppard PE, Gottlieb DJ. Epidemiology of obstructive sleep apnea: a population health perspective. Am J Respir Crit Care Med. 2002;165:1217–39.
139. Young T, Finn L, Peppard PE, et al. Sleep disordered breathing and mortality: eighteen-year follow-up of the Wisconsin sleep cohort. Sleep. 2008;31:1071–8.

4 Protective Effects of Chronic Intermittent Hypoxia Against Myocardial Ischemia/Reperfusion Injury

Huang-Tian Yang, Yi Zhang, Zhi-Hua Wang,
and Zhao-Nian Zhou

Abstract

Accumulated evidence has shown that adaptation to chronic hypobaric intermittent hypoxia (IH) increases myocardial tolerance to the subsequent severe hypoxia, Ca^{2+} overload, or ischemia/reperfusion (I/R) injury. Attractively, this form of protection is noninvasive, persists longer than ischemic preconditioning, and has less side effects such as right ventricular hypertrophy compared with the chronic continuous hypoxia. The cardioprotective effects are largely dependent on the degree and duration of IH. Therefore, to identify suitable cycle length, the number of hypoxic episodes per day, degree, and duration of chronic hypobaric IH is important for clinical application. In addition, elucidation of the mechanisms underlying chronic IH-induced cardioprotection is of basic and clinical importance. To address these issues, this chapter focuses primarily on the cardioprotective effects of chronic hypobaric IH in the improvement of myocardial contractile dysfunction and in the reduction of arrhythmias due to Ca^{2+} overload or I/R injury. The recent progresses in the understanding of the mechanisms, especially related to the cellular adaptation, are discussed. The knowledge we have got from this area should provide new insights into the understanding of the intrinsic defensive mechanism and have impact on the exploring of new therapeutic approaches in the protection of the heart against ischemic heart diseases and other stress.

H.-T. Yang (✉)
Laboratory of Molecular Cardiology, Institute of Health Sciences,
Shanghai Institutes for Biological Sciences (SIBS),
Chinese Academy of Sciences (CAS) and Shanghai Jiao Tong
University School of Medicine (SJTUSM),
Shanghai 200025, China
e-mail: htyang@sibs.ac.cn

Key Laboratory of Stem Cell Biology,
Shanghai Institutes for Biological Sciences (SIBS),
Chinese Academy of Sciences (CAS), Shanghai, China

Y. Zhang
Department of Physiology, Hebei Medical University,
Shijiazhuang 050017, China

Z.-H. Wang
Laboratory of Molecular Cardiology, Institute of Health Sciences,
Shanghai Institutes for Biological Sciences (SIBS),
Chinese Academy of Sciences (CAS) and Shanghai Jiao Tong
University School of Medicine (SJTUSM),
Shanghai 200025, China

Z.-N. Zhou
Physiological Laboratory of Hypoxia, SIBS, CAS,
Shanghai 200031, China

L. Xi, T.V. Serebrovskaya (eds.), *Intermittent Hypoxia and Human Diseases*,
DOI 10.1007/978-1-4471-2906-6_4, © Springer-Verlag London 2012

Abbreviations

AP	Action potential
APD	Action potential duration
AT1	Angiotensin II type 1
ATP	Adenosine triphosphate
$[Ca^{2+}]_i$	Intracellular free Ca^{2+} concentration
CaMKII	Ca^{2+}/calmodulin-dependent kinase II
CF	Coronary flow
ERP	Effective refractory period
ET-1	Endothelin-1
GS I	Glycogen synthase I
K_{ATP}	ATP-sensitive potassium
HAH	High-altitude hypoxia
IH	Intermittent hypoxia
I_{ca-L}	L-type calcium channel
$I_{Na/Ca}$	NCX currents
I_{to}	Outward potassium channel
IPC	Ischemic preconditioning
I/R	Ischemia/reperfusion
MPTP	Mitochondrial permeability transition pore
NCX	Na^+/Ca^{2+} exchanger
OSA	Obstructive sleep apnea
PKA	Protein kinase A
PKC	Protein kinase C
PLB	Phospholamban
RP	Resting potential
RyR	Ryanodine receptor
SERCA2	Sarcoplasmic reticulum Ca^{2+}-ATPase isoforms 2
SR	Sarcoplasmic reticulum
VEGF	Vascular endothelial growth factor

4.1 Introduction

Ischemic heart disease is a leading cause of cardiovascular mortality in advanced countries. It is essential to restore the blood supply by early reperfusion to prevent the progression of myocardial necrosis and thus to limit the infarct size. This process, however, may injure the heart with three main characteristics: reperfusion arrhythmias, myocardial stunning, and lethal myocyte injury [1]. This paradox is clinically important with the advent of thrombolytic treatment and primary coronary angioplasty for acute myocardial infarction. Thus, there are urgent needs to explore new approaches to reduce ischemia/reperfusion (I/R) injury and to understand underlying intrinsic cardioprotective mechanisms.

Hypoxia is a life-threatening stress that occurs as a natural consequence or in various clinical diseases. As many species live with hypoxia as an everyday occurrence, the organism develops multiple endogenous adaptive responses to minimize the injurious effects of hypoxia. It has been well documented that ischemic preconditioning (IPC) is a powerful way to trigger intrinsic adaptive responses to protect the heart against subsequent I/R injury since the first description in 1986 by Murry and colleagues [2]. In fact, as early as 1960, the epidemiological observation revealed lower incidence of myocardial infarction in people living at high altitude (Peru, 4,000 m) [3]. This long-term acclimatization to high-altitude hypoxia (HAH)-induced myocardial tolerance to ischemic injury was also observed in experimental studies using a simulated model of HAH in a hypobaric chamber in 1958 [4] and 1966 [5], and led to the development of animal models of chronic hypobaric intermittent hypoxia (IH) to mimic the physiological adaptation to altitude and the cardioprotective effect in the laboratory in early 1970s [6]. Since then, this form of cardioprotection has been well confirmed to be reproducible in improving postischemic recovery of contractile function, reducing the incidence and severity of arrhythmias, and limiting the infarct size [6–13]. It has the merits that the cardioprotection persists longer compared with IPC and has less adverse effects such as right ventricular hypertrophy compared with the chronic continuous hypoxia [9, 14–16]. The other model is chronic short-cycle intermittent hypoxia, representative by obstructive sleep apnea (OSA), to reproduce the pattern of intermittent hypoxia (IH)-related pathologies [17]. Thus, the effect of IH on the I/R heart largely depends on the IH protocols, such as cycle length, number of hypoxic episodes per day, number of exposure days, and the degree and duration of hypoxic exposure [18, 19]. In addition, recent researches in this area have provided more knowledge of the mechanisms underlying the protective effects of chronic hypobaric IH.

To address these issues, this chapter focuses primarily on the cardioprotective effects of chronic hypobaric IH in the myocardial contractile dysfunction and the arrhythmias due to Ca^{2+} overload or I/R injury. The underlying mechanisms, such as ion channels, intracellular Ca^{2+} homeostasis, myofilament Ca^{2+} sensitivity, and energy metabolism, as well as signal transduction pathways involved are also discussed. The findings in this area have provided new insights into the understanding of the intrinsic defensive mechanism and are significant in the development of new approaches to protect the heart against I/R injury.

4.2 Antiarrhythmic Effects of Chronic Hypobaric IH During Myocardial Ischemic Injury

It has been proved by the laboratory researches that prior adaptation to chronic hypobaric IH definitely protects the heart against ischemic arrhythmia [20, 21]; however, the antiarrhythmic effect from the limited studies of chronic

Table 4.1 Summary of animal models of chronic intermittent hypobaric hypoxia for the antiarrhythmic and electrophysiological researches

Authors (years)	Species	Samples	Simulated altitude (m)	Daily exposure (h)	Total duration (days)	Effects
Vovc (1998) [25]	Rat	Isolated hearts and papillary muscles	4,000	5	40	Antiarrhythmic effect; limitation of rest and action potentials decreasing and maintenance of action potential duration
Asemu et al. (1999) [9]	Rat	Isolated hearts	5,000	4	10–30	Antiarrhythmic effect
Zhou et al. (1999) [30]	Rat	Isolated ventricular myocytes	3,500	6	28–42	Ito adapted change
Asemu et al. (2000) [27]	Rat	Whole body or isolated hearts	5,000 or 7,000	4 or 8	7–42	Anti/proarrhythmic effect
Zhang et al. (2000) [21]	Rat	Whole body	5,000	6	14–42	Antiarrhythmic effect
Zhang et al. (2000) [29]	Rat	Papillary muscles	5,000	6	14–42	Prolongation of action potential duration and effective refractory period
Naryzhnaia et al. (2009) [24]	Rat	Whole body	5,000 or 7,000	6 or 8	42–49	Antiarrhythmic effect
Zhang et al. (2010) [31]	Rat	Isolated ventricular myocytes	5,000	6	28–42	Antagonize the decrease of peak I_{ca-L} and the change of inactivation dynamics

hypobaric IH is not entirely consistent, and the electrophysiological mechanisms underlying are not clear. One earlier experiment in rats showed that chronic hypobaric IH (7,000 m, 4 h/day for 24 days) protects the heart against acute myocardial ischemia-induced arrhythmia. This protective effect is pronounced in conscious animals, less pronounced in anesthetized animals, and absent in the isolated heart [22]. However, chronic hypobaric IH seems to have equal prophylactic effects in the reperfusion-induced arrhythmia either in conscious and anesthetized animals or in isolated hearts [22]. Another earlier study reported that adaptation to chronic hypobaric IH (5,000 m, 6 h/day for 30 days) reduces the duration of severe ventricular arrhythmias in acute ischemia and reperfusion, while adaptation to chronic continuous hypoxia simulating at an altitude of 5,000 m (6 h/day for 30 days) has a similar protective effect only in ischemic arrhythmias and promotes the development of reperfusion arrhythmias [23]. However, some contradictory evidences were reported recently showing that the antiarrhythmia effect of chronic hypobaric IH (5,000 and 7,000 m) does not exist in the isolated rat heart [24], while others observed that chronic hypobaric IH at 4,000 and 5,000 m has the antiarrhythmic effect in isolated rat hearts [25]. It was reported that the incidence of delay after depolarization and of trigger activity in isolated rat hearts is diminished after chronic hypobaric IH exposure [23]. Adaptation to chronic hypobaric IH could prevent the post-stress fall of the electrical threshold of heart fibrillation. The number of fibrillation episodes and the death rate of preadapted animals are 2–3-fold lower than that in the controls. Our previous studies showed that chronic hypobaric IH induces significant resistance to both ischemia- or reperfusion-induced arrhythmia in anesthetized rats [21] and enhances the antiarrhythmic effect of estradiol [26]. Similarly, the antiarrhythmic effect of chronic hypobaric IH is also dependent on the degree and duration of hypoxic exposure; for example, adaptation to 5,000 m for 4 h/day decreases the total number of premature ventricular beats, while extending the daily exposure to 8 h and/or increasing the altitude to 7,000 m promotes ventricular arrhythmia [27]. Table 4.1 summarizes the antiarrhythmic effect of chronic hypobaric IH and electrophysiological mechanisms in various animal models.

4.3 Electrophysiological Mechanisms Underlying the Antiarrhythmic Effects

It has been reported that adaptation to chronic hypobaric IH effectively prevents ischemia-induced fall of resting potential (RP), action potential (AP), and action potential duration (APD) of isolated hearts subjected to global I/R [28]. The experiment performed by Vovc [25] showed that adaptation to chronic hypobaric IH limits RP and AP decreases during hypercalcium perfusion and maintains the APD. Our study showed that chronic hypobaric IH adaptation (simulated 5,000 m, 6 h/day for 28 days) induces the prolongation of APD and effective refractory period (ERP) in normoxia in a time-dependent manner and efficiently prevents the inhibition of AP and contraction in ventricular papillary muscle during the simulated ischemia [29]. Taken together, the effect of chronic hypobaric IH on the AP under normoxic and simulated I/R conditions may be one of the electrophysiological bases for the antiarrhythmic effect of chronic hypobaric IH.

It is well known that the activities of ionic channels constitute to the basis of bioelectricity in cardiomyocytes in physiological condition and are involved in the occurrence of arrhythmia under pathological situation. So far only a few studies have been performed to explore the effect of chronic hypobaric IH on ionic channels of cardiomyocytes. It was reported that opening of ATP-sensitive potassium (K_{ATP}) channels, especially mitochondrial K_{ATP} channels, plays an important role in the antiarrhythmic effect in chronic hypobaric IH-adapted rats [9]. A recent report showed that adaptation to two different regimes of chronic hypobaric IH, 5,000 m, 6 h/day for 6 weeks or 7,000 m, 8 h/day for 7 weeks, increases cardiac tolerance to arrhythmogenic impact of acute ischemia. Their study also demonstrated that the opening of mitochondrial (mito) K_{ATP} channels contributes to the antiarrhythmic effect of adaptation in the 7,000-m regimen, whereas both mitoK_{ATP} and sarcolemmal (sarc) K_{ATP} channels are involved in the antiarrhythmia of chronic hypobaric IH in the 5,000-m regimen [24]. We used whole-cell parch-clamp technique to investigate the effect of chronic hypobaric IH adaptation on the transient outward potassium channel (I_{to}) and L-type calcium channel (I_{ca-L}) in rat ventricular myocytes. The I_{to} displays an adapted change, i.e., the density of I_{to} in the myocytes from the right ventricle rather than the left ventricle increases dramatically after the exposure of rats to 28-day (6 h/day) chronic hypobaric IH, but it returns to normal after 42-day exposure [30]. We recently found that the current density and voltage dependence of activation and inactivation of I_{ca-L} remain unchanged in ventricular myocytes of chronic hypobaric IH rats, but the decrease of peak I_{ca-L} and a positive shift of the steady-state inactivation curve under simulated ischemic condition that occurred in control myocytes do not exist in the myocytes from chronic hypobaric IH group [31]. These results suggest that adaptation to chronic hypobaric IH might increase the tolerability of cardiac myocytes to ischemic insults through preventing electrophysiological remodeling of the Ca^{2+} channel. On the whole, the understanding of the mechanism for antiarrhythmic effects of chronic hypobaric IH, even though some progress has been made, is far more behind, and further investigation is needed.

4.4 Effects of Chronic Hypobaric IH on the Myocardial Contractile Dysfunction due to I/R

A great number of studies have proved that chronic hypobaric IH, similar to IPC and long-term continuous HAH adaptation, has significant protective effects on the heart against I/R injury, including improving the postischemic recovery of contractile function. Since Kopecky and Daum [4] firstly demonstrated the cardioprotection of simulated HAH in hypobaric chambers (24 h every 2 days, 6 weeks, 7,000 m) on the animal model in 1958, the protective effect of chronic hypobaric IH on the heart against I/R injury has been extensively studied using various animal models. The early studies from Poupa [5], McGrath [32], Widimsky [7], and Meerson [6, 20] suggested that IH in relative short time (4–6 h/day, 24–45 days) or relative low altitude (5,000 m) has similar protective effects on the heart. The results from our studies showed that rats subjected to 28–42 days of chronic hypobaric IH (6 h/day, 5,000 m) display obvious cardioprotective effects against myocardial contractile dysfunction in both global and regional I/R [33–36] or in Ca^{2+} paradox model [16], but it does not affect myocardial contractile function during baseline perfusion. In addition, the reperfusion-induced cardiac contracture is significantly attenuated by chronic hypobaric IH via protein kinase A (PKA)- and Ca^{2+}/calmodulin-dependent kinase II (CaMKII)-independent pathways, manifested by delayed time and reduced amplitude of the maximum contracture during ischemia in isolated rat hearts [11]. Because ischemic contracture may be due to a lock in the rigor state as a result of a decrease in myocardial ATP or an increase in ADP [37], chronic hypobaric IH may attenuate the I/R-induced myocardial contracture by the preservation of cytosolic ATP content at higher levels compared with those in control hearts through accelerating the restoration of creatine phosphate, ATP, and creatine phosphokinase activity in reoxygenated myocardium [38].

Though some groups have already attempted to explore the clinical application of chronic hypobaric IH either in the prevention or in the treatment of ischemic heart diseases, the optimum degree of chronic hypobaric IH and duration of acclimatization for cardioprotection have not yet been clarified. Asemu et al. [27] found that adaptation of the rats to an altitude of 5,000 m slightly decreases the body weight, but does not induce hypertrophy, which is consistent with our observations at this altitude (6 h/day, 42 days) [16, 31]. However, adaptation of the rats to an altitude of 7,000 m markedly decreases the body weight and induces right ventricular hypertrophy [27, 39]. In our studies, the body weight and heart weight are similar between the rats in normoxic condition and in chronic hypobaric IH adaptation. Therefore, the ventricle to body weight ratio and the left/right ventricle to body weight ratio remain unchanged in chronic hypobaric IH as compared with those in normoxic group [29, 33]. However, some studies showed that the relative weight of the right ventricle slightly increases in the same altitude (4 h/day, 5–6 weeks), and this change is more pronounced in severe hypoxia of 7,000-m group (8 h/day, 5–6 weeks) [27]. The different effects of

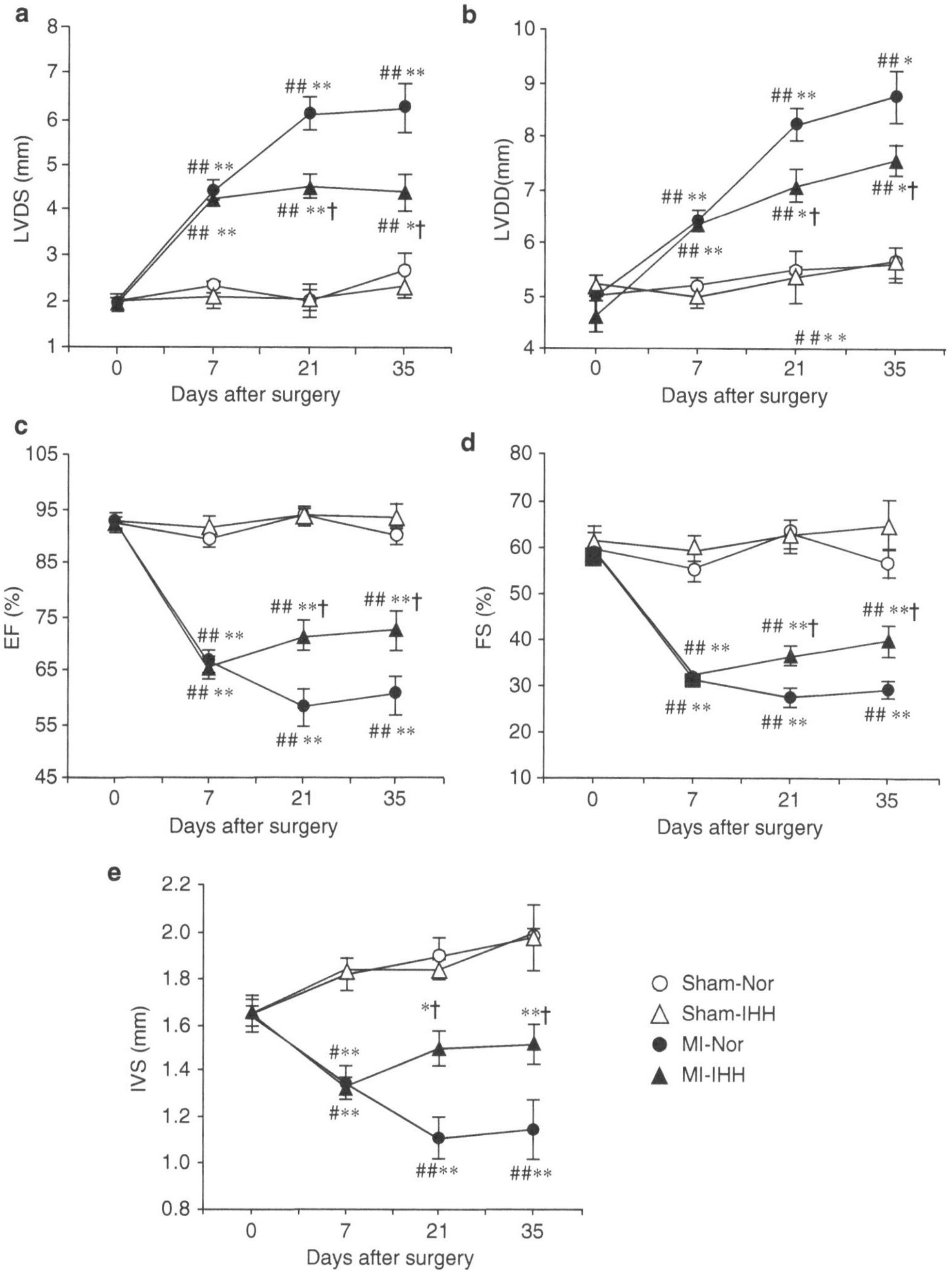

Fig. 4.1 Time course of in vivo LV dimensions and function on days 0, 7, 21, and 35 after surgery examined by echocardiography. (**a**) LV end-systolic diameter (*LVDS*); (**b**) LV end-diastolic diameter (*LVDD*); (**c**) ejection fraction (*EF%*); (**d**) fractional shortening (*FS%*); (**e**) septum thickness (*IVS*). On day 0 and day 7 of surgery, $n=12$ each in Sham-normoxic (Nor) and Sham-IH groups, and $n=32$ each in myocardial infarction (MI)-Nor and MI-IH groups. On days 21 and 35 of surgery, $n=6$ each in Sham-Nor and Sham-IH groups, and $n=16$ each in MI-Nor and MI-IHH groups. $^*P<0.05$ and $^{**}P<0.01$ versus corresponding Sham groups; $^\dagger P<0.05$ versus corresponding MI-Nor; $^\#P<0.05$ and $^{\#\#}P<0.01$ versus corresponding day 0 values (Cited from Xu et al. [40])

chronic hypobaric IH on the body weight and ventricular hypertrophy may be affected by several factors, such as the hypoxic degree and duration and the environment of hypobaric chambers (the size, ventilation, etc.).

Recent studies in our group also revealed a therapeutic effect of chronic hypobaric IH on rat myocardial infarction generated by permanent coronary artery ligation [40]. Exposure to 14 or 28 days of chronic hypobaric IH after 7 days of myocardial infarction significantly improved myocardial viability, reduction in scar area, and attenuated left ventricular dysfunction (Figs. 4.1 and 4.2). These effects appear to be at least associated with the antiapoptotic effect

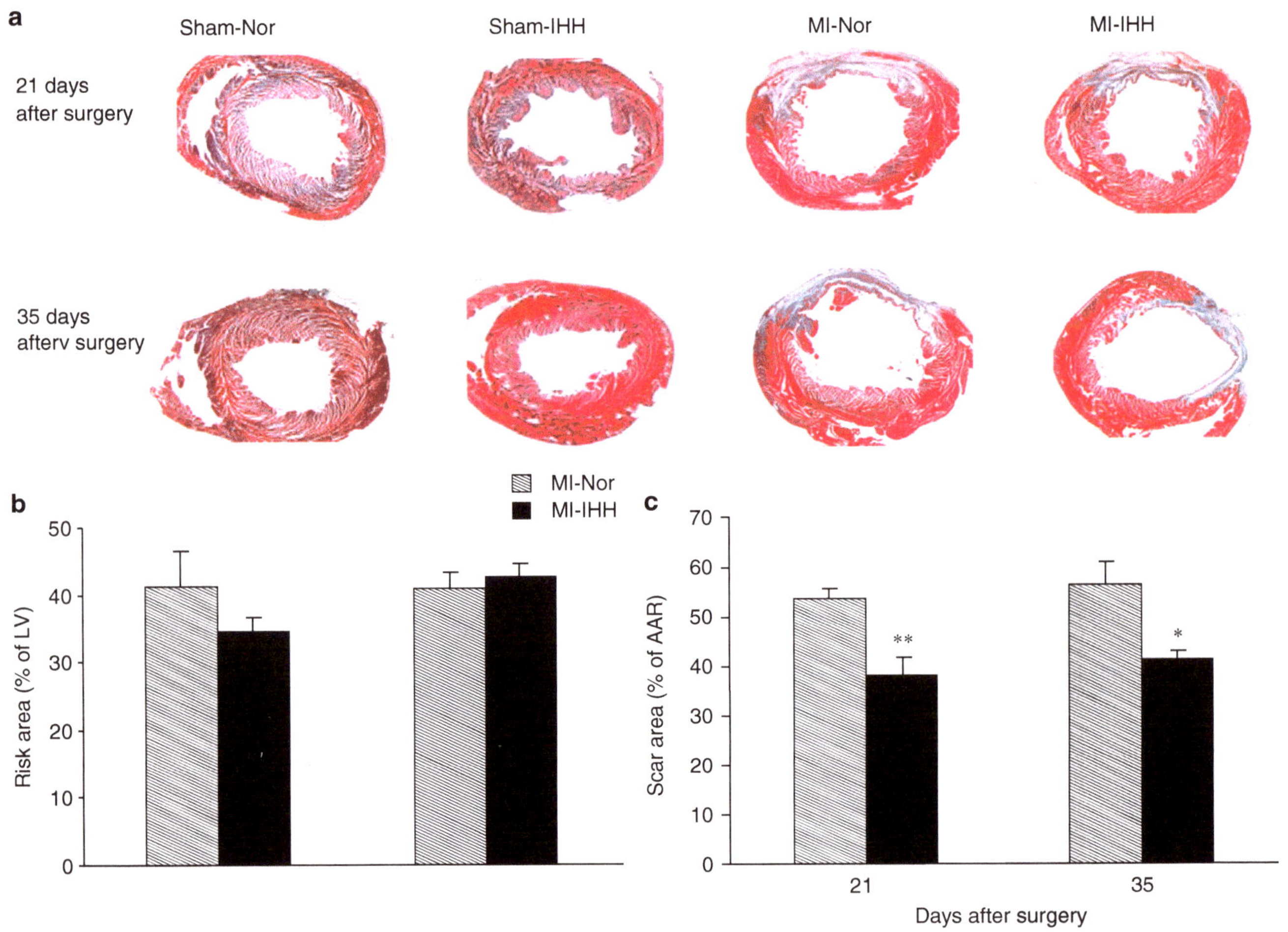

Fig. 4.2 Morphometric analysis of midventricular slices stained with Masson's trichrome at 21 and 35 days post-MI. (**a**) Representative photomicrographs of histological midventricular sections (magnification, ×1). (**b**) The area at risk (AAR) expressed as percentage of LV. (**c**) The scar area expressed as percentage of AAR. $*P<0.05$ and $**P<0.01$ versus the corresponding MI-Nor group ($n=5$ each) (Cited from Xu et al. [40])

in the infarcted myocardium and with the improvement of coronary flow via increasing in vascular endothelial growth factor (VEGF) expression and capillary density in the peri-infarct region. The latter mechanism supports the observation showing that chronic hypobaric IH improves myocardial perfusion in patients with severe coronary heart diseases [41]. Although further studies are required to confirm this therapeutic effect and to dissect the mechanisms underlying, these data raise the intriguing possibility that a relatively simple intervention—intermittent exposure to simulated altitude, initiated days after coronary artery occlusion—may offer profound benefit to patients with acute myocardial infarction, as commented by Przyklenk and Whittaker [42].

The immature heart is generally thought to be more resistant to oxygen deprivation than the adult heart, possibly as a consequence of its greater capability for anaerobic glycolysis [43]. Therefore, the cardioprotective effect of chronic hypobaric IH in the myocardial contractile function may be affected by age. We showed that exposure of postnatal rats to chronic hypobaric IH (6 h/day, 60 days, 5,000 m) significantly improved postischemic recovery of cardiac contractile function [44]. This is consistent with other reports that the hearts of neonatal rats subjected to chronic hypobaric IH are protected from I/R injury [45, 46]. However, the protective phenomenon seems to appear only at the first few days after birth, because prenatal exposure to chronic hypobaric IH does not show cardioprotection [46]. More recently, Zhang et al. [47] reported that the I/R-suppressed cardiac performance is aggravated by chronic hypobaric IH at 5,000-m altitude (6 h/day, 28 days, 56 days) but is conquered by chronic hypobaric IH at 3,000 m. In addition, chronic hypobaric IH at 5,000-m altitude leads to developmental retardance and right ventricular hypertrophy, which are not observed in 3,000-m group [44, 47], although these side effects are not observed in adult rats under the similar chronic hypobaric IH conditions [33]. The more significant growth retardance induced by chronic hypobaric IH in developing rats than in adult ones is also observed in other laboratory [45], although the low body weight alone seems to not influence cardiac tolerance to I/R injury in neonatal rats [48]. The effect of prenatal chronic hypobaric IH stress on the cardiac contractile function and responsiveness to calcium was studied in rats during the perinatal period from days 14–18 of pregnancy [49]. Body and heart weights are significantly lower in chronic hypobaric IH than in matched control rats starting from postnatal day 1. The contractile performance in chronic hypobaric IH group does not differ from the control, but the inotropic response to increasing Ca^{2+} concentrations is, however, significantly reduced on prenatal day 22 and postnatal day 7 in IHH group. These results suggest that prenatal maternal hypoxia affects the cardiac inotropic responsiveness to Ca^{2+} even postnatally.

It has been shown that chronic hypobaric IH (8 h/day, 5 days/week, stepwise up to 7,000 m, total 24 exposures) induces similar chronic pulmonary hypertension and right ventricular hypertrophy and enhances the resistance to oxygen deficiency in both male and female rats, although the myocardium of control female rats is more resistant to oxygen deficiency and chronic hypobaric IH females, but not males, maintain normal body weight [50].

Hypoxic reactivity is known to vary widely between species. Generally, cattle and pigs are the most vulnerable to hypoxia, while goats and dogs show high resistance. Rats and rabbits are intervenient between them [51, 52]. Thus, the cardioprotective effects of chronic hypobaric IH may also vary between species. The relationship between the hypoxic extent and cardiovascular responsiveness in different species needs further investigation.

4.5 Cardioprotective Mechanisms of Chronic Hypobaric IH on the Improvement of Postischemic Contractile Function

As chronic hypobaric IH influences various organs and systems and multiple cells and molecules, the cardioprotective mechanisms of chronic hypobaric IH may involve multiple aspects.

Several mechanisms in the heart seem to be involved in the cardioprotective effect of chronic hypobaric IH on the improvement of postischemic contractile function. The limitation of infarct size and antiarrhythmic effects by chronic hypobaric IH would contribute to the improvement of postischemic contractile performance [6, 9, 12, 20, 21, 27]. Another factor contributing to the cardioprotection is enhancement of coronary flow (CF) during I/R. It is noteworthy that the chronic hypobaric IH significantly enhances the CF in both physiological condition and Ca^{2+} paradox in animal models [11, 16, 33], which will restore myocardial perfusion. More recently, it has been shown that chronic hypobaric IH training (4 h/session, 14 sessions in total, from 2,400 to 4,200 m) markedly improves myocardial perfusion in patients with severe coronary heart disease [41]. Moreover, these patients do not show any evidence of impairment of myocardial perfusion after the treatment. This phenomenon may be related to a decrease in coronary circulation resistance and/or to an increase in myocardial capillary density in hypoxic/ischemic hearts [53, 54]. However, there are contradictory reports about whether chronic hypobaric IH stimulates myocardial capillary density. Rakuson et al. [55] observed no alterations in myocardial capillary density and distribution in the rat heart exposed to intermittent normobaric hypoxia, while we found that the myocardial capillary density increases significantly after exposure to chronic hypobaric IH (6 h/day, 5,000 m) for both 28 and 42 days [33]. Recently, Rakuson et al. [56] found that chronic hypobaric IH (8 h/day, 5,000 m, 10 days) increases capillary supply in both right and left ventricles but increases arteriolar supply only in the left ventricle of neonate rats. This angiogenic response is completely prevented by irbesartan, an inhibitor of angiotensin II type 1 (AT1) receptor. Moreover, the chronic hypobaric IH-improved postischemic recovery of myocardial contractile function during reperfusion is abolished by irbesartan, indicating that the AT1 receptor pathway plays an important role in the chronic hypobaric IH-improved coronary angiogenesis and postischemic contractile performance.

4.6 Cellular and Molecular Protective Mechanisms of Chronic Hypobaric IH on the Improvement of Postischemic Contractile Function

4.6.1 Maintenance of Ca^{2+} Homeostasis

Cytosolic free Ca^{2+} concentration ($[Ca^{2+}]_i$) plays a crucial role in determining cardiac contraction and relaxation in both physiological and pathophysiological conditions. Intracellular Ca^{2+} overload due to abnormal Ca^{2+} homeostasis in cardiomyocytes is one of the main factors involved in I/R injury resulting in cell death by causing cardiac hypercontracture and mitochondrial permeability transition pore (MPTP) opening [1]. This is thought to be a result of sarcolemmal-membrane damage and sarcoplasmic reticulum (SR) dysfunction, particularly the impairment of Na^+/Ca^{2+} exchanger (NCX) and SR Ca^{2+} release channels/ryanodine receptors (RyRs) and SR Ca^{2+}-pump ATPase (SERCA2) [1, 57]. We found that chronic hypobaric IH (5,000 m, 6 h/day, 42 days) markedly suppressed I/R-induced cytosolic Ca^{2+} overload [11, 58]. To determine whether this is a critical mechanism of chronic hypobaric IH-afforded cardioprotection, we then tested the effect of chronic hypobaric IH on the lethal myocardial injury induced by severe Ca^{2+} overload, such as Ca^{2+} paradox, to imitate and exaggerate the pathomechanisms of severe I/R injury [59]. We demonstrated that chronic hypobaric IH markedly protects the rat heart against the lethal myocardial injury, such as severe contractile dysfunction and myocyte death, caused by severe Ca^{2+} overload [62]. The dynamic analysis of Ca^{2+} transients and cell shortening during preischemia and I/R in ventricular cardiomyocytes further revealed that chronic hypobaric IH does not affect the preischemic dynamics of Ca^{2+} transients and cell shortening, but it significantly improves I/R-suppressed amplitude and rise as well as decay of Ca^{2+} transients and cell shortening [10, 58]. The chronic hypobaric IH-maintained $[Ca^{2+}]_i$ homeostasis during I/R has been confirmed to play a critical role in the improvement of I/R-suppressed myocardial contractile function [13] and myocyte contraction as well as relaxation [10, 58].

This protective mechanism involves the main Ca^{2+}-handling proteins and organelles: (1) 20 min of ischemia in control isolated rat myocytes significantly decreases both the inward and outward directed NCX currents ($I_{Na/Ca}$) and shifts the apparent reversal potential to a positive direction. Chronic hypobaric IH does not change the $I_{Na/Ca}$ in the cardiac myocytes compared with the control ones. However, it totally reserves these changes, with the similar apparent reversal potential between the preischemia and 20 min of ischemia [58]; (2) it (5,000 m, 6 h/day, 42 days) significantly attenuates I/R-induced depression of the protein contents [58], but not in shorter chronic hypobaric IH (5,000 m, 6 h/day, 7 days) [60], and activities of SR RyR2 and SERCA2 and thereby improves SR Ca^{2+} release and uptake during I/R; (3) phosphorylation of phospholamban (PLB) relieves SERCA2 from inhibition. We demonstrated that the chronic hypobaric IH-improved SERCA2 activity during I/R is at least related to the improvement of PLB phosphorylation at Ser^{16} during the end of ischemia and beginning of reperfusion and Thr^{17} at 30 min of reperfusion in the rat heart, but it does not affect the expression of total PLB protein [13, 61]; and (4) chronic hypobaric IH suppresses I/R-induced mitochondrial Ca^{2+} overload and enhances the mitochondrial tolerance to Ca^{2+} overload by prolonging the time taken to open MPTP and to induce rigor contracture when myocytes are subjected to oxidative stress [10]. Opening of MPTP by atractyloside and inhibiting mitoK_{ATP} by 5-HD abolish chronic hypobaric IH-afforded suppression of Ca^{2+} overload. It seems that limitation of mitochondrial Ca^{2+} overload plays a key role in the cardioprotection because the attenuation of cytosolic Ca^{2+} overload is more likely a secondary effect in the cardioprotection [60, 62–64].

Various protein kinases play important roles in the mechanisms of cardioprotection. It has been demonstrated that during those protective processes, the activities of PKA during the end of ischemia and early reperfusion, CaMK II during the reperfusion, and protein kinase C (PKC) are significantly improved by chronic hypobaric IH [13, 35, 60]. The improved activities of PKA and CaMKII by chronic hypobaric IH contribute to the improved SR function during I/R through regulation of the SR key Ca^{2+}-handling proteins, such as PLB [13, 16]. More recently, chronic hypobaric IH was found to inhibit the ischemia-induced acidosis through a PKC-dependent way [65]. This may be related to the maintenance of Ca^{2+} homeostasis and cardiac function during I/R because high intracellular H^+ could induce the influx of Ca^{2+} via Na^+/H^+ exchanger and NCX and aggravate the Ca^{2+} overload [66].

4.6.2 Regulation of Myofilament Ca^{2+} Sensitivity

Besides the Ca^{2+} overloading, the decrease of myofilament Ca^{2+} sensitivity characterizes myocardial stunning during I/R injury [67]. It has been reported that IH associated with sleep apnea increases circulating concentrations of the vasoconstrictor peptide endothelin-1 (ET-1) and eucapnic-IH increases the ET-1-induced Ca^{2+} sensitization in small pulmonary arteries through Rho kinase-independent mechanisms [68]. However, there are few data related to the effect of chronic hypobaric IH on the cardiac myofilament Ca^{2+} sensitization either in physiological conditions or in I/R. Rats living continuously in a hypobaric hypoxic condition for 5 weeks with aerobic training sessions show depressed myofilament response to Ca^{2+} compared with those training at sea level [69]. We observed that I/R has a heavier suppression in the cell contraction than that in Ca^{2+} transients. Moreover, chronic hypobaric IH restores the cell contraction more significantly than the Ca^{2+} transients, suggesting that chronic hypobaric IH may improve I/R-suppressed myofilament Ca^{2+} sensitivity [58]. This is supported by the observations that Ca^{2+} overload directly decreases the Ca^{2+} sensitivity of the myofilaments and depresses contractility during reperfusion [70, 71]. In addition, chronic hypobaric

IH-reduced ischemic acidosis [65] and restored mitochondrial function [10] are supposed to improve acidosis-induced depression of myofilament Ca^{2+} sensitivity, maximum force [72], and the function of myofibrillar enzymes [73]. Therefore, the chronic hypobaric IH-improved postischemic contraction may be resulted from the suppression of Ca^{2+} overload and the restoration of myofilament Ca^{2+} sensitivity. The contribution of restoration of myofilament Ca^{2+} sensitivity during reperfusion in the beneficial effect of chronic hypobaric IH requires further study in the future.

4.6.3 Adaptation of Energy Metabolism

The effect of chronic hypoxia on the energy metabolism has been intensively investigated over 20 years. The adaptation changes in myocardial energy metabolism have been observed in chronic hypobaric IH animals to let the heart work more economically under hypoxia or I/R. Adaption to chronic hypobaric IH (4 h/day, 4,000 m, 40 days) significantly accelerates the restoration of creatine phosphate, adenosine triphosphate (ATP), and creatine kinase activity in myocardium in reoxygenation following acute anoxia [38]. This effect reduces the competition of H^+ with Ca^{2+} in myofibrils to improve the energy supply and to accelerate the restoration of myocardial contractile function in reoxygenation. It has also been reported that glucose-utilizing capacity (hexokinase) and capacity for the synthesis and degradation of lactate increase significantly in both ventricles during acclimatization to chronic hypobaric IH (4–8 h/day, 5 days a week, stepwise up to 7,000 m), while other enzyme activities associated with anaerobic glycolysis (triosephosphate dehydrogenase, glyceraldehyde-3-phosphate dehydrogenase) and those linked up in aerobic metabolism (malate dehydrogenase, citrate synthase) remain unchanged. On the other hand, the ability to break down fatty acids (β-hydroxyacyl-CoA dehydrogenase) decreases significantly [74]. All the above changes in the enzyme profile are found after only 24 4-h-exposures in both the hypertrophic right ventricle and the unenlarged left ventricle. When the length of daily exposure is raised from 4–8 h, the above changes are not intensified, and 45 days after the last exposure to IH, none of the given activity values differed from those estimated in the corresponding control animals. In addition, during hypoxia, the heart consumes glycogen to generate ATP. In intact rats, chronic hypobaric IH reduces myocardial glycogen by approximately 30% and increases both the fraction of glycogen synthase I (GS I) in its physiologically active (GS I) form and glycogen synthesis. Moreover, chronic hypobaric IH increases GS I activity in the perfused heart in vitro only under conditions where glycogen is consumed. This suggests myocardial glycogen synthase is activated by systemic hypoxia and catalyzes rapid post-hypoxic glycogen synthesis [75]. Furthermore, it facilitates the preference transition of energy substrate from free fatty acid to glycogen [76]. Such transformation is thought to maintain the energy homeostasis in hepatocytes and cardiomyocytes [76] and to be cardioprotective during I/R injury [77].

Mitochondria contribute 90% of the ATP utilized by myocardium during normal metabolism. Chronic hypobaric IH significantly attenuates the ultrastructural damage of mitochondria [16] and reduces the deprivation of mitochondrial membrane potential during myocardial I/R injury [10]. We also found that chronic hypobaric IH significantly recovers the decreases of ATP contents induced by both ischemia and reperfusion (unpublished data). Taken together, these data suggest that chronic hypobaric IH confers the cardioprotection via preservation of mitochondrial energy metabolism. The elaborate regulation of chronic hypobaric IH in the energy metabolism during I/R needs to be investigated.

In cerebral cortex, Lukyanova et al. [78] compared the different mitochondrial metabolic responses of prescreened low hypoxia-resistant and high hypoxia-resistant rats to normobaric IH. It was observed that normobaric IH significantly increased the K_m and V_{max} for rotenone-sensitive NADH-cytochrome C reductase (complexes I + III). While decreased K_m for succinate-cytochrome C reductase (complexes II + III), reflecting the increase in enzyme affinity for the substrate (succinate), was observed in normobaric IH group, K_m and for cytochrome C oxidase during this period (complex IV) showed no significant changes. These data suggest that mitochondrial complexes play a role in the response to hypoxic conditioning and are closely related to the development of resistance. The responses of kinetic properties of mitochondrial enzymes in the heart need to be further elucidated.

Figure 4.3 shows a schematic representation of cellular and molecular mechanisms underlying chronic hypobaric IH-afforded cardioprotective effects in improving recovery of contractile function during reperfusion. Other cellular and molecular mechanisms underlying cardioprotective effects of chronic hypobaric IH were summarized recently by Belaidi et al. [19, 79]. It has been shown that cardioprotective effects of chronic hypobaric IH (8 h/day, 5 days/week, 24–30 exposures, stepwise to 7,000 m), evaluated by infarct size and incidence, duration, and number of episode for arrhythmias, are not additive to the effect of IPC [80], suggesting that the mechanisms of cardioprotection conferred by chronic hypobaric IH and IPC may share the same signaling pathways. However, the long-lasting protective effects after stop of the exposures [46, 81] and the alterations in key protein abundances [58] suggest that the chronic

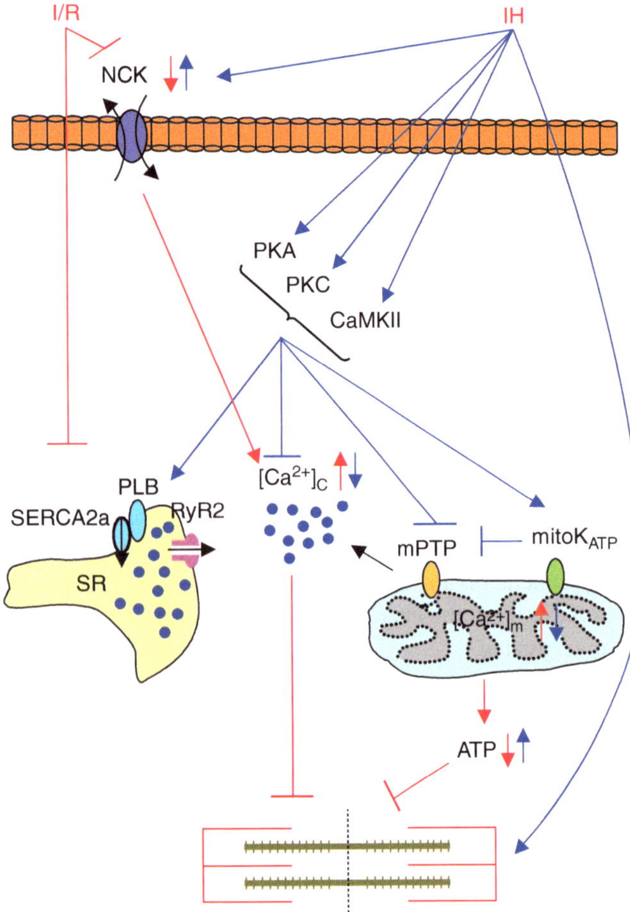

Fig. 4.3 Schematic representation of cellular and molecular mechanisms underlying chronic hypobaric intermittent hypoxia (*IH*)-afforded cardioprotective effects in improving recovery of contractile function during reperfusion. Myocardial ischemia, characteristic of oxygen deprivation, leads to intracellular Ca^{2+} overload, which results from the suppression of activities of Na^+/Ca^{2+} exchanger (*NCX*), sarcoplasmic reticulum (*SR*) ryanodine receptor 2 (RyR2), and SR Ca^{2+} ATPase (*SERCA2a*). The activity of SERCA2a is regulated by phosphorylation of phospholamban (*PLB*) which relieves SERCA2 from the inhibition. Reperfusion following ischemia causes abrupt increases in cytosolic free Ca^{2+} concentration $[Ca^{2+}]_c$ and mitochondrial free Ca^{2+} concentration $[Ca^{2+}]_m$, which constitute as main factors for the reperfusion injury. The ischemia/reperfusion (I/R)-induced mitochondrial Ca^{2+} overload and subsequent opening of the mitochondrial permeability transition pore (mPTP) can further exacerbate the intracellular Ca^{2+} overload. Adaptation to chronic hypobaric IH induces adaptive changes in the Ca^{2+}-handling proteins in cardiomyocytes, i.e., increasing activities of NCX, RyR2, and SERCA2a and upregulation of PLB phosphorylation during I/R. In addition, chronic hypobaric IH inhibits activation of mitochondrial K_{ATP} channels (mito K_{ATP}) that subsequently inhibits the opening of mPTP. These adaptive regulations inhibit $[Ca^{2+}]_c$ and $[Ca^{2+}]_m$ overload and preserves ATP, resulting in the improvement of myocardial contractile function during I/R through the activation of protein kinase A (*PKA*), protein kinase C (*PKC*), and Ca^{2+}/calmodulin-dependent kinase II (*CaMKII*). *Red lines* indicate the effects of I/R injury, while *blue* ones indicate the effects of chronic hypobaric IH

hypobaric IH may have direct effects on gene and protein regulations.

Conclusion

The experimental data obtained during the last 40 years have demonstrated that adaptation to chronic hypobaric IH increases cardiac tolerance to I/R and stress injury, such as improvement of postischemic contractile dysfunction. The cardioprotection of chronic hypobaric IH is affected by the degree, cycle number and length, and duration of IH. It is also altered by some factors, such as age, species, and situation of animals and patients. Therefore, the adaptation protocols for chronic hypobaric IH to sufficiently enhance the cardiac tolerance to I/R and other stress through triggering intrinsic defensive mechanisms but cause minimal injuries need to be optimized. For the clinical practice of chronic hypobaric IH, the suitable candidates of patients suffering from ischemic heart disease need to be identified. Recently, advanced studies have revealed more cellular and molecular mechanisms underlying the cardioprotective effect of chronic hypobaric IH. However, our knowledge on the cardioprotective mechanisms of chronic hypobaric IH against I/R is much less compared with that on the IPC or ischemic postconditioning. The usage of advanced molecular techniques in this research area should provide new insight into the mechanisms, especially, related to the transcriptional, posttranslational changes, and epigenetic regulations. More importantly, the potential exploitation of chronic hypobaric IH in the prevention and treatment of patients suffering from ischemic heart diseases needs to be explored upon the development of basic researches.

Acknowledgments Some of the studies were supported partially by grants from Major State Basic Research Development Program of People's Republic of China (2006CB504106; 2007CB512100) and Knowledge Innovation Program of the CAS (KSCX2-YW-R-75).

References

1. Yellon DM, Hausenloy DJ. Myocardial reperfusion injury. N Engl J Med. 2007;357:1121–35.
2. Murry CE, Jennings RB, Reimer KA. Preconditioning with ischemia: a delay of lethal cell injury in ischemic myocardium. Circulation. 1986;74:1124–36.
3. Hurtado A. Some clinical aspects of life at high altitudes. Ann Intern Med. 1960;53:247–58.
4. Kopecky M, Daum S. Adaptation of the myocardium to altitude anoxia. Cesk Fysiol. 1958;7:218–9 [In Czech].
5. Poupa O, Krofta K, Prochazka J, et al. Acclimation to simulated high altitude and acute cardiac necrosis. Fed Proc. 1966;25:1243–6.
6. Meerson FZ, Gomzakov OA, Shimkovich MV. Adaptation to high altitude hypoxia as a factor preventing development of myocardial ischemic necrosis. Am J Cardiol. 1973;31:30–4.

7. Widimsky J, Urbanova D, Ressl J, et al. Effect of intermittent altitude hypoxia on the myocardium and lesser circulation in the rat. Cardiovasc Res. 1973;7:798–808.
8. McGrath JJ, Prochazka J, Pelouch V, et al. Physiological responses of rats to intermittent high-altitude stress: effects of age. J Appl Physiol. 1973;34:289–93.
9. Asemu G, Papousek F, Ostadal B, et al. Adaptation to high altitude hypoxia protects the rat heart against ischemia-induced arrhythmias. Involvement of mitochondrial KATP channel. J Mol Cell Cardiol. 1999;31:1821–31.
10. Zhu WZ, Xie Y, Chen L, et al. Intermittent high altitude hypoxia inhibits opening of mitochondrial permeability transition pores against reperfusion injury. J Mol Cell Cardiol. 2006;40:96–106.
11. Zhu HF, Dong JW, Zhu WZ, et al. ATP-dependent potassium channels involved in the cardiac protection induced by intermittent hypoxia against ischemia/reperfusion injury. Life Sci. 2003;73: 1275–87.
12. Neckar J, Markova I, Novak F, et al. Increased expression and altered subcellular distribution of PKC-delta in chronically hypoxic rat myocardium: involvement in cardioprotection. Am J Physiol Heart Circ Physiol. 2005;288:H1566–72.
13. Xie Y, Zhu Y, Zhu WZ, et al. Role of dual-site phospholamban phosphorylation in intermittent hypoxia-induced cardioprotection against ischemia-reperfusion injury. Am J Physiol Heart Circ Physiol. 2005;288:H2594–602.
14. Leon-Velarde F, Monge CC, Vidal A, et al. Serum immunoreactive erythropoietin in high altitude natives with and without excessive erythrocytosis. Exp Hematol. 1991;19:257–60.
15. Zhuang J, Zhou Z. Protective effects of intermittent hypoxic adaptation on myocardium and its mechanisms. Biol Signals Recept. 1999;8:316–22.
16. Xie Y, Zhu WZ, Zhu Y, et al. Intermittent high altitude hypoxia protects the heart against lethal Ca^{2+} overload injury. Life Sci. 2004;76:559–72.
17. McGuire M, Bradford A. Chronic intermittent hypoxia increases haematocrit and causes right ventricular hypertrophy in the rat. Respir Physiol. 1999;117:53–8.
18. Beguin PC, Joyeux-Faure M, Godin-Ribuot D, et al. Acute intermittent hypoxia improves rat myocardium tolerance to ischemia. J Appl Physiol. 2005;99:1064–9.
19. Belaidi E, Ramond A, Joyeux-Faure M, et al. Contrasting effects of intermittent hypoxia on myocardial ischemic tolerance. In: Xi L, Serebrovskaya TV, editors. Intermittent hypoxia: from molecular mechanisms to clinical applications. New York: Nova; 2009. p. 3–18.
20. Meerson FZ, Ustinova EE, Orlova EH. Prevention and elimination of heart arrhythmias by adaptation to intermittent high altitude hypoxia. Clin Cardiol. 1987;10(12):783–9.
21. Zhang Y, Zhong N, Zhu HF, et al. Antiarrhythmic and antioxidative effects of intermittent hypoxia exposure on rat myocardium. Sheng Li Xue Bao. 2000;52:89–92 [In Chinese].
22. Meerson FZ, Ustinova EE, Manukhina EB. Prevention of cardiac arrhythmias by adaptation to hypoxia: regulatory mechanisms and cardiotropic effect. Biomed Biochim Acta. 1989;48:S83–8.
23. Meerson FZ, Beloshitskii PV, Vorontsova EI, et al. Effect of adaptation to continuous and intermittent hypoxia on heart resistance to ischemic and reperfusion arrhythmias. Patol Fiziol Eksp Ter. 1989; May-June (3):48–50 [In Russian].
24. Naryzhnaia NV, Neckar J, Maslov LN, et al. The role of sarcolemmal and mitochondrial K_{ATP}-channels in realization of the cardioprotection and antiarrhythmic effect of different regimens of hypobaric adaptation. Ross Fiziol Zh Im I M Sechenova. 2009;95: 837–49 [In Russian].
25. Vovc E. The antiarrhythmic effect of adaptation to intermittent hypoxia. Folia Med (Plovdiv). 1998;40:51–4.
26. Zhang Y, Zhong N, Zhou ZN. Estradiol potentiates antiarrhythmic and antioxidative effects of intermittent hypoxic rat heart. Acta Pharmacol Sin. 2000;21:609–12.
27. Asemu G, Neckar J, Szarszoi O, et al. Effects of adaptation to intermittent high altitude hypoxia on ischemic ventricular arrhythmias in rats. Physiol Res. 2000;49:597–606.
28. Meerson FZ, Vovk VI. Effects of adaptation to stress exposure and periodic hypoxia on bioelectric activity of cardiomyocytes of isolated heart in ischemia and reperfusion. Biull Eksp Biol Med. 1991;112:573–5 [In Russian].
29. Zhang Y, Zhong N, Zhou ZN. Effects of intermittent hypoxia on action potential and contraction in non-ischemic and ischemic rat papillary muscle. Life Sci. 2000;67:2465–71.
30. Zhou J, Tian M, Zhang Y, et al. Effects of intermittent hypoxia on transient outward current in rat ventricular myocytes. Sheng Li Xue Bao. 1999;51:187–92 [In Chinese].
31. Zhang Y, Zhong N, Zhou ZN. Effects of chronic intermittent hypobaric hypoxia on the L-type calcium current in rat ventricular myocytes. High Alt Med Biol. 2010;11:61–7.
32. McGrath JJ, Bullard RW. Altered myocardial performance in response to anoxia after high-altitude exposure. J Appl Physiol. 1968;25:761–4.
33. Zhong N, Zhang Y, Zhu HF, et al. Myocardial capillary angiogenesis and coronary flow in ischemia tolerance rat by adaptation to intermittent high altitude hypoxia. Acta Pharmacol Sin. 2002;23: 305–10.
34. Ding HL, Zhu HF, Dong JW, et al. Inducible nitric oxide synthase contributes to intermittent hypoxia against ischemia/reperfusion injury. Acta Pharmacol Sin. 2005;26:315–22.
35. Yu Z, Wang ZH, Yang HT. Calcium/calmodulin-dependent protein kinase II mediates cardioprotection of intermittent hypoxia against ischemic-reperfusion-induced cardiac dysfunction. Am J Physiol Heart Circ Physiol. 2009;297:H735–42.
36. Ding HL, Zhu HF, Dong JW, et al. Intermittent hypoxia protects the rat heart against ischemia/reperfusion injury by activating protein kinase C. Life Sci. 2004;75:2587–603.
37. Ventura-Clapier R, Veksler V. Myocardial ischemic contracture. Metabolites affect rigor tension development and stiffness. Circ Res. 1994;74:920–9.
38. Kopylov I, Golubeva LI. Effect of adaptation to periodic hypoxia on the resistance of the indicators of energy metabolism and myocardial contraction in acute anoxia and reoxygenation. Biull Eksp Biol Med. 1991;111:22–5 [In Russian].
39. Kolar F, Jezkova J, Balkova P, et al. Role of oxidative stress in PKC-delta upregulation and cardioprotection induced by chronic intermittent hypoxia. Am J Physiol Heart Circ Physiol. 2007;292:H224–30.
40. Xu WQ, Yu Z, Xie Y, et al. Therapeutic effect of intermittent hypobaric hypoxia on myocardial infarction in rats. Basic Res Cardiol. 2011;106:329–42.
41. del Pilar V, Garcia-Godos F, Woolcott OO, et al. Improvement of myocardial perfusion in coronary patients after intermittent hypobaric hypoxia. J Nucl Cardiol. 2006;13:69–74.
42. Przyklenk K, Whittaker P. Cardioprotection via adaptation to hypoxia: expanding the timeline and targets? Basic Res Cardiol. 2011;106:325–8.
43. Ostadal B, Ostadalova I, Dhalla NS. Development of cardiac sensitivity to oxygen deficiency: comparative and ontogenetic aspects. Physiol Rev. 1999;79:635–59.
44. Zhu WZ, Dong JW, Ding HL, et al. Postnatal development in intermittent hypoxia enhances resistance to myocardial ischemia/reperfusion in male rats. Eur J Appl Physiol. 2004;91:716–22.
45. Ostadal B, Kolar F, Pelouch V, et al. Ontogenetic differences in cardiopulmonary adaptation to chronic hypoxia. Physiol Res. 1995; 44:45–51.

46. Ostadalova I, Ostadal B, Jarkovska D, et al. Ischemic preconditioning in chronically hypoxic neonatal rat heart. Pediatr Res. 2002;52: 561–7.
47. Zhang H, Yang CY, Wang YP, et al. Effects of different modes of intermittent hypobaric hypoxia on ischemia/reperfusion injury in developing rat hearts. Sheng Li Xue Bao. 2007;59:660–6.
48. Chvojkova Z, Ostadalova I, Ostadal B. Low body weight and cardiac tolerance to ischemia in neonatal rats. Physiol Res. 2005;54:357–62.
49. Ostadalova I, Ostadal B, Kolar F. Effect of prenatal hypoxia on contractile performance and responsiveness to Ca^{2+} in the isolated perinatal rat heart. Physiol Res. 1995;44:135–7.
50. Ostadal B, Prochazka J, Pelouch V, et al. Comparison of cardiopulmonary responses of male and female rats to intermittent high altitude hypoxia. Physiol Bohemoslov. 1984;33:129–38.
51. Wauthy P, Pagnamenta A, Vassalli F, et al. Right ventricular adaptation to pulmonary hypertension: an interspecies comparison. Am J Physiol Heart Circ Physiol. 2004;286:H1441–7.
52. Zhang Y, Yang HT, Zhou ZN. The cardioprotection of intermittent hypoxic adaptation. Sheng Li Xue Bao. 2007;59:601–13 [In Chinese].
53. Kayar SR, Banchero N. Myocardial capillarity in acclimation to hypoxia. Pflugers Arch. 1985;404:319–25.
54. Reller MD, Morton MJ, Giraud GD, et al. Maximal myocardial blood flow is enhanced by chronic hypoxemia in late gestation fetal sheep. Am J Physiol. 1992;263:H1327–9.
55. Rakusan K, Chvojkova Z, Oliviero P, et al. The effect of intermittent normobaric hypoxia on myocardial structure in rats. Hypoxia Med J. 1997;5:3–8.
56. Rakusan K, Chvojkova Z, Oliviero P, et al. ANG II type 1 receptor antagonist irbesartan inhibits coronary angiogenesis stimulated by chronic intermittent hypoxia in neonatal rats. Am J Physiol Heart Circ Physiol. 2007;292:H1237–44.
57. Leblanc N, Hume JR. Sodium current-induced release of calcium from cardiac sarcoplasmic reticulum. Science. 1990;248:372–6.
58. Chen L, Lu XY, Li J, et al. Intermittent hypoxia protects cardiomyocytes against ischemia-reperfusion injury-induced alterations in Ca^{2+} homeostasis and contraction via the sarcoplasmic reticulum and Na^{+}/Ca^{2+} exchange mechanisms. Am J Physiol Cell Physiol. 2006;290:C1221–9.
59. Piper HM. The calcium paradox revisited: an artefact of great heuristic value. Cardiovasc Res. 2000;45:123–7.
60. Yeung HM, Kravtsov GM, Ng KM, et al. Chronic intermittent hypoxia alters Ca^{2+} handling in rat cardiomyocytes by augmented Na^{+}/Ca^{2+} exchange and ryanodine receptor activities in ischemia-reperfusion. Am J Physiol Cell Physiol. 2007;292:C2046–56.
61. Said M, Vittone L, Mundina-Weilenmann C, et al. Role of dual-site phospholamban phosphorylation in the stunned heart: insights from phospholamban site-specific mutants. Am J Physiol Heart Circ Physiol. 2003;285:H1198–205.
62. Miyamae M, Camacho SA, Weiner MW, et al. Attenuation of postischemic reperfusion injury is related to prevention of $[Ca^{2+}]_m$ overload in rat hearts. Am J Physiol. 1996;271(5 Pt 2):H2145–53.
63. Cao CM, Yan WY, Liu J, et al. Attenuation of mitochondrial, but not cytosolic, Ca^{2+} overload reduces myocardial injury induced by ischemia and reperfusion. Acta Pharmacol Sin. 2006;27:911–8.
64. Gao H, Chen L, Yang HT. Activation of alpha1B-adrenoceptors alleviates ischemia/reperfusion injury by limitation of mitochondrial Ca^{2+} overload in cardiomyocytes. Cardiovasc Res. 2007;75:584–95.
65. Li J, Zhang H, Zhu WZ, et al. Preservation of the pHi during ischemia via PKC by intermittent hypoxia. Biochem Biophys Res Commun. 2007;356:329–33.
66. Piper HM, Garcia-Dorado D, Ovize M. A fresh look at reperfusion injury. Cardiovasc Res. 1998;38:291–300.
67. Carrozza Jr JP, Bentivegna LA, Williams CP, et al. Decreased myofilament responsiveness in myocardial stunning follows transient calcium overload during ischemia and reperfusion. Circ Res. 1992;71:1334–40.
68. Snow JB, Kanagy NL, Walker BR, et al. Rat strain differences in pulmonary artery smooth muscle ca entry following chronic hypoxia. Microcirculation. 2009;16:603–14.
69. Cazorla O, Ait MY, Goret L, et al. Effects of high-altitude exercise training on contractile function of rat skinned cardiomyocyte. Cardiovasc Res. 2006;71:652–60.
70. Kusuoka H, Porterfield JK, Weisman HF, et al. Pathophysiology and pathogenesis of stunned myocardium. Depressed Ca^{2+} activation of contraction as a consequence of reperfusion-induced cellular calcium overload in ferret hearts. J Clin Invest. 1987;79:950–61.
71. Gao WD, Atar D, Backx PH, et al. Relationship between intracellular calcium and contractile force in stunned myocardium: direct evidence for decreased myofilament Ca^{2+} responsiveness and altered diastolic function in intact ventricular muscle. Circ Res. 1995;76: 1036–48.
72. Kentish JC, Allen DG. Is force production in the myocardium directly dependent upon the free energy change of ATP hydrolysis? J Mol Cell Cardiol. 1986;18:879–84.
73. Piper HM, Abdallah Y, Schafer C. The first minutes of reperfusion: a window of opportunity for cardioprotection. Cardiovasc Res. 2004;61:365–71.
74. Bass A, Ostadal B, Prochazka J, et al. Intermittent high altitude-induced changes in energy metabolism in the rat myocardium and their reversibility. Physiol Bohemoslov. 1989;38:155–61.
75. McNulty PH, Ng C, Liu WX, et al. Autoregulation of myocardial glycogen concentration during intermittent hypoxia. Am J Physiol. 1996;271:R311–9.
76. Lebkova NP, Chizhov AI, Bobkov I. The adaptational intracellular mechanisms regulating energy homeostasis during intermittent normobaric hypoxia. Ross Fiziol Zh Im I M Sechenova. 1999;85:403–11 [In Russian].
77. Ashrafian H, Frenneaux MP, Opie LH. Metabolic mechanisms in heart failure. Circulation. 2007;116:434–48.
78. Lukyanova LD, Germanova EL, Kopaladze RA. Development of resistance of an organism under various conditions of hypoxic preconditioning: role of the hypoxic period and reoxygenation. Bull Exp Biol Med. 2009;147:400–4.
79. Samaja M, Veicsteinas A, Milano G. Effects of intermittent versus chronic hypoxia on myocardial ischemic tolerance. In: Xi L, Serebrovskaya TV, editors. Intermittent hypoxia: from molecular mechanisms to clinical applications. New York: Nova; 2009. p. 19–52.
80. Neckar J, Papousek F, Novakova O, et al. Cardioprotective effects of chronic hypoxia and ischaemic preconditioning are not additive. Basic Res Cardiol. 2002;97:161–7.
81. Milano G, Corno AF, Lippa S. Chronic and intermittent hypoxia induce different degrees of myocardial tolerance to hypoxia-induced dysfunction. Exp Biol Med. 2002;227:389–97.

Role of Mitochondrial Permeability Transition Pore in Intermittent Hypoxia-Induced Cardiac and Neuronal Protection

5

Galina Vavilova, Tatyana Shimanskaya, Nataliya Strutynska, Sergey Talanov, and Vadim Sagach

Abstract

We have investigated protective effects of intermittent hypoxic training (IHT) in three experimental models. In experiments on isolated hearts from adult and old guinea pigs, perfused under Langendorff mode, the effect of the intermittent hypoxia on reperfusion injury and activation of mitochondrial permeability transition pore (mPTP) was studied. It was shown that 7-day course of the IHT led to decrease of mitochondrial permeability transition, increased efficiency of the heart in both adult and old animals. Cardiac reperfusion was followed by an increased cardiac contractility and decrease of an oxygen cost of myocardial work. On the heart mitochondria from adult and old rats subjected to IHT, we studied the sensitivity of mPTP opening to its inductor, phenylarsine oxide (PAO). We have found that IHT used in regime II (8% O_2 gas mixture) resulted in a twofold decrease as compared with the control in the PAO-induced adult rat heart mitochondria swelling, which was completely abolished in the presence of an inhibitor – cyclosporin A (10^{-5} mol/l). We have estimated the sensitivity of mPTP opening based on two parameters: alterations of mitochondrial swelling and release of mitochondrial substances (mitochondrial factor). We have demonstrated that old rat heart mitochondria are more sensitive to PAO (that induces the CsA-sensitive mPTP opening and mPTP-dependent release of mitochondrial factor) than adult rat heart mitochondria. Therefore, we have observed protective effect of IHT on PAO-induced mPTP-opening and mPTP-dependent factor release from old rat heart mitochondria. In experiments on the rat hemiparkinsonian model induced by 6-hydroxydopamine (6-OHDA), we have demonstrated that the used IHT course prevented pharmacologically induced unilateral dopaminergic neuronal loss. The most significant neuroprotective effect was observed in case when IHT course carried out prior and after 6-OHDA injection. Prevention of DAergic nigral neurons apoptosis upon the action of 6-OHDA is apparently due to the protective effect of IHT on mPTP opening. By reference to the obtained data, we conclude that IHT, due to its cardio- and neuroprotective effects, can be used as a protective procedure preventing mPTP opening in aging, in a number of chronic pathologies induced by oxidative stress, and also in neurodegenerative diseases.

G. Vavilova • T. Shimanskaya • N. Strutynska (✉) • S. Talanov
V. Sagach
Department of Blood Circulation, Bogomoletz Institute of Physiology,
National Academy of Sciences of Ukraine,
Kiev, Ukraine
e-mail: na-strutynska@biph.kiev.ua

L. Xi, T.V. Serebrovskaya (eds.), *Intermittent Hypoxia and Human Diseases*,
DOI 10.1007/978-1-4471-2906-6_5, © Springer-Verlag London 2012

Abbreviations

A	Absorbance
Apo	Apomorphine
CsA	Cyclosporin A
DA	Dopamine
IHT	Intermittent hypoxia training
IV	Index Veragut
LVP	Left ventricle pressure
mPTP	Mitochondrial permeability transition pore
NO	Nitric oxide
OCMW	Oxygen cost of myocardial work
6-OHDA	6-hydroxydopamine
PAO	Phenylarsine oxide
PD	Parkinson's disease
ROS	Reactive oxygen species

5.1 Introduction

In recent decades, it has been demonstrated that mitochondria are not only the main suppliers of energy in cells but they also play a central role in the induction of apoptotic cell death under both physiological and pathological conditions. Opening of the mitochondrial megachannel (also called mitochondrial permeability transition pore, mPTP) is known to be a critical event, which is realized in the cell and leads to its death. The mPTP opening allows a number of solutes with molecular weights up to 1.5 kDa (including cytochrome *c*, apoptosis-inducing factor, Ca^{2+}, etc.) to be released into the cytosol [8, 15, 35]. Just cytochrome *c* released into the cytosol increases the activity of caspases that, in turn, destroy protein structures and genetic apparatus of the cell [13]. In addition to the above solutes, adenine nucleotide metabolites can also be released from the mitochondria [27, 39]. It was demonstrated that the appearance of adenine nucleotide metabolites in the outflowing solution observed in experiments on isolated organs (in particular on isolated animal hearts) [41, 43] or in the blood of experimental animals [41] correlates with the mPTP opening [26]; the mPTP-dependent release of mitochondrial factors is considered as an index of the mPTP opening. Such specific method for detecting the mPTP opening was successfully used in our studies carried out in cardiological clinic and enabled us to find a close correlation between the appearance of adenine nucleotide metabolites in the patient's blood and disorders of cardiac activity in these persons [38].

Numerous experimental studies carried out on isolated organs or cells indicate that an increase in the sensitivity of mPTP to inducers of its opening is accompanied by dysfunction of the studied tissues [63, 64]. Inhibitors of the mPTP opening are frequently used for prevention of dysfunction of various organs under ischemia reperfusion. Recently, we have demonstrated that the increased mPTP sensitivity to inducers is typical for old animals [44] and animals with Parkinson's disease (PD) model [54]. Preconditioning state and physical trainings decrease the sensitivity of mPTP to inducers of its opening and improve the heart functioning [7, 15].

Intermittent hypoxic training (IHT) is successfully used for the complex adaptation of the entire organism and also for the improvement of the functional state of the cardiovascular system [18, 34]. Training of the organism with the use of short-term normobaric intermittent hypoxic stimuli can be taken equal (by the effect per se) to hypoxic preconditioning. Based on the fact that IHT exerts protective effects on different functional disorders, our research work was aimed at studying the effects of IHT in the sensitivity's changes of mPTP opening to its inductor PAO and also at elucidating the role of mPTP in IHT-induced protection against both functional injuries of the heart and development of neurodegenerative process in PD.

5.2 Animal Models

Experiments were carried out on isolated guinea-pig heart, rat heart mitochondria, and a rat hemiparkinsonian model induced by 6-hydroxydopamine (6-OHDA).

All experiments were carried out in accordance with the existing norm of the "European Convention on the Protection of Vertebrate Animals Used for Experimental and Other Scientific Purposes". Animal species, age, IHT modalities, and drug intervention are presented in Tables 5.1 and 5.2.

The rats were kept daily in an airproof normobaric chamber. We used a ventilated chamber where the corresponding hypoxic gas mixture ($O_2 + N_2$, %) could be injected. To eliminate CO_2 and water vapors from the chamber, an absorbent was used.

As it can be seen from Table 5.1, in experimental series dealing with the mitochondria isolated from the rat hearts, two groups of adult animals were subjected to the IHT course carried out in two regimes. Animals of the first group were subjected to soft but long-term IHT sessions (regime I), 15 min of hypoxia 12% O_2/15 min of breathing with normal atmospheric air, while animals of the second group were subjected to more severe but shorter IHT sessions (regime II), 5 min of hypoxia 8% O_2/15 min of breathing with normal atmospheric air. Such sessions were carried out five times daily during 14 days. Old rats were also subjected to IHT sessions (five times daily during 7 days): 10 min of hypoxia 10% O_2/10 min of breathing with normal atmospheric air.

Table 5.1 Experimental paradigm of examination of protective effects of IHT

	IHT sessions				
Animal groups	Hypoxic dose (O_2, %)	Time of hypoxia (min)	Time of break (min)	Number of sessions per day	Number of training days
	Isolated heart				
Guinea pigs					
Adult (6 month old), n =10	12	15	15	5	7
Old (24 month old), n = 10	12	15	15	5	7
	Isolated heart mitochondria				
Wistar rats					
Adult (6 month old), n = 10	12	15	15	5	14
Adult (6 month old), n = 10	8	5	15	5	14
Old (24 month old), n = 10	10	10	10	5	7

Table 5.2 Experimental paradigm of examination of protective effects of IHT. Testing of IHT-induced neuronal protection on the 6-OHDA-induced hemiparkinsonian model

	IHT sessions					
Animal groups	Hypoxic dose (O_2, %)	Time of hypoxia (min)	Time of air break (min)	Number of sessions per day	Number of training days	IHT sessions combined with 6-OHDA injection
Wistar rats (3 month old)						
Group 1: control, adult (n = 197)	–	–	–	–	–	6-OHDA injection
Group 2: adult (n = 7)	12	15	15	5	30	6-OHDA injection 1 day after 30-day IHT
Group 3: adult (n = 12)	12	15	15	5	30	6-OHDA injection 1 day prior to 3-day IHT
Group 4: adult (n = 16)	12	15	15	5	30 + 3	6-OHDA injection 1 day after 30-day IHT course with subsequent 3 days of IHT

In experimental series dealing with the hearts isolated from adult and old guinea pigs (Table 5.1), as well as with the 6-OHDA-induced hemiparkinsonian rat model (Table 5.2), animals were subjected to IHT carried out five times daily in the following regime: 15 min isobaric hypoxia 12%/15 min normoxia.

A rat hemiparkinsonian model was induced by the dopamine (DA) neurotoxin 6-OHDA. Rats were divided into four groups. Animals from the group 1 were subjected to unilateral damage to DAergic neurons using stereotaxic injection of 4 μg of the selective neurotoxin 6-OHDA into the left forebrain lateral bundle; rats from the group 1 served as the control. Rats from groups 2–4 were injected with 6-OHDA in the same manner as animals from the control group but 1 day after 30-day IHT course (group 2), 1 day prior to 3-day IHT (group 3), and 6-OHDA injection 1 day after 30-day IHT course with subsequent 3-day IHT (group 4). Since pharmacologically induced neurodegeneration of DA-synthesizing cells and unilateral hypersensitivity to DA developed 7 days after 6-OHDA injection, all animal groups were subjected to systemic injections of an agonist of DA receptors, apomorphine (Apo, 0.5 mg/kg, i.p.) 7 days after injection of the above neurotoxin. This standard behavioral Apo test allowed us to find the degree of 6-OHDA-induced neurodegeneration of the nigrostriatal DAergic system in the toxin-injected hemisphere, which clearly correlated with the intensity of the Apo-induced motor activity (intense rotational movements). Taking into account that 30 days of IHT carried out prior to 6-OHDA injection is an optimal time interval for the development of clearly pronounced neuroprotective effect of IHT and that neurodegeneration is more intense within 3 days after injection of neurotoxin [21], we used such regime of training. The obtained data were processed using the χ^2 test.

Other experimental procedures were performed according to techniques described in detail earlier [42, 43].

5.3 Effects of IHT on the Heart Reperfusion Injury and mPTP Opening

Adaptation to hypoxia (hypoxic preconditioning) is widely used for prophylaxis and therapies of cardiovascular diseases, an increase in the organism resistance to O_2 insufficiency. It has been demonstrated that intermittent hypoxia activates intracellular protective systems and can decrease the arrhythmia development [17, 23, 28]. The mechanism of cardioprotective effect of hypoxic preconditioning has been widely discussed [3, 30]. A number of confirmations were obtained on that reperfusion myocardial dysfunction associated with mPTP and action of factors that are released from mitochondria and stimulate the apoptosis [12, 29, 40]. We hypothesize that any changes in myocardial cell metabolism, leading to mobilization of protective mechanisms and therefore to inhibition of the opening of these nonselective mitochondrial channels will be accompanied by decrease in the heart reperfusion injuries. It seems that a similar effect is observed in the process of adaptation to hypoxia. The aim of our study was to assess the effects of intermittent hypoxia on reperfusion injuries of myocardium contractile function and mPTP opening.

In experiments on guinea-pig hearts isolated by the Langendorff mode, it was shown that 7-day course of interval hypoxic training in adult and old animals led to an increased efficiency of the heart: myocardial relaxation of old guinea-pig hearts (d*P*/d*t* min) improved significantly to 1,026 ± 44 mmHg/s as compared with untrained animals 885 ± 40 mmHg/s and myocardial contractility index (IV) value increased by 1.5 times. Oxygen consumption of old guinea-pig hearts decreased significantly, while the effectiveness of O_2 consumption (OCMW) increased by 38 ± 10%. The earlier data indicate that hypoxic preconditioning has a considerable endogenous cardioprotective potential [23, 31]. Our data on the effectiveness of old animal hypoxic training agree with the other researchers results: moderate hypobaric hypoxic preconditioning resulted in an increase in the endurance to physical loading in elderly humans (both in healthy persons and in patients with cardiac pathology) [5].

Reperfusion injuries of the adult and old animals hearts subjected to the IHT, that observed on the 40 min of the flow recovery (20-min total ischemia), were less significant than those in control hearts (Fig. 5.1). Thus, intermittent hypoxia activated some links of intracellular signal systems responsible for the increase in the myocardial resistance to ischemia reperfusion. By the end of the observation period, the recovery of left ventricle development pressure (LVP) in old animals was 89 ± 4% (in control old animals – 75 ± 3%, $P < 0.05$) and the rate of myocardial contraction dP/dt max – 104 ± 6.0% (as in control rats – 84 ± 6.5%, $P < 0.05$). Dynamics of the end-diastolic pressure during reperfusion confirmed the conclusion of the relaxation improvement in myocardial adaptation to hypoxia. In adult animals, cardioprotective effect of interval hypoxic training during ischemia-reperfusion occurred to a much greater extent (Fig. 5.2). We observed the hypoxia-induced optimization of O_2 exchange in the hearts of trained guinea pigs of both age group. Unlike the control animals, the oxygen cost of myocardial work did

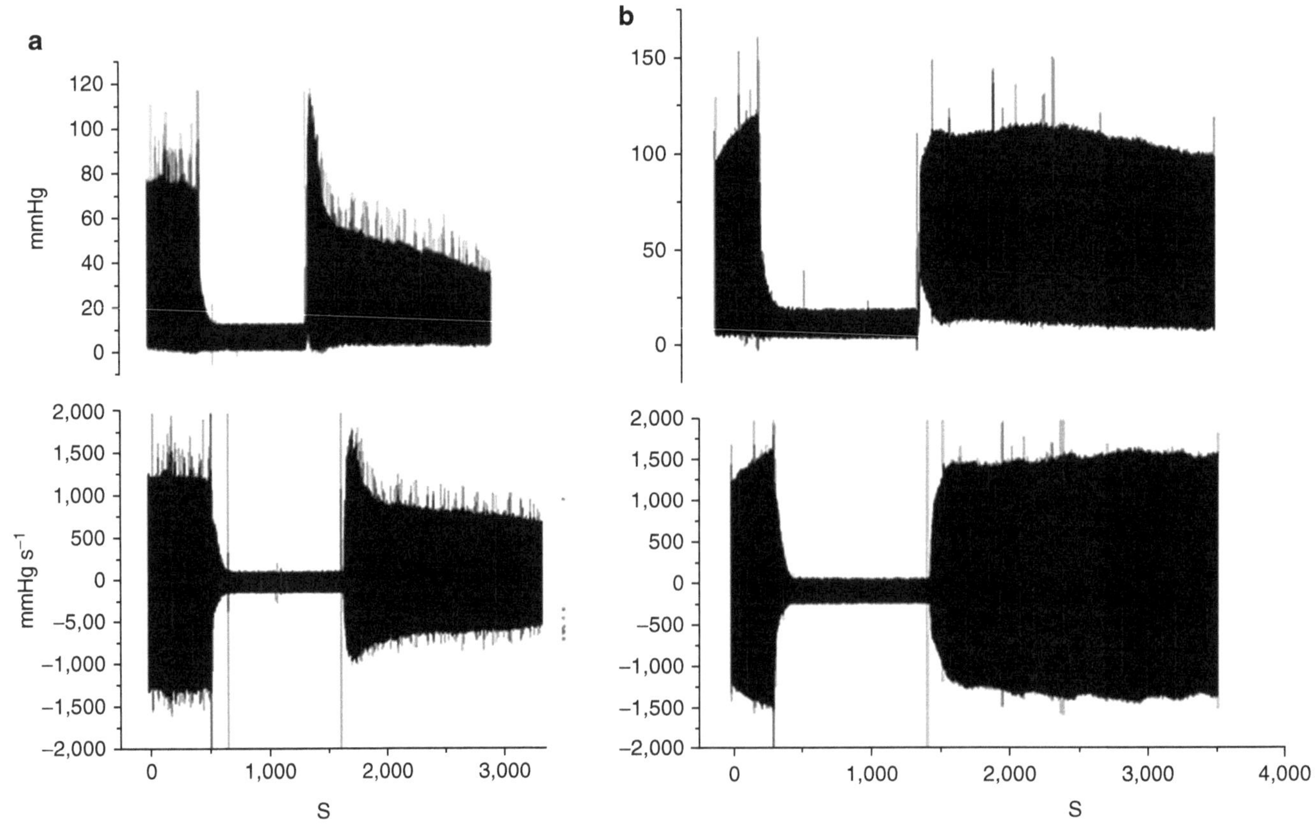

Fig. 5.1 Left ventricle pressure (LVP) and myocardial contractility during reperfusion in adult guinea pigs in control (**a**) and after intermittent hypoxic training (**b**)

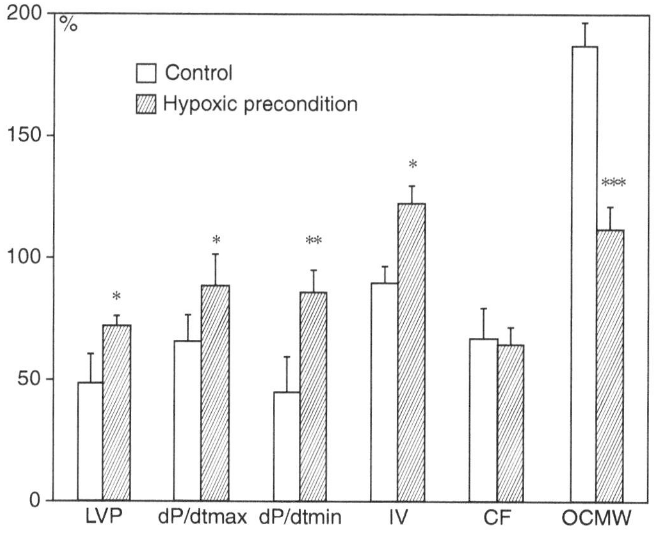

Fig. 5.2 Effect of IHT on heart function recovery to 40 min of reperfusion in adult guinea pigs. $*P<0.05$, $**P<0.01$, and $***P<0.001$, as compared with the control

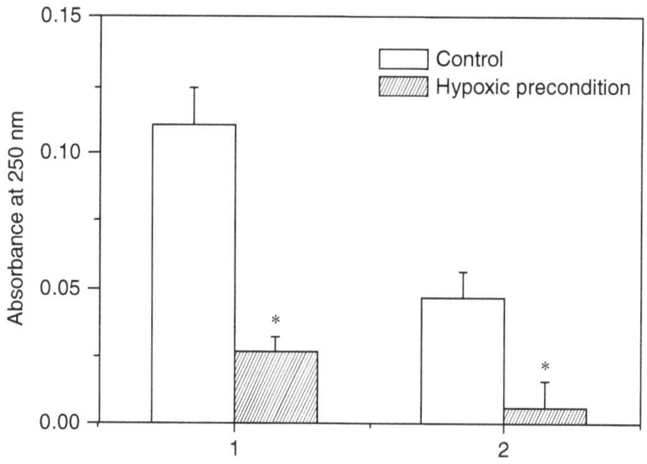

Fig. 5.3 Effect of IHT on the absorbance spectra of coronary effluents collected during postischemic reperfusion from adult – *1* and old – *2* guinea-pig hearts. $*P<0.05$, as compared with the control

not change significantly during reperfusion, while in control adult animals not subjected to adaptation to hypoxia, it increased by 82±9%.

The question arises about the mechanisms of protective effect of intermittent hypoxia. In earlier reports [27, 41–43], the activation of mPTP during heart reperfusion was accompanied by the release of low-molecular compounds of intramitochondrial solutes into the coronary flow. It was experimentally proved that inhibitors of mPTP, cyclosporine A (CsA), trolox, sanglifehrin A, and melatonin, as well as stimulation of NO synthesis, led to a decrease in both the level of reperfusion heart injuries and the mPTP-dependent release of mitochondrial compounds [40, 50]. These compounds so-called mitochondrial factor, recorded spectrophotometrically in the wavelength 230–260 nm in the ultraviolet spectrum. The appearance of such compounds in the outflowing solution can serve as a marker of the mPTP opening in experiments in situ and in vivo. In the clinic, we used the definition of this marker of mitochondrial damage in the blood serum as a diagnostic method of ischemic-reperfusion myocardial injury in humans [37]. Spectrophotometric analysis showed that increase of absorbance of the solution collected on the 1st min of reperfusion was significantly smaller in hearts from adult guinea pigs after IHT than that in control hearts (0.026±0.006 vs. 0.11±0.014, $P<0.001$), while in old hearts, this increment was practically absent (Fig. 5.3). Thus, it has been shown that the ability of heart mitochondria to activate mPTP decreased significantly after the IHT course in both adult and old guinea pigs. This conclusion is confirmed by the data obtained in studies on the effects of adaptation to hypoxia on contractile function of the heart and its O_2 exchange during ischemia reperfusion.

Our experiments showed that the reperfusion injuries of the guinea-pig hearts after IHT were significantly smaller than those observed in the control. In addition, a significant reduction in increase of the absorbance of the coronary effluent under reperfusion is indicating the inhibition of mPTP opening. Therefore, cardioprotective effect of intermittent hypoxia is due to a decrease in the ability of the heart mitochondria to opening mPTP.

5.4 Effect of IHT on Sensitivity of Phenylarsine Oxide-Induced mPTP Opening in the Rat Heart

In previous section, the data on positive effects of IHTs on indices of the functional state of the heart with reperfusion injuries caused by formation of pores in the mitochondria of cardiomyocytes are presented. Taking into account these data, we aimed at clarifying whether IHT influences the sensitivity of mPTP (as target of cardioprotection) to the inductor phenylarsine oxide (PAO). For this purpose, we studied the effects of different regimes of IHT on sensitivity of the PAO-induced mPTP opening in adult rats.

To model oxidative stress on the heart mitochondria in vitro and also to estimate the sensitivity of mPTP to inductor, we used a modifier of sulfhydric protein groups, PAO oxidant. Figure 5.4a shows typical curves of PAO-induced swelling of adult rat heart mitochondria. PAO used in the concentration of 10^{-5}or 10^{-4} mol/l led to a significant drop, as compared with the control (with no action of PAO), in the value of absorption (A) of mitochondrial suspension. This was indicative of an increase in mitochondrial swelling with $\Delta\%=17$, $P<0.05$, where $\Delta\%$ is the difference (expressed in percents) of the values of mitochondrial swelling measured

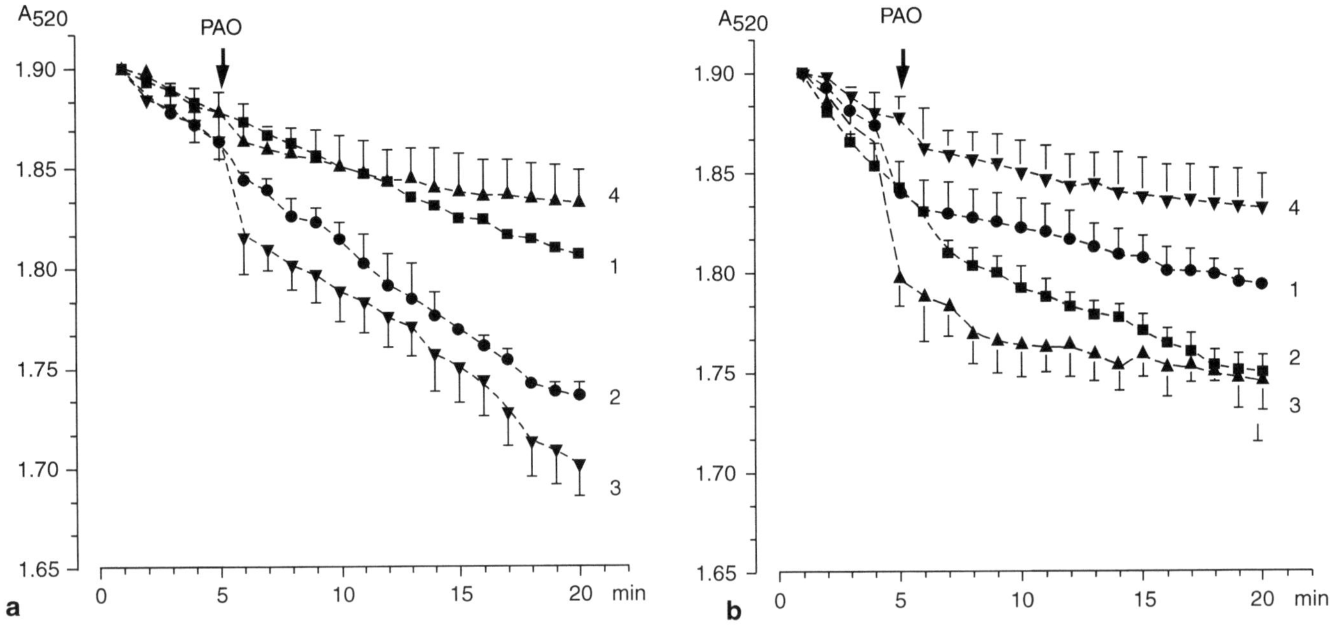

Fig. 5.4 Swelling of the mitochondria isolated from the hearts of adult rats (**a**) and rats preliminary subjected to IHT in regime II (**b**). *1* – Control (with no action of PAO); *2* and *3* – upon the action of PAO 10–5 and 10–4 mol/l, respectively; and *4* – preincubation with cyclosporin A 10–5 mol/l, upon the action of PAO 10–5 mol/l (Adapted from [58] with permission)

between the 1st and 20th min using a spectrophotometric technique. A classic inhibitor of the mPTP opening, CsA, used in the concentration of 10^{-5} mol/l prevented PAO-induced mitochondrial swelling, which was indicative of direct dependence of swelling of these organelles on the mPTP opening (Fig. 5.4a, curve 4) [58].

After trainings of adult rats in regime I (with higher O_2 content), significant changes with respect to the PAO-induced mPTP opening, as compared with the control, were not observed. Upon the action of the above inductor (10^{-5} mol/l), the values of mitochondrial swelling demonstrated no significant changes and were similar to those in control rats.

After trainings of rats in regime II, we observed a twofold decrease in the values of mitochondrial swelling upon the action of 10^{-5} mol/l PAO, as compared with the control ($\Delta\% = 10$, $P < 0.05$), which is indicative of a drop in the sensitivity of mPTP opening to the inductor used (Fig. 5.4b). The level of changes in the PAO-induced mPTP opening was estimated by alteration of the value of mitochondrial swelling upon the action of 10^{-5} mol/l PAO. The effect of decreased sensitivity of mPTP to the inductor was preserved 45 days after IHT carried out in regime II, i.e., the mitochondria acquired resistance to the action of PAO [48, 58].

Therefore, we have found the protective effect of 14-day-long IHT carried out in severe regime, which was manifested in a decrease in the sensitivity to PAO-induced mPTP opening in the studied adult heart. Our data are in agreement with findings described in the previous section with respect to a drop in the level of reperfusion heart injuries and also indicate that mPTP plays a role of the target of cardioprotection.

Despite the fact that the mechanisms underlying hypoxic and ischemic preconditioning are extensively investigated on various organs under both in vitro and in vivo conditions, it is believed that both types of effects are accompanied by synthesis of novel RNA and proteins [33, 57]. In addition, our own data on the biochemical parameters of free-radical oxidation and activity of antioxidant enzymes indicate that IHT carried out in more severe regime II (as compared with regime I) resulted in intensification of the processes of free-radical oxidation and also in a more expressed increase in the activity of superoxide dismutase accompanied by a decrease in the activity of catalase [32, 58]. Thus, in the case of more severe hypoxia, intermittent trainings result in stimulation of the activity of enzymes responsible for antioxidant protection. This, in turn, leads to the formation of protective mechanisms that prevent further activation of free-radical processes in the organism. It was reported [32] that IHT, in contrast to chronic hypoxia, is more influential and inertial factor and causes prolonged systemic activation.

Our data are in agreement with the findings obtained by other researchers [49, 62] with respect to the fact that protective effect of hypoxic preconditioning depends on the O_2 content (8–9%) in hypoxic mixture. In our experiments, where we studied the PAO-induced mPTP opening in the hearts from adult rats preliminary subjected to IHT in severe regime (8% O_2), we observed decreased sensitivity of mPTP to PAO.

Intensified production of free radicals observed in experiments where we used IHT in regime II, which resulted in accumulation of products of lipid peroxidation, can serve as a trigger mechanism of antioxidant protection at the expense of an increase in the activity of the corresponding enzymes. Therefore, based on our own data, we can conclude that severe regime of hypoxic trainings is the most influential factor of a rise in the resistance of the mitochondrial membrane to the inductor of mPTP opening in adult hearts.

As it was described in the previous section, low-molecular compounds of a mitochondrial nature, the appearance of which is related to the mPTP opening, are released into coronary flow during reperfusion of the myocardium. Based on these data, the goal of our further studies on adult and old rats was to investigate the effects of IHT on the sensitivity of PAO-induced mPTP opening and also on the mPTP-dependent release of mitochondrial factor into cardiac tissues. Free radicals (which are accumulated with aging and exert toxic effect on the organism) are one of the main inductors of the mPTP opening in general and in aging in particular. Our own biochemical studies of the content of reactive oxygen species (ROS), as well as the corresponding investigations of other researchers [19, 20, 36], confirm that the development of oxidative stress in the old hearts is intensified. We have shown earlier that the sensitivity of PAO-induced mPTP opening is increased in the old hearts; such increase is accompanied by release of the mitochondrial factor [44].

Figure 5.5 shows the data obtained in studies on the effects of IHT on the mitochondrial swelling and mPTP-dependent release of unidentified mitochondrial factor in old rat hearts upon the action of PAO. We have found protective effects of IHT with respect to the mPTP opening and release of the

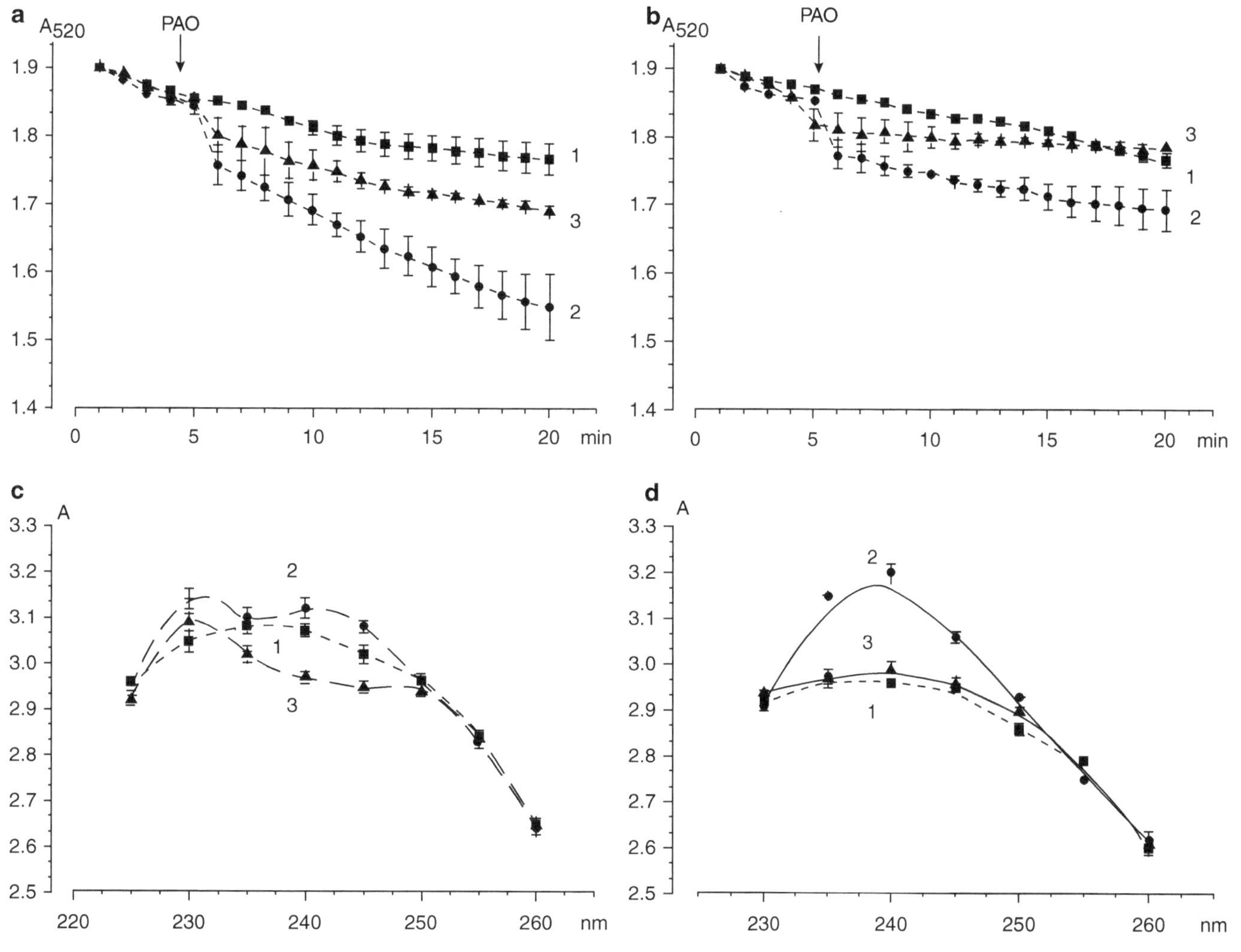

Fig. 5.5 Mitochondrial swelling and mPTP-dependent release of unidentified factor from the old rat heart mitochondria (**a**, **c**) and old rats subjected to IHT (**b**, **d**). *1* – Control (with no action of *PAO*), *2* – upon the action of PAO 10–5 mol/l, and *3* – preincubation with cyclosporin A 10–5 mol/l, upon the action of PAO 10–5 mol/l (Adapted from [36] with permission)

mitochondrial factor in old rat heart (Fig. 5.5b, d). Such effects in old rat heart mitochondria, in contrast to control old rat heart mitochondria, were manifested, first of all, in a decrease in the sensitivity of PAO-induced mPTP opening. In particular, in old rat heart mitochondria subjected to IHT, the mitochondrial swelling upon the action of 10^{-5} mol/l PAO decreased (Fig. 5.5b) and became nearly the same as that observed in adult rats (Fig. 5.4a) [37].

It should be noted that the mPTP opening in the adult rat heart mitochondria was suppressed by the classic mPTP inhibitor CsA (10^{-5} mol/l) completely (Fig. 5.4a), while in old rat heart mitochondria, such suppression was partial (Fig. 5.5a). As a result, we observed the release of mitochondrial factor from old rat heart upon the action of PAO (10^{-5} mol/l) with the maximum of absorption (A) at two wavelengths: CsA-insensitive release at $\lambda=230$ nm (I peak) and CsA-sensitive release at $\lambda=245$ nm (II peaks) (Fig. 5.5c). These data indicate that a partial formation of the nonspecific CsA-insensitive pore occurs along with formation of classic mPTP in the old rat heart mitochondria [37, 44].

We observed the recovery of protective action of CsA (10^{-5} mol/l) with respect to the mitochondrial swelling and also the CsA-sensitive release of the mitochondrial factor from subjected to IHT old rats heart mitochondria (Fig. 5.5b, d). The absence of the CsA-insensitive component of the mitochondrial factor is indicative of the protective role of IHT with respect to the development of mitochondrial dysfunction in aging.

Using the mPTP inductor PAO, we found that the mitochondrial factor is released from the mitochondria of both adult and old rat hearts, which can be considered an index of the mPTP opening [42]. It was also found that a factor of the mitochondrial nature is stably released during ischemia reperfusion and is revealed in the blood serum of animals and humans [38, 41]; this factor also can be used as a marker of the mPTP opening for determination of ischemic injuries of the myocardium in humans. Therefore, the early detection of markers of ischemic heart injuries in the blood enables one to provide timely diagnostics and also to increase the effectiveness of therapies [37].

In addition, we showed that the protective effect of IHT on the PAO-induced mPTP opening in the old rat hearts is accompanied by a decrease in the content of markers of oxidative stress, namely, of ROS (stable metabolite of active O_2, hydrogen peroxide, and hydroxylic radicals) [36]. The protective effect of IHT with respect to a decrease in the sensitivity of mPTP opening to oxidants observed in our experiments can be explained by a drop in the content of ROS in the old rat heart, which significantly decreases oxidative stress loading. It seems probable that, under such conditions, antioxidant enzymes are triggered due to the increased expression of their genes induced by substrates of these enzymes (free O_2 radicals). It is hypothesized that inhibition of complexes I and IV of mitochondrial electron-transport chain is one of the sources of IHT-induced accumulation of ROS [32, 60]. At the same time, IHT not only results in accumulation of ROS but also causes an increase in the functional activity of enzymes responsible for antioxidant protection. Published data indicate that dosed intermittent hypoxic stimuli positively influence the processes of antioxidant protection and prevent destroying effects of free radicals, in particular during episodes of acute hypoxia [22, 47].

The above data may be summed as follows: We have found the protective effect of IHT, which was manifested in a decrease in the sensitivity of the PAO-induced mPTP opening and also in prevention of the release of mitochondrial factor in the old rat heart. These findings are in agreement with the data obtained on isolated guinea-pig heart during ischemia reperfusion in particular, with respect to a decrease in the mPTP-dependent release of mitochondrial factor measured in the flowing-out solution.

5.5 IHT Presents Degeneration of DAergic Neurons via Inhibition of mPTP

Selective death of dopaminergic neurons of the *substantia nigra* and insufficiency of cerebral DA underlie pathogenesis of PD. A large body of studies showed that the PD-related death of dopaminergic nigral neurons is realized mostly through apoptosis [4, 24, 25]. This process is determined mostly by disturbance of the functional state of the mitochondria; dysfunction of these cellular organelles results in the mPTP opening and release of compounds, which trigger a cascade of apoptotic processes, into the cytosol.

A decrease in the activity of mitochondrial complex I in DAergic neurons [4, 45], which results in a weakening of cell respiration and also in a drop in ATP production, is typical of PD. An inhibition of the complex I leads to a decrease in the membrane potential and its loss [6, 46] and, therefore, to the mPTP opening [6, 61]. We have shown earlier [54] that, under conditions of insufficiency of cerebral DA, the sensitivity of mPTP to Ca^{2+} also increases in cardiac tissues, which can be the reason for apoptotic death of cardiomyocytes and, therefore, for the development of cardiac pathologies in patients suffering from PD.

In experiments on rats, the death of DA-synthesizing neurons was induced by injections of the selective neurotoxin 6-OHDA (which is known to be the natural metabolite of DA) into the lateral ascending forebrain bundle [1, 9]. In such rat 6-OHDA-induced hemiparkinsonian model, as well as in patients suffering from PD, dysfunction of the mitochondria is observed, and neuronal death is realized by apoptotic type [51, 59].

After death of a considerable number of DAergic neurons accompanied by a significant drop in the level of cerebral

DA, target neurons demonstrate hypersensitivity to this neurotransmitter. It should be noted that DA-synthesizing cells of the *substantia nigra* send no projections to the opposite cerebral hemisphere. This is why the DA level decreases only in one hemisphere under conditions of unilateral 6-OHDA injection and, correspondingly, unilateral damage to the DAergic system (hemiparkinsonian animal model); hypersensitivity to DA is also developed only in one (denervated) hemisphere.

The level of unilateral degeneration of the DAergic system is easily estimated with the use of behavioral Apo test [52]. After systemic injections of this agonist of DA receptors, rats demonstrated Apo-induced rotational movements toward the side contralateral with respect to the 6-OHDA-injected hemisphere. It should be noted that the intensity of such rotational movements corresponds to the intensity of cell death. According to our morphological studies [52], intense rotations (more than 180 rotations within 30-min-long intervals after Apo injection) indicate that 90% of DAergic neurons of the *substantia nigra* (on the side of 6-OHDA injection) are damaged. Our broad experience (experiments on 197 animals) has shown that unilateral injection of 6-OHDA resulted in significant damage to the DAergic system, which was manifested in an intense rotational movements in the Apo test in 42.6% of rats. A decrease in the number of animals with clearly pronounced motor asymmetry in the Apo test after 6-OHDA injection upon the action of any factor can be indicative of its neuroprotective effect.

Recently, it was demonstrated that IHT is capable of exerting inhibitory effect on mPTP [36, 58]. Taking into account the importance of mPTP opening in the induction of apoptotic death of DAergic neurons, we studied the effects of IHTs on 6-OHDA-induced degeneration of the DAergic system.

In our experiments, in control rats (group 1) subjected to the Apo test, intense rotational movements toward the side contralateral to 6-OHDA injections were observed in 42.6% of the cases (i.e., in 84 animals of the 197 studied rats). In rats of group 2, the level of pharmacologically induced degeneration of DAergic neurons remained unchanged: intense rotational movements after systemic Apo injections were observed in three (42.9%) rats of the seven studied animals. In group 3, we observed the Apo-initiated intense rotational movements in one rat of 12 the studied animals (8.3%; $P<0.05$). In group 4, none of 16 rats ($P<0.001$) demonstrated rotational movements upon injection of agonist of DA receptors (Fig. 5.6). These data indicate that IHT effectively prevented 6-OHDA-induced apoptotic death of DAergic nigral neurons. It should be noted that IHT exerted positive effects after neurotoxin injection; the maximum neuroprotective effect of IHT was observed in animals of group 4.

It is well known that oxidative stress is the main factor of mPTP opening [44]; hypoxic training results in intensification

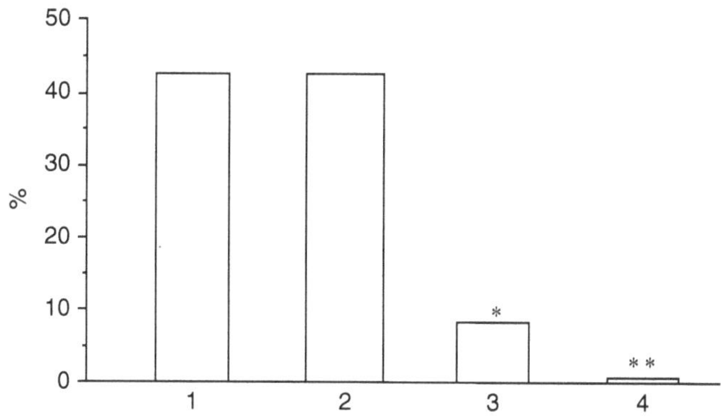

Fig. 5.6 Neuroprotective effect of IHT. Vertical scale: relative number (%) of rats with intense rotational movements induced by systemic apomorphine injection, which was indicative of mass (more than 90%) 6-hydroxydopamine (6-OHDA)-caused degeneration of the dopaminergic system. *1* – Control (injection of 6-OHDA without IHT), *2* – 30 days of IHT carried out prior to injection of 6-OHDA, *3* – 3 days of IHT carried out after injection of 6-OHDA, and *4* – 30 days prior to 6-OHDA injection with subsequent 3 days of IHT. *$P<0.05$ and **$P<0.001$, as compared with the control (Adapted from [55] with permission)

of the activity of enzymes of antioxidant system and, therefore, exerts positive effect on the processes of antioxidant protection [10, 47]. Intermittent hypoxic training demonstrates more expressed and longer effect than chronic hypoxia [32]. Hypoxic preconditioning increases the time necessary for mPTP opening [16], which plays a considerable role in the protective effect of preconditioning [2]. It was also found that hypoxic postconditioning exerts inhibitory effect on the mPTP opening and, therefore, can be used against the effects of different disturbing factors [2, 11]. In addition, IHT significantly decreases calcium loading in the cell [56], which is one of the important factors responsible for suppression of mPTP opening and also for weakening of tissue damage under in vivo conditions [14].

Recently [52, 53], we have shown that melatonin, the well-known antioxidant and inhibitor of mPTP, also significantly prevents 6-OHDA-induced apoptotic death of DA-synthesizing neurons of the *substantia nigra*. These data indirectly confirm that neuroprotective effect of IHT, observed in our experiments, is most probably realized via inhibition of mPTP [55].

The data described above indicate that IHT can to a significant extent prevent the 6-OHDA-induced death of DAergic neurons of the *substantia nigra* via inhibition of the mPTP.

Conclusion

Our studies on hearts from adult and old guinea pigs subjected to 7-day-long IHT have shown that such training resulted in a decrease in the level of reperfusion injury of the heart and also in a significant decrease in the level of mitochondrial factor released into the coronary flow under test ischemia of this organ. In addition, we found the protective effect of IHT with respect to the PAO-induced mPTP opening and also the release of mitochondrial factor in adult and old hearts, which can, in the future, be used as protective means of prevention of the mPTP opening in aging and also in a number of chronic pathological states of the organism (in particular in Parkinson's disease). Our data confirm that the use of IHT (that exerts moderate oxidative stress) opens up new prospects for prophylaxis of different pathologies of the cardiovascular system and/or also for therapies for cardiovascular diseases.

In experiments on hemiparkinsonian animal model, we demonstrated that the used IHT course prevented the 6-OHDA-caused death of DAergic neurons of the *substantia nigra*. The most significant neuroprotective effect of IHT was observed under conditions of the 34-day-long combined action of IHT and 6-OHDA injection (in the case where 30-day-long IHT course was performed 1 day prior to 6-OHDA injection and 3-day-long IHT course was performed 1 day after injection of this neurotoxin). Prevention of apoptosis of DAergic nigral neurons upon the action of 6-OHDA is apparently due to the protective effect of IHT on the PTP opening. The mechanisms underlying the protective effects of IHT, which possess, probably, common signal pathways with ischemic preconditioning, need further investigation.

References

1. Andrew R, Watson DG, Best SA. The determination of hydroxydopamines and other trace amines in the urine of parkinsonian patients and normal controls. Neurochem Res. 1993;18:1175–7.
2. Argaud L, Gateau-Roesch O, Muntean D, et al. Specific inhibition of the mitochondrial permeability transition prevents lethal reperfusion injury. J Mol Cell Cardiol. 2005;38:367–74.
3. Bertuglia S. Intermittent hypoxia modulates nitric oxide-dependent vasodilation and capillary perfusion during ischemia-reperfusion-induced damage. Am J Physiol. 2008;294:H1914–22.
4. Bowling AC, Beal MF. Bioenergetic and oxidative stress in neurodegenerative diseases. Life Sci. 1995;56:1151–71.
5. Burtscher M, Pachinger O, Ehrenbourg I, et al. Intermittent hypoxia increases exercise tolerance in elderly men with and without coronary artery disease. Int J Cardiol. 2004;96:247–54.
6. Cassarino DS, Bennett Jr JP. An evaluation of the role of mitochondria in neurodegenerative diseases: mitochondrial mutations and oxidative pathology, protective nuclear responses, and cell death in neurodegeneration. Brain Res Rev. 1999;29:1–25.
7. Chorna SV, Talanov SO, Strutynska NA, et al. The functional state of the rat heart during ischemia-reperfusion, the sensitivity of calcium-induced NO-dependent mitochondrial permeability transition pore opening and the uncoupling protein 3 expression under long exercise training. Fiziol Zh. 2010;56:13–21 [In Ukrainian].
8. Crompton M. Mitochondria and aging: a role for the permeability transition? Aging Cell. 2004;3:3–6.
9. Curtius HC, Wolfensberger M, Steinmann B, et al. Mass fragmentography of dopamine and 6-hydroxydopamine. Application to the determination of dopamine in human brain biopsies from the caudate nucleus. J Chromatogr. 1974;99:529–40.
10. El'chaninova SA, Smagina IV, Koreniak NA, et al. The influence of interval hypoxic training on lipid peroxidation and antioxidant enzyme activity. Fiziol Cheloveka. 2003;29:72–5 [In Russian].
11. Feng J, Lucchinetti E, Ahuja P, et al. Isoflurane postconditioning prevents opening of the mitochondrial permeability transition pore through inhibition of glycogen synthase kinase 3beta. Anesthesiology. 2005;103:987–95.
12. Griffiths E, Halestrap A. Mitochondrial non-specific pores remain closed during cardiac ischemia but open upon reperfusion. Biochem J. 1995;307:93–8.
13. Halestrap AP. A pore way to die: the role of mitochondria in reperfusion injury and cardioprotection. Biochem Soc Trans. 2010; 38:841–60.
14. Halestrap AP, Clarke SJ, Javadov SA. Mitochondrial permeability transition pore opening during myocardial reperfusion - a target for cardioprotection. Cardiovasc Res. 2004;61:372–85.
15. Halestrap AP, Pasdois P. The role of the mitochondrial permeability transition pore in heart disease. Biochim Biophys Acta. 2009;1787:1402–15.
16. Hausenloy DJ, Yellon DM, Mani-Babu S, et al. Preconditioning protects by inhibiting the mitochondrial permeability transition. Am J Physiol. 2004;287:H841–9.
17. Jung ME, Simpkins JW, Wilson AM, et al. Intermittent hypoxia conditioning prevents behavioral deficit and brain oxidative stress in ethanol-withdrawn rats. J Appl Physiol. 2008;105:510–7.
18. Kolchinskaya AZ, Cyganova TN, Ostapenko LA. Normobaric intermittent hypoxic training in medicine and sport. Moscow: Medicine; 2003 [In Russian].
19. Leeuwenburgh C, Phaneuf S. Cytochrome c release from mitochondria in the aging hear: a possible mechanism for apoptosis with age. Am J Physiol Regul Integr Comp Physiol. 2002;282: R423–30.
20. Lesnefsky EJ, Hoppel CL. Ischemia-reperfusion injury in the aged heart: role of the mitochondria. Arch Biochem Biophys. 2003;420:287–97.
21. Lin AM, Chen CF, Ho LT. Neuroprotective effect of intermittent hypoxia on iron-induced oxidative injury in rat brain. Exp Neurol. 2002;176:328–35.
22. Malyshev IY, Manuhina EB. Stress, adaptation and nitric oxide. Biochemistry. 1998;67:992–1006 [In Russian].
23. Meerson FZ. Essentials of adaptive medicine: protective effects of adaptation, hypoxia. Moscow: Hypoxia Medical LTD; 1994.
24. Mochizuki H, Goto K, Mori H, et al. Histochemical detection of apoptosis in Parkinson's disease. J Neurol Sci. 1996;137:120–3.
25. Mochizuki H, Mori H, Mizuno Y. Apoptosis in neurodegenerative disorders. J Neural Transm. 1997;50:125–40.
26. Nadtochiy SM, Bohuslavs'kyĭ AI, Sagach VF. Determination of the stable mitochondrial factor in vivo. Fiziol Zh. 2003;49:25–30 [In Ukrainian].
27. Nadtochiy SM, Nauduri D, Shimanskaya TV, et al. Purine release: a protective signaling mechanism of the mitochondrial permeability transition pore in ischemia. Fiziol Zh. 2008;54:5–14.
28. Naghshin J, McGaffin KR, Witham WG, et al. Chronic intermittent hypoxia increases left ventricular contractility in C57BL/6J mice. J Appl Physiol. 2009;107:787–93.
29. Nazareth W, Yafei N, Crompton M. Inhibition of anoxia-induced injury in heart myocytes by cyclosporin A. J Mol Cell Cardiol. 1991;23:1351–4.
30. Park AM, Suzuki YJ. Effects of intermittent hypoxia on oxidative stress-induced myocardial damage in mice. J Appl Physiol. 2007;102:1806–14.
31. Pilar Valle M, García-Godos F, Woolcott OO, et al. Improvement of myocardial perfusion in coronary patients after intermittent hypobaric hypoxia. J Nucl Cardiol. 2006;13:69–74.

32. Prabhakar NR, Kumar GK. Oxidative stress in the systemic and cellular responses to intermittent hypoxia. Biol Chem. 2004;385:217–21.
33. Prabhakar NR, Kumar GK, Nanduri J. Intermittent hypoxia augments acute hypoxic sensing via HIF-mediated ROS. Respir Physiol Neurobiol. 2010;174:230–4.
34. Prabhakar NR, Peng YJ, Kumar GK, et al. Long-term regulation of carotid body function: acclimatization and adaptation. Adv Exp Med Biol. 2009;648:307–17.
35. Rasola A, Sciacovelli M, Pantic B, et al. Signal transduction to the permeability transition pore. FEBS Lett. 2010;584:1989–96.
36. Rudyk OV, Vavilova HL, Strutyns'ka NA, et al. Sensitivity of phenylarsineoxide-induced mitochondrial permeability transition pore opening in the heart of old rats during intermittent hypoxic training. Fiziol Zh. 2004;50:29–37 [In Ukrainian].
37. Sagach VF, Dmitrieva AV, Bubnova IuO, et al. Diagnostics method of myocardium ischemia-reperfusion injury and the mitochondrial permeability transition pore opening. 2007; Patent of utility model № 26385. Bul.№15 of 25.09.2007.
38. Sagach VF, Dmytrieva AV, Bubnova IuO, et al. Using marker of the mitochondrial pore opening in diagnostics of patients with myocardial ischemic lesions. Fiziol Zh. 2009;55:12–8 [In Ukrainian].
39. Sagach VF, Maksymenko VB, Dmytrieva AV, et al. Early marker of myocardial injury of the ischemia-reperfused heart in dogs and during operations with artificial circulation in humans. Fiziol Zh. 2006;52:3–8 [In Ukrainian].
40. Sagach VF, Shimanskaya TV, Nadtochiy SM. Protection of heart from reperfusion injury and ineffective oxygen consumption by inhibitors of the mitochondrial permeability transition pore. Fiziol Zh. 2002;48:3–9 [In Ukrainian].
41. Sagach VF, Shimanskaya TV, Nadtochiy SM. Factor, released under the isolated heart reperfusion may be the marker of the opening the mitochondrial permeability transition pore. Fiziol Zh. 2003;49:7–13 [In Ukrainian].
42. Sagach VF, Vavilova HL, Rudyk OV, et al. Release of unidentified mitochondrial substance – evidence for mitochondrial permeability transition pore opening in heart mitochondria of rats. Fiziol Zh. 2003;49:3–12 [In Ukrainian].
43. Sagach VF, Vavilova HL, Strutynska NA, et al. Effect of inductors and inhibitors of the mitochondrial permeability transition pore on its opening and release of unidentified mitochondrial factor. Fiziol Zh. 2003;49:3–12 [In Ukrainian].
44. Sagach VF, Vavilova HL, Strutynska NA, et al. The aging-related increase of sensitivity of the mitochondrial permeability transition pore opening to inductors in rat heart. Fiziol Zh. 2004;50:49–63 [In Ukrainian].
45. Schapira AH, Gu M, Taanman JW, et al. Mitochondria in the etiology and pathogenesis of Parkinson's disease. Ann Neurol. 1998;44:S89–98.
46. Schulz JB, Matthews RT, Klockgether T, et al. The role of mitochondrial dysfunction and neuronal nitric oxide in animal models of neurodegenerative diseases. Mol Cell Biochem. 1997;174:193–7.
47. Serebrovs'ka TV, Kurgaliuk NM, Nosar VI, et al. Intermittent hypoxic training with exogenous nitric oxide improves rat liver mitochondrial oxidation and phosphorylation during acute hypoxia. Fiziol Zh. 2001;47:85–92 [In Ukrainian].
48. Serebrovskaya TV, Vavilova GL, Rudyk OV, et al. Different regimen of intermittent hypoxia training (IHT) as modulator of mitochondrial membrane permeability transition pore in rat heart. In: Mitochondrial physiology. MiP2005, Schröcken, Vorarlberg, Austria, p.29–30.
49. Sharp FR, Ran R, Lu A, et al. Hypoxic preconditioning protects against ischemic brain injury. NeuroRx. 2004;1:26–35.
50. Shimanskaya T, Dobrovolsky F, Vavilova G, et al. NO-dependent modulation of the sensitivity of the mitochondrial permeability transition pore opening under ischemia-reperfusion of the isolated heart. I M Sechenov Physiol J. 2009;95:28–37 [In Russian].
51. Singh S, Kumar S, Dikshit M. Involvement of the mitochondrial apoptotic pathway and nitric oxide synthase in dopaminergic neuronal death induced by 6-hydroxydopamine and lipopolysaccharide. Redox Rep. 2010;15:115–22.
52. Talanov SA, Oleshko NN, Tkachenko MN, et al. Pharmacoprotective influences on different links of the mechanism underlying 6-hydroxydopamine-induced degeneration of nigro-striatal dopaminergic neurons. Neurophysiology. 2006;38:150–6.
53. Talanov SA, Sahach VF. Antioxidants prevent experimental hemiparkinsonism in rats. Fiziol Zh. 2008;54:23–9 [In Ukrainian].
54. Talanov SA, Timoshchuk SV, Rudyk OV, et al. An increased sensitivity of the mitochondrial permeability transition pore to calcium in the heart of rats with chronic deficiency of nigrostriatal dopamine. Fiziol Zh. 2009;55:3–8 [In Ukrainian].
55. Talanov SO, Sahach VF, Oleshko MM, et al. Inhibitors of mitochondrial permeability transition pore prevent apoptosis of dopaminergic neurons in the mesencephalon. Fiziol Zh. 2006;52:13–8 [In Ukrainian].
56. Tatton WG, Chalmers-Redman RM, Ju WY, et al. Apoptosis in neurodegenerative disorders: potential for therapy by modifying gene transcription. J Neural Transm Suppl. 1997;49:245–68.
57. Vannucci RC, Towfighi J, Vannucci SJ. Hypoxic preconditioning and hypoxic-ischemic brain damage in the immature rat: pathologic and metabolic correlates. J Neurochem. 1998;71:1215–20.
58. Vavilova GL, Serebrovskaya TV, Rudyk OV, et al. Influence of the intermittent hypoxia training on the sensitivity of phenylarsineoxide-induced mitochondrial permeability transition pore in rat heart. Fiziol Zh. 2005;51:3–12 [In Ukrainian].
59. Wang T, Liu YY, Yang N, et al. Relationship of oxidative DNA damage and expression of mitochondrial apoptotic proteins in rat striatum induced by 6-hydroxydopamine. Zhonghua Yi Xue Za Zhi. 2010;90:2074–7 [In Chinese].
60. Yuan G, Adhikary G, McCormick AA, et al. Role of oxidative stress in intermittent hypoxia-induced immediate early gene activation in PC12 cells. J Physiol. 2004;157:773–83.
61. Zamzami N, Susin SA, Marchetti P, et al. Mitochondrial control of nuclear apoptosis. J Exp Med. 1996;183:1533–44.
62. Zhu W-Z, Xie Y, Chen L, et al. Intermittent high altitude hypoxia inhibits opening of mitochondrial permeability transition pores against reperfusion injury. J Mol Cell Cardiol. 2006; 40:96–106.
63. Zorov DB, Filburn CR, Klotz LO, et al. Reactive oxygen species (ROS)-induced ROS release: a new phenomenon accompanying induction of the mitochondrial permeability transition in cardiac myocytes. J Exp Med. 2000;192:1001–14.
64. Zorov DB, Juhaszova M, Yaniv Y, et al. Regulation and pharmacology of the mitochondrial permeability transition pore. Cardiovasc Res. 2009;83:213–25.

Intermittent Hypoxia Alters the Function of Cardiovascular Neurons and Reflex Pathways in the Brainstem

6

David D. Kline and David Mendelowitz

Abstract

Obstructive sleep apnea, and the animal model of this disease, chronic intermittent hypoxia, alters autonomic balance and many different neurobiological functions in the brainstem that likely play an important role in both the initiation and progression of cardiovascular diseases associated with obstructive sleep apnea including hypertension and arrhythmia. Current research suggests the targets of chronic intermittent hypoxia include increased release of the excitatory neurotransmitter glutamate from baroreceptor sensory neurons, likely via altered presynaptic calcium homeostasis and increased spontaneous release of neurotransmitters from these baroreceptor sensory neurons onto brainstem neurons in the nucleus tractus solitarius. Additionally, acute exposures to hypoxia diminish excitatory and enhance inhibitory neurotransmission to parasympathetic cardiac neurons in the nucleus ambiguus that control heart rate and cardiac excitability. Future targets for restoring autonomic balance and increasing survival in these cardiorespiratory diseases require a more thorough understanding of the alterations of synaptic neurotransmission and receptor activation in the brainstem that occur with chronic intermittent hypoxia and obstructive sleep apnea.

Abbreviations

5-HT	5-Hydroxytryptamine, serotonin
AP	Action potential
CIH	Chronic intermittent hypoxia
CPAP	Continuous positive airway pressure
CVLM	Caudal ventrolateral medulla
DA	Dopamine
EPSCs	Excitatory postsynaptic currents
IPSCs	Inhibitory postsynaptic currents
NA	Nucleus ambiguus
NMDA	*N*-methyl-D-aspartate
NO	Nitric oxide
NTS	Nucleus tractus solitarius
OSA	Obstructive sleep apnea
RVLM	Rostral ventrolateral medulla
TH	Tyrosine hydroxylase

6.1 Introduction

The autonomic nervous system is vital for the maintenance of homeostasis and the reflex responses to a variety of stressors. Heart rate, sympathetic activity, and mean arterial pressure are controlled in a beat-to-beat manner by precise reflex pathways and their related nuclei in the brainstem. These cardiorespiratory reflexes are essential for responding to challenges such as alterations in blood pressure, demands of exercise, and hypoxia. Measures of these ongoing, tonic, and

D.D. Kline
Department of Biomedical Sciences,
Dalton Cardiovascular Research Center, University of Missouri,
134 Research Park Dr., Columbia, MO 65211, USA

D. Mendelowitz (✉)
Department of Pharmacology and Physiology,
The George Washington University,
2300 Eye St. N.W., Washington, DC 20037, USA
e-mail: dmendel@gwu.edu

L. Xi, T.V. Serebrovskaya (eds.), *Intermittent Hypoxia and Human Diseases*,
DOI 10.1007/978-1-4471-2906-6_6, © Springer-Verlag London 2012

rapid adjustments in sympathetic, and especially parasympathetic activity (e.g., heart rate variability), are indicators of cardiac health and, when absent, can predict an important risk of cardiac sudden death.

Heart rate in healthy individuals is determined mainly by the tonic and reflex control of parasympathetic activity that innervates the heart. In conscious and anesthetized animals, there is an endogenous cardiac-pulse rhythmic parasympathetic activity to the heart and minimal sympathetic activity at rest, as described in humans [1], dogs [2], cats [3], and rats [4, 5]. During increases in arterial pressure, the initial reflex-induced slowing of the heart is caused primarily, if not exclusively, by increases in parasympathetic activity to the heart [2, 5]. During decreases in arterial pressure, the reflex-induced tachycardia is caused mostly by decreases in parasympathetic, in addition to increases in sympathetic cardiac nerve activity [2, 6, 7]. When both parasympathetic and sympathetic activities are present, parasympathetic activity generally dominates the control of heart rate. Increases in parasympathetic activity evoke a bradycardia that is more pronounced when there is a high level of sympathetic firing [8]. During moderate or high level of parasympathetic activity, changes in sympathetic firing elicit negligible changes in heart rate [8].

The sympathetic nervous system innervates almost every tissue in the body, including the adrenal gland, kidneys, heart, and arteriole blood vessels. There is a tonic rhythmic discharge of sympathetic activity to the arteriole blood vessels to maintain vasomotor tone and total peripheral resistance [9]. This sympathetic tone has a dominant role in both the short- and long-term control of blood pressure. Increases in basal and reflex-mediated sympathetic activity result in a rise of peripheral resistance in the circulation increasing blood pressure. The sympathetic nervous system also innervates the heart and modulates myocardial contractility and heart rate. Increases in sympathetic activity therefore increase blood pressure via increases in contractility, heart rate, and vascular resistance. Increases in sympathetic activity also evoke release of vasoactive hormones including vasopressin, angiotensin, and aldosterone.

Levels of parasympathetic and sympathetic activity are determined in large part from the function of the arterial baroreceptor reflex. The baroreflex is a classic negative feedback reflex in which increases in arterial blood pressure activate mechanosensitive arterial baroreceptors in the carotid sinus and aortic arch that trigger reflex responses that ultimately act to restore arterial blood pressure to control levels. The discharge of arterial baroreceptors is conducted through cranial nerve axons (IX and X) projecting directly into the brainstem to neurons in the nucleus tractus solitarius (NTS) where they make the first synapse in the baroreflex pathway [10]. Processed afferent signals exit the NTS to activate premotor cardiac vagal neurons located primarily in the nucleus ambiguus (NA) that in turn project to cardioinhibitory parasympathetic ganglia in the fat pads of the heart. Activation of NTS neurons by baroreceptor activity also activates sympathoinhibitory neurons, located in the caudal ventrolateral medulla (CVLM), which in turn inhibit presympathetic neurons in the rostral ventrolateral medulla (RVLM) [11]. Perturbations such as increases in arterial pressure are then corrected via dual cardiovascular pathways that produce negative feedback control by (1) increased release of acetylcholine by parasympathetic postganglionic neurons evoking a bradycardia and (2) decreased release of norepinephrine by sympathetic postganglionic neurons eliciting reduced vasoconstriction and peripheral resistance.

In the resting, conscious state, midcollicular decerebration does not alter the gain or sensitivity of the baroreflex, suggesting that brainstem mechanisms are sufficient for reflex function. Although brain structures above the medulla are not required, information from the forebrain and other higher CNS sites modulates the baroreflex during various behaviors including stressful emotional responses. Thus, the core heart rate baroreflex circuit appears to reside below the pons and contains both short and longer latency pathways and includes at a minimum three vital components: (1) baroreceptors and (2) neurons in the NTS that receive this sensory information and relay this information to (3) parasympathetic cardiac vagal neurons in the NA. Such a parasympathetic reflex pathway is responsible for relatively short-latency (<100 ms) cardiovascular-cardiac reflexes that adjust heart rate within one cardiac cycle. Likewise, the core circuit for baroreflex control of sympathetic activity involves peripheral baroreceptors and NTS, followed by activation of sympathoinhibitory neurons in the CVLM which inhibit the activity of presympathetic neurons in the RVLM. Projections from the RVLM to the spinal preganglionic sympathetic neurons complete the efferent sympathetic pathway within the autonomic nervous system.

However, parasympathetic activity to the heart is attenuated or unresponsive in many disease states in which there is a decrease in baroreflex sensitivity and diminished cardiac vagal activity [12–16]. Parasympathetic withdrawal is associated with ventricular arrhythmias, sudden cardiac death [17], and congestive heart failure [18]. Diminished heart rate recovery after exercise due to blunted parasympathetic outflow is an independent predictor of mortality in chronic heart failure [19]. Reestablishment of parasympathetic outflow is associated with increased recovery in ischemia and reperfusion-induced arrhythmias, as well as myocardial infarction, and restoring proper parasympathetic outflow is suggested as a therapeutic target to reduce mortality and sudden death [20–23].

Sympathetic activity is not only important for transient blood pressure control but also long-term arterial blood pressure regulation. Elevated sympathetic nervous system activity is characteristic of numerous cardiovascular diseases, including left ventricular hypertrophy, hypertension, heart failure, sudden death, and arrhythmias [24]. Elevated sympathetic activity is also associated with obesity, diabetes, metabolic syndrome, and the increased mortality accompanying these diseases [25].

6.2 Alterations in Baroreceptor Reflex Function with Obstructive Sleep Apnea

A very prevalent cardiorespiratory disease is obstructive sleep apnea (OSA). OSA, and accompanying episodic hypoxia, is a significant health risk occurring in as many as ~24% of males and 9% of females (between 30 and 60 years of age) within the United States population [26, 27]. Severe OSA increases cardiovascular mortality fourfold, and even when corrected for other risk factors, severe OSA increases cardiovascular mortality threefold [28].

OSA is associated with elevated cardiovascular risk. OSA can participate in both the initiation and progression of several cardiovascular diseases including hypertension, arrhythmias, myocardial ischemia, and stroke [29, 30]. The reader is referred to several excellent clinical reviews [29, 30], and as such, only a brief discussion on the association of OSA and cardiovascular disease is presented here. For instance, OSA is an independent risk factor for hypertension as 50% of individuals with sleep disordered breathing are also hypertensive. It is estimated that 11–37% of heart failure patients also possess OSA. Arrhythmias are commonly observed in OSA patients along with a high incidence of bradyarrhythmias (including vagal-mediated sinus bradycardia, sinus arrest, and atrioventricular block), ventricular arrhythmias (especially during sleep), and atrial fibrillation. Further, OSA was recently shown to be an independent risk factor for coronary artery disease with the risk of nocturnal sudden death increasing with OSA severity. In addition, there is a strong relationship with OSA and the incidence of stroke. OSA patients have an increased incidence of silent brain infarctions, prestroke cerebrovascular disease, and poststroke mortality.

Clinical studies suggest that activation of the carotid body chemoreceptors plays a key role in initiating the cardiovascular abnormalities during OSA [31, 32]. Specifically, sleep apnea patients exhibit increased chemoreflex sensitivity and hypertension [33] even when other factors are eliminated. Ventilatory depression caused by brief hyperoxia, a measure of peripheral chemosensitivity, is more pronounced in OSA [34]. Further, apneic patients who have had their carotid bodies removed for unrelated purposes do not develop hypertension [35].

Treatment of OSA is primarily continuous positive airway pressure (CPAP). This treatment is marginally effective in reducing elevated arterial pressure (~2 mmHg) [26] and sympathetic nerve activity [33, 36, 37] and partially restoring chemoreflex [33] and baroreflex sensitivity [38]. CPAP may also improve the outcome and well-being of patients with heart failure, arrhythmias, coronary artery disease, and cerebrovascular disease [29]. However, CPAP is intrusive, poorly tolerated, and often discontinued despite the continued health risks of OSA [26].

6.3 Chronic Intermittent Hypoxia Alters the Function of Sensory Cardiovascular Neurons and Synapses

Chronic exposure to intermittent hypoxia during the nocturnal period in animals mimics the repetitive episodes of apneas and hypoxia that occurs in humans with OSA. Chronic intermittent hypoxia, in both animal models and humans, decreases baroreflex sensitivity, elevates blood pressure and sympathetic activity, and diminishes parasympathetic activity to the heart [12–16]. While chronic intermittent hypoxia decreases the baroreflex control of heart rate and diminishes parasympathetic activity to the heart, these changes are not due to changes in parasympathetic innervation of the sinoatrial node or function within the cardiac ganglia but are rather most likely due to changes in the activity of the major cardiovascular neurons in the brainstem including neurons in the NTS and premotor parasympathetic cardiac vagal neurons in the NA.

Baroreceptor encoded information synapse upon neurons within dorsal medial portions of the caudal NTS as the central first step of the medullary baroreceptor reflex. Sensory inputs from baroreceptor afferent neurons release glutamate as their primary neurotransmitter to activate non-*N*-methyl-D-aspartate (NMDA) receptors on second-order NTS neurons. As the first site of information processing for cardiorespiratory reflexes, it is not unexpected that the NTS is also the first site where such processing is modulated by chronic intermittent hypoxia [39]. Following 10 days of chronic intermittent hypoxia (repetitive series of alterations from 21% O_2 for 5 min to 6% O_2 for 45 s; 8 h/day), more NTS neurons exhibit spontaneous discharge compared to normoxic control NTS neurons. In spontaneously active cells exposed to chronic intermittent hypoxia, the number of action potentials observed is also elevated. Stimulation of the solitary tract, which contains the main sensory fibers to these neurons, evoked discharge in both chronic intermittent hypoxia and normoxia-exposed NTS cells. However, in cells exposed to chronic intermittent hypoxia, following the synchronous burst of activity that coincides with afferent stimulation, discharge activity remained elevated whereas activity in normoxic cells rapidly returned to baseline. Taken together, these results indicate that chronic intermittent hypoxia increases and exaggerates overall activity in NTS cells as well as their response to afferent input.

Surprisingly, however, the increased activity of NTS neurons is not due to enhanced neurotransmitter release from sensory neurons during an action potential. In horizontal slices from normoxic and chronic intermittent hypoxia-conditioned rats, solitary tract stimulation elicited glutamatergic excitatory postsynaptic currents (EPSCs) which were blunted after 10 and 30 days of intermittent hypoxia. This diminished transmission from sensory afferents to NTS neurons likely results from a decrease in transmitter release at this first synapse of the baroreceptor reflex pathway. The diminished neurotransmission to NTS neurons that occurred with chronic intermittent hypoxia reversed when chronic intermittent hypoxia terminated and the normal respiratory conditions were restored.

The question then remains, if sensory information is not enhanced, but is rather inhibited, what is responsible for the increases activity of NTS neurons following chronic intermittent hypoxia? Data suggests chronic intermittent hypoxia increases spontaneous excitatory neurotransmission to NTS neurons under baseline conditions and following an evoked event and that this spontaneous release of neurotransmitters onto NTS neurons overcompensates for diminished evoked sensory neurotransmission. The asynchronous activity after chronic intermittent hypoxia in NTS neurons is indicative of exaggerated neurotransmitter release from the afferent synaptic terminal. Interestingly, asynchronous EPSC activity is sufficient to significantly increase action potential discharge in neurons both from normoxic and animals exposed to chronic intermittent hypoxia. Two likely mechanisms responsible for the decreased evoked EPSC and increased asynchronous EPSC activity in NTS neurons following chronic intermittent hypoxia are alterations in the calcium homeostasis and protein kinases that mediate release of neurotransmitters from the presynaptic terminal. The increase in asynchronous release from the solitary tract might also be caused by chronic intermittent hypoxia-induced preferential activation of unmyelinated C fiber discharge, rather than changes in myelinated A fiber baroreceptor activity [40].

Other studies in primary dissociated NTS cells suggest chronic intermittent hypoxia may also induce postsynaptic changes in glutamatergic receptor function. Following 7 days of chronic intermittent hypoxia (alternating cycles of 3 min at 10% O_2 followed by 3 min at 21% O_2, for 8 h/day), NTS neurons exhibited enhanced postsynaptic non-NMDA yet decreased NMDA receptor currents when exposed to brief agonist application [41]. Ion channels, such as potassium channels which exert strong control over membrane excitability, may also be altered by chronic intermittent hypoxia. One channel recently shown to be reduced by chronic intermittent hypoxia is the ATP-sensitive potassium channel [42]. A reduction in the function of this channel will increase neuronal discharge. Whether other channels or receptors are altered by chronic intermittent hypoxia in NTS neurons are still unknown.

In addition to the role of ATP-gated potassium channel function and glutamatergic neurotransmission at the first synapse of the baroreflex in the NTS, several additional neurotransmitters and modulators may be involved. Chronic intermittent hypoxia alters tyrosine hydroxylase (TH) expression and/or function in the carotid body, brainstem, and forebrain [43, 44]. Dopamine is also released from afferent fibers upon activation of the chemoreflex [45], and its receptors have also been localized in the brainstem, including the NTS, where they are upregulated by chronic hypoxia [46]. Dopamine is also elevated following chronic intermittent hypoxia in the carotid body [44], brainstem [43], and hypothalamus [47]. Dopamine is tonically released from chemoreceptor and vagal afferents and attenuates neurotransmission from sensory fibers to neurons in the NTS [48]. However, the increased release of dopamine or activation of its receptor following chronic intermittent hypoxia does not appear to be responsible for the attenuated sensory neurotransmission to NTS neurons and is unlikely to mediate the increased spontaneous excitatory synaptic input to NTS neurons that occurs with chronic intermittent hypoxia [49].

Additional neuromodulators may play a role in chronic intermittent hypoxia adaptations in the NTS. The role for nitric oxide (NO) has recently been explored based on its known involvement in autonomic control and NTS neuronal and synaptic activity. However, following chronic intermittent hypoxia (cycles of 21% O_2 for 5 min, 6% O_2 for 40 s; 8 h/day) there is not an alteration in the neuronal isoform of nitric oxide synthase, which produces NO, or NO production when determined by fluorescence indicators [50]. Additional work is clearly needed to establish the mechanisms for increased activation of NTS neurons postchronic intermittent hypoxia, and likely candidates include a wide range of accessory transmitters including peptides such as ATP, substance P, and calcitonin gene-related peptide. Hypothesized changes that occur with chronic intermittent hypoxia to the first synapse of the baroreflex pathway in the NTS are illustrated in Fig. 6.1.

6.4 Hypoxia Alters Parasympathetic Cardiac Neuron Activity and Synaptic Inputs

Proceeding from the first synapse of the baroreflex, as discussed previously, projections from the NTS to other brainstem nuclei play an essential role in maintaining the balance of autonomic motor control, both sympathetic and parasympathetic activity. Stimulation of the NTS evokes a glutamatergic pathway that activates both NMDA and non-NMDA postsynaptic currents in cardiac vagal neurons [51, 52]. NTS neurons also project to the CVLM and RVLM, the

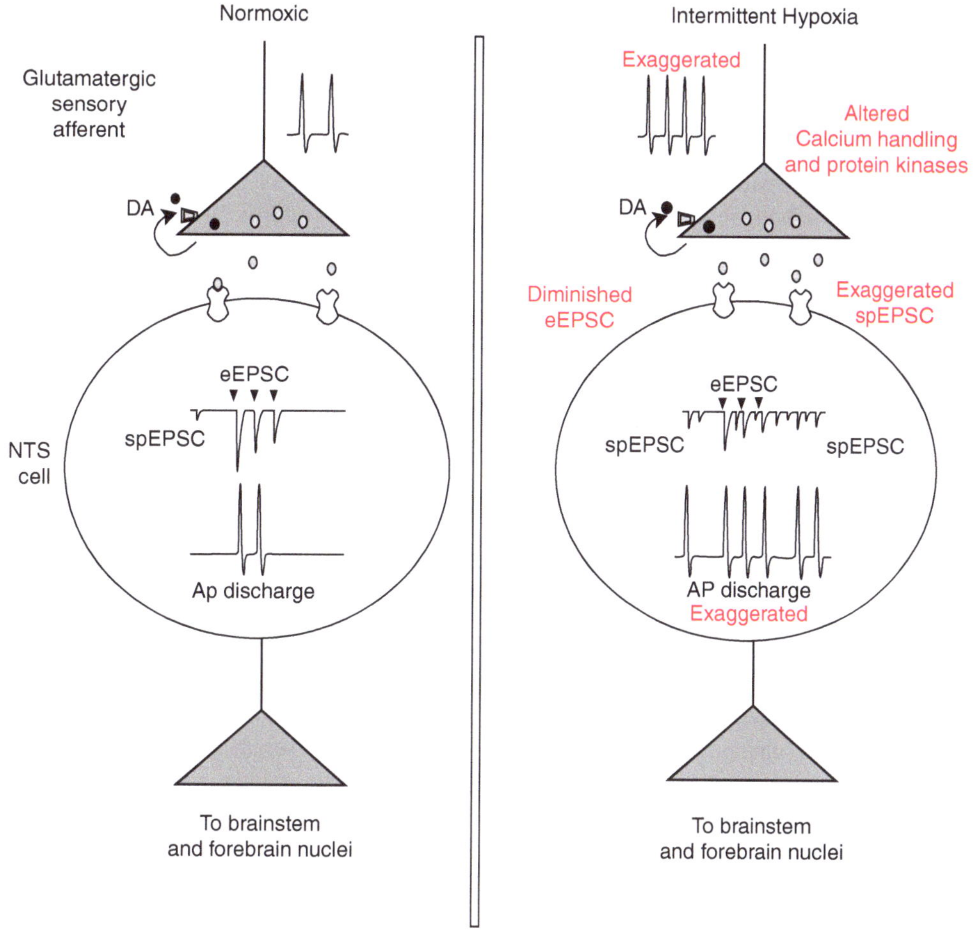

Fig. 6.1 Proposed model for synaptic signaling alterations in the NTS after CIH. Schematic representation of synaptic transmission in a normoxic (*left*) and CIH (*right*) NTS synapse. Under normoxia, sensory afferent action potential discharge increases presynaptic calcium in the synaptic terminal to release glutamate and produce evoked (*e*) EPSCs in the NTS cell. The *arrowhead* in the NTS cell represents afferent stimulation which produces EPSCs. Dopamine (*DA*) is also released from the sensory fiber and through its retrograde signaling onto D2 receptors, decreases glutamate release. This activity, in addition to spontaneous (*sp*) EPSCs, results in action potential (*AP*) discharge in the NTS cell. Following CIH (*right*), the exaggerated action potential discharge in the sensory afferent axon leads to an altered calcium handling and protein kinases to reduce evoked, synchronous transmitter release and augment spontaneous and asynchronous EPSCs from the synaptic terminal. The increase in spEPSCs and asynchronous activity, coupled with synchronous release (although reduced), results in exaggerated AP discharge in NTS cells. Dopamine release and activation of presynaptic D2 receptors continue to play a role following CIH. In normoxia and CIH conditions, the balance of inhibitory and excitatory neurotransmitter release, and ion channel properties, is responsible for postsynaptic activity which is subsequently sent to other cardiorespiratory nuclei in the forebrain and brainstem

sites for control and generation of sympathetic nerve activity [11, 53–55]. These pathways likely constitute the essential links between increases in blood pressure and afferent baroreceptor activity, which activates neurons in the NTS, and the reflex compensatory decrease in heart rate caused by increases in efferent parasympathetic cardioinhibitory cardiac vagal activity as well as inhibition of brainstem presympathetic activity.

GABAergic neurons that project to cardiac vagal neurons have recently been localized to populations within specific areas immediately medial and ventral to the NA and in close proximity to the NTS [56]. The GABAergic pathway from the NTS can be activated upon both electrical and photo-uncaging excitation of these neurons [56, 57]. Stimulation of afferents in the central end of a sectioned vagus nerve evokes both GABAergic and glutamatergic responses in cardiac vagal neurons [58]. Capsaicin, which inactivates C-fibers, increased the latency of the GABAergic response without changing the latency of the glutamatergic responses [58]. It is likely that this inhibitory GABAergic pathway evoked from vagal nerve or NTS stimulation is involved in patterning cardiac vagal activity which is bursting and synchronous with the cardiac cycle.

In addition to control from baroreceptors and NTS activity, cardiac vagal neurons are profoundly influenced by inputs from the respiratory system. There are two well-known physiological interactions between the respiratory system and cardiac vagal neuron activity. The respiratory system influences cardiovascular reflexes by modulating the baroreceptor and chemoreceptor input to cardiac vagal neurons. In both animals and humans, the baroreceptor and chemoreceptor reflexes are inhibited during inspiration and are facilitated during post-inspiration and expiration or during a maintained phase of post-inspiration and apnea [59–61]. This respiratory modulation of both reflexes persists after pulmonary denervation, and ventilatory paralysis, suggesting that this "gating" of the baroreceptor and chemoreceptor reflexes occurs within the brainstem [62, 63]. A number of studies indicate respiratory inputs do not alter baroreceptor and chemoreceptor synapses at their first synapse in the NTS [6, 7] suggesting that respiratory influences on baroreceptor and chemoreceptor reflexes occur beyond the NTS in these brainstem reflex pathways.

In addition to respiratory modulation of baro- and chemoreflexes, the most ubiquitous cardiorespiratory interaction is respiratory sinus arrhythmia. During each respiratory cycle, the heart slows during expiration and heart rate increases during inspiration. Respiratory sinus arrhythmia helps match pulmonary blood flow to lung inflation and maintain the appropriate diffusion gradient for oxygen in the lungs [64].

Many factors influence the changes in heart rate in response to respiration. These include sensory input related to lung inflation, changes in the activity of atrial stretch-sensitive receptors (due to variations in venous return produced by intrathoracic pressure changes), and activation of baroreceptors in the aortic arch and carotid sinus (also due to variations in venous return) [64–67]. While feedback from pulmonary stretch receptors, direct respiratory-related changes in venous return and cardiac stretch can evoke respiratory-related changes in heart rate, the dominant source of respiratory sinus arrhythmia originates from the brainstem [68]. Respiratory sinus arrhythmia persists when the lungs are stationary (caused by muscle paralysis or constant flow ventilation), and the respiratory modulation of heart rate remains synchronized with brainstem respiratory rhythms even if artificial ventilation of the lungs, and chemoreceptor activation, occurs at different intervals [7, 69–72]. In both animals and humans, respiratory sinus arrhythmia is mediated via cardiac vagal activity. Respiratory sinus arrhythmia persists in animals upon sectioning sympathetic pathways and in quadriplegic patients with spinal cord injury and sympathetic dysfunction [69–73]. Furthermore, respiratory sinus arrhythmia persists after blocking sympathetic activity to the heart by administration of the beta-adrenergic antagonist propanolol and after sectioning of sympathetic fibers [8, 71, 74]. Blocking parasympathetic activity with atropine, however, significantly reduces respiratory sinus arrhythmia, indicating that this cardiorespiratory interaction is predominantly mediated by the activity of cardiac vagal neurons [66, 71, 75].

To mediate respiratory sinus arrhythmia, cardiac vagal neurons fire most rapidly in post-inspiration and are often silent in inspiration [3, 6, 61]. Unfortunately, obtaining information concerning the transmitters and neurons responsible for this cardiorespiratory interaction in vivo is extremely difficult. The low probability of finding and recording from the sparse number of cardiac vagal neurons (~200/animal) and the difficulty of the necessary task of identifying these neurons by antidromic stimulation of the cardiac branch of the vagus nerve make in vivo recordings particularly challenging. More recent in vitro work has characterized the respiratory inputs to cardiac vagal neurons that mediate respiratory sinus arrhythmia. In brain slices that generate rhythmic, inspiratory phase motor discharge, the frequency of both spontaneous GABAergic and glycinergic synaptic events in cardiac vagal neurons significantly increases with each inspiratory burst [76]. The GABA -mediated inhibition of cardiac vagal neurons during inspiration is inhibited by curare, indicating that the increase in GABAergic frequency is mediated by the activation of nicotinic receptors [76]. This increase in GABAergic frequency is unaffected by α-bungarotoxin, demonstrating that it is not mediated by the activation of α7 nicotinic receptors [76]. A β2-selective concentration of dihydro-beta-erythroidine, however, abolishes the GABAergic inhibition of cardiac vagal neurons during inspiration, indicating that activation of β2 containing nicotinic receptors by endogenous acetylcholine drives the GABAergic inhibition in this cardiorespiratory interaction [76]. The facilitation of GABAergic inhibition of cardiac vagal neurons by activation of nicotinic receptors is consistent with previous work which has shown that spontaneous GABAergic inhibition of cardiac vagal neurons is enhanced by the activation of β2 receptors presumably located in the presynaptic terminals of GABAergic neurons [57, 77]. This study also indicates that the nicotinic receptors responsible for the increased GABAergic activity during inspiration are in close proximity to the cardiac vagal neurons since focal application of the nicotinic antagonist DHβE abolished this increase. In contrast, greater concentrations of DHβE did not significantly alter the respiratory-related increase in glycinergic synaptic frequency in cardiac vagal neurons [76]. Interestingly, previous studies have shown that spontaneous glycinergic inputs to cardiac vagal neurons are also enhanced by activation of β2 nicotinic receptors in glycinergic presynaptic terminals [77]. This suggests that although glycinergic inputs to cardiac vagal neurons likely possess presynaptic nicotinic receptors, these receptors are apparently not involved with the inspiratory-evoked increase in glycinergic synaptic input to cardiac vagal neurons.

Challenges such as hypoxia evoke strong coordinated responses from the cardiovascular and respiratory systems. Hypoxia initially elicits a transient increase, followed by a sustained decrease in respiratory frequency, and eventually cessation of breathing [78]. In addition, respiration changes from the normal pattern of eupneic breathing to gasping in response to hypoxia, which increases the chance of autoresuscitation [78].

Heart rate also exhibits a biphasic response to hypoxia. Hypoxia evokes a transient tachycardia, followed by a parasympathetically mediated bradycardia, and ultimately, cessation of cardiac contractions [79–81]. Studies in humans have shown that hypoxia-induced bradycardia can be blocked by atropine and is absent in heart transplant recipients [82–86] and in animals, application of atropine to block parasympathetic outflow prevents bradycardia during hypoxia [87–95]. Further, vagotomy prevents bradycardia during hypoxia [92, 96]. Bradycardia during hypoxia increases animal survival, as atropine sharply decreases survival under hypoxia [97]. The changes in parasympathetic cardiac activity in response to hypoxia are due to changes in medullary activity since the discharge of cardiac efferent fibers in the central end of the transected vagus nerve is increased during hypoxia [98]. Although peripheral chemoreceptors may also be involved, the hypoxia-induced bradycardia persists after section of both the carotid sinus and aortic nerves indicating chemoreceptors within the central nervous system can activate pathways that increase the activity of cardiac vagal neurons [99].

Recent work has delineated the changes in synaptic neurotransmission to cardiac vagal neurons evoked during hypoxia (15–20 min of acute hypoxia). Hypoxia evokes a biphasic change in inhibitory neurotransmission to cardiac vagal neurons [100]. In response to hypoxia, GABAergic inhibition of cardiac vagal neurons changes in a biphasic fashion, initially increasing and then significantly decreasing during hypoxia [100]. Similarly, in response to hypoxia, there is a biphasic change in glycinergic inhibition comprised initially of an increase followed by a depression of spontaneous and inspiratory-evoked glycinergic activity [100].

In addition to changes in GABA neurotransmission, serotonin (5-hydroxytryptamine, 5-HT) receptors and signaling in the brainstem play an important role in central cardiorespiratory responses to hypoxia. Hypoxia induces Fos-like immunoreactivity in 5-HT neurons in the nucleus raphe pallidus, the nucleus raphe magnus, and along the ventral medullary surface [101, 102]. Within the ventral respiratory, group 5-HT levels significantly increase and reach a maximum after 9 min of hypoxia and then gradually decline posthypoxia [103]. 5-HT acting on 5-HT1A receptors in the nucleus raphe magnus plays no role under normal conditions but modulates breathing during hypoxia [104]. In the anteroventral preoptic region, both 5-HT1A and 5-HT7 receptors are involved in the inhibitory modulation of the hypoxic ventilatory response [105]. Activation of central 5-HT2A receptors is required to sustain hypoxic gasping and to restore respiratory activity during posthypoxia [106, 107]. Central 5-HT2A receptors are also critical for long-term facilitation in respiratory activity followed by intermittent hypoxia [106, 108, 109].

5-HT receptors and pathways are recruited in the response of cardiac vagal neurons to hypoxia. Within the NA, premotor neurons receive a large number of axosomatic 5-HT contacts, and the 5-HT synaptic density on neurons in the NA is among the highest in the brainstem [110]. 5-HT fibers also specifically surround cardiac vagal neurons, which have been described as "ensheathed in 5-HT immunoreactive axonal boutons" [111]. Under normoxic conditions, excitatory synaptic inputs to cardiac vagal neurons are nearly completely blocked by application of NMDA and AMPA/kainate glutamatergic receptor antagonists, while blocking 5-HT3 and purinergic receptors has no effect [112]. However, hypoxia recruits an additional 5-HT-mediated excitation of cardiac vagal neurons which can be blocked with the 5-HT3 receptor antagonist, ondansetron. This serotonergic pathway is spontaneously active and is not inspiratory-related. This direct activation of 5-HT3 receptors on cardiac vagal neurons, in combination with glutamatergic receptor activation, provides excitatory input and helps maintains parasympathetic cardiac activity during hypoxia [112]. In addition, during hypoxia, 5-HT2 receptors on cardiac vagal neurons are also recruited and act to sustain excitation of cardiac vagal neuron activity during hypoxia via facilitation of 5-HT3 receptor activation [113]. 5-HT receptors may also be responsible for the withdrawal of GABAergic and glycinergic neurotransmission to cardiac vagal neurons during hypoxia. Although this has not yet been tested, previous work has demonstrated that activation of 5-HT1A/7 receptors, as well as repetitive activation of 5-HT2B receptors exerts an inhibitory action on both spontaneous and inspiratory-related GABAergic inputs to cardiac vagal neurons [114, 115]. Therefore, a combination of two mechanisms, disinhibition of cardiac vagal neurons via withdrawal of GABAergic and glycinergic neurotransmission and excitation of cardiac vagal neurons via activation of postsynaptic glutamatergic and 5-HT3 receptors, is likely important in the increase in cardiac vagal neuron activity and the resultant bradycardia during hypoxia.

Hypoxia not only evokes a biphasic tachycardia followed by a bradycardia, but in the recovery following hypoxia, a strong bradycardia persists during the recovery period [116, 117]. Pronounced excitatory inspiratory-related synaptic pathways are recruited to excite cardiac vagal neurons posthypoxia [118]. During recovery from hypoxia, spontaneous and respiratory-related excitatory events are generated mainly by the recruitment of glutamatergic and purinergic pathways [112, 119]. 5-HT2 receptors not only play a role by maintaining excitatory neurotransmission to cardiac vagal neurons during hypoxia, as previously discussed, but activation of 5-HT2 receptors diminishes the subsequent inspiratory-related excitatory neurotransmission to cardiac vagal neurons that is recruited during the recovery from hypoxia likely by exerting an inhibitory action on inspiratory-related purinergic signaling [113].

Brief (5 min) and intermittent hypoxic episodes (3 bouts of 3 min of hypoxia over 15 min) incrementally recruit a respiratory-related glutamatergic neurotransmission that occurs during respiratory bursts and becomes increasingly robust in successive hypoxic episodes [120]. Likely, as a result of the successive recovery periods that occur with repeated periods of hypoxia, reactive oxygen species are produced [120]. Inspiratory-synchronous glutamatergic inputs to cardiac vagal neurons during repeated bouts of hypoxia are blocked by application of reactive oxygen species scavengers, and visualization of reactive oxygen species generation indicates they are incrementally produced in the ventrolateral medulla during each hypoxic period [120].

The reactive oxygen species-dependent cardiorespiratory plasticity induced by intermittent hypoxia likely involves serotonergic synaptic mechanisms. Central respiratory responses to repeated hypoxia are serotonin dependent, and the respiratory plasticity evoked by intermittent hypoxia can be mimicked with intermittent application of serotonin 5-HT_{2A} agonists [121, 122]. Taken together with the serotonin-dependent increases in glutamatergic neurotransmission to cardiac vagal neurons elicited during single hypoxic insults, this suggests that reactive oxygen species may enhance serotonergic pathways to induce inspiratory-related excitatory inputs during repeated hypoxias.

As noted previously, chronic intermittent hypoxia, in both animal models and humans, decreases baroreflex sensitivity, elevates blood pressure and sympathetic activity, and diminishes parasympathetic activity to the heart [12–16]. While chronic intermittent hypoxia decreases the baroreflex control of heart rate and diminishes parasympathetic activity to the heart, these changes are not due to changes in parasympathetic innervation of the sinoatrial node or function within the cardiac ganglia but are rather most likely due to changes in the activity of premotor parasympathetic cardiac vagal neurons in the brainstem. Although anatomical work has shown a decrease in efferent cardiac vagal innervation, ganglia size, and density of axonal terminals within the cardiac ganglia after chronic intermittent hypoxia [123, 124], heart rate responses to vagal efferent stimulation are not diminished, but rather enhanced [125–127]. These results indicate a central dysregulation of premotor cardiac vagal neuronal activity, but not cardiac ganglia function, is responsible for the impaired parasympathetic control of heart rate that occurs with chronic intermittent hypoxia. The bradycardia evoked upon microinjection of glutamate [127] as well as NMDA and AMPA [128] into the NA is diminished by chronic intermittent hypoxia. However, beyond alterations in glutamate receptor density, little is known how chronic intermittent hypoxia impairs cardiac vagal neuron function and whether these changes include alterations in GABA, glycine, glutamate, 5-HT and purinergic pathways and receptors known to be essential in the responses of cardiac vagal neurons to acute hypoxic challenges.

Given the synaptic pathways and brainstem neurotransmission activated in response to acute hypoxia, one hypothesis is that chronic intermittent hypoxia exaggerates the GABAergic and/or glycinergic neurotransmission to cardiac vagal neurons, particularly in response to additional exposures of hypoxia. Another worthwhile hypothesis, yet to be tested, is that excitatory hypoxia-evoked input to cardiac vagal neurons is blunted after chronic intermittent hypoxia and that this dysfunction may involve the normally recruited excitatory purinergic, serotonin, and glutamatergic neurotransmission to parasympathetic cardiac vagal neurons. A third, and not mutually exclusive, hypothesis is that chronic intermittent hypoxia impairs the synaptic neurotransmission from the NTS to brainstem parasympathetic cardiac neurons, and these changes would be responsible for diminished baroreceptor reflex activation of premotor cardiac vagal neurons. Hypothesized changes that occur with chronic intermittent hypoxia to the neurotransmission that controls the activity of parasympathetic cardiac vagal neurons in the nucleus ambiguus are illustrated in Fig. 6.2. The chronic intermittent hypoxia-induced alterations of the synaptic pathways from the NTS and changes in the function of CVLM and RVLM neurons that mediate brainstem presympathetic activity remain unknown.

6.5 OSA, Central Nervous System Mechanisms, and Potential Therapeutic Targets

As discussed above, CPAP is poorly tolerated. Given the important role of neurochemicals and receptors in brainstem cardiorespiratory function, several pharmacological approaches have been recently assessed to alleviate OSA. Therapeutic targets have been proposed or tested to either alter ventilatory drive, sleep state, or the number of apneas during sleep. A number of agents have been studied, including utilizing sex hormones, acetazolamide, opioid antagonists, nicotine, antihypertensive drugs (β-blockers and ACE inhibitors), glutamate antagonists, serotonergic agents, or serotonin-specific reuptake inhibitors (SSRIs). However, these studies have had varying success in reducing the frequency of apneic episodes, stabilizing the upper airway, or patient tolerance [129–132]. The inconsistent outcome of pharmacotherapies on OSA is likely due to a lack of specificity of the drug's site of action and understanding the mechanisms of OSA-induced complications. Clearly, additional studies are required to identify the mechanisms and cellular targets for pharmacotherapeutic strategies in OSA and the central mechanisms altered by chronic intermittent hypoxia.

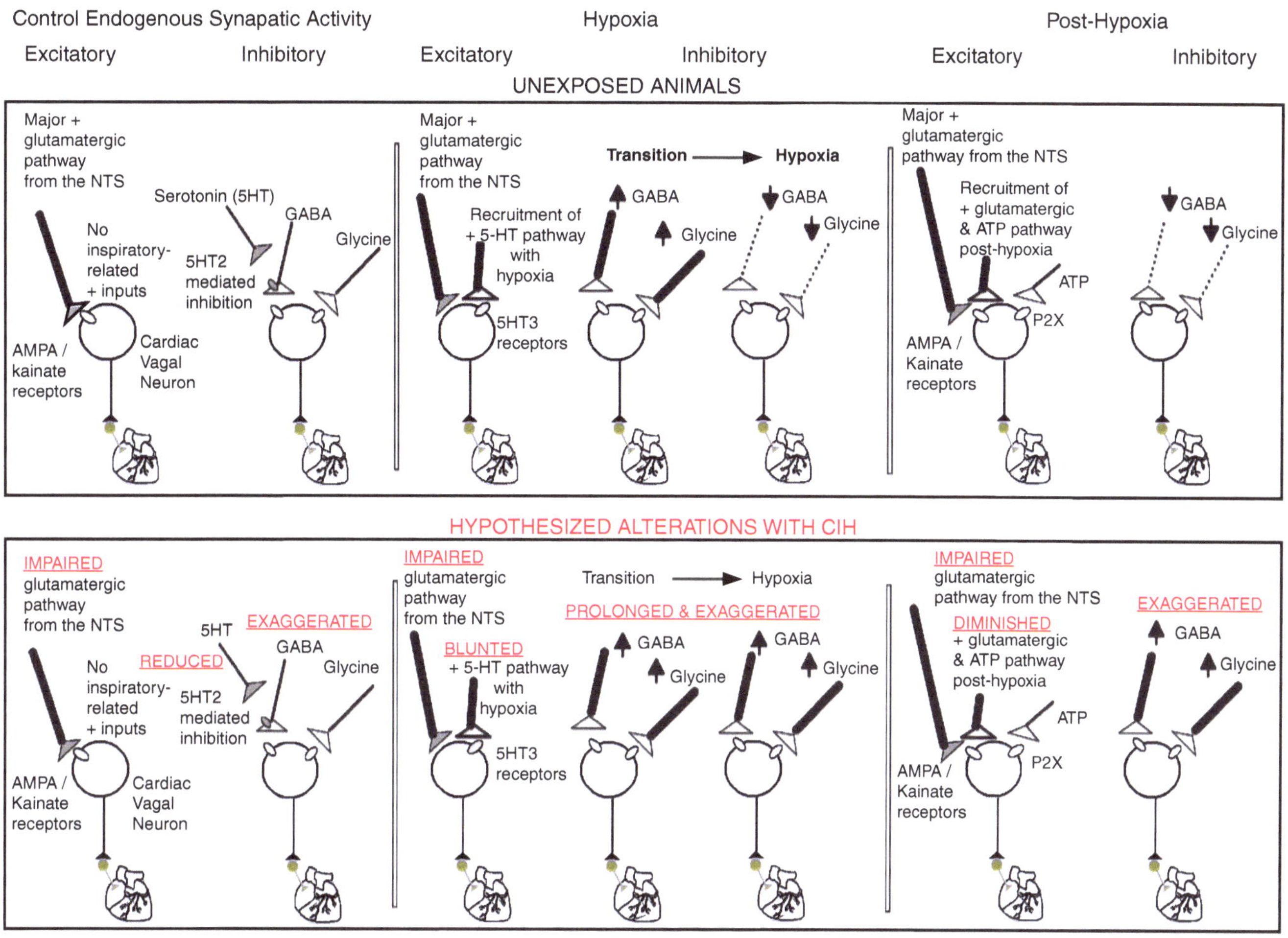

Fig. 6.2 Major pathways to CVNs include an excitatory glutamatergic pathway from the NTS that likely mediates the baroreflex and inspiratory-related increases in inhibitory GABAergic and glycinergic pathways that are likely responsible for respiratory sinus arrhythmia. Hypoxia evokes a biphasic change in inhibitory GABAergic and glycinergic neurotransmission to cardiac vagal neurons. In response to hypoxia, GABAergic and glycinergic inhibition of CVNs initially increase and then significantly decrease during hypoxia. 5-HT receptors and pathways are recruited and play an important role in the responses of cardiac vagal neurons to hypoxia. Under normoxic conditions, excitatory synaptic inputs to cardiac vagal neurons are nearly completely blocked by application of NMDA and AMPA/kainate glutamatergic receptor antagonists, while blocking 5-HT3 and purinergic receptors has no effect. However, hypoxia recruits an additional 5-HT-mediated excitation of cardiac vagal neurons which can be blocked with the 5-HT3 receptor antagonist, ondansetron. The recruited 5-HT pathway and activation of 5-HT3 receptors on cardiac vagal neurons provides excitatory input and increases parasympathetic cardiac activity during hypoxia. In addition, during hypoxia, 5-HT2 receptors are also involved and act to sustain excitation of cardiac vagal neuron activity during hypoxia via facilitation of 5-HT3 receptor activation. Pronounced excitatory synaptic pathways are recruited to excite cardiac vagal neurons posthypoxia. During recovery from hypoxia, spontaneous and respiratory-related excitatory events are generated mainly by the recruitment of glutamatergic and purinergic pathways activating postsynaptic AMPA/kainate and P2X receptors, respectively. It is proposed that chronic intermittent hypoxia alters the endogenous and spontaneously active pathways and neurobiological responses in cardiac vagal neurons that occur in response to acute hypoxia challenges and furthermore impairs essential reflex activation and excitation of premotor cardiac vagal neurons originating from the NTS. More specifically, chronic intermittent hypoxia may impair the excitatory pathway from the NTS that mediates the baroreflex, exaggerate the GABAergic inhibition of cardiac vagal neurons that occurs with hypoxia, blunt the recruited serotonergic pathway during hypoxia, and impair excitatory glutamatergic and purinergic neurotransmission to cardiac vagal neurons posthypoxia

6.6 Summary

Over the past 10 years, there have been many significant advances in our understanding of the neural control of heart rate and blood pressure. Recent work indicates obstructive sleep apnea and chronic intermittent hypoxia increase the spontaneous activation of NTS neurons and blunt the activity of parasympathetic cardiac vagal neurons in the NA. Likely, mechanisms for these alterations include altered calcium homeostasis and increased spontaneous release of neurotransmitters in the NTS and blunted excitatory and enhanced inhibitory neurotransmission to parasympathetic cardiac neurons, including the pathways from the NTS. Further work is necessary to determine, at the cellular level, alterations in receptor function and synaptic transmission that occur in chronic cardiorespiratory diseases such as OSA. Identification of these changes will provide a clear understanding of brainstem cardiovascular dysfunction as well as provide future targets for restoring autonomic balance and increasing survival in these cardiorespiratory diseases.

Acknowledgments Supported by NIH grants HL49965, HL59895, and HL72006 to D.M. and HL085108 to DDK.

References

1. Pickering TG, Gribbin B, Petersen ES, et al. Effects of autonomic blockade on the baroreflex in man at rest and during exercise. Circ Res. 1972;30:177–85.
2. Scher AM, Young AC. Reflex control of heart rate in the unanesthetized dog. Am J Physiol. 1970;218:780–9.
3. Kunze DL. Reflex discharge patterns of cardiac vagal efferent fibres. J Physiol. 1972;222:1–15.
4. Coleman TG. Arterial baroreflex control of heart rate in the conscious rat. Am J Physiol. 1980;238:H515–20.
5. Stornetta RL, Guyenet PG, McCarty RC. Autonomic nervous system control of heart rate during baroreceptor activation in conscious and anesthetized rats. J Auton Nerv Syst. 1987;20:121–7.
6. Spyer KM. Neural organisation and control of the baroreceptor reflex. Rev Physiol Biochem Pharmacol. 1981;88:24–124.
7. Spyer KM, Gilbey MP. Cardiorespiratory interactions in heart-rate control. Ann N Y Acad Sci. 1988;533:350–7.
8. Levy MN, Zieske H. Autonomic control of cardiac pacemaker activity and atrioventricular transmission. J Appl Physiol. 1969;27:465–70.
9. Guyenet PG. The sympathetic control of blood pressure. Nat Rev Neurosci. 2006;7:335–46.
10. Andresen MC, Kunze DL. Nucleus tractus solitarius – gateway to neural circulatory control. Annu Rev Physiol. 1994;56:93–116.
11. Schreihofer AM, Guyenet PG. The baroreflex and beyond: control of sympathetic vasomotor tone by GABAergic neurons in the ventrolateral medulla. Clin Exp Pharmacol Physiol. 2002;29:514–21.
12. Carlson JT, Hedner JA, Sellgren J, Elam M, Wallin BG. Depressed baroreflex sensitivity in patients with obstructive sleep apnea. Am J Respir Crit Care Med. 1996;154:1490–6.
13. Bonsignore MR, Parati G, Insalaco G, et al. Baroreflex control of heart rate during sleep in severe obstructive sleep apnoea: effects of acute CPAP. Eur Respir J. 2006;27:128–35.
14. Bonsignore MR, Parati G, Insalaco G, et al. Continuous positive airway pressure treatment improves baroreflex control of heart rate during sleep in severe obstructive sleep apnea syndrome. Am J Respir Crit Care Med. 2002;166:279–86.
15. Lai CJ, Yang CC, Hsu YY, et al. Enhanced sympathetic outflow and decreased baroreflex sensitivity are associated with intermittent hypoxia-induced systemic hypertension in conscious rats. J Appl Physiol. 2006;100:1974–82.
16. Narkiewicz K, Somers VK. Sympathetic nerve activity in obstructive sleep apnoea. Acta Physiol Scand. 2003;177:385–90.
17. Hull Jr SS, Vanoli E, Adamson PB, et al. Do increases in markers of vagal activity imply protection from sudden death? The case of scopolamine. Circulation. 1995;91:2516–9.
18. Ferguson DW, Berg WJ, Sanders JS. Clinical and hemodynamic correlates of sympathetic nerve activity in normal humans and patients with heart failure: evidence from direct microneurographic recordings. J Am Coll Cardiol. 1990;16:1125–34.
19. Nishime EO, Cole CR, Blackstone EH, et al. Heart rate recovery and treadmill exercise score as predictors of mortality in patients referred for exercise ECG. JAMA. 2000;284:1392–8.
20. Routledge HC, Chowdhary S, Townend JN. Heart rate variability – a therapeutic target? J Clin Pharm Ther. 2002;27:85–92.
21. Eckberg DL, Drabinsky M, Braunwald E. Defective cardiac parasympathetic control in patients with heart disease. N Engl J Med. 1971;285:877–83.
22. La Rovere MT, Specchia G, Mortara A, et al. Baroreflex sensitivity, clinical correlates, and cardiovascular mortality among patients with a first myocardial infarction. A prospective study. Circulation. 1988;78:816–24.
23. Vanoli E, De Ferrari GM, Stramba-Badiale M, et al. Vagal stimulation and prevention of sudden death in conscious dogs with a healed myocardial infarction. Circ Res. 1991;68:1471–81.
24. Esler M. The sympathetic system and hypertension. Am J Hypertens. 2000;13:99S–105.
25. Straznicky NE, Eikelis N, Lambert EA, et al. Mediators of sympathetic activation in metabolic syndrome obesity. Curr Hypertens Rep. 2008;10:440–7.
26. Bazzano LA, Khan Z, Reynolds K, et al. Effect of nocturnal nasal continuous positive airway pressure on blood pressure in obstructive sleep apnea. Hypertension. 2007;50:417–23.
27. Punjabi NM. The epidemiology of adult obstructive sleep apnea. Proc Am Thorac Soc. 2008;5:136–43.
28. Marin JM, Carrizo SJ, Vicente E, et al. Long-term cardiovascular outcomes in men with obstructive sleep apnoea-hypopnoea with or without treatment with continuous positive airway pressure: an observational study. Lancet. 2005;365:1046–53.
29. Bradley TD, Floras JS. Obstructive sleep apnoea and its cardiovascular consequences. Lancet. 2009;373:82–93.
30. Kato M, Adachi T, Koshino Y, et al. Obstructive sleep apnea and cardiovascular disease. Circ J. 2009;73:1363–70.
31. Narkiewicz K, van de Borne PJ, Montano N, et al. Contribution of tonic chemoreflex activation to sympathetic activity and blood pressure in patients with obstructive sleep apnea. Circulation. 1998;97:943–5.
32. Narkiewicz K, van de Borne PJ, Pesek CA, et al. Selective potentiation of peripheral chemoreflex sensitivity in obstructive sleep apnea. Circulation. 1999;99:1183–9.
33. Spicuzza L, Bernardi L, Balsamo R, et al. Effect of treatment with nasal continuous positive airway pressure on ventilatory response to hypoxia and hypercapnia in patients with sleep apnea syndrome. Chest. 2006;130:774–9.
34. Tafil-Klawe M, Thiele AE, Raschke F, et al. Peripheral chemoreceptor reflex in obstructive sleep apnea patients; a relationship between ventilatory response to hypoxia and nocturnal bradycardia during apnea events. Pneumologie. 1991;45 Suppl 1:309–11.
35. Somers VK, Abboud FM. Chemoreflexes – responses, interactions and implications for sleep apnea. Sleep. 1993;16:S30–3.
36. Narkiewicz K, Kato M, Phillips BG, et al. Nocturnal continuous positive airway pressure decreases daytime sympathetic traffic in obstructive sleep apnea. Circulation. 1999;100:2332–5.
37. Doherty LS, Kiely JL, Swan V, et al. Long-term effects of nasal continuous positive airway pressure therapy on cardiovascular outcomes in sleep apnea syndrome. Chest. 2005;127:2076–84.
38. Parati G, Lombardi C, Narkiewicz K. Sleep apnea: epidemiology, pathophysiology, and relation to cardiovascular risk. Am J Physiol Regul Integr Comp Physiol. 2007;293:R1671–83.
39. Kline DD, Ramirez-Navarro A, Kunze DL. Adaptive depression in synaptic transmission in the nucleus of the solitary tract after in vivo chronic intermittent hypoxia: evidence for homeostatic plasticity. J Neurosci. 2007;27:4663–73.

40. Peters JH, McDougall SJ, Fawley JA, et al. Primary afferent activation of thermosensitive TRPV1 triggers asynchronous glutamate release at central neurons. Neuron. 2010;65:657–69.
41. de Paula PM, Tolstykh G, Mifflin S. Chronic intermittent hypoxia alters NMDA and AMPA-evoked currents in NTS neurons receiving carotid body chemoreceptor inputs. Am J Physiol Regul Integr Comp Physiol. 2007;292:R2259–65.
42. Zhang W, Carreno FR, Cunningham JT, et al. Chronic sustained and intermittent hypoxia reduce function of ATP-sensitive potassium channels in nucleus of the solitary tract. Am J Physiol Regul Integr Comp Physiol. 2008;295:R1555–62.
43. Raghuraman G, Rai V, Peng YJ, et al. Pattern-specific sustained activation of tyrosine hydroxylase by intermittent hypoxia: role of reactive oxygen species-dependent downregulation of protein phosphatase 2A and upregulation of protein kinases. Antioxid Redox Signal. 2009;11:1777–89.
44. Hui AS, Striet JB, Gudelsky G, et al. Regulation of catecholamines by sustained and intermittent hypoxia in neuroendocrine cells and sympathetic neurons. Hypertension. 2003;42:1130–6.
45. Goiny M, Lagercrantz H, Srinivasan M, et al. Hypoxia-mediated in vivo release of dopamine in nucleus tractus solitarii of rabbits. J Appl Physiol. 1991;70:2395–400.
46. Huey KA, Powell FL. Time-dependent changes in dopamine D_2-receptor mRNA in the arterial chemoreflex pathway with chronic hypoxia. Brain Res Mol Brain Res. 2000;75:264–70.
47. Li R, Bao G, el-Mallakh RS, et al. Effects of chronic episodic hypoxia on monoamine metabolism and motor activity. Physiol Behav. 1996;60:1071–6.
48. Kline DD, Takacs KN, Ficker E, et al. Dopamine modulates synaptic transmission in the nucleus of the solitary tract. J Neurophysiol. 2002;88:2736–44.
49. Kline DD, Hendricks G, Hermann G, et al. Dopamine inhibits N-type channels in visceral afferents to reduce synaptic transmitter release under normoxic and chronic intermittent hypoxic conditions. J Neurophysiol. 2009;101:2270–8.
50. Pajolla GP, Accorsi-Mendonca D, Lunardi CN, et al. Immunoreactivity for neuronal NOS and fluorescent indication of NO formation in the NTS of juvenile rats submitted to chronic intermittent hypoxia. Auton Neurosci. 2009;148:55–62.
51. Mendelowitz D. Advances in parasympathetic control of heart rate and cardiac function. News Physiol Sci. 1999;14:155–61.
52. Neff RA, Mihalevich M, Mendelowitz D. Stimulation of NTS activates NMDA and non-NMDA receptors in rat cardiac vagal neurons in the nucleus ambiguus. Brain Res. 1998;792:277–82.
53. Koshiya N, Guyenet PG. NTS neurons with carotid chemoreceptor inputs arborize in the rostral ventrolateral medulla. Am J Physiol. 1996;270:R1273–8.
54. Accorsi-Mendonca D, Bonagamba LG, Leao RM, et al. Are L-glutamate and ATP cotransmitters of the peripheral chemoreflex in the rat nucleus tractus solitarius? Exp Physiol. 2009;94:38–45.
55. Kline DD, King TL, Austgen JR, et al. Sensory afferent and hypoxia-mediated activation of nucleus tractus solitarius neurons that project to the rostral ventrolateral medulla. Neuroscience. 2010;167:510–27.
56. Frank JG, Jameson HS, Gorini C, et al. Mapping and identification of GABAergic neurons in transgenic mice projecting to cardiac vagal neurons in the nucleus ambiguus using photo-uncaging. J Neurophysiol. 2009;101:1755–60.
57. Wang J, Irnaten M, Mendelowitz D. Characteristics of spontaneous and evoked GABAergic synaptic currents in cardiac vagal neurons in rats. Brain Res. 2001;889:78–83.
58. Evans C, Baxi S, Neff RA, et al. Synaptic activation of cardiac vagal neurons by capsaicin sensitive and insensitive sensory neurons. Brain Res. 2003;979:210–5.
59. Davidson NS, Goldner S, McCloskey DI. Respiratory modulation of barareceptor and chemoreceptor reflexes affecting heart rate and cardiac vagal efferent nerve activity. J Physiol. 1976;259:523–30.
60. Eckberg DL, Orshan CR. Respiratory and baroreceptor reflex interactions in man. J Clin Invest. 1977;59:780–5.
61. McAllen RM, Spyer KM. The baroreceptor input to cardiac vagal motoneurones. J Physiol. 1978;282:365–74.
62. Eckberg DL. The human respiratory gate. J Physiol. 2003;548:339–52.
63. Loewy AD, Spyer KM. Central regulation of autonomic functions. New York: Oxford University Press; 1990.
64. Anrep G, Pascual F, Rossler R. Respiratory variations of the heart rate II – the central mechanism of the respiratory sinus arrythmia and the inter-relations between the central and the reflex mechanisms. Proc R Soc. 1936;119:218–32.
65. Richter DW, Spyer KM. Cardiorespiratory control. In: Spyer KM, editor. Central regulation of autonomic function. New York: Oxford University Press; 1990. p. 189–207.
66. Berne RM, Levy MN. Cardiovascular physiology. 7th ed. St. Louis: Mosby; 1997.
67. Anrep G, Pascual F, Rossler R. Respiratory variations of the heart rate I – the reflex mechanism of the respiratory sinus arrhythmia. Proc R Soc. 1936;119:191–217.
68. Anrep GVPW, Rossler R. Respiratory variations of the heart rate II – the central mechanism of the respiratory arrhythmia and the inter-relationships between the central and reflex mechanisms. Proc R Soc. 1935;119:218–31.
69. Daly MD. Some reflex cardioinhibitory responses in the cat and their modulation by central inspiratory neuronal activity. J Physiol. 1991;439:559–77.
70. Elghozi JL, Laude D, Girard A. Effects of respiration on blood pressure and heart rate variability in humans. Clin Exp Pharmacol Physiol. 1991;18:735–42.
71. Hrushesky WJ. Quantitative respiratory sinus arrhythmia analysis. A simple noninvasive, reimbursable measure of cardiac wellness and dysfunction. Ann N Y Acad Sci. 1991;618:67–101.
72. Shykoff BE, Naqvi SS, Menon AS, et al. Respiratory sinus arrhythmia in dogs. Effects of phasic afferents and chemostimulation. J Clin Invest. 1991;87:1621–7.
73. Inoue K, Miyake S, Kumashiro M, et al. Power spectral analysis of heart rate variability in traumatic quadriplegic humans. Am J Physiol. 1990;258:H1722–6.
74. Kollai M, Koizumi K. Reciprocal and non-reciprocal action of the vagal and sympathetic nerves innervating the heart. J Auton Nerv Syst. 1979;1:33–52.
75. Warner MR, deTarnowsky JM, Whitson CC, et al. Beat-by-beat modulation of AV conduction. II. Autonomic neural mechanisms. Am J Physiol. 1986;251:H1134–42.
76. Neff RA, Wang J, Baxi S, et al. Respiratory sinus arrhythmia: endogenous activation of nicotinic receptors mediates respiratory modulation of brainstem cardioinhibitory parasympathetic neurons. Circ Res. 2003;93:565–72.
77. Wang J, Wang X, Irnaten M, et al. Endogenous acetylcholine and nicotine activation enhances GABAergic and glycinergic inputs to cardiac vagal neurons. J Neurophysiol. 2003;89:2473–81.
78. Guntheroth WG, Kawabori I. Hypoxic apnea and gasping. J Clin Invest. 1975;56:1371–7.
79. Deshpande P, Khurana A, Hansen P, et al. Failure of autoresuscitation in weanling mice: significance of cardiac glycogen and heart rate regulation. J Appl Physiol. 1999;87:203–10.
80. Schuen JN, Bamford OS, Carroll JL. The cardiorespiratory response to anoxia: normal development and the effect of nicotine. Respir Physiol. 1997;109:231–9.
81. Taylor EW, Butler PJ. Nervous control of heart rate: activity in the cardiac vagus of the dogfish. J Appl Physiol. 1982;53:1330–5.

82. Baird TM. Clinical correlates, natural history and outcome of neonatal apnoea. Semin Neonatol. 2004;9:205–11.
83. Madden BP, Shenoy V, Dalrymple-Hay M, et al. Absence of bradycardic response to apnea and hypoxia in heart transplant recipients with obstructive sleep apnea. J Heart Lung Transplant. 1997;16:394–7.
84. Berk JL, Levy MN. Profound reflex bradycardia produced by transient hypoxia or hypercapnia in man. Eur Surg Res. 1977;9:75–84.
85. Somers VK, Dyken ME, Mark AL, et al. Parasympathetic hyperresponsiveness and bradyarrhythmias during apnoea in hypertension. Clin Auton Res. 1992;2:171–6.
86. Martin RJ, Abu-Shaweesh JM, Baird TM. Apnoea of prematurity. Paediatr Respir Rev. 2004;5:S377–82.
87. O'Donnell CP, Bower EA. Heart rate changes evoked by hypoxia in the anaesthetized, artificially ventilated cat. Exp Physiol. 1992;77:271–83.
88. de Burgh DM, Elsner R, Angell-James JE. Cardiorespiratory control by carotid chemoreceptors during experimental dives in the seal. Am J Physiol. 1977;232:H508–16.
89. Daly MB, Korner PI, Angell-James JE, et al. Cardiovascular-respiratory reflex interactions between carotid bodies and upper-airways receptors in the monkey. Am J Physiol. 1978;234:H293–9.
90. Lewis AB, Donovan M, Platzker AC. Cardiovascular responses to autonomic blockade in hypoxemic fetal lambs. Biol Neonate. 1980;37:233–42.
91. Cohn HE, Piasecki GJ, Jackson BT. The effect of fetal heart rate on cardiovascular function during hypoxemia. Am J Obstet Gynecol. 1980;138:1190–9.
92. Przybylski J, Trzebski A, Przybyszewski A. Circulatory responses to acute hypoxia in spontaneously hypertensive and normotensive rats. Acta Physiol Pol. 1980;31:463–8.
93. Yu ZY, Lumbers ER, Gibson KJ, et al. Effects on hypoxaemia on foetal heart rate, variability and cardiac rhythm. Clin Exp Pharmacol Physiol. 1998;25:577–84.
94. Ikenoue T, Martin Jr CB, Murata Y, et al. Effect of acute hypoxemia and respiratory acidosis on the fetal heart rate in monkeys. Am J Obstet Gynecol. 1981;141:797–806.
95. Hayashi M, Nagasaka T. Hypoxic tachycardia in hypoxia-acclimated rats. Jpn J Physiol. 1982;32:149–52.
96. Boddy K, Dawes GS, Fisher R, et al. Foetal respiratory movements, electrocortical and cardiovascular responses to hypoxaemia and hypercapnia in sheep. J Physiol. 1974;243:599–618.
97. Scremin AM, Scremin OU, Brechner T. Survival under hypoxia. Age dependence and effect of cholinergic drugs. Stroke. 1980;11:548–52.
98. Potter EK, McCloskey DI. Effects of hypoxia on cardiac vagal efferent activity and on the action of the vagus nerve at the heart in the dog. J Auton Nerv Syst. 1986;17:325–9.
99. Serani A, Lavados M, Zapata P. Cardiovascular responses to hypoxia in the spontaneously breathing cat: reflexes originating from carotid and aortic bodies. Arch Biol Med Exp (Santiago). 1983;16:29–41.
100. Neff RA, Simmens SJ, Evans C, et al. Prenatal nicotine exposure alters central cardiorespiratory responses to hypoxia in rats: implications for sudden infant death syndrome. J Neurosci. 2004;24: 9261–8.
101. Erickson JT, Millhorn DE. Hypoxia and electrical stimulation of the carotid sinus nerve induce Fos-like immunoreactivity within catecholaminergic and serotoninergic neurons of the rat brainstem. J Comp Neurol. 1994;348:161–82.
102. Teppema LJ, Veening JG, Kranenburg A, et al. Expression of c-fos in the rat brainstem after exposure to hypoxia and to normoxic and hyperoxic hypercapnia. J Comp Neurol. 1997;388:169–90.
103. Richter DW, Schmidt-Garcon P, Pierrefiche O, et al. Neurotransmitters and neuromodulators controlling the hypoxic respiratory response in anaesthetized cats. J Physiol. 1999;514:567–78.
104. Nucci TB, Branco LG, Gargaglioni LH. 5-HT1A, but not 5-HT2 and 5-HT7, receptors in the nucleus raphe magnus modulate hypoxia-induced hyperpnoea. Acta Physiol (Oxf). 2008;193: 403–14.
105. Gargaglioni LH, Bicego KC, Nucci TB, et al. Serotoninergic receptors in the anteroventral preoptic region modulate the hypoxic ventilatory response. Respir Physiol Neurobiol. 2006;153: 1–13.
106. Tryba AK, Pena F, Ramirez JM. Gasping activity in vitro: a rhythm dependent on 5-HT2A receptors. J Neurosci. 2006;26: 2623–34.
107. St-John WM, Leiter JC. Maintenance of gasping and restoration of eupnea after hypoxia is impaired following blockers of α-1 adrenergic receptors and serotonin 5HT2 receptors. J Appl Physiol. 2008;104:665–73.
108. Fuller DD, Zabka AG, Baker TL, et al. Physiological and genomic consequences of intermittent hypoxia selected contribution: phrenic long-term facilitation requires 5-HT receptor activation during but not following episodic hypoxia. J Appl Physiol. 2001;90:2001–6.
109. McGuire M, Zhang Y, White DP, et al. Serotonin receptor subtypes required for ventilatory long-term facilitation and its enhancement after chronic intermittent hypoxia in awake rats. Am J Physiol Regul Integr Comp Physiol. 2004;286:R334–41.
110. Takeuchi Y, Kojima M, Matsuura T, et al. Serotonergic innervation on the motoneurons in the mammalian brainstem. Light and electron microscopic immunohistochemistry. Anat Embryol (Berl). 1983;167:321–33.
111. Izzo PN, Deuchars J, Spyer KM. Localization of cardiac vagal preganglionic motoneurones in the rat: immunocytochemical evidence of synaptic inputs containing 5-hydroxytryptamine. J Comp Neurol. 1993;327:572–83.
112. Dergacheva O, Kamendi H, Wang X, et al. The role of 5-HT3 and other excitatory receptors in central cardiorespiratory responses to hypoxia: implications for sudden infant death syndrome. Pediatr Res. 2009;65:625–30.
113. Dergacheva O, Kamendi H, Wang X, et al. 5-HT2 receptors modulate excitatory neurotransmission to cardiac vagal neurons within the nucleus ambiguus evoked during and after hypoxia. Neuroscience. 2009;164:1191–8.
114. Dergacheva O, Griffioen KJ, Wang X, et al. 5-HT2 receptor subtypes mediate different long-term changes in GABAergic activity to parasympathetic cardiac vagal neurons in the nucleus ambiguus. Neuroscience. 2007;149:696–705.
115. Wang X, Dergacheva O, Kamendi H, et al. 5-Hydroxytryptamine 1A/7 and 4alpha receptors differentially prevent opioid-induced inhibition of brain stem cardiorespiratory function. Hypertension. 2007;50:368–76.
116. Pichot V, Roche F, Gaspoz JM, et al. Relation between heart rate variability and training load in middle-distance runners. Med Sci Sports Exerc. 2000;32:1729–36.
117. Roche F, Reynaud C, Garet M, et al. Cardiac baroreflex control in humans during and immediately after brief exposure to simulated high altitude. Clin Physiol Funct Imaging. 2002;22:301–6.
118. Evans C, Wang J, Neff R, et al. Hypoxia recruits a respiratory-related excitatory pathway to brainstem premotor cardiac vagal neurons in animals exposed to prenatal nicotine. Neuroscience. 2005;133:1073–9.
119. Griffioen KJ, Gorini C, Jameson H, et al. Purinergic P2X receptors mediate excitatory transmission to cardiac vagal neurons in the nucleus ambiguus after hypoxia. Hypertension. 2007;50: 75–81.
120. Griffioen KJ, Kamendi HW, Gorini CJ, et al. Reactive oxygen species mediate central cardiorespiratory network responses to acute intermittent hypoxia. J Neurophysiol. 2007;97:2059–66.

121. Feldman JL, Mitchell GS, Nattie EE. Breathing: rhythmicity, plasticity, chemosensitivity. Annu Rev Neurosci. 2003;26:239–66.
122. Bocchiaro CM, Feldman JL. Synaptic activity-independent persistent plasticity in endogenously active mammalian motoneurons. Proc Natl Acad Sci USA. 2004;101:4292–5.
123. Soukhova-O'Hare GK, Cheng ZJ, Roberts AM, et al. Postnatal intermittent hypoxia alters baroreflex function in adult rats. Am J Physiol Heart Circ Physiol. 2006;290:H1157–64.
124. Lin M, Ai J, Li L, et al. Structural remodeling of nucleus ambiguus projections to cardiac ganglia following chronic intermittent hypoxia in C57BL/6J mice. J Comp Neurol. 2008;509:103–17.
125. Gu H, Lin M, Liu J, et al. Selective impairment of central mediation of baroreflex in anesthetized young adult Fischer 344 rats after chronic intermittent hypoxia. Am J Physiol Heart Circ Physiol. 2007;293:H2809–18.
126. Lin M, Liu R, Gozal D, et al. Chronic intermittent hypoxia impairs baroreflex control of heart rate but enhances heart rate responses to vagal efferent stimulation in anesthetized mice. Am J Physiol Heart Circ Physiol. 2007;293:H997–1006.
127. Yan B, Soukhova-O'Hare GK, Li L, et al. Attenuation of heart rate control and neural degeneration in nucleus ambiguus following chronic intermittent hypoxia in young adult Fischer 344 rats. Neuroscience. 2008;153:709–20.
128. Yan B, Li L, Harden SW, et al. Chronic intermittent hypoxia impairs heart rate responses to AMPA and NMDA and induces loss of glutamate receptor neurons in nucleus ambiguous of F344 rats. Am J Physiol Regul Integr Comp Physiol. 2009;296:R299–308.
129. Smith IE, Quinnell TG. Pharmacotherapies for obstructive sleep apnoea: where are we now? Drugs. 2004;64:1385–99.
130. Carley DW, Olopade C, Ruigt GS, et al. Efficacy of mirtazapine in obstructive sleep apnea syndrome. Sleep. 2007;30:35–41.
131. Veasey SC. Serotonin agonists and antagonists in obstructive sleep apnea: therapeutic potential. Am J Respir Med. 2003;2:21–9.
132. Grunstein RR, Hedner J, Grote L. Treatment options for sleep apnoea. Drugs. 2001;61:237–51.

Part II

Intermittent Hypoxia and Respiratory Disorders

Effect of Intermittent Hypoxia on Breathing Stability in Individuals with Sleep Apnea

7

Jason H. Mateika

Abstract

There is much speculation that respiratory motor long-term facilitation may have a significant impact on apnea severity in individuals with sleep apnea because this disorder is characterized by exposure to intermittent hypoxia, one stimulus known to initiate long-term facilitation. It has been suggested that activation of long-term facilitation may serve to mitigate apnea by facilitating minute ventilation and, perhaps more importantly, upper airway muscle activity. The less discussed but equally plausible situation is that exposure to intermittent hypoxia might ultimately lead to the promotion of apnea. There are at least two scenarios in which apnea might be promoted following exposure to intermittent hypoxia. In both scenarios, long-term facilitation of upper airway muscle activity is initiated but ultimately rendered ineffective because of muscle fatigue or the initiation of other forms of respiratory plasticity, more specifically progressive augmentation of the hypoxic ventilatory response. The primary goal of this chapter is to discuss whether the complex interactions of various forms of respiratory motor neuronal plasticity have a beneficial or a detrimental impact on breathing stability in individuals with sleep apnea. The overall conclusion is that exposure to intermittent hypoxia should not be considered exclusively beneficial or detrimental to breathing stability in individuals with sleep apnea. Rather, the beneficial or detrimental outcomes of exposure to intermittent hypoxia are likely dependent on a variety of circumstances and the complex interactions between various forms of respiratory motor plasticity.

7.1 Introduction

This chapter is designed to examine the impact that intermittent hypoxia (IH) has on breathing stability in individuals with sleep apnea. The chapter will focus primarily on the role that two basic phenomena, progressive augmentation (PA) of the hypoxic ventilatory response and long-term facilitation (LTF) of respiratory motor activity, initiated by exposure to IH, have in altering breathing stability in individuals with sleep apnea. Although this chapter will provide a brief overview of the phenomena, it will not focus on reviewing all the literature pertaining to these forms of respiratory plasticity. Instead, the reader is referred to comprehensive reviews that have carefully examined all aspects of these phenomena including the various factors that influence their initiation and magnitude [16, 39, 43, 50]. The intention of this chapter is to highlight, based on the published literature, that exposure to IH should not be considered exclusively beneficial or detrimental to breathing stability in individuals with sleep apnea. Rather, the discussion below promotes the notion that beneficial or detrimental outcomes of exposure to IH are likely dependent on the complex interaction between

J.H. Mateika
Department of Physiology,
Wayne State University School of Medicine,
Detroit, MI 48201, USA

Department of Internal Medicine,
Wayne State University School of Medicine,
Detroit, MI 48201, USA

John D. Dingell Veterans Affairs Medical Center,
Division of Research and Development,
Detroit, MI 48201, USA
e-mail: jmateika@med.wayne.edu

L. Xi, T.V. Serebrovskaya (eds.), *Intermittent Hypoxia and Human Diseases*,
DOI 10.1007/978-1-4471-2906-6_7,

PA of the hypoxic ventilatory response and LTF of respiratory motor activity.

7.2 Progressive Augmentation and Long-Term Facilitation

Progressive augmentation of the hypoxic ventilatory response is characterized by a gradual increase in the magnitude of the response from the initial to the final hypoxic episode of an IH protocol (Fig. 7.1). The increase in the hypoxic ventilatory response can be sustained for minutes to hours after exposure to IH [25, 41]. Although the carotid bodies likely contribute to PA, given their role in other time-dependent ventilatory responses to hypoxia [64, 72], this form of plasticity (i.e., PA) probably originates from a variety of sites within the respiratory system including the phrenic motor neurons, respiratory premotor neurons (i.e., at the level of the medulla), and carotid bodies. The relative contribution of each site to PA in animals and humans has not been well differentiated to date, and consequently the reader should be cognizant of this gap in the literature while reading the discussion below. Likewise, PA of upper airway muscle activity might reflect integration of both carotid body and hypoglossal motor neuronal plasticity.

Independent of the site of plasticity, it should be recognized that measurement of the hypoxic ventilatory response is dependent on the isocapnic partial pressure of carbon dioxide that is maintained during measurement of the response, as well as the threshold and central ventilatory response to carbon dioxide (Fig. 7.2). The reader is referred to Duffin's review [21] of this concept for a detailed discussion. The impact of carbon dioxide on the hypoxic ventilatory response is important because PA of the hypoxic response (Fig. 7.2 – left hand graph – dashed vertical arrow labeled PA) may be due to alterations in the response threshold to carbon dioxide otherwise known as the apneic threshold. The apneic threshold demarcates the point at which ventilation ceases (i.e., 0 L/min in Fig. 7.2) in response to a reduction in carbon dioxide below resting values (i.e., the normal

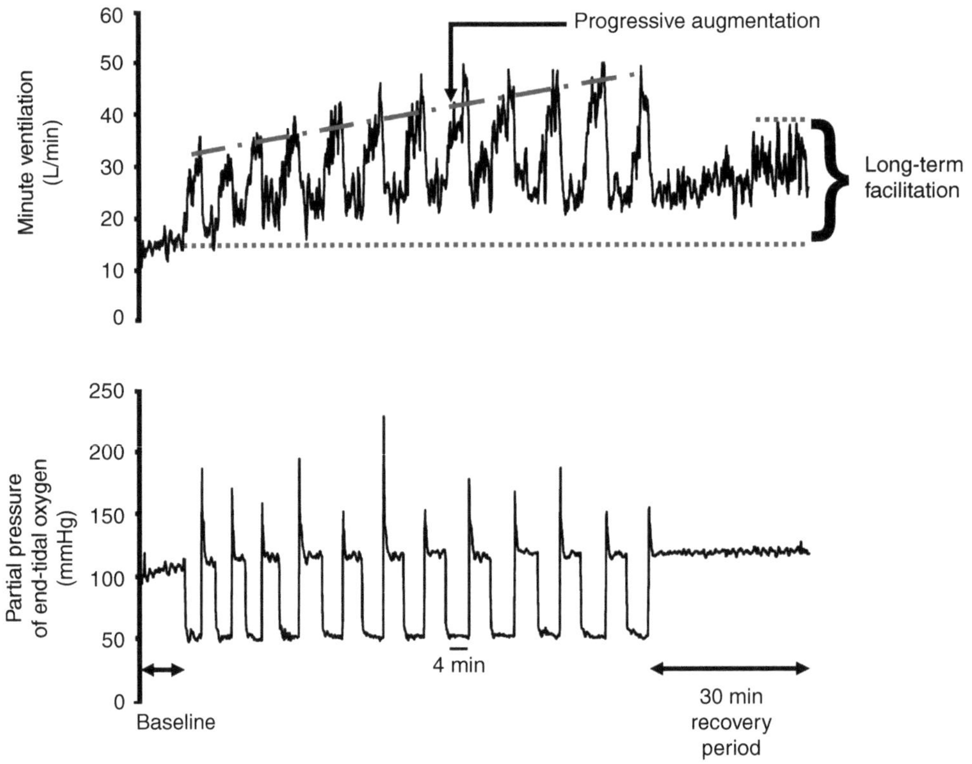

Fig. 7.1 A recording of breath-by-breath minute ventilation values recorded from a human participant before, during, and following exposure to 12 episodes of hypoxia. Each hypoxic episode and subsequent recovery period was 4 min in duration with the exception of the last recovery period, which was 30 min in duration. Each hypoxic episode was induced by the inhalation of a gas mixture comprised of 8% oxygen balance nitrogen. One hundred percent supplemental oxygen was added when required to maintain the partial pressure of end-tidal oxygen at 50 mmHg during each hypoxic episode. Throughout the entire protocol, the partial pressure of end-tidal carbon dioxide was maintained 3 mmHg above baseline levels. Note that during exposure to intermittent hypoxia, the ventilatory response to hypoxia gradually increased from the initial to the final hypoxic episode. This phenomenon is referred to as progressive augmentation. Also note that during exposure to intermittent hypoxia, minute ventilation gradually increased during the normoxic recovery periods so that it was substantially higher during the final recovery period compared with baseline. This phenomenon is referred to as long-term facilitation

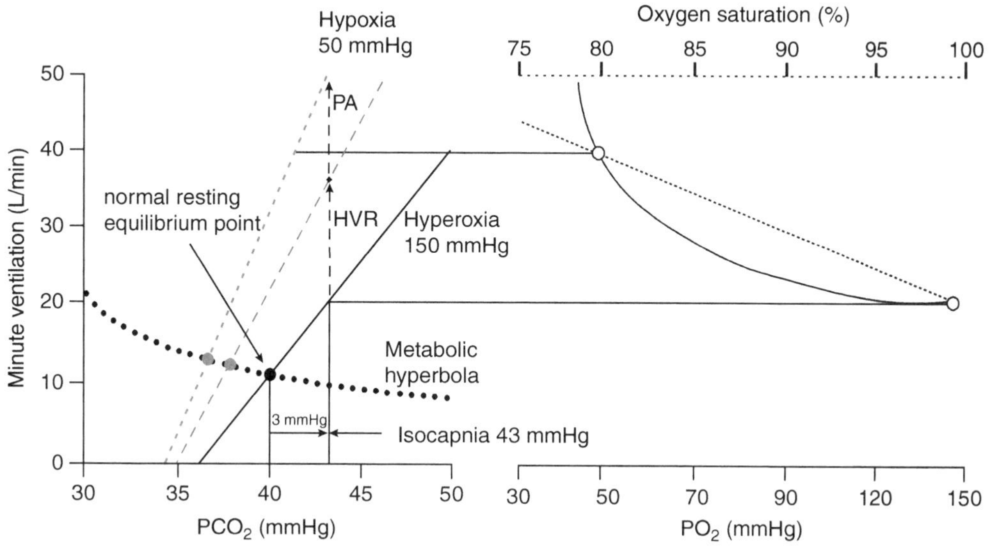

Fig. 7.2 The measurement of the hypoxic ventilatory response is dependent on the level of carbon dioxide that is sustained throughout the intermittent hypoxia protocol. At a chosen isocapnic partial pressure of carbon dioxide (set to 3 mmHg above resting in this example), the ventilation increase from the hyperoxic carbon dioxide response line (*black line* – assumed to reflect the central chemoreflex response) to the hypoxic carbon dioxide response line (*gray solid line* – assumed to reflect the sum of central and peripheral chemoreflex responses) is the value measured for the hypoxic ventilatory response (*arrowed labeled HVR*). Progressive augmentation (*PA*) of the hypoxic ventilatory response (*gray dotted line*) during exposure to intermittent hypoxia may be the result of changes in either the apneic threshold or ventilatory sensitivity. However, at a given isocapnic partial pressure of carbon dioxide (43 mmHg in this case), the mechanisms (change in slope or threshold) responsible for the hypoxic response are indistinguishable from one another. Definitions: PCO_2 partial pressure of carbon dioxide, PO_2 partial pressure of oxygen; oxygen saturation, arterial hemoglobin saturation with oxygen

resting equilibrium point in Fig. 7.2). Figure 7.2 shows that a shift in the apneic threshold leftward (i.e., from the solid gray line to the dashed gray line) could result in an increase in ventilation for a given partial pressure of carbon dioxide and oxygen. Progressive augmentation may also be due to increases in the ventilatory sensitivity to changes in oxygen and carbon dioxide levels. Ventilatory sensitivity is determined by measuring the slope of the minute ventilation vs. end-tidal carbon dioxide relationship, which is linear above the apneic threshold. Figure 7.2 shows that an increase in ventilatory sensitivity (left hand graph – from the solid gray to the dashed gray line) to oxygen and carbon dioxide results in an increase in minute ventilation for a given partial pressure of carbon dioxide and oxygen. For example, minute ventilation at a $P_{ET}O_2$ of 50 mmHg and a $P_{ET}CO_2$ of 43 mmHg is greater when measured from the dashed gray compared to the solid gray line.

The potential impact of altering the threshold or sensitivity on PA is mentioned at this point because altering one or both of these variables impacts on breathing stability. The role of the apneic threshold and/or ventilatory sensitivity in maintaining or exacerbating breathing is related primarily to the impact that these variables have on the carbon dioxide reserve [17–19]. The carbon dioxide reserve is defined as the difference between the partial pressure of carbon dioxide associated with breathing at rest (Fig. 7.3 – black circle) and the partial pressure of carbon dioxide that demarcates the apneic threshold (Fig. 7.3 – vertical black arrow) [17–19]. If the apneic threshold (more specifically the $P_{ET}CO_2$ that demarcates the apneic threshold) (Fig. 7.3 – dashed gray line) or sensitivity decreases (Fig. 7.3 – solid gray line), the carbon dioxide reserve will increase (Fig. 7.3 – dashed gray and solid gray horizontal arrows). This increase would tend to promote breathing stability since a greater decease in carbon dioxide would be required to exceed the apneic threshold. In contrast, if the apneic threshold or sensitivity increases (Fig. 7.4 – solid gray and dashed gray lines), the carbon dioxide reserve decreases (Fig. 7.4 – solid gray and dashed gray horizontal arrows), which would tend to exacerbate breathing instability.

Long-term facilitation is a form of neuronal plasticity that is characterized by a progressive increase in respiratory motor output during periods of normoxia that are separated by hypoxic episodes and by a sustained elevation in respiratory motor activity for up to 90 min following exposure [43, 51] (Fig. 7.1). Exposure to IH for the first time will initiate LTF at most sites which display phasic respiratory activity, including the hypoglossal nucleus (and the genioglossus muscle that is innervated by the hypoglossal nerve) [10, 14, 26, 28, 40, 48], brainstem respiratory nuclei [53], phrenic motoneurons [5, 49], and minute ventilation (and its components tidal volume and/or breathing frequency) [4, 28, 35,

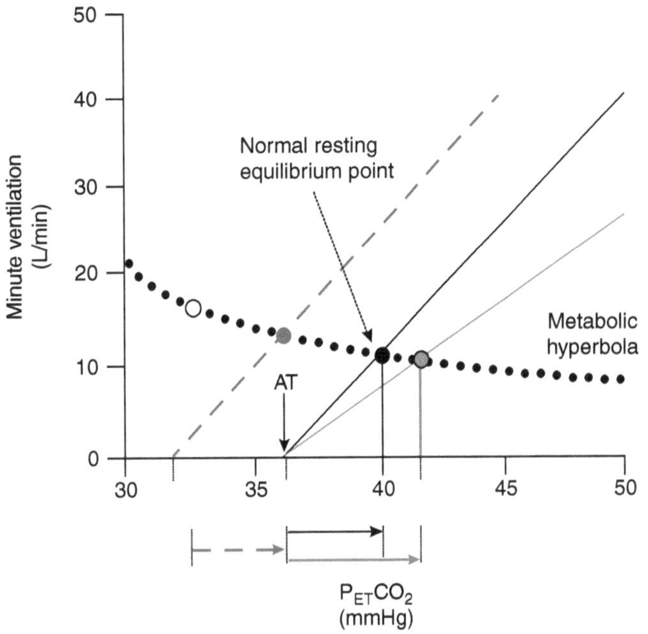

Fig. 7.3 Schematic representation of the control of breathing and the possible beneficial impact of exposure to intermittent hypoxia. *Dotted black line* (labeled metabolic hyperbola) represents the impact of the efferent arm of the respiratory control loop on arterial blood gases (i.e., carbon dioxide levels), and the *solid black line* represents chemoreflex afferent feedback. The *blacked filled circle* represents the calculated normal resting equilibrium point (i.e., normal resting minute ventilation and the concomitant level of carbon dioxide), and the vertical *black arrow* represents the apneic threshold (V_T). The *horizontal black arrow* represents the carbon dioxide reserve (the difference between the carbon dioxide levels that correspond to normal resting breathing and the ventilatory threshold). The *solid gray circle* represents an increase in normal resting breathing (ventilatory long-term facilitation) while the *gray dashed line* represents a shift in the apneic threshold that might occur as a consequence of exposure to intermittent hypoxia. The *dashed horizontal gray arrow* represents the increase in the carbon dioxide reserve that would occur as a consequence of these alterations, ultimately resulting in increased breathing stability. The *solid gray line* represents a reduction in ventilatory sensitivity to carbon dioxide following exposure to intermittent hypoxia. This alteration would be independent of ventilatory long-term facilitation since it is accompanied by a decrease in normal resting breathing (*light gray circle*). The *solid gray horizontal arrow* represents the calculated increase in the carbon dioxide reserve that would occur. Lastly, the *white circle* represents an increase in normal resting breathing following exposure to intermittent hypoxia that is independent of changes in chemoreflex properties (i.e., ventilatory threshold and sensitivity)

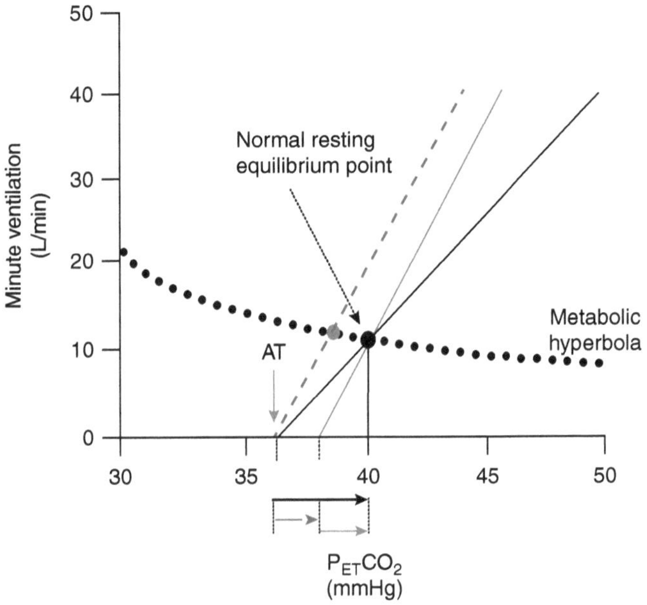

Fig. 7.4 Schematic representation of the control of breathing and the possible detrimental impact of exposure to intermittent hypoxia. *Dotted black line* (labeled metabolic hyperbola) represents the impact of the efferent arm of the respiratory control loop on arterial blood gases (i.e., carbon dioxide levels), and the *solid black line* represents chemoreflex afferent feedback. The *blacked filled circle* represents the calculated normal resting equilibrium point (i.e., normal resting minute ventilation and the concomitant level of carbon dioxide) (*black circle*), and the *vertical gray arrow* represents the ventilatory threshold (*AT*). The *horizontal black arrow* represents the carbon dioxide reserve (the difference between the carbon dioxide levels that correspond to normal resting breathing and the apneic threshold). The *solid gray circle* represents an increase in normal resting breathing (ventilatory long-term facilitation) while the *gray dashed line* represents an increase in ventilatory sensitivity that might occur as a consequence of exposure to intermittent hypoxia. The *dashed horizontal gray arrow* represents the decrease in the carbon dioxide reserve that would occur as a consequence of these alterations, ultimately resulting in increased breathing instability. The *solid gray line* represents an increase in ventilatory sensitivity and threshold to carbon dioxide following exposure to intermittent hypoxia. This alteration would be independent of ventilatory long-term facilitation since it is accompanied by unchanged resting breathing (*black circle*). The *solid gray horizontal arrow* represents the calculated decrease in the carbon dioxide reserve

55, 56, 73]. The magnitude of LTF can be enhanced by repeated daily exposure to IH (i.e., chronic IH) in a variety of animal species including humans with sleep apnea [27, 36, 45, 47, 60, 79]. However, it should be noted that studies completed to date have not clearly established that repeated daily exposure to IH enhances LTF in healthy humans since measures of resting minute ventilation following exposure to chronic IH have not been found to be statistically significant from baseline [24, 62]. Exposure to chronic IH also initiates a unique form of LTF. Long-term facilitation of carotid sensory nerve activity is not activated following a first-time exposure to IH but is initiated following repeated daily exposure to IH [59, 61].

7.3 Respiratory Plasticity and Sleep Apnea

Sleep apnea is characterized by episodes of breathing cessation accompanied by hypoxemia and hypercapnia [19, 75]. Given that individuals with sleep apnea are exposed to IH throughout the night, it is possible that PA and LTF are initiated at various sites within the respiratory system of these individuals. Indeed, as outlined below, some studies completed in individuals with sleep apnea support this contention [1, 4, 27, 35], although additional studies are required to support the possibility. If one accepts that these phenomena are initiated in individuals with sleep apnea following exposure to IH, the question remains as to whether or not the interaction between PA and LTF is beneficial or a detriment to breathing stability. In other words, it is of interest to speculate how PA and LTF might interact to promote or mitigate apnea over a selected time period (i.e., hours, days, months, or years).

In the discussion below (see Sect. 7.3.1), the role of PA, ventilatory LTF (vLTF) and long-term facilitation of upper airway muscle activity (LTF_{ua}) in mitigating or promoting apnea is addressed since these measures are typically obtained in healthy humans and humans suffering from obstructive sleep apnea. Throughout the discussion, vLTF is assumed to be initiated by LTF of phrenic nerve activity. However, the possibility that LTF of respiratory premotor neurons or LTF of carotid sensory nerve activity is in part responsible for vLTF is not ruled out. Likewise, alterations in the apneic threshold and/or sensitivity responsible for PA of the hypoxic ventilatory response are assumed to be a manifestation of LTF of carotid sensory nerve activity; however, the potential contribution of other forms of plasticity (i.e., LTF of phrenic nerve or medullary respiratory motoneurons) to alterations in the threshold and sensitivity of the hypoxic ventilatory response is recognized. Lastly, changes in the apneic threshold and sensitivity to both hypoxia and hypercapnia are both assumed to have a role in PA of the hypoxic ventilatory response (see Sect. 7.2 for further discussion of this issue).

Initially, the hypothesis that alterations in LTF_{ua}, vLTF, and PA following exposure to IH may be beneficial in the promotion of breathing stability in humans is presented. This hypothesis focuses on the importance of upper airway muscle plasticity in maintaining airway patency and the importance of vLTF in preventing centrally initiated apnea. The hypothesis also focuses on the role that the apneic threshold and sensitivity to hypoxia might have in the prevention of hypocapnia and how this may contribute to the effectiveness of upper airway muscle plasticity in mitigating apnea. The second hypothesis presented examines the potentially detrimental impact that exposure to IH may have on upper airway muscle function. More specifically, the potentially detrimental influence that vLTF and chemoreflex plasticity following exposure to IH has in promoting central apnea and its impact on upper airway muscle function will be examined. In the presentation of the two hypotheses, all other variables (e.g., sleep stage, arousal threshold, and anthropometric factors) that impact on breathing stability are assumed to remain constant. The presentation of each hypothesis (see Sect. 7.3.1), which are principally theoretical in nature, will be followed by a discussion of outcome measures that support the hypothesis along with a brief summary of the subsection.

7.3.1 Beneficial Impact of Intermittent Hypoxia on Breathing Stability

7.3.1.1 Upper Airway Function

LTF can occur at many sites within the central nervous system. However, it might be argued that the most important site, as it pertains to breathing stability during sleep, is at the level of brainstem upper airway motor nuclei since obstructive sleep apnea is characterized by collapse of the upper airway [19, 75]. Numerous studies in rats have shown that IH initiates LTF of the hypoglossal nerve [9, 25, 26]. Likewise, either direct measures of genioglossus muscle activity from healthy humans [14, 28] or measures of upper airway resistance in individuals suffering from sleep apnea [1] indicate that LTF of the genioglossus muscle can be activated following exposure to IH. Moreover, short periods of sustained hypoxia have also been shown to activate both the genioglossus muscle and retractor muscles of the tongue in healthy humans [42]. If LTF_{ua} is indeed initiated throughout the night in individuals with sleep apnea, this phenomenon would likely serve to protect against collapse of the upper airway.

7.3.1.2 Ventilatory Long-Term Facilitation

If vLTF is initiated in individuals with sleep apnea independent of alterations in chemoreflex plasticity (i.e., changes in ventilatory sensitivity and the apneic threshold), this would serve to promote breathing stability. This possibility is supported by studies completed in my laboratory which showed that vLTF can be initiated in individuals with sleep apnea during wakefulness following exposure to 12 episodes of hypoxia that were 4 min in duration [27, 35] and by other studies which demonstrated that vLTF is evident during sleep following a similar number of episodes that were shorter in duration (i.e., 1 min) [4]. However, maintenance of carbon dioxide levels at or slightly above baseline levels (i.e., 3 mmHg) was required for the initiation of vLTF in these studies.

The role that carbon dioxide has in the initiation of vLTF is likely important since vLTF would probably be most effective in promoting breathing stability in individuals with sleep apnea if the phenomenon persists in the presence of hypocapnia. If this was the case, resting breathing would increase (Fig. 7.3 – white circle on resting metabolic hyperbola), and carbon dioxide levels would potentially be reduced below the apneic threshold (Fig. 7.3 – vertical black arrow indicating apneic threshold – AT). As a consequence of ventilation persisting in the presence of hypocapnia, central apnea would not ensue during sleep. Demonstrating that vLTF is initiated independent of chemoreflex plasticity and persists in the presence of carbon dioxide levels that are below the apneic threshold is difficult to demonstrate in humans. However, one would expect that levels of minute ventilation during completion of Duffin's modified rebreathing protocol [20–22] would be increased below the apneic threshold following exposure to

IH if vLTF was initiated independent of chemoreflex plasticity and hypocapnia. However, this increase was not observed in previous studies [32, 41]. More importantly, studies have indicated that the manifestation of vLTF is impacted by the presence of hypocapnia. In rats, the magnitude of vLTF is reduced in the presence of hypocapnia [56]. More importantly, studies in humans during wakefulness have clearly shown that vLTF does not manifest itself in the presence of iso/hypocapnia [28, 30, 32, 41, 44] using an identical IH protocol that initiated vLTF in the presence of sustained hypercapnia. Whether or not hypocapnia prevents the manifestation of vLTF during sleep in humans has not yet been adequately determined; however, Badr and colleagues did speculate that the absence of vLTF in some studies may have been due to a reduction in carbon dioxide levels [63]. Nevertheless, if both vLTF and LTF_{ua} persist in the presence of hypocapnia, vLTF would serve to reduce central apnea, and LTF_{ua} would assist in the reduction of obstructive apneic events.

7.3.1.3 Chemoreflex Plasticity

Specific alterations associated with PA of the hypoxic ventilatory response could contribute to breathing stability. More specifically, reductions in the apneic threshold could occur following exposure to IH. A reduction in the apneic threshold (Fig. 7.2 – dashed gray line) would not only contribute to PA of the hypoxic ventilatory response (see Fig. 7.2 – dotted vertical arrow between the solid gray and dashed gray line) but it could contribute to stabilization of breathing. As shown in Fig. 7.3, if a reduction in the apneic threshold (see dark gray dashed line) occurred concomitantly with an increase in baseline breathing (gray circle), as a consequence of vLTF, this would result in an increase in the carbon dioxide reserve (dark gray horizontal dashed arrow below *x*-axis). As discussed earlier, increases in the carbon dioxide reserve should promote breathing stability because a greater reduction in carbon dioxide would be required to reduce carbon dioxide levels below the threshold. The possibility that the apneic threshold is reduced following exposure to IH has received support from some studies. One study completed in rats showed that the apneic threshold decreased following a one-time exposure to IH [38]. In contrast, we have found in most studies that the apneic threshold is not significantly altered by exposure to acute IH in humans [2, 32, 41, 52]. However, decreases in the apneic threshold have been observed in humans following repeated daily exposure to IH [33]; thus, repeated exposure may be required before alterations in the threshold are evident. If indeed the apneic threshold decreases following exposure to IH, the increase in carbon dioxide reserve coupled with LTF_{ua} and vLTF that persists in the presence of both iso- and hypocapnia would be the ideal conditions for the promotion of breathing stability.

It should also be noted that a reduction in chemoreflex sensitivity would also serve to promote breathing stability. As shown in Fig. 7.3 (light grey solid line), if the apneic threshold remained unchanged but the sensitivity was reduced, this would result in an increase in the carbon dioxide reserve (see light gray solid horizontal arrow below the *x*-axis). There is support for this hypothesis since Katayama and colleagues showed in dogs that the ventilatory sensitivity to carbon dioxide below eupnea progressively decreased from the first to the third week of exposure to chronic IH [31]. This decrease resulted in a widening of the carbon dioxide reserve. It should be noted that in this study, vLTF was not observed (i.e., no change in eupneic air breathing was observed) following chronic IH [31]. Indeed, it is unlikely that a reduction in chemoreflex sensitivity would be coupled with vLTF since on the one hand the depression of ventilatory sensitivity would likely be accompanied by no change or a decrease in baseline breathing, while on the other hand vLTF by definition is associated with increases in baseline minute ventilation.

Exposure to IH could have a differential effect on those motor neurons innervating chest wall muscles compared to brainstem motor neurons innervating upper airway muscles. If this was the case, it is possible that LTF_{ua} could be initiated in the absence of vLTF and in the presence of reduced or unchanged chemoreflex sensitivity. Although this possibility has not been fully established, studies in rats and cats have shown that the magnitude of hypoglossal LTF (or genioglossus LTF) compared to phrenic LTF (or diaphragm LTF) varies [40, 77, 78], indicating that the degree of LTF may be dependent on the motor neuronal pool. Likewise, there is some evidence in individuals with sleep apnea that exposure to IH initiates LTF_{ua} in the absence of LTF of chest wall muscle activity [1, 70].

7.3.1.4 Beneficial Outcome Measures in Humans After Exposure to Intermittent Hypoxia

Few beneficial outcomes after the initiation of respiratory plasticity have been identified primarily because final outcome measures (e.g., apnea/hypopnea index) have not been typically examined in the studies completed. One investigation did show that the induction of LTF decreases the variability of expiratory time in both spontaneously breathing anesthetized cats and in healthy human participants [54]. Likewise, we recently showed that although the apnea/hypopnea index increased above baseline following acute exposure to 12 episodes of hypoxia (see Sect. 7.3.2.4 for further discussion of this finding), this increase was mitigated after 10 days of exposure to the protocol. This finding is similar to that previously reported in healthy individuals sojourning to high altitude [66]. On the initial day of exposure to hypoxia at high altitude, apnea severity relative to baseline was greatest. Although severity on subsequent days remained above sea level baseline measures, the severity tended to be less compared to the initial day of exposure to hypoxia. Perhaps,

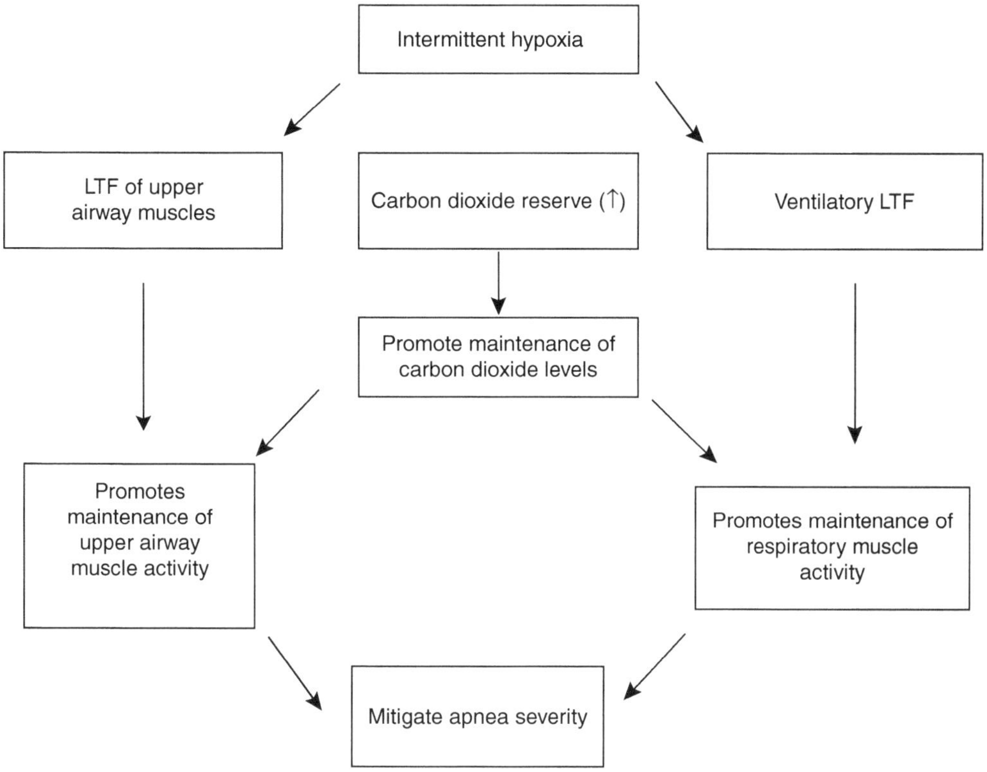

Fig. 7.5 Beneficial influence of intermittent hypoxia on apnea severity. The ideal situation is presented in which exposure to intermittent hypoxia promotes breathing stability. In this scenario, exposure to intermittent hypoxia leads to long-term facilitation of upper airway muscle activity, promoting the maintenance of upper airway patency. In addition, the carbon dioxide reserve is increased because of the initiation of ventilatory long-term facilitation and a decrease in the apneic threshold (see Fig. 7.3 for additional details regarding the relationship between ventilatory long-term facilitation and the carbon dioxide reserve). The increase in the carbon dioxide reserve promotes the maintenance of carbon dioxide levels, ensuring that hypocapnia does not develop, which could restrain the manifestation of long-term facilitation of upper airway muscle activity and minute ventilation. Ultimately, this integrated response promotes breathing stability and potentially mitigates apnea severity

under certain circumstances, the detrimental forms of plasticity are more relevant on an acute time cycle, and the beneficial forms of plasticity tend to manifest after exposure over a longer duration of time, given that all other variables are constant.

Given the scarcity of beneficial outcome measures, additional well-designed studies on specific phenotypic groups (e.g., young male/female with mild to moderate apnea versus older male and females with severe apnea) are required to fully establish whether or not initiation of respiratory plasticity improves breathing stability. Moreover, studies designed to expose participants with sleep apnea to IH during sleep in the presence of hypocapnia and hypercapnia will provide important information as to whether or not carbon dioxide levels impact on the initiation and maintenance of vLTF and LTF_{ua} and ultimately specific outcome measures during sleep.

7.3.1.5 Summary

There is some experimental evidence to suggest that LTF_{ua}, vLTF, and reductions in the apneic threshold occur in response to exposure to IH. Nevertheless, there is little evidence to date to confirm that all these modifications occur concurrently in individuals exposed to IH and that these modifications lead to improvement in outcome measures. Nevertheless, if vLTF, LTF_{ua}, and increases in the carbon dioxide reserve were to occur simultaneously as proposed, this would certainly contribute to breathing stability (Fig. 7.5). Moreover, if vLTF and LTF_{ua} persisted in the presence of hypocapnia, the role of carbon dioxide reserve could play a potentially lesser role in the maintenance of breathing stability.

7.3.2 Detrimental Impact of Intermittent Hypoxia on Breathing Stability

7.3.2.1 Upper Airway Function

It is important to recognize that exposure to IH and the subsequent initiation of LTF of upper airway motor neurons might not always translate into sustained increases in upper airway muscle activity and force production. It is possible that exposure to mild hypoxia particularly over an acute period of time initiates LTF of hypoglossal motor neurons and that this translates to sustained increases in genioglossus muscle activity and force production in humans [28]. Chronic exposure to mild hypoxia over a longer period of time might also induce a similar response, although this is not established in humans. However, exposure to severe levels of hypoxia over many hours, days, months, or years is likely to impair hypoglossal motoneuronal and/or upper airway muscle function, resulting in the loss of capacity to develop the force necessary to overcome a resistive load applied to the upper airway. Whether the loss of muscle function is myogenic or non-myogenic in nature is not fully established. Studies in rats have shown that exposure to CIH initiated changes in both structure and function of the pharyngeal dilator muscles (geniohyoid and sternohyoid) [11]. Specifically, CIH led to increased fatigability of pharyngeal dilator muscles [11, 46]. In contrast, Ray and colleagues [65] reported that fatigability of the sternohyoid muscle was not altered by CIH indicating that non-myogenic rather than myogenic mechanisms might contribute at least in part to the absence of LTF of hypoglossal nerve activity and reduced muscle function following chronic exposure to severe levels of hypoxia. Independent of the site of impairment, reduced muscle function following long-term exposure to IH might ultimately occur as a consequence of the accumulation of reactive oxygen species either at the level of the muscle [11] or the hypoglossal motor nucleus [74]. If upper airway dysfunction ensues (i.e., LTF of hypoglossal nerve activity or LTF_{ua} is not evident and/or overt upper airway muscle impairment is evident) following exposure to CIH, this could have a significant impact on the promotion of apnea. This impairment of upper airway muscle function could ultimately overpower any stabilizing influence that alterations in ventilatory sensitivity or the apneic threshold might have on apnea severity. For example, exposure to severe hypoxia over a prolonged period of time might dampen ventilatory sensitivity which could mitigate apnea (see Sect. 7.3.1.3). However, in the presence of upper airway muscle fatigue, alterations in chemoreflex properties may have little impact. Likewise, the impact of upper airway muscle fatigue could be further pronounced if a simultaneous increase in ventilatory sensitivity and the apneic threshold (i.e., a reduction in the carbon dioxide reserve) was initiated by exposure to chronic IH.

7.3.2.2 Ventilatory Long-Term Facilitation

It is possible that the initiation of vLTF could lower carbon dioxide below the apneic threshold. If vLTF is not sustained in the presence of hypocapnia, as suggested by published findings, the subthreshold levels of carbon dioxide could result in the promotion of a central apnea (Fig. 7.3 – see white circle located on the metabolic hyperbola). Likewise, the induction of hypocapnia could also result in the formation of an obstructive event as a consequence of disfacilitation of upper airway motor neuron activity (for further discussion involving the role of carbon dioxide in the maintenance of upper airway patency, see Sect. 7.3.2.3).

7.3.2.3 Chemoreflex Plasticity

In contrast to the potential beneficial impact of reducing the apneic threshold, PA induced by increases in chemoreflex sensitivity (Fig. 7.4 – dashed dark gray line and solid light gray line) could result in a reduction in the carbon dioxide reserve (Fig. 7.4 – dark gray and light gray horizontal arrow on *x*-axis). The reduction in carbon dioxide reserve could occur as a consequence of alterations in chemoreflex sensitivity independent of whether (Fig. 7.4 – light gray line) or not (Fig. 7.4 – dark gray dashed line) the apneic threshold was altered. Consequently, small decreases in carbon dioxide would reduce values below the apneic threshold. Likewise, the increase in chemoreflex sensitivity could result in inappropriate responses to chemical stimuli (hypoxia and hypercapnia) which in addition to the reduced carbon dioxide reserve would promote reductions in carbon dioxide levels below the apneic threshold. This development of hypocapnia could occur following an apneic event. The peripheral chemoreflex and possibly the central chemoreflex are activated as a consequence of hypoxia and hypercapnia developed during an apnea. Increases in chemoreflex sensitivity as a consequence of repeated exposure to IH throughout the night could result in an inappropriate response to these chemical stimuli inducing carbon dioxide levels below the apneic threshold. The induction of hypocapnia would be of little consequence if vLTF and LTF_{ua} persisted in the presence of hypocapnia. However, if this is not the case, the induction of hypocapnia could have a significant influence on breathing stability. The induction of carbon dioxide levels below the apneic threshold would result in the development of a central apnea in the absence of vLTF. Likewise, the induction of a central apnea as a consequence of hypocapnia might be followed by occlusion of the airway, as shown in a variety of studies [6, 8, 29, 57]. This may occur in part because of a reduction in upper airway muscle activity reduced as a consequence of the induction of hypocapnia [6, 7]. This possibility might ultimately explain the ineffectiveness of LTF_{ua} in mitigating apnea following exposure to IH since even if the phenomenon exists, it may not manifest itself in the presence of severe hypocapnia (Fig. 7.6).

There is a good deal of evidence to support the contention that ventilatory sensitivity to hypoxia/hypercapnia is increased in humans in response to exposure to AIH and CIH [32, 33, 37, 41, 68] during wakefulness. Likewise, Chowdhuri and colleagues showed that the ventilatory sensitivity to reductions in carbon dioxide during sleep was increased following exposure to IH [15]. Most applicable to the topic of this chapter, Salloum and colleagues revealed that ventilatory sensitivity was greater in patients with sleep

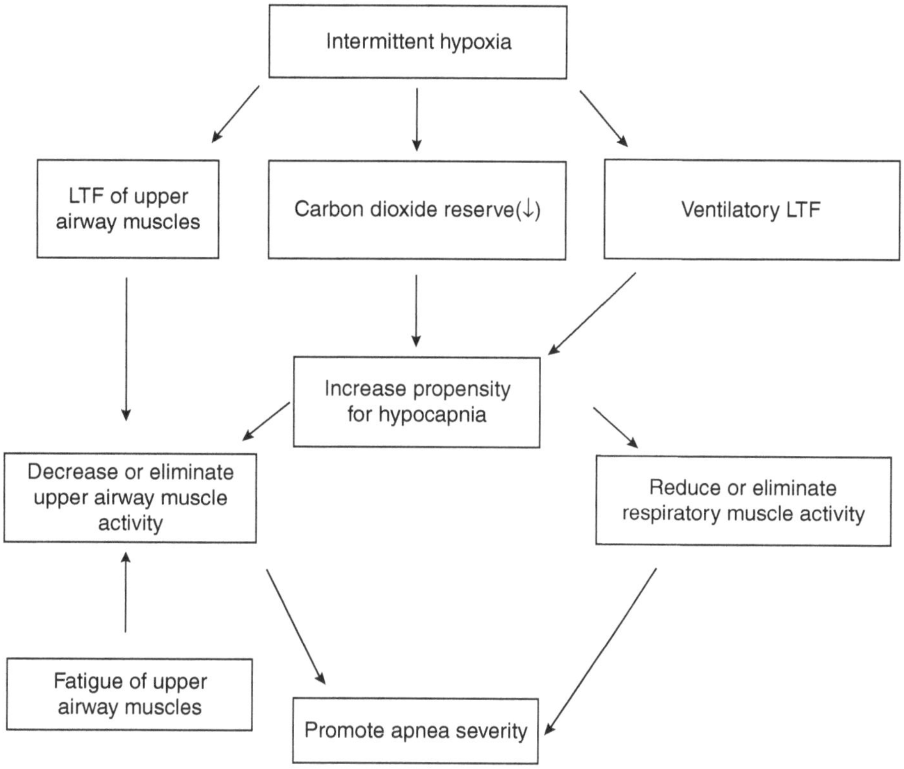

Fig. 7.6 Detrimental influence of intermittent hypoxia on apnea severity. In this scenario, long-term facilitation is induced in upper airway muscles following exposure to intermittent hypoxia but ultimately is ineffective in mitigating apnea because increases in ventilatory sensitivity that ultimately result in decreases in the carbon dioxide reserve increase the propensity for developing hypocapnia. The induced hypocapnia restrains LTF of upper airway muscle activity and respiratory muscle activity, ultimately resulting in the promotion of apnea. Likewise, the function of upper airway muscle activity could be diminished because of fatigue of the upper airway muscles induced following prolonged exposure to intermittent hypoxia

apnea compared to matched controls and that the ventilatory sensitivity decreased in these patients 1 month following treatment with continuous positive airway pressure [67]. Although, the mechanism responsible for this alteration was not investigated specifically, it is viable that the increase in sensitivity was caused by nightly exposure to IH and that the subsequent decrease in sensitivity occurred once this exposure was eliminated by treatment with continuous positive airway pressure. In contrast, the results regarding changes in apneic threshold are more equivocal with decreases reported in animals after AIH [38] and no alterations reported in humans [2, 32, 41, 52].

7.3.2.4 Detrimental Outcome Measures in Humans After Exposure to Intermittent Hypoxia

Individuals with sleep apnea are exposed to IH over short (nightly) and long periods of time (repeated nightly exposure over days, months, and years). Thus, examining outcome measures over these time periods might provide clues as to whether or not exposure to IH has a beneficial or detrimental impact on breathing stability. Findings to date suggest that the impact may be predominantly detrimental since clinical studies have revealed that apnea number [23, 69] and duration [12, 13, 69] increase throughout the night independent of other factors (i.e., sleep stage, circadian rhythms) that could be responsible for this phenomenon. Whether or not upper airway muscle fatigue, or disfacilitation of LTF_{ua} and vLTF via hypocapnia induced by PA, played a role in promoting apnea severity in these studies is speculative since these forms of plasticity were not quantified.

Some clinical studies have also examined whether or not apnea severity increases with age, which potentially addresses the impact that long-term exposure to IH has on apnea severity [3, 34, 58, 76]. These studies were cross-sectional in nature; thus, establishing direct physiological links between exposure to IH and apnea severity were difficult given the myriad of physiological alterations that could impact on apnea severity during the aging process. Nevertheless, published results have revealed that apnea severity increases with age in both individuals that suffer from obesity and other comorbidities linked to sleep apnea [58, 76], as well as nonobese individuals without symptoms or signs of obstructive sleep apnea [58]. It was intriguing to note that age was negatively correlated to minimum oxygen saturation in those individuals without signs of symptoms associated with sleep apnea [58], suggesting that exposure to hypoxia might be responsible in part for the increase in apnea severity that was reported with age. Nonetheless, additional studies are required to establish whether or not short or long-term exposure to hypoxia is directly responsible for the increase in apnea severity that has been linked with age.

In contrast to these indirect findings, two studies have shown directly that exposure to IH can lead to increases in the apnea/hypopnea index. Tamisier and colleagues showed that exposure to IH for 8 h each night over a 2-week period resulted in a significant increase in central hypopneas in healthy individuals [71], although this finding must be considered carefully given the nature of the paradigm that was employed (i.e., participants were exposed to sustained hypoxia for 8 h and cyclic reoxygenation occurred for 15 s every 2 min) and the type of hypopneas observed (most hypopneas were not spontaneous but rather occurred upon reoxygenation). Nevertheless, we also showed recently that exposure to 12 episodes of hypoxia during wakefulness, that were 4 min in duration, led to increases in the apnea/hypopnea index during a sleep study completed by young males with moderate sleep apnea immediately after exposure. This finding was replicated after daily exposure to the protocol for 10 days, although the increase in apnea severity was not as great on the tenth day compared to the initial day (see Sect. 7.3.1.4 for further discussion of this finding). Interestingly, a significant correlation between the magnitude of the hypoxic ventilatory response during exposure to IH and apnea severity during sleep was evident, while the magnitude of vLTF was not correlated with the apnea/hypopnea index.

Conclusion

The impact of IH on breathing stability is likely a consequence of the complex interaction between LTF_{ua}, vLTF, and alterations in ventilatory sensitivity and the apneic threshold that contribute to PA. Consequently, final outcome measures (e.g., breathing stability) are likely dependent on which forms of plasticity (i.e., beneficial vs. detrimental) predominate. Presently, the literature suggests that if respiratory plasticity is initiated during sleep, the outcome is primarily detrimental at least on an acute basis. Thus, alterations in chemoreflex properties associated with PA appear to override any beneficial effects that vLTF and LTF_{ua} may have on breathing stability. The conditions under which the beneficial forms of plasticity prevail remain to be determined. My laboratory has clearly shown that vLTF during wakefulness only manifests itself in the presence of carbon dioxide levels that are slightly above resting values [28, 41, 52]. Thus, vLTF, as well as LTF_{ua}, may be ineffective in reducing apnea severity during sleep in the presence of hypocapnia, which often is evident during repetitive apneic events. Perhaps, the maintenance of elevated carbon dioxide levels during sleep might not only ensure that carbon dioxide levels remain above the apneic threshold but will also ensure that both vLTF and LTF_{ua} contribute to the maintenance of breathing stability. Likewise, the predominance of beneficial forms of plasticity resulting in increases in breathing stability might prevail under other conditions related to the duration (i.e., exposure over a single night vs. repeated daily exposure over days, months, or years) and intensity of exposure to hypoxia, as well as the age and sex of a given individual. However, further work is required to establish if beneficial forms of plasticity predominate under specific physiological constraints. Thus, these issues must be considered in future studies in order to fully explore the potential impact of IH and respiratory plasticity on breathing stability.

Acknowledgments This work was supported by a grant from the National Heart, Lung, and Blood Institute and a VA Merit Award.

References

1. Aboubakr SE, Taylor A, Ford R, et al. Long-term facilitation in obstructive sleep apnea patients during NREM sleep. J Appl Physiol. 2001;91:2751–7.
2. Ahuja D, Mateika JH, Diamond MP, et al. Ventilatory sensitivity to carbon dioxide before and after episodic hypoxia in women treated with testosterone. J Appl Physiol. 2007;102:1832–8.
3. Ancoli-Israel S, Kripke DF, Klauber MR, et al. Sleep-disordered breathing in community-dwelling elderly. Sleep. 1991;14:486–95.
4. Babcock MA, Badr MS. Long-term facilitation of ventilation in humans during NREM sleep. Sleep. 1998;21:709–16.
5. Bach KB, Mitchell GS. Hypoxia-induced long-term facilitation of respiratory activity is serotonin dependent. Respir Physiol. 1996;104:251–60.
6. Badr MS. Effect of ventilatory drive on upper airway patency in humans during NREM sleep. Respir Physiol. 1996;103:1–10.
7. Badr MS, Kawak A, Skatrud JB, et al. Effect of induced hypocapnic hypopnea on upper airway patency in humans during NREM sleep. Respir Physiol. 1997;110:33–45.
8. Badr MS, Toiber F, Skatrud JB, et al. Pharyngeal narrowing/occlusion during central sleep apnea. J Appl Physiol. 1995;78:1806–15.
9. Baker-Herman TL, Bavis RW, Dahlberg JM, et al. Differential expression of respiratory long-term facilitation among inbred rat strains. Respir Physiol Neurobiol. 2010;170:260–7.
10. Behan M, Zabka AG, Thomas CF, et al. Sex steroid hormones and the neural control of breathing. Respir Physiol Neurobiol. 2003;136:249–63.
11. Bradford A, McGuire M, O'Halloran KD. Does episodic hypoxia affect upper airway dilator muscle function? Implications for the pathophysiology of obstructive sleep apnoea. Respir Physiol Neurobiol. 2005;147:223–34.
12. Cala SJ, Sliwinski P, Cosio MG, et al. Effect of topical upper airway anesthesia on apnea duration through the night in obstructive sleep apnea. J Appl Physiol. 1996;81:2618–26.
13. Charbonneau M, Marin JM, Olha A, et al. Changes in obstructive sleep apnea characteristics through the night. Chest. 1994;106:1695–701.
14. Chowdhuri S, Pierchala L, Aboubakr SE, et al. Long-term facilitation of genioglossus activity is present in normal humans during NREM sleep. Respir Physiol Neurobiol. 2008;160:65–75.
15. Chowdhuri S, Shanidze I, Pierchala L, et al. Effect of episodic hypoxia on the susceptibility to hypocapnic central apnea during NREM sleep. J Appl Physiol. 2010;108:369–77.
16. Dale-Nagle EA, Hoffman MS, Macfarlane PM, et al. Spinal plasticity following intermittent hypoxia: implications for spinal injury. Ann N Y Acad Sci. 2010;1198:252–9.
17. Dempsey JA. Crossing the apnoeic threshold: causes and consequences. Exp Physiol. 2005;90:13–24.
18. Dempsey JA, Smith CA, Przybylowski T, et al. The ventilatory responsiveness to CO_2 below eupnoea as a determinant of ventilatory stability in sleep. J Physiol. 2004;560:1–11.

19. Dempsey JA, Veasey SC, Morgan BJ, et al. Pathophysiology of sleep apnea. Physiol Rev. 2010;90:47–112.
20. Duffin J. The role of the central chemoreceptors: a modeling perspective. Respir Physiol Neurobiol. 2010;173:230–43.
21. Duffin J. Measuring the ventilatory response to hypoxia. J Physiol. 2007;584:285–93.
22. Duffin J, Mohan RM, Vasiliou P, et al. A model of the chemoreflex control of breathing in humans: model parameters measurement. Respir Physiol. 2000;120:13–26.
23. Fanfulla F, Patruno V, Bruschi C, et al. Obstructive sleep apnoea syndrome: is the "half-night polysomnography" an adequate method for evaluating sleep profile and respiratory events? Eur Respir J. 1997;10:1725–9.
24. Foster GE, McKenzie DC, Milsom WK, et al. Effects of two protocols of intermittent hypoxia on human ventilatory, cardiovascular and cerebral responses to hypoxia. J Physiol. 2005;567:689–99.
25. Fuller DD. Episodic hypoxia induces long-term facilitation of neural drive to tongue protrudor and retractor muscles. J Appl Physiol. 2005;98:1761–7.
26. Fuller DD, Baker TL, Behan M, et al. Expression of hypoglossal long-term facilitation differs between substrains of Sprague–Dawley rat. Physiol Genomics. 2001;4:175–81.
27. Gerst III DG, Yokhana SS, Carney LM, et al. The hypoxic ventilatory response and ventilatory long-term facilitation are altered by time of day and repeated daily exposure to intermittent hypoxia. J Appl Physiol. 2011;110:15–28.
28. Harris DP, Balasubramaniam A, Badr MS, et al. Long-term facilitation of ventilation and genioglossus muscle activity is evident in the presence of elevated levels of carbon dioxide in awake humans. Am J Physiol Regul Integr Comp Physiol. 2006;291:R1111–9.
29. Hudgel DW, Chapman KR, Faulks C, et al. Changes in inspiratory muscle electrical activity and upper airway resistance during periodic breathing induced by hypoxia during sleep. Am Rev Respir Dis. 1987;135:899–906.
30. Jordan AS, Catcheside PG, O'Donoghue FJ, et al. Long-term facilitation of ventilation is not present during wakefulness in healthy men or women. J Appl Physiol. 2002;93:2129–36.
31. Katayama K, Smith CA, Henderson KS, et al. Chronic intermittent hypoxia increases the CO_2 reserve in sleeping dogs. J Appl Physiol. 2007;103:1942–9.
32. Khodadadeh B, Badr MS, Mateika JH. The ventilatory response to carbon dioxide and sustained hypoxia is enhanced after episodic hypoxia in OSA patients. Respir Physiol Neurobiol. 2006;150: 122–34.
33. Koehle MS, Sheel AW, Milsom WK, et al. Two patterns of daily hypoxic exposure and their effects on measures of chemosensitivity in humans. J Appl Physiol. 2007;103:1973–8.
34. Lavie P. Incidence of sleep apnea in a presumably healthy working population: a significant relationship with excessive daytime sleepiness. Sleep. 1983;6:312–8.
35. Lee DS, Badr MS, Mateika JH. Progressive augmentation and ventilatory long-term facilitation are enhanced in sleep apnoea patients and are mitigated by antioxidant administration. J Physiol. 2009; 587:5451–67.
36. Ling L, Fuller DD, Bach KB, et al. Chronic intermittent hypoxia elicits serotonin-dependent plasticity in the central neural control of breathing. J Neurosci. 2001;21:5381–8.
37. Lusina SJ, Kennedy PM, Inglis JT, et al. Long-term intermittent hypoxia increases sympathetic activity and chemosensitivity during acute hypoxia in humans. J Physiol. 2006;575:961–70.
38. Mahamed S, Mitchell GS. Respiratory long-term facilitation: too much or too little of a good thing? Adv Exp Med Biol. 2008; 605:224–7.
39. Mahamed S, Mitchell GS. Is there a link between intermittent hypoxia-induced respiratory plasticity and obstructive sleep apnoea? Exp Physiol. 2007;92:27–37.
40. Mateika JH, Fregosi RF. Long-term facilitation of upper airway muscle activities in vagotomized and vagally intact cats. J Appl Physiol. 1997;82:419–25.
41. Mateika JH, Mendello C, Obeid D, et al. Peripheral chemoreflex responsiveness is increased at elevated levels of carbon dioxide after episodic hypoxia in awake humans. J Appl Physiol. 2004;96:1197–205.
42. Mateika JH, Millrood DL, Kim J, et al. Response of human tongue protrudor and retractors to hypoxia and hypercapnia. Am J Respir Crit Care Med. 1999;160:1976–82.
43. Mateika JH, Narwani G. Intermittent hypoxia and respiratory plasticity in humans and other animals: does exposure to intermittent hypoxia promote or mitigate sleep apnoea? Exp Physiol. 2009;94:279–96.
44. McEvoy RD, Popovic RM, Saunders NA, et al. Effects of sustained and repetitive isocapnic hypoxia on ventilation and genioglossal and diaphragmatic EMGs. J Appl Physiol. 1996;81:866–75.
45. McGuire M, Ling L. Ventilatory long-term facilitation is greater in 1- vs. 2-mo-old awake rats. J Appl Physiol. 2005;98:1195–201.
46. McGuire M, MacDermott M, Bradford A. The effects of chronic episodic hypercapnic hypoxia on rat upper airway muscle contractile properties and fiber-type distribution. Chest. 2002;122:1400–6.
47. McGuire M, Zhang Y, White DP, et al. Chronic intermittent hypoxia enhances ventilatory long-term facilitation in awake rats. J Appl Physiol. 2003;95:1499–508.
48. McKay LC, Janczewski WA, Feldman JL. Episodic hypoxia evokes long-term facilitation of genioglossus muscle activity in neonatal rats. J Physiol. 2004;557:13–8.
49. Millhorn DE, Eldridge FL, Waldrop TG. Prolonged stimulation of respiration by a new central neural mechanism. Respir Physiol. 1980;41:87–103.
50. Mitchell GS, Baker TL, Nanda SA, et al. Invited review: intermittent hypoxia and respiratory plasticity. J Appl Physiol. 2001;90: 2466–75.
51. Mitchell GS, Johnson SM. Neuroplasticity in respiratory motor control. J Appl Physiol. 2003;94:358–74.
52. Morelli C, Badr MS, Mateika JH. Ventilatory responses to carbon dioxide at low and high levels of oxygen are elevated after episodic hypoxia in men compared with women. J Appl Physiol. 2004;97: 1673–80.
53. Morris KF, Baekey DM, Shannon R, et al. Respiratory neural activity during long-term facilitation. Respir Physiol. 2000;121: 119–33.
54. Morris KF, Gozal D. Persistent respiratory changes following intermittent hypoxic stimulation in cats and human beings. Respir Physiol Neurobiol. 2004;140:1–8.
55. Nakamura A, Olson Jr EB, Terada J, et al. Sleep state dependence of ventilatory long-term facilitation following acute intermittent hypoxia in Lewis rats. J Appl Physiol. 2010;109:323–31.
56. Olson Jr EB, Bohne CJ, Dwinell MR, et al. Ventilatory long-term facilitation in unanesthetized rats. J Appl Physiol. 2001;91:709–16.
57. Onal E, Burrows DL, Hart RH, et al. Induction of periodic breathing during sleep causes upper airway obstruction in humans. J Appl Physiol. 1986;61:1438–43.
58. Pavlova MK, Duffy JF, Shea SA. Polysomnographic respiratory abnormalities in asymptomatic individuals. Sleep. 2008;31:241–8.
59. Peng YJ, Overholt JL, Kline D, et al. Induction of sensory long-term facilitation in the carotid body by intermittent hypoxia: implications for recurrent apneas. Proc Natl Acad Sci USA. 2003;100: 10073–8.
60. Peng YJ, Prabhakar NR. Reactive oxygen species in the plasticity of respiratory behavior elicited by chronic intermittent hypoxia. J Appl Physiol. 2003;94:2342–9.
61. Peng YJ, Yuan G, Ramakrishnan D, et al. Heterozygous HIF-1alpha deficiency impairs carotid body-mediated systemic responses and reactive oxygen species generation in mice exposed to intermittent hypoxia. J Physiol. 2006;577:705–16.

62. Pialoux V, Hanly PJ, Foster GE, et al. Effects of exposure to intermittent hypoxia on oxidative stress and acute hypoxic ventilatory response in humans. Am J Respir Crit Care Med. 2009;180: 1002–9.
63. Pierchala LA, Mohammed AS, Grullon K, et al. Ventilatory long-term facilitation in non-snoring subjects during NREM sleep. Respir Physiol Neurobiol. 2008;160:259–66.
64. Powell FL, Milsom WK, Mitchell GS. Time domains of the hypoxic ventilatory response. Respir Physiol. 1998;112:123–34.
65. Ray AD, Magalang UJ, Michlin CP, et al. Intermittent hypoxia reduces upper airway stability in lean but not obese Zucker rats. Am J Physiol Regul Integr Comp Physiol. 2007;293:R372–8.
66. Reite M, Jackson D, Cahoon RL, et al. Sleep physiology at high altitude. Electroencephalogr Clin Neurophysiol. 1975;38:463–71.
67. Salloum A, Rowley JA, Mateika JH, et al. Increased propensity for central apnea in patients with obstructive sleep apnea: effect of nasal continuous positive airway pressure. Am J Respir Crit Care Med. 2010;181:189–93.
68. Serebrovskaya TV, Swanson RJ, Karaban IN, et al. Intermittent hypoxia alters hypoxic ventilatory responses. Fiziol Zh. 1999;45: 9–18.
69. Sforza E, Krieger J, Petiau C. Nocturnal evolution of respiratory effort in obstructive sleep apnoea syndrome: influence on arousal threshold. Eur Respir J. 1998;12:1257–63.
70. Shkoukani M, Babcock MA, Badr MS. Effect of episodic hypoxia on upper airway mechanics in humans during NREM sleep. J Appl Physiol. 2002;92:2565–70.
71. Tamisier R, Gilmartin GS, Launois SH, et al. A new model of chronic intermittent hypoxia in humans: effect on ventilation, sleep, and blood pressure. J Appl Physiol. 2009;107:17–24.
72. Teppema LJ, Dahan A. The ventilatory response to hypoxia in mammals: mechanisms, measurement, and analysis. Physiol Rev. 2010;90:675–754.
73. Terada J, Nakamura A, Zhang W, et al. Ventilatory long-term facilitation in mice can be observed during both sleep and wake periods and depends on orexin. J Appl Physiol. 2008;104:499–507.
74. Veasey SC, Zhan G, Fenik P, et al. Long-term intermittent hypoxia: reduced excitatory hypoglossal nerve output. Am J Respir Crit Care Med. 2004;170:665–72.
75. White DP. Pathogenesis of obstructive and central sleep apnea. Am J Respir Crit Care Med. 2005;172:1363–70.
76. Young T, Palta M, Dempsey J, et al. The occurrence of sleep-disordered breathing among middle-aged adults. N Engl J Med. 1993; 328:1230–5.
77. Zabka AG, Behan M, Mitchell GS. Long term facilitation of respiratory motor output decreases with age in male rats. J Physiol. 2001;531:509–14.
78. Zabka AG, Mitchell GS, Behan M. Ageing and gonadectomy have similar effects on hypoglossal long-term facilitation in male Fischer rats. J Physiol. 2005;563:557–68.
79. Zabka AG, Mitchell GS, Olson Jr EB, et al. Selected contribution: chronic intermittent hypoxia enhances respiratory long-term facilitation in geriatric female rats. J Appl Physiol. 2003;95: 2614–23.

Activation of Inflammatory Circulating Factors by Intermittent Hypoxia in Sleep Apnea Syndrome

8

Larissa Dyugovskaya and Andrey Polyakov

Abstract
Obstructive sleep apnea syndrome (OSAS), characterized by intermittent and recurrent pauses in respiration during sleep, constitutes an independent risk factor for cardiovascular morbidity. Intermittent hypoxia (IH) is the hallmark of OSAS. A large number of clinical studies, cell culture, and animal models utilizing IH delineate the central role of oxidative stress in OSAS. These facilitate increased interactions of blood leukocytes with endothelial cells, resulting in endothelial injury and dysfunction. Such events can promote the development of cardiovascular morbidities in OSAS. IH can activate several global signaling pathways and various transcription factors such as nuclear factor κB and hypoxia-inducible factor 1α, which play a key role in mediating the inflammatory and cardiovascular consequences in OSAS. This chapter summarized the current literature and our own data on phenotype, functional changes, and inflammatory responses of various blood cells exposed to IH in vivo and in vitro. We focus on the causal relationships between IH and atherogenic transformation of monocytes, lymphocytes, and neutrophils in OSAS patients and on the molecular mechanisms of the cell dysfunctions developed under IH conditions.

Abbreviations

OSAS	Obstructive sleep apnea syndrome
IH	Intermittent hypoxia
nCPAP	Nasal continuous positive air pressure
HIF	Hypoxia-inducible factor
AHI	Apnea-hypopnea index
ROS	Reactive oxygen species
ECs	Endothelial cells
EPO	Erythropoietin
VEGF	Vascular endothelial growth factor
MAPK	Mitogen-activated protein kinase
ERK	Extracellular signal-regulated kinase
DCs	Dendritic cells
Ox-LDL	Oxidized low-density lipoprotein
PMA	Phorbol myristate acetate
HUVEC	Human umbilical vein endothelial cells
HCAEC	Human coronary artery endothelial cells
NA	Neutrophil apoptosis
IHD	Ischemic heart disease
TNF	Tumor necrotic factor

L. Dyugovskaya (✉) • A. Polyakov
The Lloyd Rigler Sleep Apnea Research Laboratory, Unit of Anatomy and Cell Biology, The Bruce Rappaport Faculty of Medicine, Technion-Israel Institute of Technology, Haifa, Israel
e-mail: larissa@tx.technion.ac.il

8.1 Introduction

Sleep-disordered breathing is a widespread phenomenon detected during sleep in at least 24% of adult males and 9% of adult females [99, 190]. In 4% of adult men and 2% of adult women, recurrent pauses in respiration during sleep are accompanied by characteristic symptoms, such as excessive daytime sleepiness, chronic fatigue, or neurocognitive decline [190], an association that defines the obstructive

L. Xi, T.V. Serebrovskaya (eds.), *Intermittent Hypoxia and Human Diseases*,
DOI 10.1007/978-1-4471-2906-6_8, © Springer-Verlag London 2012

sleep apnea syndrome (OSAS) [88]. The syndrome is also associated with male gender, smoking, obesity, and a postmenopausal status in women [190]. Intermittent hypoxia (IH), which results from a cyclic fall in oxygen saturation, due to repetitive airway occlusions during sleep, is one of the main features of OSAS [2, 21, 81, 88, 138].

The most common criteria of OSAS severity is the apnea-hypopnea index (AHI), which denotes the number of apneic and/or hypopneic events per hour of sleep and the percent sleep time patients spend below 90% arterial oxyhemoglobin saturation [99, 190]. Apneas are complete cessations of breathing for at least 10 s duration, and hypopneas are partial cessations for the same duration. These intermittent breathing arrests during sleep are considered analogous to repetitive hypoxia/reperfusion injury [80, 82, 122]. Continuous IH can be reproduced in animal models in rats [12, 20, 47, 78, 196] and mice [27, 131, 137, 174, 183, 193, 194] as well as in cell culture systems to investigate fundamental mechanisms [146, 147, 191].

It is now well documented that OSAS is strongly associated with increased cardiovascular morbidity and mortality [81, 102, 122, 126, 157, 164] and even constitutes an independent risk factor for cardiovascular pathology [106, 127]. It makes OSAS a public health problem [86]. Moreover, OSAS patients without overt cardiovascular diseases showed subclinical signs of atherosclerosis both on the structure (increased intima-media thickness, arterial plaque formation, calcified artery atheromas) [5, 31, 49, 66, 111] and functional (endothelial dysfunction) levels [65, 73]. The last one is a key component of atherogenesis and a predictor of future cardiovascular morbidity [3, 86]. During the last few years, there has been a fundamental challenge in understanding the underlying mechanisms responsible for the development of cardiovascular pathology in OSAS patients. One of these mechanisms is increased oxidative stress due to chronic IH [70, 80, 82, 83, 164, 185], evidence of which in OSAS was shown both in plasma and in various types of cells [7, 35, 89, 155]. It was demonstrated that OSAS directly affects the vascular endothelium by promoting oxidative stress and inflammation while decreasing NO bioavailability and repair capacity [67]. Rodent models of IH reinforce and expand these findings by showing increased oxidative stress with activation of NADPH oxidase in tissues such as the brain, carotid bodies, myocardium, and the liver [20, 71, 78, 130, 193].

Oxidative stress results in an imbalance between oxidant-producing systems and antioxidant defense mechanisms, resulting in excessive formation of reactive oxygen species (ROS). Normally, this is a tightly regulated balance to maintain homeostasis (redox balance), and at low levels, ROS molecules participate in essential physiologic signaling functions. However, excess ROS mediate cellular damage by functionally modifying various cell structures such as membranes, lipids, proteins, and DNA [32, 82, 86, 171]. IH, which triggers mitochondrial dysfunctions, results in increased ROS formation [129]. In OSAS as well, mitochondrial dysfunction and changes in cytochrome oxidase redox state during the obstructive apneas support increased ROS production from mitochondria [104]. Other sources include various ROS-producing enzymes such as xanthine oxidase, endothelial NO synthase, and NADPH oxidase from primed endothelial cells (ECs) and leukocytes [80]. In parallel, decreased antioxidant capacities were also reported in OSAS [6, 22, 89], further disrupting the tightly regulated cellular oxidation-reduction (redox) state.

Apart from their injurious nature, ROS molecules are also key activators of redox-sensitive gene expression via control of numerous redox-sensitive transcription factors, contributing to the expression of various inflammatory cytokines, chemokines, growth factors, and adhesion molecules [159] and thus eliciting either inflammatory or adaptive mechanisms. Of these, as shown in Fig. 8.1a, nuclear factor (NF)-κB activates inflammatory signaling pathways, whereas hypoxia-inducible factor (HIF)-1α activates downstream genes adaptive to hypoxia [32, 82, 171]. It is proposed that NF-κB is more sensitive to activation by IH than SH and conversely that HIF-1α is more sensitive to activation by SH than IH [147], however possibly is dependent on the target cells and experimental conditions because the hypoxia-induced activations of transcription factors are highly cell-type-specific dependent. Furthermore, there is an extensive degree of crosstalk occurring between NF-κB and HIF-1α [17]. Thus, it was reported that NF-κB links innate immunity to the hypoxic response through transcriptional regulation of HIF-1α, and HIF-1α, in turn, activates NF-κB [144].

NF-κB is a family of proteins involved in the regulation of genes related to innate immunity, inflammation, and apoptosis. IH-mediated NF-κB activation may be an important mechanism linking OSAS and multiple cardiovascular disorders [54, 182] since it initiates inflammatory pathways and orchestrates the production of adhesion molecules and inflammatory cytokines [186]. Upregulation of NF-κB was demonstrated in neutrophils and monocytes of OSAS patients [61, 186], in cardiovascular tissues exposed to chronic IH in vivo [54], and in an in vitro model of HeLa cells [147] or neutrophils of healthy subjects treated with IH [40].

HIF-1α is another transcription factor with potentially important implications to OSAS and associated comorbidities. HIF-1α is a global regulator of oxygen homeostasis that controls hundreds of target genes, including those encoding erythropoietin (EPO), vascular endothelial growth factor (VEGF), endothelin-1, and other proteins affecting glycolysis and energy metabolism [156]. It was found that mice deficient in HIF-1α and treated by chronic IH did not increase blood pressure and oxidative stress [131]. Also, HIF-1α-deficient T lymphocytes produced more pro-inflammatory

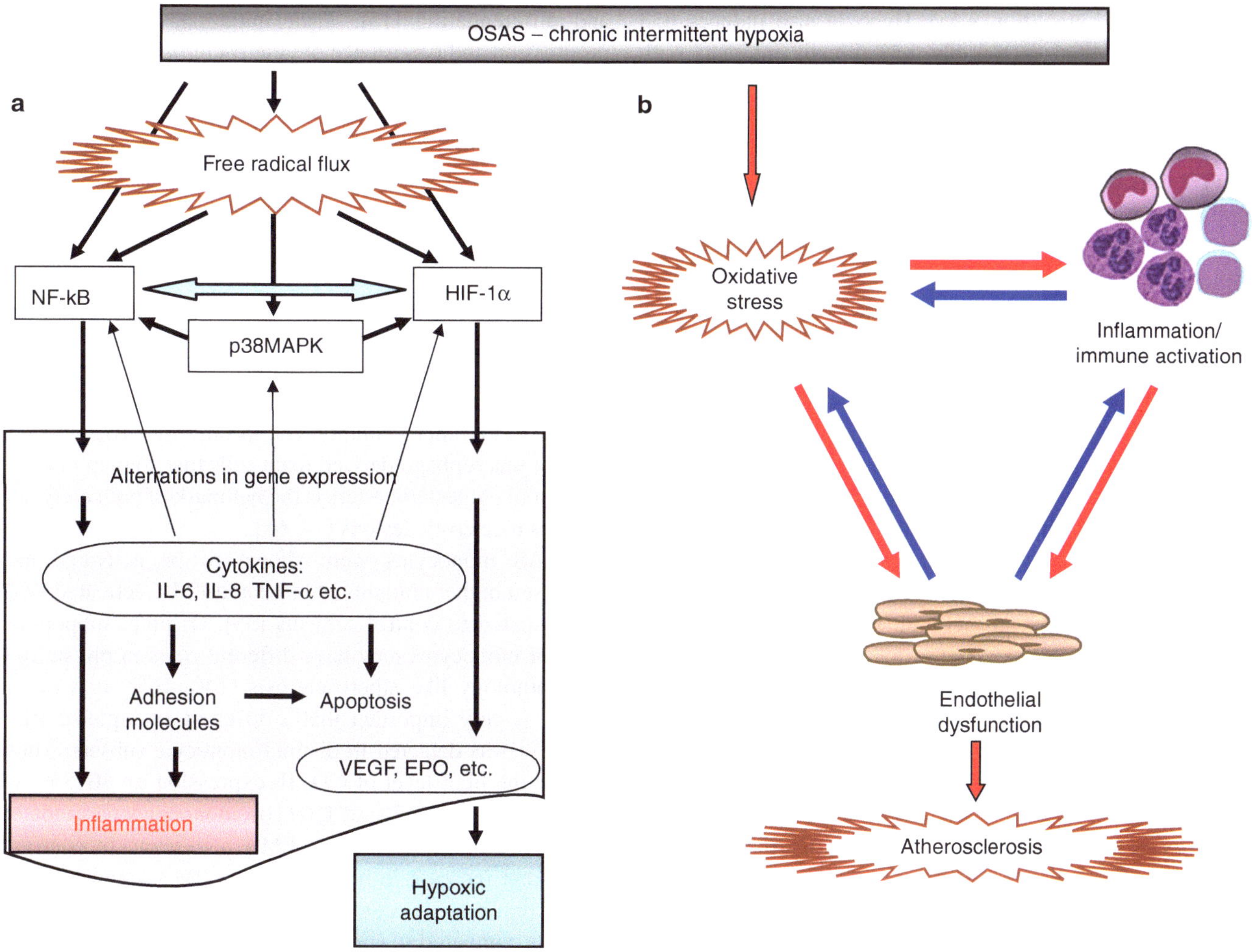

Fig. 8.1 Schematic illustration of the various molecular pathways that can be activated by IH in OSAS patients and lead to cardiovascular diseases. (**a**) Chronic IH activates both HIF-1α and NF-κB via ROS-dependent and ROS-independent pathways. NF-κB activates inflammatory signaling pathways with downstream products including TNF-α, IL-6, IL-8, adhesion molecules etc., whereas HIF-1α induces transcription of genes adaptive to hypoxia and primarily involved in glycolysis and angiogenesis (production of vascular endothelial growth factor (*VEGF*), erythropoietin (*EPO*), etc.). There is crosstalk between these two pathways: NF-κB upregulates HIF-1α through transcriptional upregulation; also, basal NF-κB is a prerequisite for constitutive HIF-1α expression. Additionally, IH can activate both HIF-1α and NF-κB via activation of p38MAPK. Nuclear transcription factors are also activated by variety of cytokines (*thin arrows*) which, in turn, can be directly regulated by IH. (**b**) We proposed that chronic IH experienced nightly by OSAS patients promotes oxidative stress which could affect ECs and the circulating inflammatory cells (such as monocytes, neutrophils, and lymphocytes) that may contribute to endothelial dysfunction and thus accentuate atherogenic processes in OSAS. Cytokines, released by activated ECs can, in turn, activate leukocytes and by that further exaggerate inflammation

cytokines compared with HIF-1α-expressing T cells [98]. On the possible adaptive role of HIF-1α in OSAS, see [85]. Interestingly, HIF-1α was also shown to exert pro-inflammatory activity by affecting inflammatory functions of monocytes/macrophages and neutrophils such as infiltration and activation in vivo [24]. Induction of the HIF-1α was documented in rodents exposed to chronic IH [12, 156] and in experimental models of IH in tissue culture. However HIF-1α accumulation in PCI2 cells was found to be regulated by NADPH oxidase [192]; in contrast, HIF-1α phosphorylation in ECs was found to be unaffected by antioxidants [169]. Also, there is a data that endogenously produced ROS do not mediate NF-κB activation [23]. So depending on the type of cells and the experimental approach, apart from being activated by oxidative stress, nuclear transcription factors may also be activated by a variety of ROS-independent signals. Interestingly, IH in vitro was shown to activate the NF-κB at least partially via activation of p38MAPK by an IκB kinase-dependent manner [146]. Furthermore, HIF-1 is a substrate for various kinase pathways including PI-3K/Akt or ERK and p38MAPK [109] which, in turn, can be regulated by IH directly or via production of growth factors, cytokines, and etc. (Fig. 8.1a). Hypoxia also induces p53 protein accumulation. Notably, p53 directly interacts with HIF-1α and limits hypoxia-induced expression of HIF-1α by promoting ubiquitination and proteasomal degradation under hypoxic conditions.

The role of other transcription factors activated by redox imbalance (activator protein (AP)-1, SREBPs, and GATA), which can be implicated in pathogenesis of OSAS and comorbidities, is discussed in [86].

We postulated that the hypoxemia experienced nightly by OSAS patients could affect the circulating inflammatory cells such as monocytes, neutrophils, and lymphocytes that may contribute to and accentuate atherogenic processes in OSAS (Fig. 8.1b). This review summarized the current literature and our own data on phenotype, functional changes, and inflammatory responses of various human blood cells exposed to IH in vivo (OSAS patients) and in vitro. Much attention has been focused on the role of chronic IH, which can lead to harmful physiological outcomes, in contrast to acute IH, which can facilitate beneficial physiological adaptations [55].

8.2 Monocytes

Monocytes are highly versatile cells able to rapidly adapt to different environmental conditions and to express distinct functional programs in response to signals of various natures [26]. Extensive work has been carried out to characterize hypoxia-mediated changes in mononuclear phagocyte gene expression and functional properties, demonstrating that oxygen availability is a critical regulator of their functional behavior [15]. Monocytes function as a key component of the innate defense mechanisms, but they are also immunoregulatory cells endowed with immunostimulatory and immunosuppressory activities [125]. Extensive monocyte extravasation is an early event in the onset of inflammation, and of various diseases, in which they exhibit a tissue-specific range of functions including phagocytosis, antigen presentation to T cells, and release of a wide array of cytokines, chemokines, growth factors, enzymes, ROS, complement components, coagulation factors, and prostaglandins [26, 115, 142]. Moreover, it was found that peripheral blood "endothelial progenitor cells" are derived from monocytes and secrete angiogenic growth factor [141]. In addition to the secretion of growth factors, the ability of monocytes to differentiate into endothelial-like cells [45, 153] may further contribute to their angiogenic effects and direct involvement in neovascularization. Monocytes can be exposed to acute hypoxia upon migration to an inflammatory site, where they can develop into macrophages or dendritic cells (DCs), and here, chronic hypoxia may affect their gene expression and differentiation [15]. Their initiation, participation in progression and persistence of atherosclerosis, is well established [94, 95]. Although the recruitment of monocytes to the arterial wall and their subsequent differentiation into macrophages may initially serve as a protective function by removing cytotoxic Ox-LDL particles and apoptotic cells, progressive accumulation of macrophages and their uptake of Ox-LDL ultimately lead to the development of atherosclerotic lesions [53]. Macrophages ingest oxidized lipoproteins via scavenger receptors, and thus as lipid-rich foam cells, they become part of the physical bulk of the disease. They also secrete inflammatory mediators that stimulate smooth muscle cell migration and proliferation and participate in plaque development, rupture, and thrombosis. The development of macrophage-derived foam cells that contain massive amount of cholesterol esters is the hallmark of both early and late atherosclerotic lesions [14, 68].

OSAS monocytes were shown to be activated and expressed higher amounts of basal and PMA-activated ROS as compared to control subjects [35]. Of note, subpopulations of monocytes may have different roles in physiology and pathology like atherosclerosis [140, 165]. In view of this, it is very important that a different example of ROS response was detected in distinct monocyte subsets. Thus, despite the high level of CD11b expression on 80–85% of monocytes, only 2–7% of CD11b+ monocytes participated in oxidation at rest and after PMA activation. In contrast, significant increase in both basal and PMA-activated ROS production was detected in CD11c+ monocytes of OSAS patients compared to controls. Finally, although basal ROS production of CD64+ monocytes did not differ significantly between patients and control subjects, PMA stimulation of this subpopulation resulted in more than a fivefold increase in ROS production in OSAS vs. control subjects. These results point to the possibility that CD64+ monocytes of OSAS patients are pre-activated. FcγRI (CD64) mediates many cellular responses crucial in host defense, including phagocytosis, cell cytotoxicity, and production and secretion of pro-inflammatory cytokines such as IL-1, IL-6, and TNF-α [44, 150].

The first step of atherosclerosis is the recruitment of monocytes from peripheral blood into the intima of the vessel wall, wherein they differentiate into macrophages, take up Ox-LDL, and transform into foam cells. To promote migration of monocytes from the circulation to the inflamed area, it is essential to adhere to the vascular endothelium via adhesion molecules [19]. We found that apart from ROS production, OSAS monocytes are associated with increased expression of adhesion molecules such as CD11c (the b-subunits of the integrins and counterreceptors for ICAM-1 on ECs responsible for firm adhesion) and the CD15 (which is a carbohydrate complex on selectins). Also, treatment of monocytes from healthy individuals with hypoxia in vitro resulted in

Table 8.1 The distribution of the main leukocyte adhesion molecules, membrane markers, and adhesion indices (±SD) in fresh whole blood cells from OSAS and controls. The effects of nCPAP treatment

	Control	OSAS	nCPAP	Cited by
		Monocytes		
CD15 (%)	1.4±0.9	20.9±10.4[a]	7.0±4.0[b]	Dyugovskaya et al. [35]
CD11c (%)	25.5±12.5	71.2±22.7[a]	58.6±20.2[b]	The same
Adhesion index	5.2±1.80	9.8±4.9[a]	5.6±4.1[b]	The same
CD11c (%) participating in ROS production	57.8±10.8	72.6±19.9[a]	36.2±23.9[b]	The same
		Neutrophils		
CD15 (MFI)	1,048±370	1,484±470[a]	1,083±101[b]	Dyugovskaya et al. [38]
CD11c (%)	29.3±26.8	27.0±22.4	–	The same
CD62L (MFI)	48.3±14.7	112.3±22.0[a]	–	Lavie et al. [84]
Low-CD16 (%)apoptosis	2.8±0.9	1.0±0.6[a]	6.1±2.9[b]	Dyugovskaya et al. [38]
Superoxide (nmol/5 × 10^6 cells)	3.7±0.5	9.3±1.5[a]	–	Schulz et al. [155]
Total ROS (MFI)	1,079±355	1,482±358[a]	–	Lavie et al. [84]
		Lymphocytes		
γδ T cells/CD62L (%)	49.6±11	65.0±11.7[a]	–	Dyugovskaya et al. [36]
γδ T cells/NKB1	1.4±2.3	8.2±5.2[a]	–	The same
γδ T cells/CD56	42.0±17.8	55.9±17.4	–	The same
γδ T cells adhesion index	3.60±0.90	6.10±0.90[a]	–	The same
γδ T cells cytotoxicity	15±2.5	40±2.5[a]	–	The same
Ratio E/T 5:1				
CD8/CD40L (%)	3.4±2.5	14.4±10.5[a]	4.0±2.8[b]	Dyugovskaya et al. [37]
CD8/CD56 (%)	35.2±11.0	50.0±13.9[a]	40.7±15.2[b]	Dyugovskaya et al. [34]
CD8/NKB1 (%)	5.4±4.2	5.3±4.0	10.5±4.5[b]	The same
CD8/adhesion index	3.54±1.40	3.90±0.90	–	Lavie et al. [84]
CD8/cytotoxicity	41.1±6.4	71.1±7.0[a]	24.8±10.7[b]	Dyugovskaya et al. [34]
Ratio E/T 10:1				
CD4/CD28^{null} (%)	6.8±1.3	19.9±5.0[a]	–	Dyugovskaya et al. [37]
CD4/adhesion index	3.47±1.4	3.90±2.40	–	Lavie et al. [84]
CD4/cytotoxicity	13.5±8.0	31.96±16.8[a]	–	Dyugovskaya et al. [37]
Ratio E/T 20:1				

[a]Statistically significant between controls and OSAS
[b]Statistically significant between OSAS and OSAS treated with nCPAP; MFI – mean fluorescence intensity, denoting intensity of expression; % – the percentage of cells from the population, which express a specific molecule; ROS – reactive oxygen species. Adhesion index was determined on non-stimulated human umbilical vein endothelial cells (HUVECs) by ^{51}Cr-released assay. Cytotoxicity against non-stimulated HUVECs was determined by ^{51}Cr-released assay; *E/T* – effector/target ratio

upregulated CD15 expression, and subsequent exposure of these cells to reoxygenation further increased CD15 expression [35]. Accordingly, increased adhesion of OSAS monocytes was noted towards ECs of venous (HUVEC) and arterial origin (HCAEC). A summary of the main adhesion parameters in OSAS monocytes is depicted in Table 8.1. By utilizing antibodies that neutralize selectins (anti-CD62) and integrins (anti-CD54), adhesion of monocytes to ECs was attenuated to values comparable to controls [35]. The involvement of monocytes in atherogenesis in OSAS was further implicated by the observation that lipid uptake was increased in human macrophages that were treated with experimental IH in vitro [79]. Moreover, we found that the Ox-LDL-induced development of DCs in monocyte cultures was a 2.5-fold higher in OSAS patients compared to controls. Moreover, OSAS DCs were transformed into foam cells. The number of macrophage-derived foam cells was also higher in OSAS (Dyugovskaya et al. unpublished observations). Collectively, these finding demonstrate that OSAS monocytes exhibited a pro-atherogenic phenotype.

8.3 Neutrophils

Like monocytes, neutrophils are best known for their classical role as professional phagocytes. They are the most abundant leukocyte subpopulations, representing approximately 60% of all circulating leukocytes. They are short-lived (up to 24 h in the blood stream) cells that continuously undergo cell death by apoptosis. Apoptotic neutrophils can be recognized and removed by the specialized organs of the reticuloendothelial system (e.g., the spleen and the liver, which have a population of macrophages) in direct contact with flowing blood. Moreover, during the past few years, it was found that senescent neutrophils home back to the bone marrow in a CXCR4-dependent manner, where they are phagocytosed and destroyed by the stromal macrophages [50].

Neutrophil apoptosis (NA) is critical in protecting against tissue injury because NA limits their life span and in doing so protects surrounding tissues from their injurious compounds, i.e., ROS molecules, bactericidal proteins, lytic enzymes, and leukotrienes, which participate in inflammatory responses against invading microorganisms, foreign particles, or cellular debris [48]. Neutrophils are exposed to multiple signals and the balance between pro-apoptotic or pro-survival signals will determine their fate. Hypoxia and cytokines are of the most potent stimulants affecting NA. Neutrophils migrating to inflammatory sites are intrinsically well adapted to operate in hypoxic environments, and in contrast to other cells, hypoxia profoundly inhibits their rate of constitutive apoptosis [57, 93, 107, 178].

The key feature of neutrophil biology is their ability to express surface receptors, adhesion molecules, growth factors, inflammatory cytokines, and chemokines that modulate endothelial permeability [29] and affect endothelial and smooth muscle cell responses [139]. Contrary to the long-standing and widely accepted belief that neutrophils are of marginal relevance to atherosclerosis, evidence revealing a previously unappreciated role of neutrophils in the onset and progression of atherosclerosis is being accumulating [4]. Central to this program is the capability of neutrophils to communicate with neighboring immune and nonimmune cells, such as monocytes, T lymphocytes, and endothelial and dendritic cells [4, 29, 187]. Neutrophils were shown to infiltrate eroded or ruptured plaques obtained from patients with acute coronary syndromes [195] and to participate in the pathogenesis of lethal myocardial reperfusion [176]. Research in animal models indicates that neutrophils are present at various stages of atherosclerotic lesions and support their functional role in atherosclerosis [4]. Their involvement in amplifying cardiovascular morbidity was further established by depletion experiments which resulted in reduced myocardial infarct size and a protected myocardium [69, 76].

Investigating neutrophil life span, functions, and adhesive properties in OSAS patients (Table 8.1) revealed increased expression of ROS molecules and the selectin receptors (CD62 and CD15) [35, 155]. The upregulated CD15 expression was found OSAS severity dependent as attested by AHI. Interestingly, the expression of CD11b (Vishnevsky et al. unpublished observations) or CD11c was unaffected. This is not surprising given that adhesion of OSAS neutrophils to nonactivated ECs in vitro was also unaffected. The fact that selectins but not integrins of OSAS neutrophils were upregulated implies that the interactions involving binding and tethering with nonactivated ECs are increased but not the firm adhesion. Importantly, treatment of HUVECs with anoxia-reoxygenation leads to ROS-dependent increase in neutrophil adhesion to hypoxic HUVECs and surface expression of ICAM-1, P-selectin, and E-selectin on HUVECs correlated with cell adhesion [62]. So the possibility that in vivo-activated endothelium, due to IH and increased pro-inflammatory cytokine production, may result in exacerbated adhesiveness should be considered.

Together with increased expression of the selectin-CD15 adhesion molecules, delayed NA, a fundamental injury-limiting mechanism and a key event in the control of inflammation, was observed in OSAS. Moreover, NA was negatively correlated with CD15 expression. Notably, most neutrophil effector functions are performed in an adherent state, and selectin receptors were suggested to trigger these neutrophil functions. Furthermore, such suppressed NA may imply that the neutrophils/ECs interactions initiated by the selectins could be exacerbated and by that amplify the destructive potential of neutrophils towards the endothelium. Additionally, soluble P-selectin (sP-selectin) levels reported to be higher in OSAS patients were also negatively correlated with NA. This indicates an involvement of sP-selectin in the inhibition of NA in OSAS, which may further exacerbate neutrophil functions to injure the endothelium [38]. It should be also noted that AHI but not sleep fragmentation was identified as an independent predictor of NA. Similar to OSAS patients, decreased NA was obtained in neutrophils from healthy individuals exposed to experimental IH in vitro [38]. The last effects occurred via a caspase-3-controlled mechanism. Western blot analysis and confocal laser scanning microscopy showed that concomitantly to the survival effects, experimental IH was associated with upregulation of the anti-apoptotic protein Mcl-1 and downregulation of the pro-apoptotic Bax proteins. Moreover, IH prevented Bax redistribution to the mitochondria. Similarly in neutrophils of OSAS patients, Bax was distributed diffusely throughout the cytoplasm and was not co-localized with mitochondria [39]. We determined that IH activates several global signaling pathways in neutrophils and modifies NA by activating ERK1/2 and p38MAPK signaling, thereby inducing the stabilization and/or production of Mcl-1 and suppressing Bax redistribution to the mitochondria [39]. Additionally, IH-induced neutrophil survival is strongly associated with increased expression of survival protein IL-8, which, in turn, can be regulated via NF-κB and p38MAPK activation [39]. IL-8 was shown to increase neutrophil survival in a variety of experimental and clinical settings [33, 74].

Thus, together with increased ROS production and upregulated selectin expression, suppressed NA may promote endothelial injury in OSAS.

8.4 T Lymphocytes

It is now well documented that T cells play a significant role in plaque formation and in the development of acute coronary syndrome [58, 117, 162, 180]. T cells are among the first cells infiltrating the intima of arteries during the initial stages of atherosclerosis [43, 162], and their presence in the atherosclerotic plaques suggests a local immune response that may be directed against local antigens in plaque [158]. Of note, on activation, T cells may differentiate into effector cells with tissue-damaging potential or can secrete cytokines that may affect aspects of atherogenesis such as macrophage activation, ROS production, adhesion molecule expression, smooth muscle proliferation, and vascular contractility [177, 180]. Vascular ECs are important targets for both inflammatory cytokines, which are released by activated T cells, and for cytotoxic attack by T cells. Importantly, T cell-mediated activation of ECs may be induced by a contact-dependent manner and by that may induce EC damage via leukocyte infiltration [113]. Various lymphocyte subpopulations were shown to be prevalent in atherosclerotic lesions and to modulate atherosclerotic responses [162, 173]. There are two main distinct lineages of T cells, those expressing αβ T cell receptors (αβ TCR) and those expressing γδ T cell receptors (γδ TCR) [13, 59]. γδ T cells differ from αβ T cells with regard to tissue localization, antigen recognition, and role in inflammatory processes and tissue repair [13, 25]. Our interest in the γδ T cells originated from studies describing enhanced accumulation of these cells in atherosclerotic plaques [77, 181] and their unique migration and cytotoxic features. Thus, γδ T cells have the capacity to recognize the main pro-atherogenic antigens such as complex lipids and heat shock proteins and exhibit higher transmigratory ability through ECs than αβ CD4 and CD8 T lymphocytes [51, 136]. Moreover, in contrast to αβ T cells, they display major histocompatibility complex-unrestricted cytotoxicity against ECs [72]. Importantly, when activated, γδ T cells can induce endothelial permeability by a cytolitic process involving the participation of adhesion pathways via γδ T cells/ECs interactions [112]. Taken together, it led us to assume that they can contribute to EC damage in OSAS as well.

The various T cells expressing CD8, CD4, and γδ molecules were rigorously investigated in our laboratory in OSAS patients. Basically all T cells studied in OSAS express an activated and a cytotoxic phenotype. A summary of the main phenotypic and functional changes of these cells in OSAS is depicted in Table 8.1.

Despite the similar percentage of γδ T cells in the circulation in OSAS patients and controls, the number of γδ T cell clones which was detected in lymphocytes/HUVECs cocultures in the presence of IL-2/IL-7 cocktail was 3.8-fold higher in OSAS patients [36]. Since IL-7 is essential to the proliferation, survival, and differentiation of γδ T cells from T cell precursors [60, 63], it suggests an increase in γδ progenitor cells of OSAS patients. Moreover, this increased amount of γδ T cells observed at the sites of adhesion to ECs in culture may indicate increased accumulation of γδ T cells on the endothelium lining the blood vessels.

Assessment of γδ T cell phenotype and function revealed that expression of CD62L selectins (of the family of adhesion molecules which mediate capture and tethering) and adhesion of purified γδ T cells to nonactivated ECs were increased as compared to controls (Table 8.1). Moreover, pretreating HUVECs with antibodies against CD62E/CD62P, which block binding through selectin receptors, significantly inhibited the adhesion index of OSAS γδ T cells by 52.5%. Also, the cytotoxicity against ECs at ratio effector/target of 5:1 was 2.5-fold higher in OSAS than that for control subjects [36].

Due to the fact that there is a close association between cytotoxicity and expression of natural killer (NK) receptors [8], we examined their distributions on γδ T cells. Paradoxically, the percentage of γδ T cells expressing the inhibitory NKB1 molecules was significantly higher in OSAS patients compared to controls, even through the cytotoxicity of OSAS γδ T cells against HUVECS was increased (Table 8.1). Unlike NKB1, the percentage of γδ T cells bearing CD56 and CD16 NK receptors did not vary between OSAS and controls. In addition, depleting CD56-/CD16-bearing cells from γδ T cells resulted only in a minor decrease in HUVEC killing. Importantly, the higher avidity and cytotoxicity of OSAS γδ T cells were mainly attributed to the pro-inflammatory cytokine TNF-α since utilizing antibodies, which neutralize TNF-α, abolished the adhesion to and killing of HUVECs [36]. This data provides evidence for a potentially important pathway in which augmented TNF-α secretion at sites of γδ T cell adhesion may play a major role in injuring the endothelium. In accord with this course of events, we found an increase in the percentage of OSAS γδ T cells expressing TNF-α (see below).

Unlike in γδ T cells, adhesion of CD4 and CD8 T cells to ECs was unaffected by OSAS. However, preincubating HUVECs with OSAS but not control γδ T cells resulted in TNF-α-dependent increased adhesion of CD4 and CD8 lymphocytes to HUVECs by 2.7-fold.

The cytotoxicity towards HUVECs was expanded in CD8 of OSAS patients at ratio effector/target of 10:1. However, while EC killing by γδ T lymphocytes was primarily mediated by TNF-α, the cytotoxicity of CD8 T cells was directly depended on the presence of perforin and NK (CD56 and CD16) receptors, whose expression was significantly increased in OSAS CD8 T lymphocytes (see Table 8.1). Also, depletion of CD8 T cells co-expressing CD56 receptors and perforin greatly attenuated the cytotoxicity towards HUVECs [34]. Finally, CD8 T cells from OSAS patients expressed more than threefold of the CD40L compared to controls, which is an important T cell activation marker and implicated in T cell-mediated MHC-unrestricted cytotoxicity [151], and in activation of inflammatory cells in atherogenesis [103]. Importantly, in atherosclerotic lesions, more than 90% of DCs co-localized with T lymphocytes. These DCs clustering with T cell display high levels of CD40 [121], interaction of which with CD40L on T cells are essential for cell activation and stimulation of cytokine secretion (IL-8, IL-12, TNF-α) that may be further involved in atherogenesis.

A significant lysis of HUVECs was also noted for OSAS CD4 T cells but only at an effector/target ratio of 20:1 and with a large variability between subjects. This elevation of CD4-induced cytotoxicity in OSAS patients was due to 2.9-fold increase in CD4/CD28^{null} subsets (Table 8.1), which are distinct from classical CD4/CD28+ T cells, could be directly involved in plaque rupture, and are known to induce killing of ECs [97, 116, 154]. Thus, it should be noted that the strongest cytotoxicity against ECs cells was expressed by OSAS γδ T cells, CD8 cytotoxicity was somewhat lower, and that of CD4 T cells was the lowest. Yet each subpopulation employed different killing mechanisms to damage ECs.

Intracellular signals necessary to elicit T lymphocyte cytotoxicity are poorly understood. In OSAS however, increased cytotoxicity could result from changes in the surrounding oxygen tension. This possibility is strongly supported by the increase in lytic CD8 T lymphocytes during hypoxia in vitro [18]. Moreover, the killing abilities of CD8 T cells were found to be AHI-severity dependent [34]. Our data from the nCPAP-treated group further support this notion (see below). Another possibility that cannot be ignored is that inflammatory/immune activation of T cells is modulated by increased sympathetic activation and catecholamine release observed in OSAS patients [128]. Sympathetic activation can affect lymphocyte traffic, circulation, and proliferation and modulate their functional activities [41].

8.5 Cytokine Profile of OSAS Leukocytes

Various pro-inflammatory cytokines are affected by the redox state of the cells in which they are synthesized and actively modulate inflammatory responses. Unlike hormones, cytokines are not stored in glands as preformed molecules but are rapidly synthesized and secreted by different cells after stimulation. These multipurpose molecules regulate both the innate and adaptive immune system. Cytokines regulate macrophage activation via expression of scavenger receptors and secretion of metalloproteinases, modulate the proliferation of smooth muscle cells and the production of nitric oxide and apoptosis, and stimulate the activation of ECs, all of which are steps in the progression of atherosclerosis. Moreover, the altered cytokine balance can result in activated T cells and can lead to their differentiation into effector cells with tissue-damaging potential or with abilities to diminish inflammation. Evidently, once the inflammatory response is initiated, these cytokines can, in turn, activate NF-kB and by that can further exaggerate inflammation. The cytokines are known to be regulated by altered oxygen tension and high free radical production [56].

T cells exist in the functionally polarized populations depending on the cytokines they produced; T lymphocytes secreting type 1 cytokines (IL-2 and IFN-γ) and those secreting type 2 cytokines IL-4 (but also IL-5, IL-6, and IL-10). Importantly, Th1 cells are implicated in cardiovascular disease [160]. Based on the ratios of IL-2/IL-4, CD4 and CD8 T cells of OSAS patients without any comorbidity had increased percentage of IL-4-expressing cells than IL-2. This shift towards type 2 dominance may represent a compensatory response of the CD8 and CD4 T cells to protect from other inflammatory cells or exacerbated pro-inflammatory responses. Critically, most of OSAS patients with hypertension and ischemic heart disease (IHD) exhibited a favor of type 1. The role of IL-4 in atherogenesis is equivocal, and it may vary with the stage of disease [177]. For example, IL-4 may participate in the progression of early "inflammatory" atherosclerotic lesions [52] inducing the upregulation of P-selectin [75] and 15-lipoxygenase [91] by ECs. On the other hand, IL-4 has also been shown as an anti-atherogenic cytokine, which inhibits smooth muscle cell proliferation and macrophage adhesiveness [42]. Finally, IL-4 has pro-angiogenic properties under hypoxic conditions via the VEGF pathway [184] and can induce the differentiation of monocytes into DCs [145].

Besides the definition of type 1 and type 2, the cytokines could be also classified as pro-inflammatory and anti-inflammatory [101]. TNF-α is a pivotal cytokine in the inflammatory cascade which is directly involved in the initiation and progression of cardiovascular diseases, via effects on lipid metabolism, coagulation, insulin resistance, and endothelial function [46, 105, 143, 148, 177]. TNF-α is capable of inducing oxidative stress, expression of adhesion molecules, and stimulating cytokine production via NF-κB-dependent pathways. IL-10 is a potent inhibitor of pro-inflammatory cytokines [114]. IL-10 was reported to inhibit pro-inflammatory signal-induced NF-κB activation in peripheral T lymphocytes and to prevent the release of ROS by monocytes and/or macrophages [123, 168]. Critically, the ratio between TNF-α and IL-10 production may influence the outcome of several cardiovascular disorders [100, 134, 135, 163, 166, 177]. In OSAS patients, increases in pro-inflammatory cytokines such as IL-6 and TNF-α were found in the circulation [64, 147, 167, 175, 188]. Critically, a significant increase in the values of TNF-α can be measured immediately after the first obstructive apnea causing a SaO_2

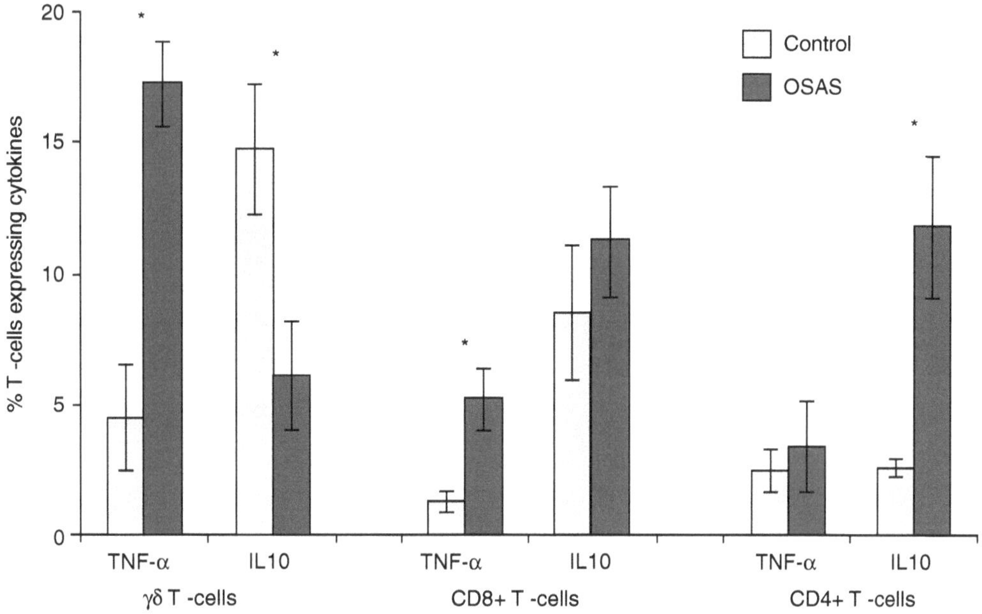

Fig. 8.2 Percentage of CD8, CD4, and γδ T cells from OSAS patients and controls expressing TNF-α and IL-10. *Statistical significance, with $p<0.001$ at least (Data adapted from Dyugovskaya et al. [36, 37] and from Lavie et al. [84])

desaturation <85% [1]. Also, elevated level of TNF-α was detected in monocytes of OSAS patients [110]. In contrast, the levels of IL-10 in serum or plasma were attenuated in OSAS [23, 111, 119]. We found that the TNF-α/IL-10 distribution among the different lymphocyte subsets varied considerably in OSAS patients (Fig. 8.2). Thus, in γδ T lymphocytes, TNF-α was increased and IL-10 was decreased, indicating the presence of a pro-inflammatory state in these cells. By contrast, in CD4 T cells, the TNF-α was unaffected by OSAS, but the expression of IL-10 was increased by 4.9-fold as compared to the control. This may represent a compensatory mechanism to downregulate TNF-α over-expression and to balance pro-inflammatory/anti-inflammatory cytokine release. The percentage of CD8 T cells expressing TNF-α was increased by 4-fold in OSAS patients whereas an incremental but not significant increase was noted for IL-10. These data indicate that each inflammatory cell has a unique pattern of pro-inflammatory/anti-inflammatory cytokine profile that may have a different damaging potential or alternatively the capacity to moderate inflammation. Despite the differences in TNF-α/IL-10 production between various T cell subsets, IL-10 expression was negatively correlated, whereas TNF-α expression was positively correlated with the severity of OSAS as evidenced by AHI [37].

Finally, the expression of IL-8, a pro-inflammatory cytokine with strong chemoattractant and activating properties was shown to increase in γδ T lymphocytes and in neutrophils of OSAS patients. Taken together, Fig. 8.3 illustrates the roles of leukocytes in endothelium injury and atherogenesis in OSAS.

8.6 Treatment with Nasal Continuous Positive Air Pressure (nCPAP)

The mainstay of therapy for OSAS remains nasal continuous positive air pressure (nCPAP). Treatment with nCPAP normalizes breathing in sleep of OSAS patients, by supplying a continuous air flow under pressure through the nostrils, preventing the collapse of the airways. A number of randomized treatment trials using a "sham CPAP" (i.e., using CPAP mask with minimal pressure) have shown reduction in blood pressure [10, 11, 118, 133] and reduced early signs of atherosclerosis [30]. Individuals using nCPAP therapy have cardiac event rates and cardiac deaths identical to controls without OSAS [102]. In contrast, untreated severe OSAS was associated with an increased in mortality from all causes including those of cardiac causes over a 10- to 20-year follow-up period [189].

To further demonstrate that sleep apnea and not any other associated variables affected leukocyte function, we compared the phenotype and some leukocyte function before and after nCPAP treatment. The main results are presented in Table 8.1. We found that (1) nCPAP treatment resulted in downregulation of the expression of adhesion molecule CD15 and CD11c on monocytes, lowered basal ROS production by CD11c+monocytes, and decreased monocyte adherence to HCAECs or HUVECs. (2) nCPAP treatment attenuated the CD15 expression in neutrophils to control levels and increased NA. (3) Due to nCPAP, the hypoxemia and apnea severity were ameliorated concomitantly with a significant decrease in CD8 T lymphocyte cytotoxicity,

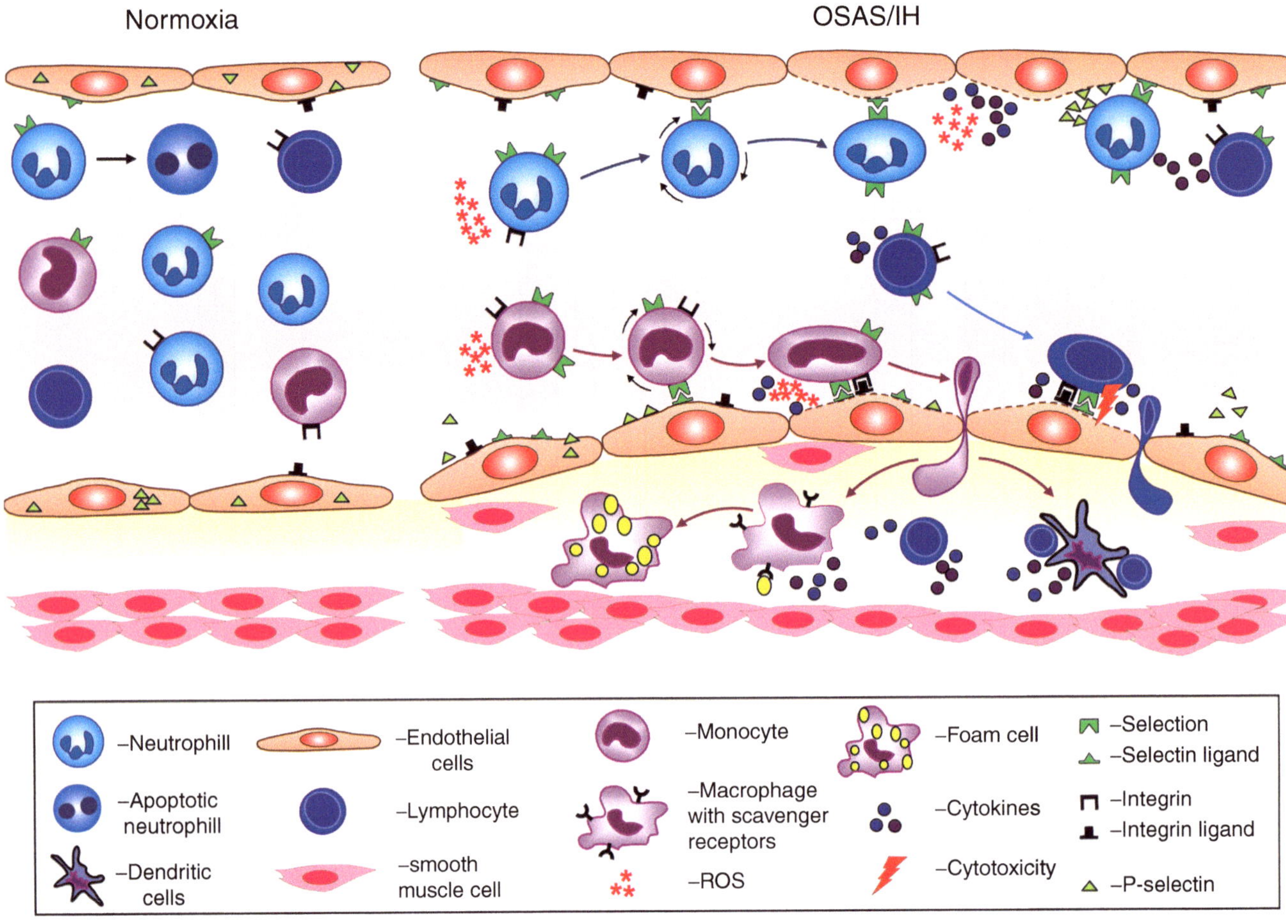

Fig. 8.3 A schematic representation of the roles of leukocytes in endothelium injury and atherogenesis in sleep apnea. In normoxia, leukocytes and ECs are nonactivated and express low levels of adhesion molecules. Neutrophils continuously die by apoptosis. Under IH, *ECs* undergo activation and upregulate adhesion molecules. In IH-activated *neutrophils*, ROS production and selectin expression are increased. After attachment, neutrophils release cytokines, ROS, proteolytic enzymes, and leukotrienes inducing EC damage. Adhesion to ECs and cytokines, released from activated leukocytes, increased neutrophil survival further exacerbates EC injury. IH-activated *monocytes* express increased amounts of selectins and integrins, ROS, and cytokines activating and damaging ECs. Adherent monocytes transmigrate into the arterial intima, differentiate into DCs and macrophages, then ingest oxidized lipoproteins, and became foam cells. IH-activated *lymphocytes* express adhesion molecules and cytokines, promoting EC damage by various cytotoxic mechanisms. Transmigrating lymphocytes cluster with DCs that result in T cell activation, proliferation, and cytokine secretion. Finally, cytokines and growth factors released from activated cells may affect the proliferation and migration of vascular smooth muscle cells into the intima, thereby potentiating atherogenesis (Reprinted with permission of the American Thoracic Society. Copyright© American Thoracic Society. Dyugovskaya et al. [38]. Official Journal of the American Thoracic Society Diane Gern, Publisher)

which correlated with decreased the percentages of CD8/CD56+ T cells, decreased CD56^{bright} receptor expression, and a 3.6-fold decrease in CD40L expression in CD8 T subset. The expression of NKB1 inhibitory receptors on CD8 T lymphocytes of nCPAP-treated patients was twofold elevated compared with either OSAS patients or controls. Thus, nCPAP treatment could have decreased the cytotoxicity of CD8 T lymphocytes either by increasing inhibitory receptor expression and/or by decreasing the expression of stimulating receptors. The frequency of IL-2-, IL-4-, and IL-10-producing T cells had no obvious change in OSAS patients treated for one night with nCPAP. However, the impact of nCPAP treatment is clearly evident as it was followed by a 2.3-fold decreased in the percentage of CD8 T cells bearing TNF-α. Taken together, all these observations clearly indicate that OSAS patients are exposed to atherogenic insult nightly. Since all these changes were observed after a single night of nCPAP treatment, this attests to a rapidly altered cellular state induced by changes in arterial oxygen tension.

8.7 Protective Mechanisms and Heterogeneity in the Biological Response

In view of the fact that many of cellular events described above are OSAS severity dependent, it could be expected that all or most patients with OSAS, in particularly those with severe

OSAS, would suffer from various cardiovascular morbidities. This, however, is not the case [84]. It is a fact that only about 50% of OSAS subjects develop hypertension [132]. Moreover, the highest risk of mortality in OSAS occurs in patients younger than 50 years, and the risk of death declines with age [90]. The question is why do some subjects with OSAS develop cardiovascular pathology while others do not? One possibility is that individuals who develop hypertension and cardiovascular disease have increased pathogenetic responses or decreased adaptive response for equivalent degrees of OSAS [2]. Such heterogeneity in response might be related to differences in protective mechanisms. Individuals vary in their antioxidant ability, which is complex. Also, the levels of anti-inflammatory molecules such as IL-10 can vary between individuals [152, 172]. It was proposed that individuals with OSAS and comorbidities may have lower IL-10 levels than those without comorbidities [2]. We found that the TNF-α/IL-10 distribution among the different lymphocyte subsets varied considerably in OSAS patients without comorbidities, and in CD4 T cells, the expression of IL-10 was increased by 4.9-fold compared to controls [37]. However, even among this group of patients, nearly 20% expressed low levels of IL-10 in CD4 T cells (personal observations). Critically, OSAS patients with hypertension and IHD showed a significant increase in TNF-α expression also in CD4 T cells that resulted in the shift of TNF-α/IL-10 ratio >1. Furthermore, despite on the high TNF-α expression in CD8 T cells, the individual analysis revealed that only a small subgroup (17.4%) was characterized by a decrease in the percentage of IL-10 and drastic increase in the percentage of TNF-α/CD8 cells [37]. Additionally, CD8 and even more so CD4 T cells can participate in protective mechanisms via a shift to type 2 cytokine secretions, as described above, and by that moderate inflammation. Increased expression of NKB1 molecules on OSAS γδ T cells may also be involved in the protective mechanisms. This type of NK receptor participates in the inhibition of cell-mediated cytotoxicity and cytokine secretion. Because the cytotoxic function is a result of a balance between activating and inhibiting signals which are delivered by the corresponding receptors [161], it is conceivable that the increased inhibitory activity of γδ T cells in OSAS provides a compensatory mechanism to avoid endothelial injury.

Other possible mechanisms, which may serve to protect some OSAS patients, include ischemic preconditioning inducing angiogenesis of newly formed heart collaterals [85]. The large interindividual differences in the angiogenic response to hypoxia that were correlated with arterial collateral formation in the heart was demonstrated. This interindividual difference in response may, at least in part, reflect genetic variants between individuals [2]. Some discrepancies can be observed at the level of HIF transcription factor and its gene products in OSAS [170, 182]. A significant variation was found within oxygen-regulation gene expression in lymphocytes of normal subjects in which induction of HIF by hypoxia can be observed [17]. There are now a great number of studies on genes conferring risk for hypertension and cardiovascular disease [149, 179]. Polymorphisms in genes affecting oxidative stress, inflammation, and sympathetic activity [92, 120] are also of high interest. There is a limited but growing number of candidate gene studies addressing the question of gene variants and their pathophysiological effect in the OSAS population [2, 9, 16, 28, 87, 96, 124].

Conclusion

As specified before, IH resulting from apnea has profound effect on redox systems and initiates oxidative stress and inflammation via activation of NF-kB, MAPKs, and downstream inflammatory/immune pathways. Consequently, upregulated expression of adhesion molecules, inflammatory cytokines, and ROS molecules are evident in various leukocyte subpopulations of OSAS patients. These induce increased avidity and cytotoxicity towards ECs. All in all, these cellular interactions in the vasculature promote endothelial dysfunction and may be involved in the early signs of atherosclerosis and exacerbate atherogenesis in OSAS patients. nCPAP treatment could ameliorate some leukocyte dysfunctions and thus block some of the atherosclerosis pathways. It can partially explain why nCPAP treatment of OSAS in cardiovascular patients is associated with a decrease in the occurrence of cardiovascular events [108].

Acknowledgments We thank Prof. Peretz Lavie for his helpful comments and suggestions. We are also indebted to Prof. Lena Lavie for her constructive comments and criticism.

References

1. Alberti A, Sarchielli P, Gallinella E, et al. Plasma cytokine levels in patients with obstructive sleep apnea syndrome: a preliminary study. J Sleep Res. 2003;12:305–11.
2. Arnardottir ES, Mackiewicz M, Gislason T, et al. Molecular signatures of obstructive sleep apnea in adults: a review and perspective. Sleep. 2009;32:447–70.
3. Atkeson A, Yeh SY, Malhotra A, et al. Endothelial function in obstructive sleep apnea. Prog Cardiovasc Dis. 2009;51:351–62.
4. Baetta R, Corsini A. Role of polymorphonuclear neutrophils in atherosclerosis: current state and future perspectives. Atherosclerosis. 2010;210:1–13.
5. Baguet JP, Hammer L, Levy P, et al. The severity of oxygen desaturation is predictive of carotid wall thickening and plaque occurrence. Chest. 2005;128:3407–12.
6. Barcelo A, Barbe F, de la Pena M, et al. Antioxidant status in patients with sleep apnoea and impact of continuous positive airway pressure treatment. Eur Respir J. 2006;27:756–60.
7. Barcelo A, Miralles C, Barbe F, et al. Abnormal lipid peroxidation in patients with sleep apnoea. Eur Respir J. 2000;16:644–7.
8. Battistini L, Borsellino G, Sawicki G, et al. Phenotypic and cytokine analysis of human peripheral blood gamma delta T cells expressing NK cell receptors. J Immunol. 1997;159:3723–30.

9. Bayazit YA, Yilmaz M, Erdal E, et al. Role of nitric oxide synthase gene intron 4 and exon 7 polymorphisms in obstructive sleep apnea syndrome. Eur Arch Otorhinolaryngol. 2009;266:449–54.
10. Bazzano LA, Khan Z, Reynolds K, et al. Effect of nocturnal nasal continuous positive airway pressure on blood pressure in obstructive sleep apnea. Hypertension. 2007;50:417–23.
11. Becker HF, Jerrentrup A, Ploch T, et al. Effect of nasal continuous positive airway pressure treatment on blood pressure in patients with obstructive sleep apnea. Circulation. 2003;107:68–73.
12. Belaidi E, Joyeux-Faure M, Ribuot C, et al. Major role for hypoxia inducible factor-1 and the endothelin system in promoting myocardial infarction and hypertension in an animal model of obstructive sleep apnea. J Am Coll Cardiol. 2009;53:1309–17.
13. Bluestone JA, Khattri R, Sciammas R, et al. TCR gamma delta cells: a specialized T-cell subset in the immune system. Annu Rev Cell Dev Biol. 1995;11:307–53.
14. Bobryshev YV. Monocyte recruitment and foam cell formation in atherosclerosis. Micron. 2006;37:208–22.
15. Bosco MC, Puppo M, Blengio F, et al. Monocytes and dendritic cells in a hypoxic environment: spotlights on chemotaxis and migration. Immunobiology. 2008;213:733–49.
16. Bostrom KB, Hedner J, Melander O, et al. Interaction between the angiotensin-converting enzyme gene insertion/deletion polymorphism and obstructive sleep apnoea as a mechanism for hypertension. J Hypertens. 2007;25:779–83.
17. Brooks JT, Elvidge GP, Glenny L, et al. Variations within oxygen-regulated gene expression in humans. J Appl Physiol. 2009;106: 212–20.
18. Caldwell CC, Kojima H, Lukashev D, et al. Differential effects of physiologically relevant hypoxic conditions on T lymphocyte development and effector functions. J Immunol. 2001;167:6140–9.
19. Carlos TM, Harlan JM. Leukocyte-endothelial adhesion molecules. Blood. 1994;84:2068–101.
20. Chen L, Einbinder E, Zhang Q, et al. Oxidative stress and left ventricular function with chronic intermittent hypoxia in rats. Am J Respir Crit Care Med. 2005;172:915–20.
21. Chiang AA. Obstructive sleep apnea and chronic intermittent hypoxia: a review. Chin J Physiol. 2006;49:234–43.
22. Christou K, Moulas AN, Pastaka C, et al. Antioxidant capacity in obstructive sleep apnea patients. Sleep Med. 2003;4:225–8.
23. Constantinidis J, Ereliadis S, Angouridakis N, et al. Cytokine changes after surgical treatment of obstructive sleep apnoea syndrome. Eur Arch Otorhinolaryngol. 2008;265:1275–9.
24. Cramer T, Yamanishi Y, Clausen BE, et al. HIF-1alpha is essential for myeloid cell-mediated inflammation. Cell. 2003;112:645–57.
25. Crowley MP, Reich Z, Mavaddat N, et al. The recognition of the nonclassical major histocompatibility complex (MHC) class I molecule, T10, by the gammadelta T cell, G8. J Exp Med. 1997;185:1223–30.
26. Crowther M, Brown NJ, Bishop ET, et al. Microenvironmental influence on macrophage regulation of angiogenesis in wounds and malignant tumors. J Leukoc Biol. 2001;70:478–90.
27. Dematteis M, Julien C, Guillermet C, et al. Intermittent hypoxia induces early functional cardiovascular remodeling in mice. Am J Respir Crit Care Med. 2008;177:227–35.
28. Diefenbach K, Kretschmer K, Bauer S, et al. Endothelin-1 gene variant Lys198Asn and plasma endothelin level in obstructive sleep apnea. Cardiology. 2009;112:62–8.
29. DiStasi MR, Ley K. Opening the flood-gates: how neutrophil-endothelial interactions regulate permeability. Trends Immunol. 2009;30:547–56.
30. Drager LF, Bortolotto LA, Figueiredo AC, et al. Effects of continuous positive airway pressure on early signs of atherosclerosis in obstructive sleep apnea. Am J Respir Crit Care Med. 2007;176:706–12.
31. Drager LF, Bortolotto LA, Lorenzi MC, et al. Early signs of atherosclerosis in obstructive sleep apnea. Am J Respir Crit Care Med. 2005;172:613–8.
32. Droge W. Free radicals in the physiological control of cell function. Physiol Rev. 2002;82:47–95.
33. Dunican AL, Leuenroth SJ, Grutkoski P, et al. TNFalpha-induced suppression of PMN apoptosis is mediated through interleukin-8 production. Shock. 2000;14:284–8; discussion 288–9.
34. Dyugovskaya L, Lavie P, Hirsh M, et al. Activated CD8+ T-lymphocytes in obstructive sleep apnoea. Eur Respir J. 2005;25: 820–8.
35. Dyugovskaya L, Lavie P, Lavie L. Increased adhesion molecules expression and production of reactive oxygen species in leukocytes of sleep apnea patients. Am J Respir Crit Care Med. 2002;165:934–9.
36. Dyugovskaya L, Lavie P, Lavie L. Phenotypic and functional characterization of blood gammadelta T cells in sleep apnea. Am J Respir Crit Care Med. 2003;168:242–9.
37. Dyugovskaya L, Lavie P, Lavie L. Lymphocyte activation as a possible measure of atherosclerotic risk in patients with sleep apnea. Ann N Y Acad Sci. 2005;1051:340–50.
38. Dyugovskaya L, Polyakov A, Lavie P, et al. Delayed neutrophil apoptosis in patients with sleep apnea. Am J Respir Crit Care Med. 2008;177:544–54.
39. Dyugovskaya L, Polyakov A, Lavie P, et al. Intermittent hypoxia-induced neutrophil survival is mediated via mitochondrial pathways by MAP kinases activation. Am J Respir Crit Care Med. 2010; A6635:181.
40. Dyugovskaya L, Polyakov A, Ginsberg D, et al. Molecular pathways of spontaneous and TNF-α-mediated neutrophil apoptosis under intermittent hypoxia. Am J Respir Cell Mol Biol. 2011;44:1–9.
41. Elenkov IJ, Wilder RL, Chrousos GP, et al. The sympathetic nerve – an integrative interface between two supersystems: the brain and the immune system. Pharmacol Rev. 2000;52:595–638.
42. Elliott MJ, Gamble JR, Park LS, et al. Inhibition of human monocyte adhesion by interleukin-4. Blood. 1991;77:2739–45.
43. Emeson EE, Robertson Jr AL. T lymphocytes in aortic and coronary intimas. Their potential role in atherogenesis. Am J Pathol. 1988;130:369–76.
44. Ericson SG, Zhao Y, Gao H, et al. Interleukin-6 production by human neutrophils after Fc-receptor cross-linking or exposure to granulocyte colony-stimulating factor. Blood. 1998;91:2099–107.
45. Fernandez Pujol B, Lucibello FC, Gehling UM, et al. Endothelial-like cells derived from human CD14 positive monocytes. Differentiation. 2000;65:287–300.
46. Ferrari R. The role of TNF in cardiovascular disease. Pharmacol Res. 1999;40:97–105.
47. Fletcher EC, Orolinova N, Bader M. Blood pressure response to chronic episodic hypoxia: the renin-angiotensin system. J Appl Physiol. 2002;92:627–33.
48. Fox S, Leitch AE, Duffin R, et al. Neutrophil apoptosis: relevance to the innate immune response and inflammatory disease. J Innate Immun. 2010;2:216–27.
49. Friedlander AH, Yueh R, Littner MR. The prevalence of calcified carotid artery atheromas in patients with obstructive sleep apnea syndrome. J Oral Maxillofac Surg. 1998;56:950–4.
50. Furze RC, Rankin SM. The role of the bone marrow in neutrophil clearance under homeostatic conditions in the mouse. FASEB J. 2008;22:3111–9.
51. Galea P, Brezinschek R, Lipsky PE, et al. Phenotypic characterization of CD4-/alpha beta TCR+ and gamma delta TCR+ T cells with a transendothelial migratory capacity. J Immunol. 1994;153:529–42.
52. George J, Shoenfeld Y, Gilburd B, et al. Requisite role for interleukin-4 in the acceleration of fatty streaks induced by heat shock protein 65 or Mycobacterium tuberculosis. Circ Res. 2000;86:1203–10.
53. Glass CK, Witztum JL. Atherosclerosis: the road ahead. Cell. 2001;104:503–16.
54. Greenberg H, Ye X, Wilson D, et al. Chronic intermittent hypoxia activates nuclear factor-kappaB in cardiovascular tissues in vivo. Biochem Biophys Res Commun. 2006;343:591–6.

55. Griffioen KJ, Kamendi HW, Gorini CJ, et al. Reactive oxygen species mediate central cardiorespiratory network responses to acute intermittent hypoxia. J Neurophysiol. 2007;97:2059–66.
56. Haddad JJ, Fahlman CS. Redox- and oxidant-mediated regulation of interleukin-10: an anti-inflammatory, antioxidant cytokine? Biochem Biophys Res Commun. 2002;297:163–76.
57. Hannah S, Mecklenburgh K, Rahman I, et al. Hypoxia prolongs neutrophil survival in vitro. FEBS Lett. 1995;372:233–7.
58. Hansson GK. Immune mechanisms in atherosclerosis. Arterioscler Thromb Vasc Biol. 2001;21:1876–90.
59. Hayday AC. [gamma][delta] cells: a right time and a right place for a conserved third way of protection. Annu Rev Immunol. 2000; 18:975–1026.
60. He YW, Malek TR. Interleukin-7 receptor alpha is essential for the development of gamma delta+T cells, but not natural killer cells. J Exp Med. 1996;184:289–93.
61. Htoo AK, Greenberg H, Tongia S, et al. Activation of nuclear factor kappaB in obstructive sleep apnea: a pathway leading to systemic inflammation. Sleep Breath. 2006;10:43–50.
62. Ichikawa H, Kokura S, Aw TY. Role of endothelial mitochondria in oxidant production and modulation of neutrophil adherence. J Vasc Res. 2004;41:432–44.
63. Ikuta K, Lee HC, Ye SK. Role of the IL-7 receptor in gamma-delta T cell development. Chem Immunol. 2001;79:29–42.
64. Imagawa S, Yamaguchi Y, Ogawa K, et al. Interleukin-6 and tumor necrosis factor-alpha in patients with obstructive sleep apnea-hypopnea syndrome. Respiration. 2004;71:24–9.
65. Itzhaki S, Lavie L, Pillar G, et al. Endothelial dysfunction in obstructive sleep apnea measured by peripheral arterial tone response in the finger to reactive hyperemia. Sleep. 2005;28:594–600.
66. Jelic S, Bartels MN, Mateika JH, et al. Arterial stiffness increases during obstructive sleep apneas. Sleep. 2002;25:850–5.
67. Jelic S, Padeletti M, Kawut SM, et al. Inflammation, oxidative stress, and repair capacity of the vascular endothelium in obstructive sleep apnea. Circulation. 2008;117:2270–8.
68. Johnson JL, Newby AC. Macrophage heterogeneity in atherosclerotic plaques. Curr Opin Lipidol. 2009;20:370–8.
69. Jolly SR, Kane WJ, Hook BG, et al. Reduction of myocardial infarct size by neutrophil depletion: effect of duration of occlusion. Am Heart J. 1986;112:682–90.
70. Jordan W, Cohrs S, Degner D, et al. Evaluation of oxidative stress measurements in obstructive sleep apnea syndrome. J Neural Transm. 2006;113:239–54.
71. Jun J, Savransky V, Nanayakkara A, et al. Intermittent hypoxia has organ-specific effects on oxidative stress. Am J Physiol Regul Integr Comp Physiol. 2008;295:R1274–81.
72. Kahaleh MB, Fan PS, Otsuka T. Gammadelta receptor bearing T cells in scleroderma: enhanced interaction with vascular endothelial cells in vitro. Clin Immunol. 1999;91:188–95.
73. Kato M, Roberts-Thomson P, Phillips BG, et al. Impairment of endothelium-dependent vasodilation of resistance vessels in patients with obstructive sleep apnea. Circulation. 2000;102:2607–10.
74. Kettritz R, Gaido ML, Haller H, et al. Interleukin-8 delays spontaneous and tumor necrosis factor-alpha-mediated apoptosis of human neutrophils. Kidney Int. 1998;53:84–91.
75. Khew-Goodall Y, Wadham C, Stein BN, et al. Stat6 activation is essential for interleukin-4 induction of P-selectin transcription in human umbilical vein endothelial cells. Arterioscler Thromb Vasc Biol. 1999;19:1421–9.
76. Kin H, Wang NP, Halkos ME, et al. Neutrophil depletion reduces myocardial apoptosis and attenuates NFkappaB activation/TNFalpha release after ischemia and reperfusion. J Surg Res. 2006;135:170–8.
77. Kleindienst R, Xu Q, Willeit J, et al. Immunology of atherosclerosis. Demonstration of heat shock protein 60 expression and T lymphocytes bearing alpha/beta or gamma/delta receptor in human atherosclerotic lesions. Am J Pathol. 1993;142:1927–37.
78. Kumar GK, Rai V, Sharma SD, et al. Chronic intermittent hypoxia induces hypoxia-evoked catecholamine efflux in adult rat adrenal medulla via oxidative stress. J Physiol. 2006;575:229–39.
79. Lattimore JD, Wilcox I, Nakhla S, et al. Repetitive hypoxia increases lipid loading in human macrophages-a potentially atherogenic effect. Atherosclerosis. 2005;179:255–9.
80. Lavie L. Obstructive sleep apnoea syndrome – an oxidative stress disorder. Sleep Med Rev. 2003;7:35–51.
81. Lavie L. Sleep apnea syndrome, endothelial dysfunction, and cardiovascular morbidity. Sleep. 2004;27:1053–5.
82. Lavie L. Intermittent hypoxia: the culprit of oxidative stress, vascular inflammation and dyslipidemia in obstructive sleep apnea. Expert Rev Respir Med. 2008;2:75–84.
83. Lavie L. Oxidative stress – a unifying paradigm in obstructive sleep apnea and comorbidities. Prog Cardiovasc Dis. 2009;51:303–12.
84. Lavie L, Dyugovskaya L, Polyakov A. Biology of peripheral blood cells in obstructive sleep apnea – the tip of the iceberg. Arch Physiol Biochem. 2008;114:244–54.
85. Lavie L, Lavie P. Ischemic preconditioning as a possible explanation for the age decline relative mortality in sleep apnea. Med Hypotheses. 2006;66:1069–73.
86. Lavie L, Lavie P. Molecular mechanisms of cardiovascular disease in OSAHS: the oxidative stress link. Eur Respir J. 2009;33: 1467–84.
87. Lavie L, Lotan R, Hochberg I, et al. Haptoglobin polymorphism is a risk factor for cardiovascular disease in patients with obstructive sleep apnea syndrome. Sleep. 2003;26:592–5.
88. Lavie L, Polotsky V. Cardiovascular aspects in obstructive sleep apnea syndrome – molecular issues, hypoxia and cytokine profiles. Respiration. 2009;78:361–70.
89. Lavie L, Vishnevsky A, Lavie P. Evidence for lipid peroxidation in obstructive sleep apnea. Sleep. 2004;27:123–8.
90. Lavie P, Herer P, Lavie L. Mortality risk factors in sleep apnoea: a matched case–control study. J Sleep Res. 2007;16:128–34.
91. Lee YW, Kuhn H, Kaiser S, et al. Interleukin 4 induces transcription of the 15-lipoxygenase I gene in human endothelial cells. J Lipid Res. 2001;42:783–91.
92. Leopold JA, Loscalzo J. Oxidative enzymopathies and vascular disease. Arterioscler Thromb Vasc Biol. 2005;25:1332–40.
93. Leuenroth SJ, Grutkoski PS, Ayala A, et al. Suppression of PMN apoptosis by hypoxia is dependent on Mcl-1 and MAPK activity. Surgery. 2000;128:171–7.
94. Libby P. Inflammation in atherosclerosis. Nature. 2002;420:868–74.
95. Libby P. Inflammatory mechanisms: the molecular basis of inflammation and disease. Nutr Rev. 2007;65:S140–6.
96. Lin L, Finn L, Zhang J, et al. Angiotensin-converting enzyme, sleep-disordered breathing, and hypertension. Am J Respir Crit Care Med. 2004;170:1349–53.
97. Liuzzo G, Goronzy JJ, Yang H, et al. Monoclonal T-cell proliferation and plaque instability in acute coronary syndromes. Circulation. 2000;101:2883–8.
98. Lukashev D, Klebanov B, Kojima H, et al. Cutting edge: hypoxia-inducible factor 1alpha and its activation-inducible short isoform I.1 negatively regulate functions of CD4+ and CD8+ T lymphocytes. J Immunol. 2006;177:4962–5.
99. Malhotra A, White DP. Obstructive sleep apnoea. Lancet. 2002;360:237–45.
100. Mallat Z, Besnard S, Duriez M, et al. Protective role of interleukin-10 in atherosclerosis. Circ Res. 1999;85:e17–24.
101. Mantovani A, Garlanda C, Introna M, et al. Regulation of endothelial cell function by pro- and anti-inflammatory cytokines. Transplant Proc. 1998;30:4239–43.
102. Marin JM, Carrizo SJ, Vicente E, et al. Long-term cardiovascular outcomes in men with obstructive sleep apnoea-hypopnoea with or without treatment with continuous positive airway pressure: an observational study. Lancet. 2005;365:1046–53.

103. Marx N, Imhof A, Froehlich J, et al. Effect of rosiglitazone treatment on soluble CD40L in patients with type 2 diabetes and coronary artery disease. Circulation. 2003;107:1954–7.
104. McGown AD, Makker H, Elwell C, et al. Measurement of changes in cytochrome oxidase redox state during obstructive sleep apnea using near-infrared spectroscopy. Sleep. 2003;26:710–6.
105. McKellar GE, McCarey DW, Sattar N, et al. Role for TNF in atherosclerosis? Lessons from autoimmune disease. Nat Rev Cardiol. 2009;6:410–7.
106. McNicholas WT, Bonsigore MR. Sleep apnoea as an independent risk factor for cardiovascular disease: current evidence, basic mechanisms and research priorities. Eur Respir J. 2007;29:156–78.
107. Mecklenburgh KI, Walmsley SR, Cowburn AS, et al. Involvement of a ferroprotein sensor in hypoxia-mediated inhibition of neutrophil apoptosis. Blood. 2002;100:3008–16.
108. Milleron O, Pilliere R, Foucher A, et al. Benefits of obstructive sleep apnoea treatment in coronary artery disease: a long-term follow-up study. Eur Heart J. 2004;25:728–34.
109. Minet E, Michel G, Mottet D, et al. Transduction pathways involved in hypoxia-inducible factor-1 phosphorylation and activation. Free Radic Biol Med. 2001;31:847–55.
110. Minoguchi K, Tazaki T, Yokoe T, et al. Elevated production of tumor necrosis factor-alpha by monocytes in patients with obstructive sleep apnea syndrome. Chest. 2004;126:1473–9.
111. Minoguchi K, Yokoe T, Tazaki T, et al. Increased carotid intima-media thickness and serum inflammatory markers in obstructive sleep apnea. Am J Respir Crit Care Med. 2005;172:625–30.
112. Mohagheghpour N, Bermudez LE, Khajavi S, et al. The VLA-4/VCAM-1 molecules participate in gamma delta cell interaction with endothelial cells. Cell Immunol. 1992;143:170–82.
113. Monaco C, Andreakos E, Young S, et al. T cell-mediated signaling to vascular endothelium: induction of cytokines, chemokines, and tissue factor. J Leukoc Biol. 2002;71:659–68.
114. Moore KW, de Waal MR, Coffman RL, et al. Interleukin-10 and the interleukin-10 receptor. Annu Rev Immunol. 2001;19:683–765.
115. Murdoch C, Giannoudis A, Lewis CE. Mechanisms regulating the recruitment of macrophages into hypoxic areas of tumors and other ischemic tissues. Blood. 2004;104:2224–34.
116. Nakajima T, Goek O, Zhang X, et al. De novo expression of killer immunoglobulin-like receptors and signaling proteins regulates the cytotoxic function of CD4 T cells in acute coronary syndromes. Circ Res. 2003;93:106–13.
117. Nakajima T, Schulte S, Warrington KJ, et al. T-cell-mediated lysis of endothelial cells in acute coronary syndromes. Circulation. 2002;105:570–5.
118. Norman D, Loredo JS, Nelesen RA, et al. Effects of continuous positive airway pressure versus supplemental oxygen on 24-hour ambulatory blood pressure. Hypertension. 2006;47:840–5.
119. Ohga E, Tomita T, Wada H, et al. Effects of obstructive sleep apnea on circulating ICAM-1, IL-8, and MCP-1. J Appl Physiol. 2003;94:179–84.
120. Olivieri F, Antonicelli R, Cardelli M, et al. Genetic polymorphisms of inflammatory cytokines and myocardial infarction in the elderly. Mech Ageing Dev. 2006;127:552–9.
121. Ozmen J, Bobryshev YV, Lord RS. CD40 co-stimulatory molecule expression by dendritic cells in primary atherosclerotic lesions in carotid arteries and in stenotic saphenous vein coronary artery grafts. Cardiovasc Surg. 2001;9:329–33.
122. Pack AI, Gislason T. Obstructive sleep apnea and cardiovascular disease: a perspective and future directions. Prog Cardiovasc Dis. 2009;51:434–51.
123. Park SH, Kim KE, Hwang HY, et al. Regulatory effect of SOCS on NF-kappaB activity in murine monocytes/macrophages. DNA Cell Biol. 2003;22:131–9.
124. Patel SR, Larkin EK, Mignot E, et al. The association of angiotensin converting enzyme (ACE) polymorphisms with sleep apnea and hypertension. Sleep. 2007;30:531–3.
125. Paulnock DM, Demick KP, Coller SP. Analysis of interferon-gamma-dependent and -independent pathways of macrophage activation. J Leukoc Biol. 2000;67:677–82.
126. Peker Y, Hedner J, Norum J, et al. Increased incidence of cardiovascular disease in middle-aged men with obstructive sleep apnea: a 7-year follow-up. Am J Respir Crit Care Med. 2002;166:159–65.
127. Peker Y, Kraiczi H, Hedner J, et al. An independent association between obstructive sleep apnoea and coronary artery disease. Eur Respir J. 1999;14:179–84.
128. Peled N, Greenberg A, Pillar G, et al. Contributions of hypoxia and respiratory disturbance index to sympathetic activation and blood pressure in obstructive sleep apnea syndrome. Am J Hypertens. 1998;11:1284–9.
129. Peng Y, Yuan G, Overholt JL, et al. Systemic and cellular responses to intermittent hypoxia: evidence for oxidative stress and mitochondrial dysfunction. Adv Exp Med Biol. 2003;536:559–64.
130. Peng YJ, Nanduri J, Yuan G, et al. NADPH oxidase is required for the sensory plasticity of the carotid body by chronic intermittent hypoxia. J Neurosci. 2009;29:4903–10.
131. Peng YJ, Yuan G, Ramakrishnan D, et al. Heterozygous HIF-1alpha deficiency impairs carotid body-mediated systemic responses and reactive oxygen species generation in mice exposed to intermittent hypoxia. J Physiol. 2006;577:705–16.
132. Peppard PE, Young T, Palta M, et al. Prospective study of the association between sleep-disordered breathing and hypertension. N Engl J Med. 2000;342:1378–84.
133. Pepperell JC, Ramdassingh-Dow S, Crosthwaite N, et al. Ambulatory blood pressure after therapeutic and subtherapeutic nasal continuous positive airway pressure for obstructive sleep apnoea: a randomised parallel trial. Lancet. 2002;359:204–10.
134. Perez Fernandez R, Kaski JC. Interleukin-10 and coronary disease. Rev Esp Cardiol. 2002;55:738–50.
135. Pinderski LJ, Fischbein MP, Subbanagounder G, et al. Overexpression of interleukin-10 by activated T lymphocytes inhibits atherosclerosis in LDL receptor-deficient Mice by altering lymphocyte and macrophage phenotypes. Circ Res. 2002;90:1064–71.
136. Poggi A, Zocchi MR, Carosio R, et al. Transendothelial migratory pathways of V delta 1+ TCR gamma delta+ and V delta 2+ TCR gamma delta+ T lymphocytes from healthy donors and multiple sclerosis patients: involvement of phosphatidylinositol 3 kinase and calcium calmodulin-dependent kinase II. J Immunol. 2002;168:6071–7.
137. Polotsky VY, Li J, Punjabi NM, et al. Intermittent hypoxia increases insulin resistance in genetically obese mice. J Physiol. 2003;552:253–64.
138. Prabhakar NR, Kumar GK, Nanduri J, et al. ROS signaling in systemic and cellular responses to chronic intermittent hypoxia. Antioxid Redox Signal. 2007;9:1397–403.
139. Raines EW, Ferri N. Thematic review series: the immune system and atherogenesis. Cytokines affecting endothelial and smooth muscle cells in vascular disease. J Lipid Res. 2005;46:1081–92.
140. Randolph GJ. The fate of monocytes in atherosclerosis. J Thromb Haemost. 2009;7 Suppl 1:28–30.
141. Rehman J, Li J, Orschell CM, et al. Peripheral blood "endothelial progenitor cells" are derived from monocyte/macrophages and secrete angiogenic growth factors. Circulation. 2003;107:1164–9.
142. Ribatti D, Nico B, Crivellato E, et al. Macrophages and tumor angiogenesis. Leukemia. 2007;21:2085–9.
143. Ridker PM, Rifai N, Pfeffer M, et al. Elevation of tumor necrosis factor-alpha and increased risk of recurrent coronary events after myocardial infarction. Circulation. 2000;101:2149–53.

144. Rius J, Guma M, Schachtrup C, et al. NF-kappaB links innate immunity to the hypoxic response through transcriptional regulation of HIF-1alpha. Nature. 2008;453:807–11.
145. Roy KC, Bandyopadhyay G, Rakshit S, et al. IL-4 alone without the involvement of GM-CSF transforms human peripheral blood monocytes to a CD1a(dim), CD83(+) myeloid dendritic cell subset. J Cell Sci. 2004;117:3435–45.
146. Ryan S, McNicholas WT, Taylor CT. A critical role for p38 map kinase in NF-kappaB signaling during intermittent hypoxia/reoxygenation. Biochem Biophys Res Commun. 2007;355:728–33.
147. Ryan S, Taylor CT, McNicholas WT. Selective activation of inflammatory pathways by intermittent hypoxia in obstructive sleep apnea syndrome. Circulation. 2005;112:2660–7.
148. Sack M. Tumor necrosis factor-alpha in cardiovascular biology and the potential role for anti-tumor necrosis factor-alpha therapy in heart disease. Pharmacol Ther. 2002;94:123–35.
149. Samani NJ, Erdmann J, Hall AS, et al. Genomewide association analysis of coronary artery disease. N Engl J Med. 2007;357:443–53.
150. Sanchez-Mejorada G, Rosales C. Signal transduction by immunoglobulin Fc receptors. J Leukoc Biol. 1998;63:521–33.
151. Sartorius R, D'Apice L, Barba P, et al. Induction of human NK cell-mediated cytotoxicity by CD40 triggering on antigen presenting cells. Cell Immunol. 2003;221:81–8.
152. Scarpelli D, Cardellini M, Andreozzi F, et al. Variants of the interleukin-10 promoter gene are associated with obesity and insulin resistance but not type 2 diabetes in caucasian italian subjects. Diabetes. 2006;55:1529–33.
153. Schmeisser A, Garlichs CD, Zhang H, et al. Monocytes coexpress endothelial and macrophagocytic lineage markers and form cord-like structures in Matrigel under angiogenic conditions. Cardiovasc Res. 2001;49:671–80.
154. Schmidt D, Goronzy JJ, Weyand CM. CD4+ CD7– CD28– T cells are expanded in rheumatoid arthritis and are characterized by autoreactivity. J Clin Invest. 1996;97:2027–37.
155. Schulz R, Mahmoudi S, Hattar K, et al. Enhanced release of superoxide from polymorphonuclear neutrophils in obstructive sleep apnea. Impact of continuous positive airway pressure therapy. Am J Respir Crit Care Med. 2000;162:566–70.
156. Semenza GL, Prabhakar NR. HIF-1-dependent respiratory, cardiovascular, and redox responses to chronic intermittent hypoxia. Antioxid Redox Signal. 2007;9:1391–6.
157. Shamsuzzaman AS, Gersh BJ, Somers VK. Obstructive sleep apnea: implications for cardiac and vascular disease. JAMA. 2003;290:1906–14.
158. Sharma R, Li DZ. Role of dendritic cells in atherosclerosis. Asian Cardiovasc Thorac Ann. 2006;14:166–9.
159. Soehnlein O, Lindbom L. Phagocyte partnership during the onset and resolution of inflammation. Nat Rev Immunol. 2010;10:427–39.
160. Soejima H, Irie A, Miyamoto S, et al. Preference toward a T-helper type 1 response in patients with coronary spastic angina. Circulation. 2003;107:2196–200.
161. Solana R, Mariani E. NK and NK/T cells in human senescence. Vaccine. 2000;18:1613–20.
162. Song L, Leung C, Schindler C. Lymphocytes are important in early atherosclerosis. J Clin Invest. 2001;108:251–9.
163. Stumpf C, Lehner C, Yilmaz A, et al. Decrease of serum levels of the anti-inflammatory cytokine interleukin-10 in patients with advanced chronic heart failure. Clin Sci (Lond). 2003;105:45–50.
164. Suzuki YJ, Jain V, Park AM, et al. Oxidative stress and oxidant signaling in obstructive sleep apnea and associated cardiovascular diseases. Free Radic Biol Med. 2006;40:1683–92.
165. Swirski FK, Weissleder R, Pittet MJ. Heterogeneous in vivo behavior of monocyte subsets in atherosclerosis. Arterioscler Thromb Vasc Biol. 2009;29:1424–32.
166. Tedgui A, Mallat Z. Interleukin-10: an anti-atherogenic cytokine? Eur J Clin Invest. 2001;31:1–2.
167. Teramoto S, Yamamoto H, Ouchi Y. Increased C-reactive protein and increased plasma interleukin-6 may synergistically affect the progression of coronary atherosclerosis in obstructive sleep apnea syndrome. Circulation. 2003;107:E40.
168. Terkeltaub RA. IL-10: an "immunologic scalpel" for atherosclerosis? Arterioscler Thromb Vasc Biol. 1999;19:2823–5.
169. Toffoli S, Feron O, Raes M, et al. Intermittent hypoxia changes HIF-1alpha phosphorylation pattern in endothelial cells: unravelling of a new PKA-dependent regulation of HIF-1alpha. Biochim Biophys Acta. 2007;1773:1558–71.
170. Valipour A, Litschauer B, Mittermayer F, et al. Circulating plasma levels of vascular endothelial growth factor in patients with sleep disordered breathing. Respir Med. 2004;98:1180–6.
171. Valko M, Leibfritz D, Moncol J, et al. Free radicals and antioxidants in normal physiological functions and human disease. Int J Biochem Cell Biol. 2007;39:44–84.
172. van Exel E, Gussekloo J, de Craen AJ, et al. Low production capacity of interleukin-10 associates with the metabolic syndrome and type 2 diabetes: the Leiden 85-Plus Study. Diabetes. 2002;51:1088–92.
173. Vanderlaan PA, Reardon CA. Thematic review series: the immune system and atherogenesis. The unusual suspects: an overview of the minor leukocyte populations in atherosclerosis. J Lipid Res. 2005;46:829–38.
174. Veasey SC, Davis CW, Fenik P, et al. Long-term intermittent hypoxia in mice: protracted hypersomnolence with oxidative injury to sleep-wake brain regions. Sleep. 2004;27:194–201.
175. Vgontzas AN, Papanicolaou DA, Bixler EO, et al. Sleep apnea and daytime sleepiness and fatigue: relation to visceral obesity, insulin resistance, and hypercytokinemia. J Clin Endocrinol Metab. 2000;85:1151–8.
176. Vinten-Johansen J. Involvement of neutrophils in the pathogenesis of lethal myocardial reperfusion injury. Cardiovasc Res. 2004;61:481–97.
177. von der Thusen JH, Kuiper J, van Berkel TJ, et al. Interleukins in atherosclerosis: molecular pathways and therapeutic potential. Pharmacol Rev. 2003;55:133–66.
178. Walmsley SR, Print C, Farahi N, et al. Hypoxia-induced neutrophil survival is mediated by HIF-1alpha-dependent NF-kappaB activity. J Exp Med. 2005;201:105–15.
179. Wang SS, Schadt EE, Wang H, et al. Identification of pathways for atherosclerosis in mice: integration of quantitative trait locus analysis and global gene expression data. Circ Res. 2007;101:e11–30.
180. Weyand CM, Goronzy JJ, Liuzzo G, et al. T-cell immunity in acute coronary syndromes. Mayo Clin Proc. 2001;76:1011–20.
181. Wick G, Xu Q. Atherosclerosis – an autoimmune disease. Exp Gerontol. 1999;34:559–66.
182. Winnicki M, Shamsuzzaman A, Lanfranchi P, et al. Erythropoietin and obstructive sleep apnea. Am J Hypertens. 2004;17:783–6.
183. Xu W, Chi L, Row BW, et al. Increased oxidative stress is associated with chronic intermittent hypoxia-mediated brain cortical neuronal cell apoptosis in a mouse model of sleep apnea. Neuroscience. 2004;126:313–23.
184. Yamaji-Kegan K, Su Q, Angelini DJ, et al. IL-4 is proangiogenic in the lung under hypoxic conditions. J Immunol. 2009;182:5469–76.
185. Yamauchi M, Kimura H. Oxidative stress in obstructive sleep apnea: putative pathways to the cardiovascular complications. Antioxid Redox Signal. 2008;10:755–68.
186. Yamauchi M, Tamaki S, Tomoda K, et al. Evidence for activation of nuclear factor kappaB in obstructive sleep apnea. Sleep Breath. 2006;10:189–93.
187. Yang D, de la Rosa G, Tewary P, et al. Alarmins link neutrophils and dendritic cells. Trends Immunol. 2009;30:531–7.

188. Yokoe T, Minoguchi K, Matsuo H, et al. Elevated levels of C-reactive protein and interleukin-6 in patients with obstructive sleep apnea syndrome are decreased by nasal continuous positive airway pressure. Circulation. 2003;107:1129–34.
189. Young T, Finn L, Peppard PE, et al. Sleep disordered breathing and mortality: eighteen-year follow-up of the Wisconsin sleep cohort. Sleep. 2008;31:1071–8.
190. Young T, Palta M, Dempsey J, et al. The occurrence of sleep-disordered breathing among middle-aged adults. N Engl J Med. 1993;328:1230–5.
191. Yuan G, Adhikary G, McCormick AA, et al. Role of oxidative stress in intermittent hypoxia-induced immediate early gene activation in rat PC12 cells. J Physiol. 2004;557:773–83.
192. Yuan G, Nanduri J, Bhasker CR, et al. Ca^{2+}/calmodulin kinase-dependent activation of hypoxia inducible factor 1 transcriptional activity in cells subjected to intermittent hypoxia. J Biol Chem. 2005;280:4321–8.
193. Zhan G, Serrano F, Fenik P, et al. NADPH oxidase mediates hypersomnolence and brain oxidative injury in a murine model of sleep apnea. Am J Respir Crit Care Med. 2005;172:921–9.
194. Zhu Y, Fenik P, Zhan G, et al. Selective loss of catecholaminergic wake active neurons in a murine sleep apnea model. J Neurosci. 2007;27:10060–71.
195. Zidar N, Jeruc J, Balazic J, et al. Neutrophils in human myocardial infarction with rupture of the free wall. Cardiovasc Pathol. 2005;14:247–50.
196. Zoccal DB, Bonagamba LG, Oliveira FR, et al. Increased sympathetic activity in rats submitted to chronic intermittent hypoxia. Exp Physiol. 2007;92:79–85.

Beneficial Effects of Intermittent Normobaric Hypoxic Training on Respiratory Function in Patients with Chronic Pulmonary Diseases

9

Mikhail I. Levashov

Abstract

In this chapter, we present the results of our studies regarding the INHT effects on respiratory functions in 103 high-risk chronic obstructive pulmonary disease (COPD) patients, 157 bronchial asthma (BA) patients, and 36 healthy individuals. Patients ranged in age from 21 to 59 years (women – 52.1%, men – 47.9%). INHT was carried out in "Orotron" chamber under such environmental parameters: PO_2 – 147–160 hPa, relative humidity – 60–70%, ambient temperature – 16–18°C, and content of light negative ions – up to 6,000/cm^3. All patients received daily 90 min of INHT alone or INHT in combination with conventional therapy for 2–4 weeks. Total time of hypoxic gas mixture breathing for the whole INHT course ranged from 21 to 42 h. We performed pulmonary function tests in all patients before, during, and after INHT. Results of our studies indicated that INHT increased reserves of lung ventilation and restored the physiological level of alveolar ventilation in 78% of patients with COPD, optimized regional air distribution in lung, and decreased by 25–30% the lung ventilation unevenness. INHT reduced the bronchial resistivity by 31–37% in BA patients and changed the respiratory regulation in COPD patients and healthy individuals. It contributed to more complete restoration of the optimal structure of respiratory pattern. Further investigations will allow INHT to emerge as an important nonpharmacological therapy for care and rehabilitation of patients with pulmonary diseases.

Abbreviations

BA	Bronchial asthma
CIA	Central inspiratory activity
COPD	Chronic obstructive pulmonary diseases
f	Respiratory rate
ERV	Expiratory reserve volume
FEV_1	Volume at the end of the first second of forced expiration
FEF_{max}	Maximum instantaneous flow achieved during FVC maneuver
$FEF_{25\%}$	Average flow from the point were 25% of the FVC has been exhaled
$FEF_{50\%}$	Average flow from the point were 50% of the FVC has been exhaled
$FEF_{75\%}$	Average flow from the point were 75% of the FVC has been exhaled
FRC	Functional residual capacity
FVC	Forced vital capacity
G_{aw}	Airway conductance
INHT	Intermittent normobaric hypoxic training
IRV	Inspiratory reserve volume
MVV	Maximal voluntary ventilation
MVV/V_E	Ratio of respiratory reserve
PO_2	Partial pressure of oxygen
PI_{max}	Maximal inspiratory pressure
R_{aw}	Airway resistance
t_I	Inspiratory time of one respiratory cycle
t_E	Expiratory time of one respiratory cycle

M.I. Levashov
National Academy of Sciences of Ukraine,
A.A. Bogomoletz Institute of Physiology,
Kiev, Ukraine
e-mail: levashov@biph.kiev.ua

L. Xi, T.V. Serebrovskaya (eds.), *Intermittent Hypoxia and Human Diseases*,
DOI 10.1007/978-1-4471-2906-6_9, © Springer-Verlag London 2012

t_{tot}	Total duration of respiratory cycle
t_I/t_{tot}	Proportion of inspiration phase in total duration of respiratory cycle or "useful cycle" of breathing
t_E/t_I	Time respiratory quotient
V_A	Alveolar ventilation/min
VC	Vital capacity
V_E	Expired volume/min
V_T	Tidal volume
V_I/t_I	Mean rate of inspiratory flow of one breath
V_E/t_E	Mean rate of expiratory flow of one breath
$V_{I\,max}/t_I$	Maximum rate of inspiratory flow of one breath
$V_{E\,max}/t_E$	Maximum rate of expiratory flow of one breath

9.1 Historical Aspect of the Problem

Sanogenic and healing properties of mountain climate are known since ancient times. Alpine climate has been used for treating patients with pulmonary tuberculosis, chronic obstructive pulmonary diseases, and bronchial asthma for more than two centuries. Doctors recommended mountain climate for patients suffering from "bronchial catarrh with profuse expectoration" (Meyer-Arens 1867) and considered it the best remedy for "raw asthma" (Lombard 1885) [1]. However, intensive study of various aspects of mountain climate effects on healthy and sick people began only in the twentieth century. Mass survey of mountain populations in different countries showed that some diseases among natives are extremely rare and considerably milder than in plainsmen [2]. Academician NN Sirotinin and his collaborators and followers made a great contribution to study mountain climate sanogenic and healing properties in the former USSR [3]. They have developed a detailed method of stepwise acclimation to mountain climate and proved its effectiveness in patients with several diseases.

A lot of scientific information has been accumulated about various aspects of mountain climate treatment of patients with BA, COPD, and other pulmonary diseases not only in low and middle altitudes but also in high mountains [4–8]. It was found that cough, asthma attacks, and number of wheezing in lungs significantly decreased, especially in BA patients with the mild form of disease, from the first days of adaptation to altitude. Studies of respiratory and hemodynamic functions showed a decrease in bronchial obstruction, reduction of hypoxemia and myocardial hypoxia severity, diminution of pulmonary vascular spasm, increase in alveolar ventilation and circulating blood volume, etc. Significant changes in immune system have been demonstrated at high altitude, including reduction of the skin allergy tests, B- and T-helper cell activation, decrease of the total and site-specific immunoglobulin E antibodies, and other immunological parameters. The positive effects of high-altitude treatment are most impressive in asthmatic children [9–11].

The well-defined therapeutic effect was obtained in COPD patients also [12, 13]. When these patients for some time remained at the middle altitudes, they experienced improvements in lung ventilation, respiratory tract aerodynamic properties, and ventilation-perfusion relationships in lungs. Gas exchange and pulmonary dust clearance were significantly better in patients with early-stage coal workers' pneumoconiosis and COPD at altitude of 2,300 m above sea level. These changes sustained for up to 6 months after returning to plain [14]. Despite the fact that the sanogenic and healing effects of mountain climate are well established, the widespread use of it for medical purposes is limited by a number of objective factors. The rapid changes in climatic zone when moving residents of plains to mountains may negatively affect on the patients' health status. That is why there exist a large number of medical contraindications for patients to stay in low barometric pressure and high-altitude hypoxia. It also should take into account the seasonal changes of meteorological, heliogeophysical, and other factors in mountains. As a result, the mountain climate therapy is unavailable for many healthy and sick people. That is why scientists and clinicians have attempted to simulate mountain climatic conditions on plains in order to use their sanogenic and healing properties in medical practice. Numerous studies have established that low partial pressure of oxygen (PO_2) is the most physiologically significant factor of mountain climate. Therefore, the main task for researchers was the creation of hypoxic conditions on plains. Hypobaric chamber was used for this purpose initially.

The first experience of treating BA patients in hypobaric chamber is associated with the name of academician NN Sirotinin. He attained encouraging results already in 1940–1941. Works done in the USSR in 1960s–1970s confirmed the high efficiency of this method in adults and children with BA. One of the most comprehensive studies was conducted in 650 BA patients in age from 2 to 49 years [15]. Full cessation of breathlessness and stable remission were observed after the first course of treatment in hypobaric chamber in 24.5% of children and 42.1% of adults. Treatment in hypobaric chamber had no significant effect only in 6.6% children and 14% adults. The immediate effect was even higher after repeated two or three courses of hypobaric treatment. The long-term positive effects were maintained from 1 month to several years. The most of BA patients significantly decreased the frequency of disease exacerbations, the number of breathlessness attacks, and incidence of acute respiratory infections. It was concluded that treatment in hypobaric chamber could be most efficient in children and adults with mild and moderate form of BA in phase of recovery and remission [16, 17].

Further investigation revealed that such factors as sympathoadrenal system activation, and cellular and humoral immunity normalization play important role in therapeutic mechanisms of the hypobaric treatment. These changes lead to decrease in bronchial hyperreactivity and severity of bronchoobstruction, improvement of lung ventilation, and bronchial drainage function in BA patients [18, 19].

It is obvious that sanogenic mechanisms of mountain climate and hypobaric chamber have much in common associated with exposure to low barometric pressure and PO_2. Nevertheless, the treatment in hypobaric chamber is not widely used in clinics because of the risk of serious complications associated with the combined effect of these factors.

Since 1970s, the researchers' and practitioners' attention was attracted by the possibility of using the intermittent normobaric hypoxic training (INHT) for increasing nonspecific resistance to pathological factors in healthy and sick people. The comparative analysis of people's reaction on an equal decrease in PO_2 showed that normobaric hypoxia tolerated much better than hypobaric one [20]. Initially, INHT has been used in oncology practice for protection of patients' body against exposure to ionizing radiation during radiation therapy [21]. This method was also used in patients with fibrocavernous tuberculosis before surgery [22] and later for nonpharmacological treatment and prevention of different diseases [23–29]. Hypoxic gas mixtures containing from 10% to 16% oxygen in nitrogen have been most commonly used. Gas mixtures are inhaled in intermittent regime for maximum efficiency and exclusion of side effects. In accordance with this method, patient inhales the hypoxic gas mixture for 3–5 min and then atmospheric air for 3–5 min. The numbers of such cycles vary from 1 to 10 depending on the nature of disease and individual patient's peculiarities. The cumulative time of hypoxic gas mixture inhaling could be up to 30–60 min for a session.

Various technical devices such as anesthetic machine with semiopen breathing circuit and individual hypoxycator (Fig. 9.1) have been used in outpatient and home settings for obtaining normobaric hypoxic gas mixture identical to PO_2 levels at certain height above sea level. This device uses the principle of rebreathing and absorption of exhaled carbon dioxide. More recently, devices based on selective gas separation elements have become widely available, which allow fine adjustment of the necessary volumes of hypoxic gas mixtures with a given oxygen concentration [30].

In 1987, the scientists of AA Bogomoletz Institute of Physiology, National Academy of Sciences of Ukraine under the guidance of Prof. VA Berezovskii invented the first climatic chamber for group INHT (Fig. 9.2) and apparatus "Boreus" for individual INHT (Fig. 9.3). For many years, these devices have been used for INHT in pulmonary patients. We observed high therapeutic and preventive efficacy especially in patients with mild form of BA and in high-risk COPD patients. Different regimes of INHT were developed and tested. This provides individualization of INHT and elimination of side effects [14, 31].

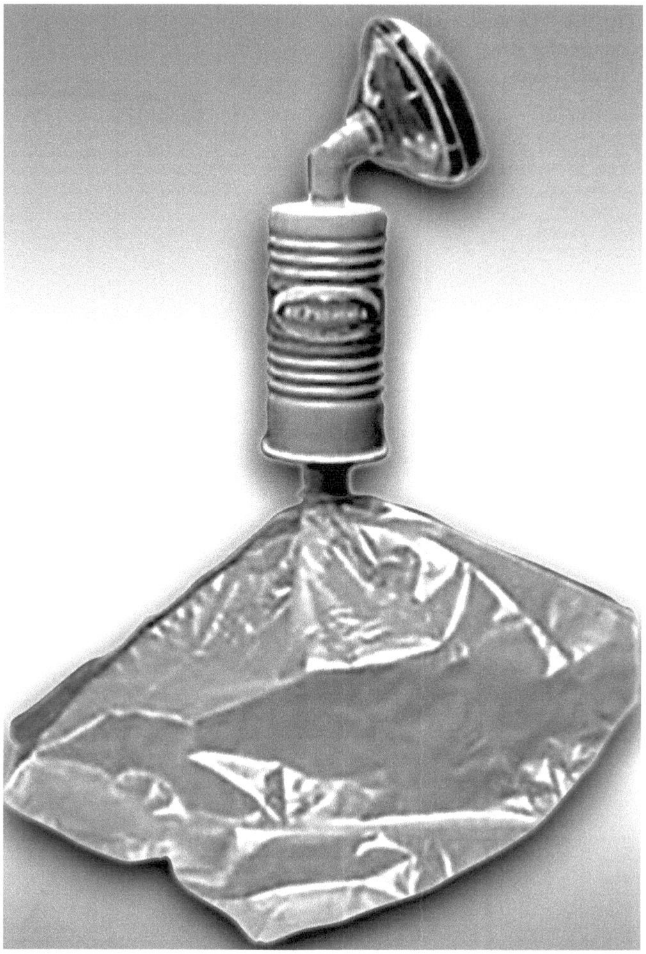

Fig. 9.1 "Vershina" – the handheld hypoxicator for individual INHT (Firm "METOM", Moscow Russia)

In this chapter, we present the results of our studies regarding the INHT effects on respiratory function in 36 healthy individuals, 103 high-risk COPD patients, and 157 BA patients. Patients ranged in age from 21 to 59 years (women – 52.1%, men – 47.9%). INHT was performed in "Orotron" chamber. Under conditions of normal atmospheric pressure, this device creates and maintains in automatic mode the following parameters: PO_2 – 147–160 kPa, relative humidity – 60–70%, ambient temperature – 16–18°C, and content of light negative ions – up to 6,000/cm^3. All patients within 2–4 weeks for 1.5 h daily received only INHT or INHT in combination with conventional therapy. The total time of hypoxic exposure in intermittent regime ranged from 21 to 42 h. Parameters of lung function were recorded in all patients before, during, and after INHT.

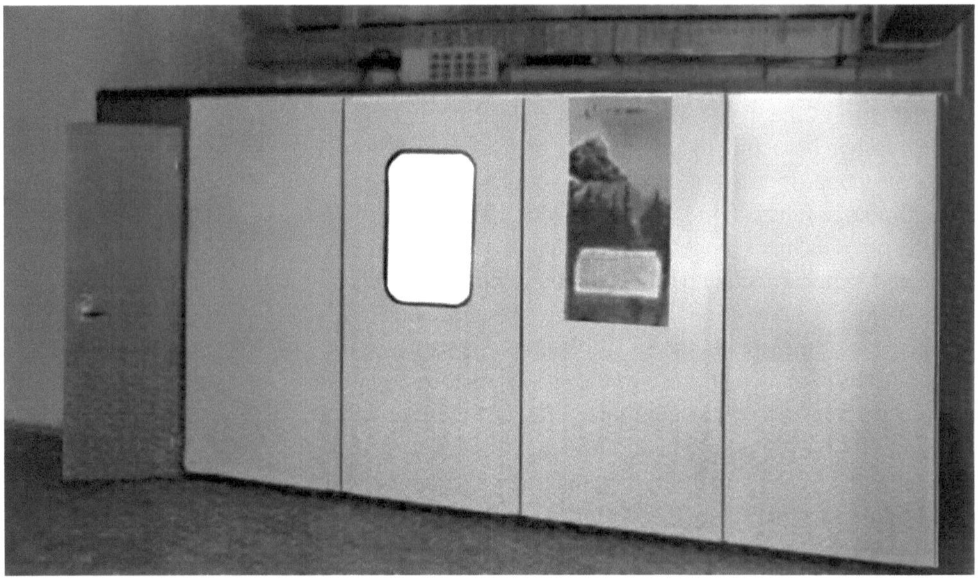

Fig. 9.2 "Orotron" – the climatic chamber for group INHT (Center "NORT," Kiev, Ukraine)

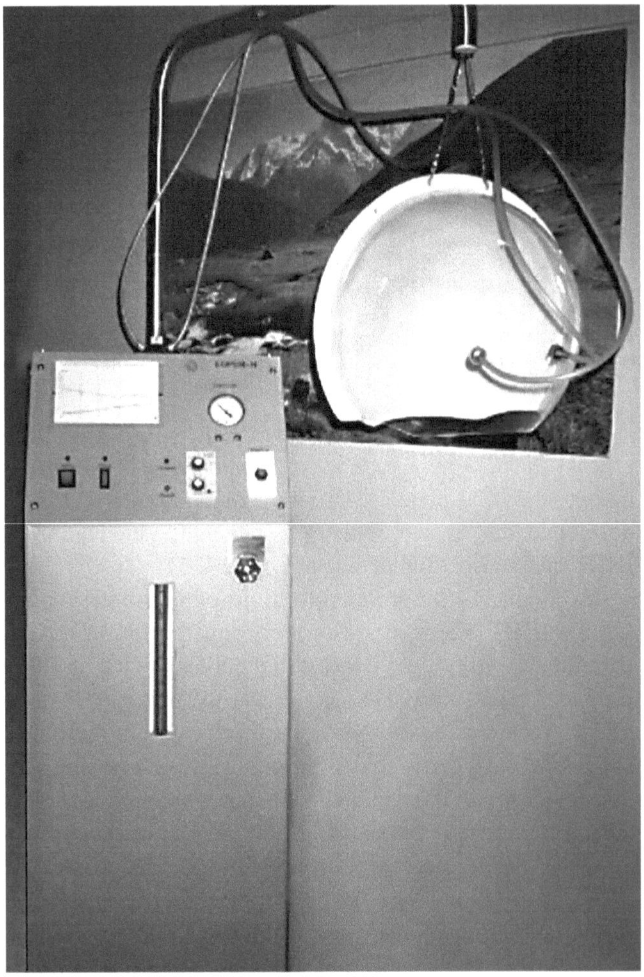

Fig. 9.3 "Boreus" – the apparatus for individual INHT (Center "NORT," Kiev, Ukraine)

9.2 INHT and Lung Ventilation in COPD and BA Patients

We studied the healthy individuals and patients with high-risk COPD and BA to clarify the nature of changes in total and alveolar lung ventilation, as well as the status of individual mechanisms that determine their effectiveness in adaptation to INHT. The methods of spirography, pneumotachography, and phonopulmography were used for investigating lung ventilation in five groups of subjects. The first group (healthy individuals) without lung diseases received only INHT. The second group – high-risk COPD patients – received conventional therapy in combination with INHT. The third group – high-risk COPD patients – received only INHT. The fourth group – patients with BA – received conventional therapy with INHT. The fifth group – patients with BA – received only conventional therapy.

Before INHT, the main parameters of lung ventilation were varied within the physiological norm in individuals who had no pulmonary diseases (Table 9.1). Minute volume of lung ventilation (V_E), tidal volume (V_T), and respiratory rate (f) did not significantly change after INHT. However, inspiratory reserve volume (IRV), maximum volume of lungs ventilation (MVV), and ratio of respiratory reserve (MVV/V_E) authentically increased. On the other hand, time of inspiration (t_I) and expiration (t_E) significantly decreased. These changes in lung ventilation were caused by adaptation of the healthy individuals to INHT. The statistically significant reduction in time of inspiration and expiration and tendency to increasing of respiratory rate in healthy peoples after INHT could be due to modifying effect of hypoxia on the respiratory regulation mechanisms [32]. This aspect will be considered in detail below.

There were no statistically significant differences in lung ventilation between the second and third groups' patients before INHT (Table 9.2). The values of vital capacity (VC), forced vital capacity (FVC), and expiratory reserve volume (ERV) increased by 9.2±2.5%, 6.1±2.9%, and 80.5±9.3%, respectively in 93.2% of high-risk COPD patients after 2 weeks of conventional therapy in combination with INHT. The volume that has been exhaled at the end of the first second of forced expiration (FEV_1) also achieved to upper limit of the physiological norm. It was characteristic that VC increased by 0.33±0.09 ($p<0.05$) mainly due to ERV.

The third group of high-risk COPD patients showed a steady tendency to increase in VC and FVC after INHT. The values of ERV increased by 0.22±0.09 l ($p<0.05$); FEV_1 did not differ from the second group of patients. Such dynamics in spirography parameters pointed to improvement of lung ventilation in 81.3% of COPD patients who received INHT alone. It was achieved by improved efficiency and increased ventilatory reserves, mainly ERV.

The most significant disturbances in lung ventilation were observed in patient groups 4 and 5 before the INHT (Table 9.3). The obstructive type of disorders was dominant. Both groups of patients showed a decrease in FEV_1, FEV_1/FVC and increase in t_E. The more considerable decrease in MVV compared with VC led to decrease in MVV/VC ratios, which also reflected the severity of lung ventilation disorders. Repeated examinations indicated the different treatment efficiency in the fourth and fifth group of patients. The statistically significant differences appeared between the main indices of lung function.

Table 9.1 Spirography indices in healthy individuals before (I) and after (II) INHT, ($n=36$)

Characteristics	I	II
V_E, l · min^{-1}	11.06±0.73	11.38±0.72
f, min^{-1}	16.6±0.8	17.7±0.9
V_T, l	0.70±0.03	0.65±0.04
t_E, s	2.27±0.12	1.91±0.13*
t_I, s	1.70±0.14	1.37±0.08*
t_E/t_I	1.42±0.08	1.57±0.08
VC, l	3.99±0.29	4.07±0.24
VC, %	99.1±4.7	102.6±3.9
IRV, l	2.51±0.32	2.90±0.22*
ERV, l	0.55±0.11	0.51±0.13
FVC, l	3.44±0.22	3.74±0.38
FEV_1, l	2.98±0.20	3.23±0.26
FEV_1, %	99.3±4.9	108.1±6.4*
FEV_1/FVC, %	85.6±2.1	88.1±1.9
MVV, l · min^{-1}	78.2±8.8	84.5±6.0
MVV, %	76.2±3.9	83.1±3.8*
MVV/VC, %	19.4±1.1	19.4±1.1
MVV/V_E	7.0±0.8	8.1±0.7*

*$p<0.05$ – values are significantly different from the initial state

Table 9.2 Spirography indices in high-risk COPD patients before (I) and after (II) INHT in combination with conventional therapy (2) and INHT only (3)

	Group of patients			
	2 ($n=57$)		3 ($n=46$)	
Characteristics	I	II	I	II
V_E, l · min^{-1}	13.28±0.93	12.57±0.76	12.02±0.85	12.29±0.73
f, min^{-1}	17.8±0.8	17.9±1.1	16.4±1.1	16.8±1.1
V_T, l	0.76±0.04	0.76±0.05	0.78±0.06	0.75±0.04
t_E, s	1.89±0.13	2.07±0.15	2.45±0.18	2.30±0.18
t_I, s	1.53±0.08	1.47±0.10	1.60±0.10	1.48±0.08
t_E/t_I	1.26±0.07	1.40±0.07	1.53±0.08	1.52±0.08
VC, l	3.33±0.19	3.66±0.21*	2.97±0.27	3.07±0.28
VC, %	87.4±4.3	96.4±3.8*	87.5±5.1	96.7±4.8
IRV, l	2.07±0.16	2.24±0.19	1.79±0.16	1.98±0.17
ERV, l	0.41±0.08	0.74±0.11*	0.51±0.11	0.73±0.13*
FVC, l	2.96±0.18	3.14±0.18*	2.69±0.26	2.85±0.25
FEV_1, l	2.50±0.13	2.75±0.16$^+$	2.12±0.21	2.46±0.22*
FEV_1, %	88.1±3.9	97.3±3.9*	82.6±5.5	96.2±5.4*
FEV_1/FVC, %	81.5±1.5	87.9±1.5*	79.3±2.5	87.8±1.6*
MVV, l · min^{-1}	65.7±5.0	69.1±5.7	59.2±5.9	60.8±6.5
MVV, %	66.1±5.6	71.7±5.5	68.0±5.7	73.9±5.9
MVV/VC, %	19.5±1.0	17.1±1.0	20.4±1.1	19.4±1.1
MVV/V_E	4.9±0.6	5.4±0.5	5.5±0.8	5.4±0.7

*$p<0.05$ – values are significantly different from the initial state

Table 9.3 Spirography indices in BA patients before (I) and after (II) INHT in combination with conventional therapy (4) and conventional therapy only (5)

	Group of patients			
	4 ($n=85$)		5 ($n=72$)	
Characteristics	I	II	I	II
V_E, l · min^{-1}	11.64±0.64	13.61±0.77	12.84±1.01	12.11±0.84
f, min^{-1}	16.8±0.8	17.0±0.9	14.8±0.9	14.5±0.6
V_T, l	0.77±0.06	0.84±0.06	0.87±0.06	0.71±0.04
t_E, s	2.21±0.15	2.40±0.19	2.39±0.19	2.10±0.17
t_I, s	1.61±0.10	1.55±0.90	1.67±0.22	1.58±0.13
t_E/t_I	2.21±0.15	2.40±0.19	2.19±0.16	2.25±0.18
VC, l	3.14±0.19	3.26±0.20	3.96±0.37	4.07±0.24
VC, %	80.6±4.1	88.2±4.2*	82.6±3.7	87.5±3.8
IRV, l	2.08±0.16	1.94±0.18	2.37±0.22	2.32±0,32
ERV, l	0.40±0.10	0.55±0.08	0.51±0.13	0.77±0.13
FVC, l	2.89±0.20	2.91±0.18	3.44±0.22	3.58±0.34
FEV_1, l	2.02±0.14	2.34±0.16**	2.81±0.27	3.07±0.21
FEV_1, %	71.8±4.5	82.2±4,8**	73.4±5,3	80.3±4.1
FEV_1/FVC, %	70.2±2.4	80.1±2.5**	68.2±1.8	74.6±1.9*
MVV, l · min^{-1}	61.2±5.4	65.3±5.4	76.9±8.6	80.1±6.1
MVV, %	64.0±4.7	66.6±4.9	69.3±5.1	71.5±5.6
MVV/VC, %	16.3±1.9	20.5±1.4*	17.4±1.7	20.3±1.2*
MVV/V_E	5.6±0.5	5.2±0.4	5.9±0.5	6.5±0.3

*$p<0.05$, **$p<0.01$ – values are significantly different from the initial state

The fourth group of patients had a significant increase in V_E from 11.64±0.64 to 13.61±0.77 l and VC from 80.6±4.1% to 88.2±4.2% ($p<0.05$). The speed characteristics of pulmonary ventilation increased more significantly. The values of FEV_1 increased by 0.32±0.08 l, FEV_1/FVC by 10.4±2.3%, and MVV/VC reached up to 20.5±1.4% ($p<0.05$). Higher rates of lung ventilation parameters after INHT in combination with conventional therapy were achieved in these patients mainly by improving the respiratory tract aerodynamic properties. There was also some positive dynamic in spirography parameters in fifth group of patients after conventional therapy. But these changes were 25–38% less ($p<0.05$) than those in patients group 4.

Thus, INHT induced the adaptive changes in lung ventilation and increased its effectiveness in healthy individuals. INHT increased the lung ventilation reserves and improved the respiratory tract aerodynamic properties in patients with COPD and BA. These effects of INHT led to efficiency gains of conventional therapy by 25–30%.

9.3 INHT and Alveolar Ventilation in COPD Patients

Given the fact that efficiency of lung ventilation is determined by not so much the total lung ventilation but the alveolar ventilation, we investigated the dynamic of alveolar ventilation (V_A) in patients with COPD before and after course of INHT in relation to changes of V_T and functional residual capacity (FRC). We used the method of pulmophonography for these purposes [33].

The patients had different ratio of V_T and FRC and, consequently, the value of V_A before INHT. The values of V_T, FRC, and alveolar ventilation were within the physiological norm in 25% of patients (Table 9.4). Enhanced alveolar hyperventilation due to increased V_T took place in 40% of patients. Alveolar hypoventilation due to significant increase in FRC and decrease in V_T were observed in 35% of patients.

The various changes of V_T and FRC were identified in all patients after 2 weeks of INHT. It was reflected in dynamics of alveolar ventilation. But the nature and severity of these changes were different. The value of V_T decreased by 0.54±0.11 ($p<0.05$), and FRC increased by 0.43±0.16 ($p<0.05$) in the first group of patients. As a result, the V_A decreased by 0.10±0.02 ($p<0.05$) and approached to the physiological level. In the second group of patients, V_T increased by 0.24±0.09 but FRC decreased by 0.16±0.05 ($p<0.05$). This led to a moderate increase in V_A. In the third group of patients, V_T and FRC significantly increased by 0.28±0.06 and 0.21±0.06 ($p<0.05$), respectively. It was accompanied by increased V_A, albeit to a lesser extent, than in the second group of patients.

Increased FRC reduced the excessive V_A in hyperventilation patients after INHT. The more significantly increased V_T led to improvement of the alveolar ventilation in hypoventilation patients. As a result of such changes of V_T and FRC, 76% of

Table 9.4 Values of V_T, FRC, and V_A measured with a pulmophonography method in high-risk COPD patients with initial alveolar hyperventilation, normoventilation, and hypoventilation before (I) and after (II) INHT

Group of patients	Stages of research	V_T, un.	FRC, un.	V_A, un.
Hyperventilation ($n=34$)	I	1.93±0.17	6.91±0.16	0.29±0.019
	II	1.38±0.11*	7.34±0.04*	0.19±0.002*
Normoventilation ($n=21$)	I	1.43±0.05	7.34±0.03	0.20±0.004
	II	1.67±0.20*	7.19±0.07*	0.24±0.003*
Hypoventilation ($n=30$)	I	0.94±0.10	7.12±0.13	0.14±0.002
	II	1.22±0.12**	7.33±0.09**	0.17±0.002*

*$p<0.05$, **$p<0.01$ – values are significantly different from the initial state

Table 9.5 Unevenness of the total and alveolar lung ventilation in high-risk COPD patients measured with a pulmophonography method before (I) and after (II) INHT, ($n=85$)

	Coefficient of unevenness, un.		
Lung ventilation	Range of physiological norm	I	II
Total ventilation of the right lung	0.53÷0.60	0.70±0.04	0.54±0.03**
Alveolar ventilation of the right lung	0.42÷0.54	0.74±0.05	0.53±0.03*
Total ventilation of the left lung	0.61÷0.78	1.08±0.05	0.82±0.04*
Alveolar ventilation of the left lung	0.49÷0.62	0.81±0.06	0.58±0.05*

*$p<0.05$, **$p<0.01$ – values are significantly different from the initial state

COPD patients with initial alveolar hyper- and hypoventilation reached up to physiological level by the end of INHT. Our results suggest that INHT could decrease or eliminate the alveolar ventilation impairment in COPD patients.

We also studied the alveolar ventilation distribution in four standard regions (i.e., superior, inferior, anterior, and posterior) of the right and left lung in COPD patients before and after INHT by means of phonopulmography method. Interesting results were obtained in hyperventilation (first group) and hypoventilation (second group) patients.

Significant disturbances in regional lung ventilation were observed in hyperventilation patients before the INHT. The total alveolar hyperventilation predominantly in posterior and superior regions was typical for the dominant lung of these patients. The alveolar hyperventilation in superior and posterior region and normal levels of alveolar ventilation in inferior and anterior regions were observed in nondominant lung. This type of regional ventilation distribution was the least favorable, since the maximum ventilation was in superior and posterior regions, which had the lowest level of perfusion even in physiological conditions. The alveolar ventilation was dramatically lower in inferior, anterior, and posterior regions of both lungs in second group of COPD patients before INHT. Disturbances of the regional ventilation were most pronounced in nondominant lung. INHT optimized the regional ventilation in the first group of patients due to significant decrease of the alveolar ventilation in posterior (by 0.23±0.06), superior (by 0.18±0.04), and, to a lesser extent, inferior (by 0.12±0.04) and anterior regions (by 0.12±0.03) of dominant lung. Changes of the alveolar ventilation in all regions of nondominant lung did not exceed 0.08–0.06. The values of regional ventilation indices approached to the physiological level in both lungs in the first group of patients by the end of INHT.

INHT moderately increased the alveolar ventilation in inferior region (by 0.04±0.01) and, to a lesser extent, in anterior and posterior regions of dominant lung in the second group of patients. Alveolar ventilation of nondominant lung increased in all regions, but maximum increase was noted in anterior (by 0.05±0.01) and posterior (by 0.04±0.01) regions.

The indices of regional ventilation unevenness were within the physiological norm in patients with normal ventilation before INHT. But adaptation to INHT was accompanied by redistribution of regional ventilation. There was a decrease of alveolar ventilation in superior and posterior regions and a moderate increase in inferior and anterior regions of dominant lung. There was a trend toward a moderate increase of alveolar ventilation in all regions of nondominant lung.

It is known that COPD patients with normal or even increased level of lung ventilation may still have severe disorders of gas exchange. Manifestations of respiratory failure are frequently associated with abnormal distribution of air in lungs or unevenness of lung ventilation. That is why we determined the degree of unevenness distribution of total and alveolar ventilation in right and left lungs in patients with COPD before and after INHT.

The total and alveolar lung ventilation unevenness was evident in all COPD patients before INHT. The highest degree of unevenness was typical for the left lung (Table 9.5). We observed a significant decrease of lung ventilation unevenness after INHT. The unevenness coefficient of total and

Table 9.6 Respiratory tract aerodynamic characteristics in high-risk COPD patients before (I) and after (II) INHT in combination with conventional therapy (1), before (III) and after (IV) INHT only (2)

	Group of patients			
	1 (n=57)		2 (n=43)	
Characteristics	I	II	III	IV
R_{awI}, mmAq · l^{-1} · s^{-1}	11.45±1.18	9.07±0.98	12.77±1.20	10.91±1.11
R_{awE}, mmAq · l^{-1} · s^{-1}	10.37±1.22	9.88±1.04	9.81±1.32	8.01±1.40
G_{awI}, mmAq^{-1} · l · s	0.11±0.02	0.22±0.05	0.14±0.03	0.20±0.06
G_{awE}, mmAq^{-1} · l · s	0.14±0.02	0.19±0.04	0.15±0.02	0.16±0.04
FEF_{max}, l · s^{-1}	5.01±0.35	5.92±0.39*	5.58±0.75	5.42±0.69*
$FEF_{25\%}$, l · s^{-1}	4.79±0.33	5.45±0.37*	4.31±0.38	5.08±0.41
$FEF_{50\%}$, l · s^{-1}	3.47±0.23	4.00±0.28*	3.90±0.34	4.87±0.23*
$FEF_{75\%}$, l · s^{-1}	1.95±0.18	2.04±0.17	2.01±0.25	2.51±0.27
$FEF_{50\%}/FEF_{75\%}$	189.2±10.3	198.8±8.9	207.6±16.5	178.1±8.7*

*$p<0.05$ – values are significantly different from the initial state

alveolar ventilation decreased by 22.9% and 21.6% in right lung and by 24.1% and 28.4% in left lung, respectively. The distribution of lung ventilation between right and left lung was improved mainly due to the increased ventilation in right lung after INHT. Consequently, the number of patients with absolute or relative dominance of right lung ventilation increased from 47% to 57%. The data indicated that the unevenness of regional lung ventilation in COPD patients was expressed more often in hyperventilation of superior and posterior regions and/or hypoventilation in inferior and anterior regions. Such changes in regional ventilation were the least favorable.

In summary, INHT improved or normalized the lung regional ventilation in 78% COPD patients. As a result, it restored the physiological level of ventilation distribution between right and left lung and reduced the severity of ventilation unevenness in each lung.

9.4 INHT and Airway Resistance in COPD and BA Patients

Bronchial obstruction is one of the important links in pathogenesis of pulmonary functional impairments in COPD and BA patients. The nature, severity, and reversibility of bronchial obstruction to a large extent determine the efficiency of therapeutic measures, as well as estimating the patient's quality of daily life and well-being. In this context, the particular interest was paid to the possibility of bronchial obstruction correction in patients with chronic pulmonary diseases by INHT. This issue was investigated in four groups of patients. The high-risk COPD patients who received conventional therapy in combination with INHT were included in group 1. The second group of COPD patients received only INHT. The third group of patients with BA received INHT in combination with conventional therapy. The fourth group of patients with BA received only conventional therapy. Investigation of airway resistance was performed by pneumotachography method.

The total airway resistance in high-risk COPD patients, who had no clinical signs of bronchial obstruction, was 11–12 mmAq · l^{-1} · s^{-1} in phase of inspiration (R_{awI}) and 9–10 mmAq · l^{-1} · s^{-1} in phase of expiration (R_{awE}). The mean values of respiratory conductance were 0.11–0.14 mmAq^{-1} · l · s (G_{awI}) and 0.14–0.15 mmAq^{-1} · l · s (G_{awE}), respectively. The maximum instantaneous flow achieved during a FVC maneuver (FEF_{max}) and the average flow from the point where 25%, 50%, and 75% of the FVC has been exhaled ($FEF_{25\%}$, $FEF_{50\%}$, $FEF_{75\%}$) did not extend beyond the lower level of physiological norm. There were no significant differences in these indices between the first and second groups of COPD patients before INHT (Table 9.6).

The values of R_{awI}, R_{awE} did not change significantly in both groups of high-risk COPD patients after INHT, but FEF_{max}, $FEF_{25\%}$, and $FEF_{50\%}$ were moderately increased. This was related to the improvement of upper respiratory tract aerodynamic properties and the increased effort of respiratory muscles. The overall changes of these parameters in COPD patients of group 1 and 2 were similar, and there was no statistically significant intergroup difference. But if the combination of INHT with the conventional therapy allowed to achieve the positive results in 91.8% of patients, whereas when only INHT was used, 78.9% of patients had such positive outcomes.

There was a significant airflow limitation in third and fourth groups of BA patients before treatment began. The airway resistance was increased up to 14–15 mmAq · l^{-1} · s^{-1}, and the value of respiratory conductance did not exceed 0.08 mmAq^{-1} · l · s. All indices of "flow-volume" curve were lower, but $FEF_{75\%}$ decreased more significantly. This indicated an increase of peripheral airways resistance (Table 9.7).

Significant improvement was found in all basic characteristics of the airway function in the third group of patients after INHT in combination with conventional therapy. Positive dynamics was significantly lower in the fourth group of patients who received only conventional therapy. Intergroup

Table 9.7 Respiratory tract aerodynamic characteristics: (1) in BA patients before (I) and after (II) INHT in combination with conventional therapy; (2) in BA patients before (III) and after (IV) INHT only (2)

	Group of patients			
	1 (n=47)		2 (n=33)	
Characteristics	I	II	III	IV
R_{awI}, mmAq · l^{-1} · s^{-1}	14.35±1.55	10.47±0.95*	15.41±1.44	13.01±0.85*
R_{awE}, mmAq · l^{-1} · s^{-1}	13.83±1.91	10.55±1.21*	14.01±1.81	12.84±1.91*
G_{awI}, mmAq^{-1} · l · s	0.08±0.01	0.11±0.02	0.07±0.01	0.10±0.01
G_{awE}, mmAq^{-1} · l · s	0.09±0.01	0.11±0.01	0.10±0.01	0.11±0.02
FEF_{max}, l · s^{-1}	4.12±0.35	4.84±0.33**	4.32±0.30	5.01±0.49*
$FEF_{25\%}$, l · s^{-1}	3.23±0.33	4.24±0.34*	3.08±0.21	3.59±0.38
$FEF_{50\%}$, l · s^{-1}	2.03±0.23	2.87±0.28*	2.11±0.32	2.65±0.56*
$FEF_{75\%}$, l · s^{-1}	0.98±0.13	1.36±0.16*	1.15±0.23	1.42±0.15*
$FEF_{50\%}/FEF_{75\%}$	262.7±39.6	213.8±15.8	263.5±34.8	212.4±28.8

*$p<0.05$, ** $p<0.01$– values are significantly different from the initial state

differences for some indices reached from 27% to 52%. These facts indicated that there was an obvious bronchodilatation effect of INHT in BA patients. This effect was more evidence in those BA patients, who received only INHT.

The efficacy of bronchodilation effect in BA patients after INHT was largely determined by duration and severity of disease, the presence of steroid dependence, and concomitant pathology. Our data show that individual selection of INHT allows to decrease the level of airflow obstruction in 88.7% of mild BA patients. Notably, the degree and duration of the positive effects of INHT on airway function and respiratory resistance in patients with chronic pulmonary diseases were not less than those achieved in mountains.

9.5 Effect of INHT on Respiratory Pattern in COPD and BA Patients

Changes in patient's respiratory pattern are very important in both diagnostic and prognostic assessment [34, 35]. It is known that frequent and shallow breathing is the least effective compensatory reaction. Development of tachypnea may be the first and only symptom of the respiratory distress syndrome and sudden death during sleep. On the other hand, the normalization in the structure and parameters of the respiratory cycle demonstrates the efficacy of therapeutic measures undertaken and the favorable course of disease.

Existing data about change in respiratory pattern in healthy men were obtained at the sea level and during high-altitude adaptation. This problem was studied also in patients during short-time adaptation to hypobaric hypoxia. The direct effects of hypoxic exposure were mainly examined in these studies. But the questions about nature and persistence of the changes in respiratory pattern during and after INHT in patients with COPD and BA remain opened [36].

We studied the dynamics of volumetric, temporal, and spatial parameters of respiratory pattern in COPD and BA patients under INHT. The following key indicators of respiratory pattern [37] were analyzed: V_E, V_T, f, t_{tot} (total duration of respiratory cycle), t_I (duration of inspiratory phase), t_E (duration of expiratory phase), t_I/t_{tot} (proportion of inspiration phase in total duration of respiratory cycle) or "useful cycle" of breathing, t_E/t_I (time respiratory quotient), V_I/t_I (mean rate of inspiratory flow), V_E/t_E (mean rate of expiratory flow), $V_{I\,max}/t_I$ (maximum rate of inspiratory flow), and $V_{E\,max}/t_E$ (maximum rate of expiratory flow).

Preliminary analysis of the initial respiratory pattern structure allowed allocating two groups of patients before INHT (Table 9.8). The values of V_E, V_T, f, and t_I were higher in the second group of patients, but $V_{E\,max}/t_E$ and t_E/t_I ratios were higher in the first group.

Changes in respiratory pattern had a stenoventilation type in the first group of patients after INHT. We found increased V_E and f by 2.21±0.74 l ($p<0.05$) and 2.6±0.7 min^{-1} ($p<0.05$), respectively. The total duration of respiratory cycle was less by 0.62±0.14 s ($p<0.05$) due to decreased t_I and to a lesser extent t_E. The t_E/t_I and t_I/t_{tot} ratios were stable because of proportional reduction in time of inspiration and expiration. The mean rate of inspiratory flow increased due to reduction of t_I while V_T remained at a constant level.

The respiratory pattern changed in isoventilation type in patients group 2 after INHT. We found a typical decrease in f by 2.46±0.46 min^{-1} ($p<0.01$) and increase in V_T by 0.13±0.06 l ($p<0.01$), whereas the value of V_E remained unchanged. The decrease in respiratory rate led to increase in t_{tot} by 0.72±0.10 s, mainly due to increase in t_E by 0.32±0.12 s ($p<0.05$) and to lesser extent t_I. The t_E/t_I and t_I/t_{tot} ratios did not change, but $V_{E\,max}/t_E$ significantly increased.

As a result of these multidirectional changes in respiratory pattern, significant differences in V_T and f values were detected between the first and second groups of patients after INHT. Respiratory pattern in group 1 patients was characterized by more frequent and less deep breathing. The similar

Table 9.8 Characteristics of stenoventilation (1) and isoventilation (2) types of adaptive changes in breathing pattern in high-risk COPD patients before (I) and after (II) INHT

	1 (n=26)		2 (n=28)	
Characteristics	I	II	I	II
V_E, l · min^{-1}	11.02±0.72	13.23±0.81*	12.68±0.53	12.86±0.69
f, min^{-1}	16.48±0.81	18.17±0.95*	17.10±0.70	14.64±0.75*
V_T, l	0.66±0.05	0.73±0.05	0.74±0.05	0.88±0.07*
t_{tot}, s	3.64±0.11	3.26±0.18*	3.76±0.17	4.15±0.12*
t_E, s	1.50±0.07	1.30±0.08*	1.63±0.08	1.70±0.11
t_I, s	2.14±0.17	1.86±0.12	2.12±0.11	2.43±0.16*
t_E/t_I	1.45±0.11	1.42±0.06	1.32±0.06	1.43±0.07
t_I/t_{tot}	0.40±0.02	0.40±0.02	0.42±0.39	0.39±0.02*
V_I/t_I, l · s^{-1}	0.49±0.04	0.60±0.05*	0.49±0.02	0.55±0.04
V_E/t_E, l · s^{-1}	0.37±0.04	0.42±0.03	0.38±0.02	0.40±0.03
$V_{I\,max}/t_I$, l · s^{-1}	0.69±0.06	1.14±0.34*	0.67±0.04	0.93±0.14*
$V_{E\,max}/t_E$, l · s^{-1}	0.66±0.39	1.13±0.33	0.54±0.17	1.03±0.16*

*p<0.05 – values are significantly different from the initial state

volume of lung ventilation in group 2 patients was achieved by deeper and fewer breaths.

The mean inspiratory flow increased much significantly in the first group of patients, but the maximum expiratory flow values were recorded in the second group. The increase in mean expiratory flow was associated with improved airway aerodynamic properties and respiratory conductance. However, the increase in mean inspiratory flow reflected not only changes in respiratory muscles efforts but also to a larger extent the changes in central respiratory regulation. The frequency of basal respiratory pattern recovery was 0.96 in COPD patients who received INHT in combination with conventional therapy. This index did not exceed 0.63 in patients who received only conventional therapy.

Our results suggested that changes in volumetric, temporal, and spatial parameters of respiratory pattern in COPD patients after INHT were different in nature. They depended on the individual characteristics of respiratory biomechanics and status of central mechanisms of respiratory regulation. Adaptation to INHT restored the basal respiratory pattern in COPD patients, which was the best in physiological and energetic sense.

9.6 INHT and Respiratory Regulation in Healthy Individuals and COPD Patients

The above-discussed investigation of lung function in healthy individuals and COPD patients led us to assume that INHT affected not only at the level of executive organs (lungs, bronchi, respiratory muscles, etc.) but also at the level of central respiratory regulation. One of the few methods to study the central control of respiration is the phase analysis of respiratory cycles [37–39].

Accordingly, we applied the method in high-risk COPD patients and in healthy individuals. The first group of COPD patients received conventional therapy in combination with INHT and the second group received INHT only. The healthy individuals also received INHT. As indicators of central inspiratory activity (CIA), the value of maximal inspiratory pressure in the airway (PI_{max}) and the mean rate of inspiratory flow (V_I/t_I) were used [40, 41]. These indicators allow obtaining information about level and intensity of respiratory chemosensory stimulation – "a respiratory drive" – which is directly proportional to CIA. Excitability threshold of the "turn off" inspiration mechanism had been determined from the "useful cycle" of respiration (t_I/t_{tot}) [42].

It was found that PI_{max} was significantly higher in both groups of COPD patients than in healthy individuals before INHT (Table 9.9). This indicated a higher initial level of the central inspiratory activity in COPD patients. But V_I/t_I, which was usually directly proportional to CIA, did not increase. The t_I/t_{tot} ratio showed a tendency to increase the excitability threshold of the "turn off" inspiration mechanism in COPD patients. Healthy individuals had the higher level of V_I/t_I than COPD patients. This pointed to a relatively higher level of respiratory chemosensory stimulation in healthy individuals before INHT.

The mean values of PI_{max} and t_I/t_{tot} were decreased and V_I/t_I was increased in all COPD patients after INHT alone or in combination with conventional therapy. No statistically significant differences in these parameters between both groups of COPD patients indicate the direct involvement of INHT in these effects. However, the differences in degree and direction of PI_{max} and V_I/t_I changes in COPD patients who had no clinical and functional signs of bronchial obstruction might be related not only to respiratory regulation mechanisms but also to latent pulmonary functional impairment.

Our results in healthy individuals confirmed the direct influence of INHT on the central respiratory regulation. There was moderate but statistically significant decrease in PI_{max} and V_I/t_I in healthy individuals after INHT. But the t_I/t_{tot} ratio and therefore level of the excitability threshold of the "turn off" inspiration mechanism remained stable.

Table 9.9 Some characteristics of respiratory regulation in high-risk COPD patients before (I) and after (II) INHT in combination with conventional therapy (1), INHT only (2), and in healthy individuals (3)

Groups of patients	Stage of research	PI_{max}, mm Aq.	V_I/t_I, $l \cdot s^{-1}$	t_I/t_{tot}
1 ($n=37$)	I	10.13±0.97	0.481±0.010	0.453±0.019
	II	7.11±0.60*	0.545±0.009*	0.411±0.008*
2 ($n=33$)	I	9.97±0.82	0.492±0.007	0.432±0.018
	II	7.08±0.55*	0.539±0.008	0.413±0.009
3 ($n=36$)	I	8.14±0.61	0.648±0.015	0.421±0.007
	II	6.50±0.49*	0.570±0.010*	0.403±0.017

*$p<0.05$ – values are significantly different from the initial state

These changes indicated the decrease in CIA level and intensity of the respiratory chemosensory stimulation after INHT.

Conclusion and Perspectives

Results of our studies indicated that INHT increased reserves of lung ventilation, restored the physiological level of alveolar ventilation in 78% of patients with COPD, optimized the regional air distribution in lungs, and decreased by 25–30% the lung ventilation unevenness. INHT also resulted in improvement of airway function due to reduction by 31–37% of bronchial resistivity in BA patients. INHT changed the functional state of central respiratory regulation in COPD patients and healthy individuals. It contributed to more complete restoration of the optimal structure of respiratory pattern, due to the normalization of respiratory biomechanics, as well as the declined level of central inspiratory activity and intensity of the respiratory chemosensory stimulation.

It is obvious that sanogenic mechanism of INHT in pulmonary patients includes the complex adaptive changes in nervous, endocrine, and humoral regulation. These changes not only increase the resistance to hypoxia but also have a marked sanogenic and healing effects [43–45]. In addition, INHT increases the overall and immunological reactivity, reduces the severity of bronchial obstruction, increases the ventilatory reserve, normalizes the level of alveolar ventilation and pulmonary microcirculation, and optimizes the ventilation-perfusion relationships and intrapulmonary gas exchange [46–50].

Duration and severity of disease, presence of comorbidity, and steroid dependence are apparently the important factors determining INHT effectiveness and expression of sanogenic effect in patients with chronic pulmonary diseases. Our analysis of INHT efficacy in patients with BA by the criterion of broncholytic effect intensity showed that if duration of disease was less than 5 years, this effect was seen in 82.3% of adult patients, from 5 to 10 years in 68.0%, and over 10 years in 57.8% of the patients. This effect was only detected in 33.4% of cases, if patients had a persistent steroid dependence. Careful definition of indications and individual selection of INHT regime could allow the positive effect reaching up to 87% of adults and 92% of children [51–55].

Finally, INHT significantly improves the health of people and reduces the morbidity with temporary disability in patients. INHT is compatible with the traditional methods of treatment and prevention of pulmonary diseases and is able to potentiate the action of other pharmacological and biophysical sanogenic factors. The further development and improvement of the methodology and technical support will allow INHT to emerge as an important nonpharmacological therapy for care and rehabilitation of patients with pulmonary diseases.

References

1. Sirotinin MM. Life at altitudes and altitude sickness. Kiev: AS of UkrSSR; 1939. pp. 225, [In Ukrainian].
2. Ado AD. Experience in conducting of bronchial asthma epidemiological studies. In: Planning and implementation of socio-hygienic and epidemiological studies of bronchial asthma. Leningrad: All-Union Sci & Research Inst of Pulm. 1973. p. 23–7 [In Russian].
3. Serebrovskaya TV. Intermittent hypoxia research in the former Soviet Union and the Commonwealth of Independent States: history and review of the concept and selected applications. High Alt Med Biol. 2002;3:205–21.
4. Brimkulov NN. The alpine climatotherapy of bronchial asthma patients. Ter Arkh. 1991;63:25–30 [In Russian].
5. Boboev AT, Gadaev AG, Razikov AA. The rehabilitation of bronchial asthma patients in a mountain climate. Vopr Kurortol Fizioter Lech Fiz Kult. 1999;1:37–8 [In Russian].
6. Cogo A, Basnyat B, Legnani D, et al. Bronchial asthma and airway hyperresponsiveness at high altitude. Respiration. 1997;64:444–9.
7. Menz G. Effect of sustained high altitude on asthma patients. Expert Rev Respir Med. 2007;1:219–25.
8. Schultze-Werninghaus G. Effects of high altitude on bronchial asthma. Pneumologie. 2008;62:170–6.
9. Yakushenko MI. Features of children adaptation to mountain climate and efficacy of bronchial asthma treatment in mountain climate. In: Alpine climatotherapy in internal medicine. Bishkek: Kyrgyz Sci & Research Inst of Cardiol. 1991. p. 90–3 [In Russian].
10. Simon HU, Grotzer M, Nikolaizik WH, et al. High altitude climate therapy reduces peripheral blood T lymphocyte activation, eosinophilia, and bronchial obstruction in children with house-dust mite allergic asthma. Pediatr Pulmonol. 1994;17:304–11.
11. Njå F, Røksund OD, Svidal B, et al. Asthma and allergy among schoolchildren in a mountainous, dry, non-polluted area in Norway. Pediatr Allergy Immunol. 2000;11:40–8.
12. Berezovskiĭ VA, Deĭnega VG, Nosar VI, et al. Effect of artificial mountain climate on respiration and circulation in coal miners with chronic dust bronchitis. Fiziol Zh. 1985;31:619–23 [In Russian].

13. Berezovskiĭ VA, Deĭnega VG. Physiological mechanisms of the mountain climate sanogenic effects. Kiev: Naukova Dumka; 1988. pp. 224, [In Ukrainian].
14. Berezovskiĭ VA, Levashov MI. Introduction to orotherapy. Kiev: Academy of Hypoxia Problems, RF; 2000. pp. 56, [In Ukrainian].
15. Bulatov PC, Uspenskaja EP, Egorov MI, et al. Immediate and long-term results of barotherapy bronchial asthma and high-risk bronchial asthma patients. In: Bronchial asthma. Leningrad: All-Union Sci & Research Inst of Pulm. 1977. p. 81–2 [In Russian].
16. Alemanova GD. Application of hypoxibarotherapy in rehabilitation of children suffering from bronchial asthma. Pediatrics. 2010;1: 67–70 [In Russian].
17. Balabolkin II, Alemanova GD. Clinical and immunological rehabilitation by application of hypobaric hypoxic stimulation in bronchial asthma child and adolescent. Pediatrics. 2010;2:90–6 [In Russian].
18. Meerson FZ, Frolov BA, Smagin EA, et al. Effect of adaptation to hypoxia on immediate and delayed type of allergic reactions. In: Adaptation and resistance of organism in mountains conditions. Kiev: Naukova Dumka 1986. p. 56–65 [In Ukrainian].
19. Bulakhov AN, Nikolaeva AG, Dotsenko EA, et al. Relaxation of the smooth muscles of bronchus under hypobaric hypoxia and its adaptation to that condition. Fiziol Zh. 2003;49:53–7 [In Ukrainian].
20. Dotsenko YI. Comparison of the effectiveness of intermittent normobaric hypoxitherapy and hypobarotherapy in clinic of chronic nonspecific lung diseases. In: Interval hypoxic training (efficacy, mechanisms of action). Kiev: State Inst of Physical Culture 1992. p. 65–8 [In Ukrainian].
21. Strelkov RB, Chizhov AI. Intermittent normobaric hypoxia in prevention, treatment and rehabilitation. Yekaterinburg: Ural Worker; 2001. pp. 400, [In Russian].
22. Radionov BV. Importance of training in preparation for pneumektomy of patients with fibro-cavernous pulmonary tuberculosis. Thesis for Ph.D. degree in Medical Science, Kiev; 1972. p. 26 [In Ukrainian].
23. Berezovskiĭ VA, Levashov MI, Gridina TN. The use of an artificial mountain climate for treating and rehabilitating chronic bronchitis patients. Vrach Delo. 1990;12:34–6 [In Ukrainian].
24. Aleksandrov OV, Struchkov PV, Vinitskaia RS, et al. Clinico-functional effect of a course of interval normobaric hypoxic therapy in patients with chronic obstructive bronchitis and bronchial asthma. Ter Arkh. 1999;71:28–32 [In Russian].
25. Serebrovska TV, Mankovska MI, Lysenko GI, et al. The method of intermittent hypoxic effects in combined treatment of patients with bronchial asthma. Lik Sprava. 1998;6:104–8 [In Ukrainian].
26. Ivanova IP, Nepomniashchikh VM, Shirinskiĭ VS, et al. Normobaric hypoxy-therapy of patients with bronchial asthma. Klin Med (Mosk). 2001;79:36–9 [In Russian].
27. Kolchinskaia AZ, Tsyganova EN, Ostapenko LA. Normobaric interval hypoxic training in medicine and sports. Moscow: Meditsina; 2003. pp. 407, [In Russian].
28. Vogtel M, Michels A. Role of intermittent hypoxia in the treatment of bronchial asthma and chronic obstructive pulmonary disease. Curr Opin Allergy Clin Immunol. 2010;10:206–13.
29. Haider T, Casucci G, Linser T, et al. Interval hypoxic training improves autonomic cardiovascular and respiratory control in patients with mild chronic obstructive pulmonary disease. J Hypertens. 2009;27:1648–54.
30. Lopata VO, Berezovskiĭ LMI, et al. Classification and review of technical devices for hypoxia therapy. Fiziol Zh. 2003;49:100–5 [In Ukrainian].
31. Berezovskiĭ VA, Levashov MI. Natural and instrumental orotherapy and rehabilitation patients with pulmonary diseases. Ukr Pulm Zh. 2005;3(suppl):15–8 [In Russian].
32. Breslav IS, Glebovskii VD. Regulation of respiration. Leningrad: Nauka; 1981. pp. 280, [In Russian].
33. Nemirovskii LI. Pulmophonography. Moscow: Meditsina; 1981. pp. 160, [In Russian].
34. McFadden JP, Price RC, Eastwood HD, et al. Raised respiratory rate in elderly patients: a valuable physical sign. Br Med J. 1982;284:626–7.
35. Gravelin TR, Weg JG. Respiratory rate as an indicator of acute respiratory dysfunction. JAMA. 1980;244:1123–5.
36. Krivoshchekov SG, Divert GM, Divert VE. Individual characteristics of external respiration during intermittent normobaric hypoxia. Fiziol Cheloveka. 2006;32:62–9 [In Russian].
37. Breslav IS. Breathing patterns: physiology, extremes conditions, and pathology. Leningrad: Nauka; 1984. pp. 206, [In Russian].
38. Grodins FS, Yamachiro SM. What is the pattern of breathing regulated for? Oxford: Centr Nerv Contr Mech Breath Proc Int Symp; 1979. p. 169–76.
39. Haas F, Distenfeld S, Axen K. Effects of perceived musical rhythm on respiratory pattern. J Appl Physiol. 1986;61:1185–91.
40. Gautier H. Control of the pattern of breathing. Clin Sci. 1980;8:343–8.
41. Gautier H, Milic-Emili J, Miserocchi G, et al. Pattern of breathing and mouth occlusion pressure during acclimatization to high altitude. Respir Physiol. 1980;40:365–77.
42. Rossi M, Maestrelli P. The effect of ventilatory drive in chronic obsrtructive lung disease. In: Clinical respiratory physiology. Bratislava: Slovak Acad of Sci. 1983. p. 44–54.
43. Kolchinskaia AZ. Mechanisms of the interval hypoxic training action. Hypoxia Med J. 1993;1:5–8 [In Russian].
44. Ksenofontova IV, Uianaeva AI, Aĭrapetova NS, et al. Interval hypoxic training as a method of prophylaxis of meteopathic reactions in patients with bronchial asthma: guide for physicians. Vopr Kurortol Fizioter Lech Fiz Kult. 2006;4:54–6 [In Russian].
45. Tlupova TG, Borukaeva IK. Application of interval hypoxitherapy for improvement of the respiratory functional system and visual functions in patients with bronchial asthma. Bull Regen Med. 2008;5:32–5 [In Russian].
46. Berezovskiĭ VA, Levashov MI. Artificial mountain climate: some mechanisms of therapeutic action. Vopr Kurortol Fizioter Lech Fiz Kult. 1993;3:23–6 [In Russian].
47. Levashov MI, Berezovskiĭ VA. Pulmonary circulation in patients with COPD under the influence of hypoxic gas mixtures and artificial mountain climate. In: Intermittent normobaric hypoxia. Reports of the Acad. of Hypoxia Problems. RF. Moscow. 1997;1:188–95 [In Russian].
48. Ragozin ON, Balykin MV, Charikova EI, et al. The analysis of a spectrum of rhythms of parameters external breath and cardiovascular system at the patients with bronchial asthma on a background normobaric hypoxitherapy. Fiziol Zh. 2001;47:36–9 [In Ukrainian].
49. Krivoshchekov SG, Divert GM, Divert VE. Effect of short-term intermittent normobaric hypoxia on the regulation of external respiration in humans. Fiziol Cheloveka. 2002;28:45–51 [In Russian].
50. Leutin VP, IaG P, Divert GM, et al. Changes in the central regulation of respiratory function after a single session of intermittent normobaric hypoxia. Fiziol Cheloveka. 2003;29:13–5 [In Russian].
51. Redzhebova OK, Chizhov AI. Results of utilization of intermittent normobaric hypoxia in patients with bronchial asthma and chronic obstructive bronchitis. Fiziol Zh. 1992;38:39–42 [In Russian].
52. Berezovskiĭ VA, Gorban EM, Levashov MI, et al. Technology to improve of the organism resistance by means of hypoxitherapy. Method Recom of the MHU. Kyiv; 2000. p. 23 [In Ukrainian].
53. Poddubnaya RY, Grineva OM, Bykov AT, et al. Intermittent normobaric hypoxytherapy in complex of sanatorium treatment and rehabilitation of persons with bronchopulmonary diseases. In: Intermittent normobaric hypoxytherapy. Reports of the Academy of Hypoxia Problems. RF. Moscow. 1999;3:215–9 [In Russian].
54. Karash YM, Strelkov RB, Chizhov AY. Normobaric hypoxia in treatment, prophylaxis and rehabilitation. Moscow: Meditsina; 1988. pp. 352, [In Russian].
55. Borukaeva IK. Effectiveness of hypoxic therapy in patients with chronic obstructive pulmonary disease. Vopr Kurortol Fizioter Lech Fiz Kult. 2009;2:16–8 [In Russian].

10 Effects of Intermittent Hypoxic Training on Exercise Tolerance in Patients with Chronic Obstructive Pulmonary Disease

Martin Burtscher

Abstract

Intermittent hypoxic training (IHT) has been suggested to increase exercise tolerance in patients with cardiovascular disease by enhancing stress resistance and/or improving oxygen delivery. This is also assumed to be true for patients with chronic obstructive pulmonary disease (COPD). This chapter discusses findings, derived from randomized controlled studies, on the effects of IHT on exercise tolerance in patients suffering from mild COPD. Three weeks of IHT increased total haemoglobin mass (+4% vs. 0%, $P<0.05$), total exercise time (+9.7% vs. 0%, $P<0.05$) and the exercise time to the anaerobic threshold (+13% vs. −7.8%, $P<0.05$) compared to controls. Changes in the total exercise time were positively related to the changes in total haemoglobin mass ($r=0.59$, $P<0.05$), and changes in the time to the anaerobic threshold were positively related to the changes in the lung diffusion capacity for carbon monoxide (DLCO) ($r=0.48$, $P<0.05$). Increases in vagal activity after IHT were related to the reduced values of heart rate and blood lactate concentration observed during submaximal exercise (6-min walk test), and changes in respiratory pattern after IHT were related to the lower ventilatory equivalents for oxygen and carbon dioxide (V_E/VO_2 and V_E/VCO_2) at the anaerobic threshold determined by incremental cycle ergometry. In conclusion, IHT can improve exercise tolerance in patients with mild COPD. IHT is considered as repeated stress training and subsequent adaptations resulting in corrections of impaired DLCO, improved ventilatory efficiency, enhancement of total haemoglobin mass and changes of the autonomic balance to higher vagal and lower sympathetic activity. Thus, IHT may be a valuable tool to complement the known beneficial effects of exercise training in patients with COPD.

Abbreviations

AT	Anaerobic threshold
CO_2-et	End-tidal CO_2
COPD	Chronic obstructive pulmonary disease
DLCO	Lung diffusion capacity for carbon monoxide
FEV1	Forced expiratory volume in 1 s
FEVC	Forced expiratory vital capacity
FiO_2	Inspiratory fraction of oxygen
HCVR	Hypercapnic ventilatory response
HIF	Hypoxia-inducible factor
HR	Heart rate
HVR	Hypoxic ventilatory response
IH	Intermittent hypoxia
IHT	Intermittent hypoxic training
NO	Nitric oxide
OSA	Obstructive sleep apnoea
RPE	Ratings of perceived exertion
SaO_2	Arterial oxygen saturation
SD	Standard deviation

M. Burtscher
Department of Sport Science, Medical Section,
University of Innsbruck,
Innsbruck, Austria
e-mail: martin.burtscher@uibk.ac.at

L. Xi, T.V. Serebrovskaya (eds.), *Intermittent Hypoxia and Human Diseases*,
DOI 10.1007/978-1-4471-2906-6_10,

V_E	Minute ventilation
VO_2	Oxygen uptake
V_E/VO_2	Ventilatory equivalent for oxygen
V_E/VCO_2	Ventilatory equivalent for carbon dioxide

10.1 Introduction

Chronic obstructive pulmonary disease (COPD) is an increasing cause of morbidity and mortality resulting in notable health and economic burden worldwide [1]. COPD represents a systemic disease which, apart from lung limitations, includes weight loss, dysfunction of skeletal muscle, increased risk of metabolic and cardiovascular diseases, osteoporosis and depression [2]. The main characteristic of patients with COPD is their inability to engage in sustained physical activity [3]. This intolerance to exercise compromises activities of daily living and quality of life [4]. Mechanisms of exercise intolerance are complex, and the respiratory, cardiovascular, metabolic and locomotor muscle systems are involved. Exercise training has been evidenced as the most effective way to improve exercise tolerance in these patients [5]. However, recent studies indicate that additional benefits may be obtained from repeated exposures to short-term hypoxia [6, 7].

Intermittent hypoxia (IH) is usually defined as repeated episodes of hypoxia interspersed with normoxic periods [6, 8]. However, the term "intermittent hypoxia" has mostly been associated with obstructive sleep apnoea (OSA) and its related adverse effects [8–10]. Experimentally repeated short-term hypoxia of approximately 5 min with normoxic intervals of a similar duration is known as interval hypoxia training which has been introduced by Russian physicians about three decades ago [11, 12]. The corresponding term predominantly used in Western literature appears to be intermittent hypoxic training (IHT). The main rationale for the clinical use of this type of hypoxic training was based on the potential cross-protective value of adaptations to one stress, which then may provide resistance to another stress [13]. Therefore, in contrast to the IH in OSA, IHT is used with the intention to improve performance and for preventive or therapeutic reasons.

IHT is typically applied as a 3-week breathing program consisting of five sessions per week [6, 7]. Each session consists of three to five hypoxic (inspiratory fraction of oxygen, FiO_2: 0.15–0.12) periods, each lasting 3–5 min with 3-min normoxic intervals (Table 10.1). Hypoxic and normoxic air is inhaled using a 2-valved face mask in a sitting position. Arterial oxygen saturation (SaO_2) and heart rate (HR) are monitored continuously by a pulse oximeter attached to a finger tip (Fig. 10.1). The program should be performed under medical supervision. This breathing protocol has been adapted to that proposed by the Clinical Research Laboratory of the Hypoxia Medical Academy in Moscow [12].

Table 10.1 Example of a typical 3-week breathing protocol of intermittent hypoxic training (IHT) [6, 7]

Days 1–5									
Duration of breathing periods (min)	3	3	3	3	3				
Fraction of oxygen (%)	15	21	15	21	15				
Days 8–12									
Duration of breathing periods (min)	4	3	4	3	4	3	4		
Fraction of oxygen (%)	13	21	13	21	13	21	13		
Days 15–19									
Duration of breathing periods (min)	5	3	5	3	5	3	5	3	5
Fraction of oxygen (%)	12	21	12	21	12	21	12	21	12

10.2 Effects of IHT on Exercise Tolerance

The presented findings are derived from recent trials (randomized, double-blind, placebo-controlled) which are among the very few studies that investigated the effects on IHT on exercise tolerance in COPD patients [6, 7]. In these studies, male and female patients over a wide range of age (33–72 years) suffering from mild COPD were randomly assigned in a double-blind fashion to receive 15 sessions of IHT (FiO_2: 0.15–0.12) or normoxia within 3 weeks as described above. Incremental cycle spiroergometry, determination of lung function and lung diffusion capacity for carbon monoxide (DLCO), testing of the autonomic cardiovascular and respiratory control, and blood analyses were performed before and after IHT for the assessment of exercise tolerance and related mechanisms.

10.2.1 Peak Performance

Peak power output and total exercise time derived from incremental exercise testing had increased by about 10% after IHT whereas no changes were observed within the control group ($P<0.05$) (Fig. 10.2). Additionally, peak SaO_2 values remained higher (~1.5%) at peak exercise after IHT compared to controls ($P<0.05$) (Fig. 10.2). No changes between groups occurred with regard to peak oxygen uptake (VO_2 peak), peak minute ventilation (V_E peak) and peak heart rate (HR peak), and maximal values of ratings of perceived exertion (RPE) [6].

10.2.2 Submaximal Performance

Exercise time to the anaerobic threshold (AT) derived from incremental exercise testing had improved after IHT (+13%) compared to controls (–7.8%) ($P<0.05$). Additionally, after IHT, SaO_2 values remained higher and the ventilatory equivalents

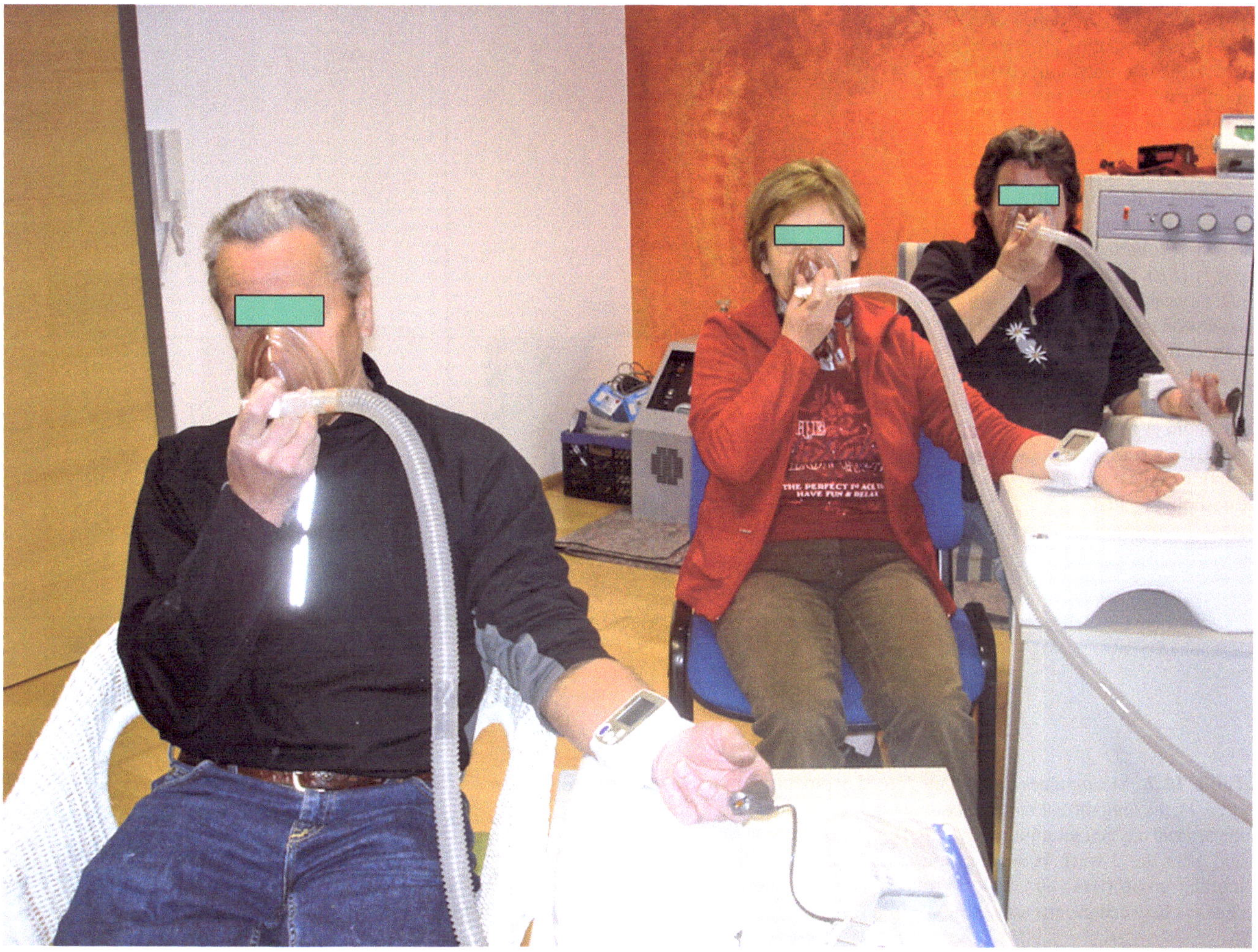

Fig. 10.1 COPD patients performing the breathing program [6, 7]

for oxygen and carbon dioxide (V_E/VO$_2$ and V_E/VCO$_2$) remained lower at the AT in comparison to controls ($P<0.05$) (Fig. 10.2). Data are reported as means (±SD).

The total distance covered during the 6-min walk test, however, did not change between groups. Changes in exercising heart rates, however, had decreased after IHT (−4 ± 14 bpm) when compared to controls (+10 ± 13 bpm) ($P<0.05$). Also, blood lactate concentrations had decreased from 2.7 ± 0.6 to 2.0 ± 0.6 mmol/l after IHT and remained unchanged within controls ($P<0.05$) [6].

10.2.3 Lung Function, DLCO, Resting Cardiorespiratory and Blood Data

Three weeks of IHT compared to control conditions effected increases in the forced expiratory volume in 1 s (FEV1: +5.1% vs. −1.7%, $P<0.05$), DLCO (+5.2% vs. −3.1%, $P<0.05$), resting SaO$_2$ values (+0.4% vs. −0.5%, $P<0.05$) and total haemoglobin mass (+4% vs. 0%, $P<0.05$) (Table 10.2). However, no changes between groups could be observed regarding the forced expiratory vital capacity (FVC), resting heart rate and blood pressure, haemoglobin concentration, haematocrit and plasma volume [6].

10.2.4 Cardiovascular and Respiratory Control

After 3 weeks of IHT, the baroreflex sensitivity increased from 6.8 ± 1.5 to 9.9 ± 2.8 ms/mmHg, $P<0.05$, in contrast to controls (normoxic air breathing), which showed an opposite trend decreasing from 5.7 ± 1.6 to 4.0 ± 0.5 ms/mmHg. The R–R intervals had significantly increased after IHT from 729 ± 49 to 852 ± 62 ms, $P<0.001$, whereas it was not significantly shortened from 751 ± 48 to 711 ± 34 ms within controls (Fig. 10.3). No significant changes were found with regard to systolic blood pressure in both groups [7].

Regarding the respiratory control, after IHT, a significant and specific increase in the hypercapnic ventilatory response (HCVR) from 1.2 ± 0.2 to 1.6 ± 0.4 l/min/mmHg of CO$_2$-et

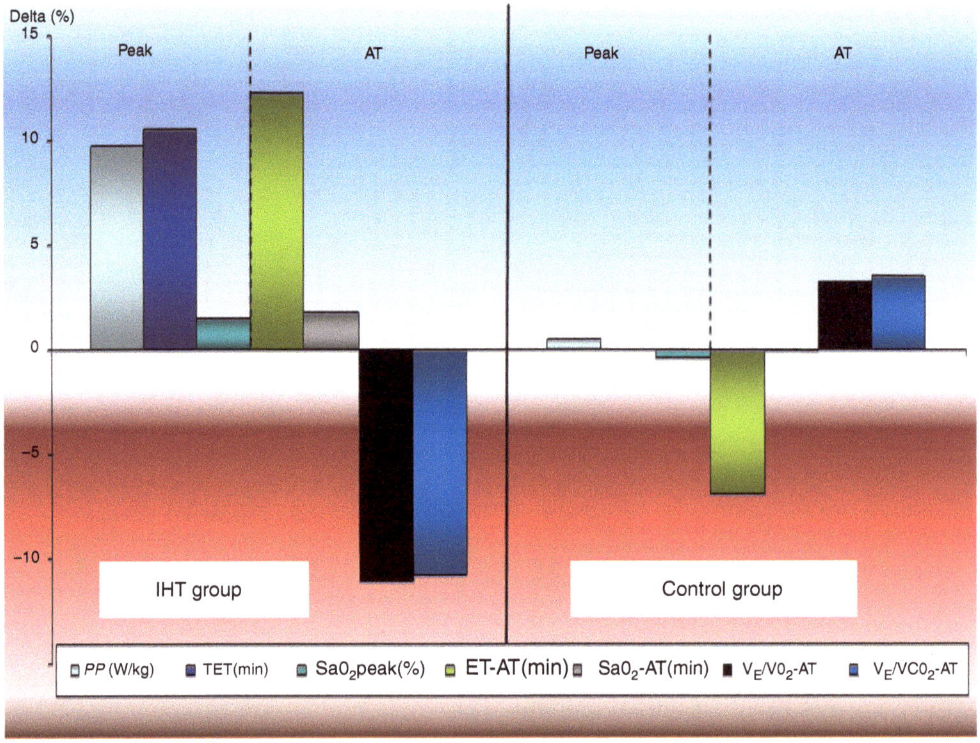

Fig. 10.2 Changes (delta) after the 3-week breathing program within the intermittent hypoxic training group (*IHT*) and the control group with regard to maximal and submaximal exercise parameters. Only variables with significant changes between groups are shown [6]. Variables: Peak power (*PP*), total exercise time (*TET*), peak arterial oxygen saturation (*SaO_2peak*), exercise time to the anaerobic threshold (*ET-AT*), ventilatory equivalent for oxygen at the anaerobic threshold (*V_E/VO_2-AT*), ventilatory equivalent for carbon dioxide at the anaerobic threshold (*V_E/VCO_2-AT*)

Table 10.2 Mean values (SD) of the forced expiratory volume in 1 s (FEV1), the lung diffusion capacity for carbon monoxide (DLCO), resting arterial oxygen saturation (SaO_2) and total haemoglobin mass before and after the 3-week breathing program of the intermittent hypoxic training group (IHT) and control group. Variables without significant changes between groups are not shown [6]

	IHT		Control group		ANOVA
	Pre	Post	Pre	Post	*P*-value
FEV_1 (l)	2.54 (0.62)	2.67 (0.60)	2.32 (0.56)	2.28 (0.53)	0.001
DLCO (% pred)	64.4 (19.2)	67.8 (16.7)	71.2 (17.3)	69.0 (15.3)	0.02
SaO_2 (%)	96.6 (0.7)	97.0 (0.9)	97.2 (0.7)	96.7 (0.7)	0.004
Total haemoglobin mass (g)	843.1 (143)	874.8 (138)	798.4 (157)	798.8 (150)	0.04

($P<0.05$) was found whereas the hypoxic ventilatory response (HVR) remained unchanged. Tidal volume tended to have increased after IHT (850 ± 89 vs. 938 ± 91 ml) which was associated with a not significantly reduced respiration rate (14.4 ± 1.4 vs. 13.1 ± 1.6 breaths/min). These changes may indicate a tendency of rearrangement toward a deeper and slower breathing [7].

10.2.5 Correlations

A positive correlation was demonstrated between changes in total exercise time and total haemoglobin mass ($r=0.59$, $P<0.05$, Fig. 10.4), and changes in total haemoglobin mass were positively related to changes in VO_2 peak ($r=0.49$, $P<0.05$) indicating that the increase in total haemoglobin mass after IHT is associated with increased exercise capacity [6]. Changes in the time to the anaerobic threshold were positively related to the changes in the DLCO ($r=0.48$, $P<0.05$, Fig. 10.5), and changes in DLCO were negatively related to the changes in V_E/VO_2 ($r=-0.75$, $P<0.01$), to changes in V_E/VCO_2 ($r=-0.55$, $P<0.05$) and to the changes in minute ventilation (V_E) at the anaerobic threshold (AT) ($r=-0.48$, $P<0.05$). These relationships indicate a role of DLCO correction particularly for improvements with regard to submaximal exercise. The increases in vagal tone after IHT were related to the reduced values of heart rate and blood lactate concentration observed during submaximal exercise (6-min walk test), and the changes in respiratory pattern after IHT were related to the lower V_E/VO_2 and V_E/VCO_2 values at the anaerobic threshold determined by incremental cycle ergometry.

10.3 Exercise Intolerance in COPD Patients and Possible Effects of IHT

Many factors contribute to exercise intolerance in COPD. The respiratory mechanisms limiting exercise include development of hypoxemia secondary to ventilation–perfusion mismatching and/or the development of dynamic hyperinflation. Airflow obstruction resulting in progressive hyperinflation is associated with activity limitation and physical deconditioning [3, 5]. The use of long-acting bronchodilators may be helpful

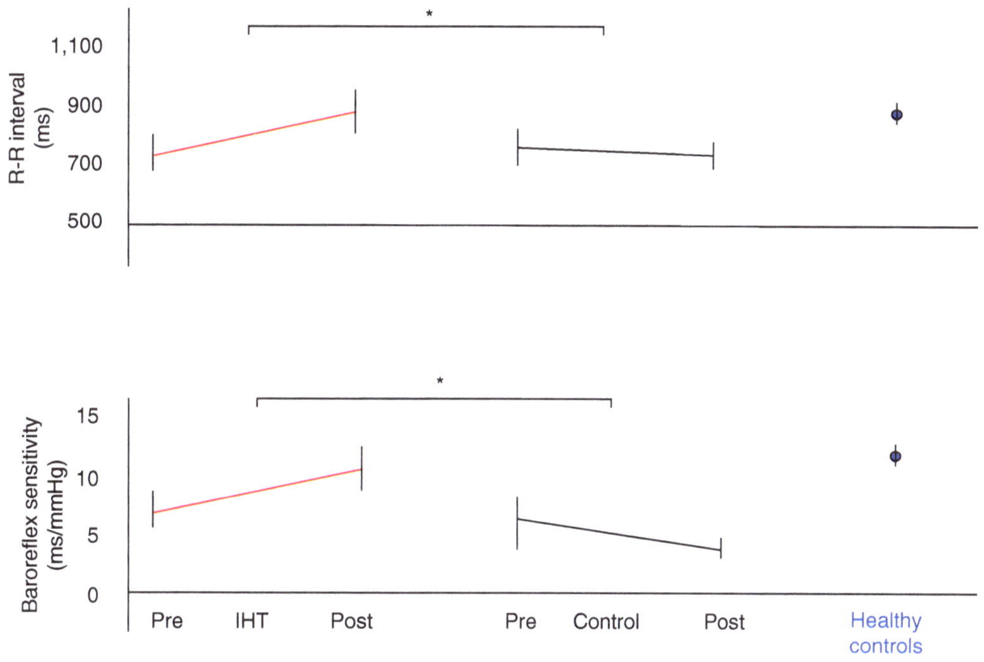

Fig. 10.3 Changes in R–R interval and baroreflex sensitivity before (pre) and after (post) the 3-week breathing program of the intermittent hypoxic training (*IHT*) and control group and comparisons to healthy controls. *Denotes significant changes between groups [7]

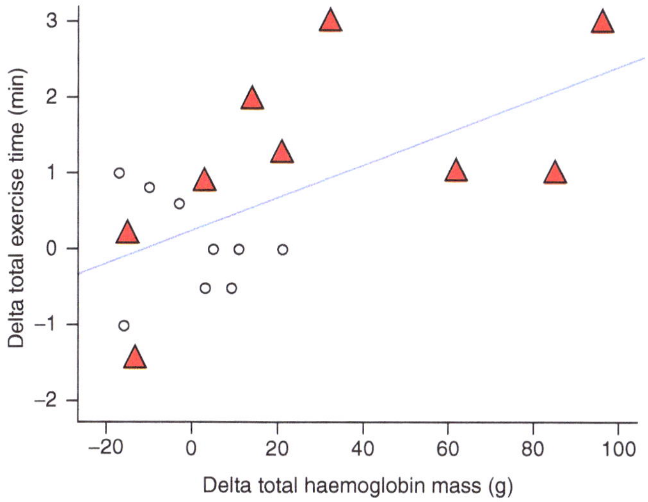

Fig. 10.4 Relationship between the changes of the total exercise time (cycle ergometry) and the changes of the total haemoglobin mass ($r=0.59$, $P<0.05$) after the 3-week breathing program. *Triangles mark* members of the intermittent hypoxic training (IHT) group, and *circles mark* members of the control group (Modified according to Ref. [6])

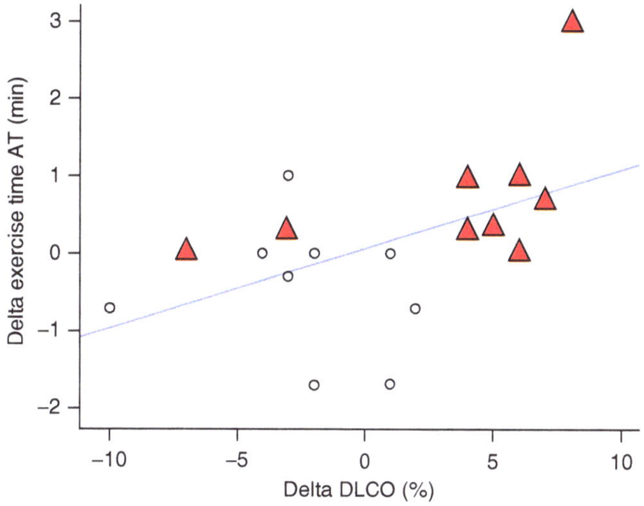

Fig. 10.5 Relationship between the changes of the exercise time (cycle ergometry) to the anaerobic threshold (*AT*) and the changes of the DLCO ($r=0.48$, $P<0.05$) after the 3-week breathing program. *Triangles mark* members of the intermittent hypoxic training (IHT) group, and *circles mark* members of the control group (Modified according to Ref. [6])

to diminish airflow obstruction and thus contribute to the improvement of exercise tolerance [14]. However, as mentioned above, there are several extrapulmonary manifestations of COPD like weight loss, dysfunction of skeletal muscle, increased risk of metabolic and cardiovascular diseases, osteoporosis and depression [2, 15] which are accounting for the majority of morbidity and mortality in patients suffering from COPD [16, 17]. Systemic inflammation is considered as a key factor for these manifestations including peripheral muscle weakness resulting in reduced performance and exercise tolerance [14, 18]. Undoubtedly, skeletal-muscle dysfunction is now recognized as an indicator of advanced COPD, and several studies have shown that exercise causes a reversal of skeletal-muscle dysfunction and other morphological and metabolic changes seen in the skeletal muscles of patients with COPD [19, 20]. In addition, physical exercise can reduce the fear of dyspnoea and improve overall quality of life. Taken together, exercise prescription and the use of bronchodilators are currently considered as the most effective therapeutic intervention to improve exercise tolerance at least in earlier COPD [20]. The question arises, how this can be complemented by IHT.

As shown above, IHT improved exercise tolerance by an increase in maximal and submaximal exercise performance. Lung function was not related to the improvements in exercise tolerance but DLCO, total haemoglobin mass and changes in the autonomic control were. These findings have also been summarized in a recent review article [21]. In addition, IHT has been found to normalize electrobiological activity of the cerebral cortex and to correct immunological reactivity [22].

10.3.1 Exercise Tolerance and Lung Function

Although IHT elicited small but significant beneficial effects on FEV1, these changes were unrelated to the improvements in exercise performance. Of course, FEV1 and FEV1/FVC are important diagnostic criteria for the degree of airway obstruction, but their relation to exercise capacity is known to be weak [20]. Similar improvements have been reported by Russian studies [23, 24]. Like them, we cannot explain the mechanisms of these improvements, but they might be related to repeated hypoxia per se or to the respiratory muscle training by hyperventilation during the hypoxic sessions [6].

10.3.2 Exercise Tolerance and DLCO

In contrast to the total exercise time, the time to the anaerobic threshold during incremental cycle ergometry was associated with improved resting DLCO indicating that improved DLCO was only beneficial during submaximal exercise [6]. Although it has been suggested that IHT might improve DLCO, the underlying mechanisms remain unclear [25]. One could speculate that the DLCO improvement after IHT was related to the changes in total blood volume [6]. Conversely, total blood volume is related to pulmonary blood volume and probably also to pulmonary capillary blood volume and in turn to DLCO [6, 26]. Nitric oxide (NO)-dependent mechanisms of adaptation to intermittent hypoxia could provide another, more speculative explanation [27]. Diminished pulmonary NO may be involved in the pathogenesis of pulmonary artery hypertension which is a well-known complication in COPD patients. Thus, an increase in NO availability after IHT should lower pulmonary artery pressure resulting in improved ventilation–perfusion mismatching and DLCO [28, 29]. The oxygenated haemoglobin is a known NO scavenger; however, a recent study demonstrated that haemoglobin generates NO by reducing nitrite to NO when deoxygenated, thereby mediating vasodilation and blood flow [30]. Therefore, the increased haemoglobin mass after IHT could also have contributed to the improved DLCO.

The significantly higher SaO_2 values during submaximal cycle exercise after IHT, despite unchanged minute ventilation, likely may result from DLCO improvement. Beside changes in autonomic cardiovascular and respiratory control, these improvements have likely contributed to the observed changes at the anaerobic threshold during cycle ergometry and those of circulatory and metabolic responses to the 6-min walk test after IHT.

10.3.3 Exercise Tolerance and Total Haemoglobin Mass

The increased maximal power output and total exercise time after IHT were positively related to the increase in the total haemoglobin mass. On the one hand, total haemoglobin mass should enhance the oxygen-carrying capacity of the blood and thus VO_2 peak and maximal power output [31]. In fact, VO_2 peak was increased after IHT [6]. However, the observed increases in total haemoglobin mass are unexpected because much longer hypoxic exposures in athletes than those applied in present IHT were insufficient to enhance erythropoiesis [32]. One could speculate that COPD patients respond more sensitively to repeated hypoxic exposure than healthy subjects or athletes. In COPD patients, the transcription factor complex HIF-1 should be up-regulated by hypoxia as well as by a broad variety of inflammatory mediators [33]. On the other hand, the larger haemoglobin mass may also have been effective by reducing oxidative stress [34] and/or enhancing the buffering capacity [35] resulting in improved endothelial function and/or reduced acidosis-related dyspnoea [6].

10.3.4 Exercise Tolerance and Autonomic Cardiovascular and Respiratory Control

Of course, the effects of IHT are complex and may much depend on the applied protocol. Modifications of the related breathing program used for IHT with regard to total hypoxia, intensity and duration of the single hypoxic cycles, the duration of normoxic pauses and the number of cycle repetitions may determine beneficial or even negative effects [7, 36]. It is well known that exposures to acute hypoxia increases ventilation and sympathetic activity [37]. Thus, IHT may be considered as a type of interval stress training resulting in improved stress tolerance during daily life of COPD patients [7] which has recently also been demonstrated in patients with coronary artery disease [38]. The tendency of an increased tidal volume with concomitant decrease in respiration rate after IHT indicates improved ventilatory efficiency also observed during submaximal exercise. These effects may be beneficial for COPD patients by the reduction of respiratory metabolic costs and probably also dyspnoea [7]. The presented results confirm previous findings of an increase in vagal and thus relatively reduced sympathetic activity after IHT even in healthy individuals [37]. The reduced sympathetic tone after IHT might also have contributed to the lower lactate formation [39] and the resulting decrease in ventilatory requirements.

10.4 Limitations

The presented data have been recorded in patients with mild COPD. Thus, the clinical relevance of the study might seem unclear because exercise limitation in patients with COPD normally develops in the later stages of the disease and progresses as the disease advances [6]. However, measures increasing exercise tolerance will decrease morbidity and mortality in patients with COPD and in healthy people as well [40, 41]. These data provide a first basis for using IHT in COPD, but they cannot be directly extended to more severe COPD patients. Besides, it is unknown how long the effects of the applied IHT are maintained [6]. One previous study in patients with coronary artery disease, however, indicated that IHT-related adaptations may actually be preserved for about 1 month without further hypoxic exposures [38].

Conclusion

IHT can improve exercise tolerance in patients with mild COPD. IHT is considered as repeated stress training and subsequent adaptations resulting in corrections of impaired DLCO, improved ventilatory efficiency, enhancement of total haemoglobin mass and changes of the autonomic balance to higher vagal and lower sympathetic tone. Thus, IHT may be a valuable tool to complement the known beneficial effects of exercise training in patients with COPD.

References

1. Mannino DM, Braman S. The epidemiology and economics of chronic obstructive pulmonary disease. Proc Am Thorac Soc. 2007;4:502–6.
2. Andreas S, Anker SD, Scanlon PD, et al. Neurohumoral activation as a link to systemic manifestations of chronic lung disease. Chest. 2005;128:3618–24.
3. O'Donnell DE, Webb KA. The major limitation to exercise performance in COPD is dynamic hyperinflation. J Appl Physiol. 2008;105:753–5.
4. Belfer MH, Reardon JZ. Improving exercise tolerance and quality of life in patients with chronic obstructive pulmonary disease. J Am Osteopath Assoc. 2009;109:268–78.
5. Casaburi R. Limitation to exercise tolerance in chronic obstructive pulmonary disease. Am J Respir Crit Care Med. 2003;168:409–10.
6. Burtscher M, Haider T, Domej W, et al. Intermittent hypoxia increases exercise tolerance in patients at risk for or with mild COPD. Respir Physiol Neurobiol. 2009;165:97–103.
7. Haider T, Casucci G, Linser T, et al. Interval hypoxic training improves autonomic cardiovascular and respiratory control in patients with mild chronic obstructive pulmonary disease. J Hypertens. 2009;27:1648–54.
8. Neubauer JA. Physiological and pathophysiological responses to intermittent hypoxia. J Appl Physiol. 2001;90:1593–9.
9. Lavie L. Oxidative stress – a unifying paradigm in obstructive sleep apnea and comorbidities. Prog Cardiovasc Dis. 2009;51:303–12.
10. O'Donnell CP. Metabolic consequences of intermittent hypoxia. Adv Exp Med Biol. 2007;618:41–9.
11. Meerson FZ, Ustinova EE, Orlova EH. Prevention and elimination of heart arrhythmias by adaptation to intermittent high altitude hypoxia. Clin Cardiol. 1987;10:783–9.
12. Tkatchouk EN, Gorbatchenkov AA, Kolchinskaya AZ, et al. Adaptation to interval hypoxia with the purpose of prophylaxis and treatment. Hypoxia Med J. 1994;11:308–28.
13. Meerson FZ, Malyshev YI, Zamotrinsky AV. Differences in adaptive stabilisation of structures in response to stress and hypoxia relate with the accumulation of hsp70 isoforms. Mol Cell Biochem. 1992;111:87–95.
14. Berton DC, Barbosa PB, Takara LS, et al. Bronchodilators accelerate the dynamics of muscle O_2 delivery and utilisation during exercise in COPD. Thorax. 2010;65:588–93.
15. Sin DD, Man SF. Skeletal muscle weakness, reduced exercise tolerance, and COPD: is systemic inflammation the missing link? Thorax. 2006;61:1–3.
16. Anthonisen NR, Connett JE, Enright PL, et al. Hospitalizations and mortality in the Lung Health Study. Am J Respir Crit Care Med. 2002;166:333–9.
17. Sin DD, Wu L, Anderson JA, et al. Inhaled corticosteroids and mortality in chronic obstructive pulmonary disease. Thorax. 2005;60:992–7.
18. Yende S, Waterer GW, Tolley EA, et al. Inflammatory markers are associated with ventilatory limitation and muscle dysfunction in obstructive lung disease in well functioning elderly subjects. Thorax. 2006;61:10–6.
19. Mador MJ, Bozkanat E. Skeletal muscle dysfunction in chronic obstructive pulmonary disease. Respir Res. 2001;2:216–24.
20. Cooper CB. Airflow obstruction and exercise. Respir Med. 2009;103:325–34.
21. Vogtel M, Michels A. Role of intermittent hypoxia in the treatment of bronchial asthma and chronic obstructive pulmonary disease. Curr Opin Allergy Clin Immunol. 2010;10:206–13.
22. Borukaeva IK. Intermittent hypoxic training in the sanatorium and spa treatment for patients with chronic obstructive pulmonary disease. Vopr Kurortol Fizioter Lech Fiz Kult. 2007;5:21–4 [In Russian].
23. Alexandrov OV, Struchkov PV, Vinitskaya RS, et al. Responses of the cardiorespiratory system to a hypoxic exposure in the course of hypoxic therapy in patients with chronic obstructive lung diseases. Hypoxia Med J. 1997;1:18–22.
24. Ehrenbourg I, Kondrykinskaya I. The efficiency of interval hypoxic training in therapy of chronic obstructive pulmonary diseases. Hypoxia Med J. 1993;1:17–8.
25. Serebrovskaya TV. Intermittent hypoxia research in the former Soviet Union and the Commonwealth of Independent States: history and review of the concept and selected applications. High Alt Med Biol. 2002;3:205–21.
26. Falch D, Stromme SB. Pulmonary blood volume and interventricular circulation time in physically trained and untrained subjects. Eur J Appl Physiol Occup Physiol. 1979;40:211–8.

27. Manukhina EB, Downey HF, Mallet R. Role of nitric oxide in cardiovascular adaptation to intermittent hypoxia. Exp Biol Med. 2006;231:343–65.
28. Clini E, Bianchi L, Vitacca M, et al. Exhaled nitric oxide and exercise in stable COPD patients. Chest. 2000;117:702–7.
29. Girgis RE, Champion HC, Diette GB, et al. Decreased exhaled nitric oxide in pulmonary arterial hypertension. Am J Respir Crit Care Med. 2005;172:352–7.
30. Crawford JH, Isbell TS, Huang Z, et al. Hypoxia, red blood cells, and nitrite regulate NO-dependent hypoxic vasodilation. Blood. 2006;107:566–74.
31. Calbet JA, Lundby C, Koskolou M, et al. Importance of haemoglobin concentration to exercise: acute manipulations. Respir Physiol Neurobiol. 2006;151:132–40.
32. Neya M, Enoki T, Kumai Y, et al. The effects of nightly normobaric hypoxia and high intensity training under intermittent normobaric hypoxia on running economy and hemoglobin mass. J Appl Physiol. 2007;103:828–34.
33. Frede S, Berchner-Pfannschmidt U, Fandrey J. Regulation of hypoxia-inducible factors during inflammation. Methods Enzymol. 2007;435:405–19.
34. Zhuang J, Zhou Z. Protective effects of intermittent hypoxic adaptation on myocardium and its mechanisms. Biol Sig Recept. 1999;8:316–22.
35. Böning D, Klarholz C, Himmelsbach B, et al. Extracellular bicarbonate and non-bicarbonate buffering against lactic acid during and after exercise. Eur J Appl Physiol. 2007;100:457–67.
36. Bernardi L. Interval hypoxic training. Adv Exp Med Biol. 2001;502:377–99.
37. Bernardi L, Passino C, Serebrovskaya Z, et al. Respiratory and cardiovascular adaptations to progressive hypoxia; effect of interval hypoxic training. Eur Heart J. 2001;22:879–86.
38. Burtscher M, Pachinger O, Ehrenbourg I, et al. Intermittent hypoxia increases exercise tolerance in elderly men with and without coronary artery disease. Int J Cardiol. 2004;96:247–54.
39. Milic-Emili J. Expiratory flow limitation: Roger S. Mitchell lecture. Chest. 2000;117:219S–23.
40. Kokkinos P, Myers J, Kokkinos JP, et al. Exercise capacity and mortality in black and white men. Circulation. 2008;117:614–22.
41. Cote CG, Pinto-Plata V, Kasprzyk K, et al. The 6-min walk distance, peak oxygen uptake, and mortality in COPD. Chest. 2007;132:1778–85.

Intermittent Hypoxia in Treatment of Bronchial Asthma in Childhood

11

Tatiana V. Serebrovskaya, Alexander N. Bakunovsky, Klaudia V. Nesvitailova, and Iryna N. Mankovska

Abstract

According to the World Health Organization, bronchial asthma (BA) is a serious public health problem with over 300 million sufferers of all ages. In this chapter, we demonstrate the possibility to treat BA in childhood with intermittent hypoxia treatment/training (IHT) programs and provide clinical evidence, adverse effects, and latest experience in IHT implementation. Particularly, it was shown that 2-week IHT resulted in a significant decline in breath shortness and feelings of chest congestion in BA children (aged 9–13 years). The cough was diminished or disappeared, and the amount of sputum was reduced and passed more easily. The attacks of asphyxia disappeared or became more occasional. Considerable augmentation of ventilatory response to hypoxic stimuli was observed as well as a diminution of heart rate (HR) reactions to increased hypoxia and an attenuated fall of SaO_2 under hypoxic conditions. Mitochondrial enzymes activity of immune cells such as succinate dehydrogenase (SDG) and alpha-glycerophosphate dehydrogenase (GPDG) increased significantly under IHT. Strong correlation between individual hypoxic sensitivity and enzymes activities was found. In conclusion, IHT represents a promising approach in prevention and treatment of bronchial asthma in childhood. The proper choice of the hypoxic dosage depending on individual's reactivity must be titrated for each patient in order to avoid negative effects of hypoxia and to augment the favorable ones.

Abbreviations

BA	Bronchial asthma
CAT	Catalase
COPD	Chronic obstructive pulmonary disease
EPO	Erythropoietin
GPDG	Alpha-glycerophosphate dehydrogenase
GST	Glutathione-s-transferase
HIF	Hypoxia-inducible factor
HR	Heart rate
HVR	Hypoxic ventilatory response
IH	Intermittent hypoxia
IHT	Intermittent hypoxia training/treatment
MEAS	Method of expert assessing scales
NO	Nitric oxide
NOS	Nitric oxide synthase
OSAS	Obstructive sleep apnea syndrome
ROS	Reactive oxygen species
SaO_2	Arterial oxygen saturation
SDG	Succinate dehydrogenase
Cu,Zn – SOD	Cu,Zn-superoxide dismutase
V_E	Minute ventilation

T.V. Serebrovskaya (✉) • A.N. Bakunovsky • K.V. Nesvitailova • I.N. Mankovska
Department of Hypoxia,
Bogomoletz Institute of Physiology,
National Academy of Sciences of Ukraine,
Kiev, Ukraine
e-mail: sereb@biph.kiev.ua

11.1 Introduction

All body cells and tissues are able to alter their functions according to changes in actual blood oxygen content. Oxygen, as two-faced Janus, is necessary for life, but this very aggressive molecule has to get into an organism in strictly dosed quantity. Intermittent hypoxia (IH) is the most frequent form

L. Xi, T.V. Serebrovskaya (eds.), *Intermittent Hypoxia and Human Diseases*,
DOI 10.1007/978-1-4471-2906-6_11, © Springer-Verlag London 2012

of hypoxia, occurring in the developing mammals. It has been widely accepted that for the majority of a population, recurrent episodes of hypoxia are more often encountered during lifetime than sustained hypoxia. During the last decades, the IH has been investigated as a procedure with notable preventative, curative, and rehabilitative potential. It has been referred as an effective stimulus evoking various respiratory, cardiovascular, metabolic, and cellular responses [45, 70].

Asthma is a global health problem affecting around 300 million individuals of all ages, ethnic groups, and countries. It is a chronic inflammatory disorder of the airways characterized by an obstruction of airflow, which may be completely or partially reversed with or without specific therapy [11]. Airflow obstruction is the main criterion of distinction between bronchial asthma (BA) and chronic obstructive pulmonary diseases (COPD) when airflow limitation is irreversible [26]. Moreover, bronchial asthma is associated with subepithelial fibroblast activation, myofibroblast hyperplasia, and hypoxia [81].

The prevalence of asthma among adults has been increasing over the last 20 years in three times. But asthma in childhood is much more serious problem for today. It is the most frequent cause of children's disability (about 90% of total number of children with disability because of COPD). According to the recent health statistics for US children [9], 14% of children aged 3–17 had ever been diagnosed with asthma. BA affects at least 12% of Canadian children, whereas in Germany, more than 10% of children suffer from this chronic disorder, which ranged 8–12% in Russia. Among them, about 20% falls in severe and moderately severe bronchial asthma and about 60% in mild forms. Severe bronchial asthma is the reason of considerable limitation of vital functions and drop in social activity of sick children, i.e., decline of their quality of life. Regular absence from classes and limitation of social and physical activity negatively influence the children's physical and intellectual growth and development.

In spite of considerable progress in understanding of BA essence and pharmaceutical success, statistical data indicate an increase of morbidity and death rate from this illness. Current drug therapy does not often achieve the target because of mass distribution of allergic reactions and common decline of body resistance to negative factors. This situation requires the development of new nonpharmacological methods for prophylaxis, medical treatment, and rehabilitation of BA. In this respect, intermittent hypoxia training/treatment (IHT) has emerged as a procedure revealing its notable preventative, curative, and rehabilitative potential. The majority of clinical investigations devoted to the use of IHT for disease treatment have been conducted by clinicians and researches from the prominent Ukrainian and Russian academic centers, who presented mostly positive clinical effects. Several thousand patients were treated during more than 30 years in different clinics.

11.2 Historical Sketch

People noticed healing properties of mountain air since olden times. Hippocrates recommended people with sick lungs and after serious illness to go to mountains for some period. Marco Polo, the famous Venetian traveler of thirteenth to fourteenth century, traveling through Asia, marked that dales men suffering from different ailments being lodged in the mountains to convalesce for a few days. There was a legend from Carpathian Mountains (Ukraine) that in an ancient village, children who suffered from asthmatic bronchitis were ranged on foot during 7 days successively on a high sacred mountain, where they were submitted to the influence of special ceremonies and drank high-altitude herbal tea. The children had recovered. One of the folk medicine recipes for patients with pant was: "When you feel the approach of asthmatic fit, close that nostril through which it is easier to breath at this moment for 15 minutes."

One of the first applications of "artificial mountain air" (i.e., hypoxic gas mixture) was carried out in Kiev Institute of Tuberculosis and Thoracic Surgery (Ukraine) in 1969 during the preparation of a patient for lung resection [5]. Numerous publications concerning the use of IHT for treatment of BA in children and adults have appeared in the Soviet Union and the CIS in the 1990s [1, 5, 13, 18, 20, 21, 46, 54, 59, 60, 62, 69, 79, 45, 70]. More detailed historical review of the papers devoted to use of IHT for treatment of BA and COPD can be found in Chap. 9 by Mikhail Levashov.

11.3 Proposed Mechanisms

The detailed mechanisms of IH impact on human organism are under intensive investigation today at different levels – from molecular to systemic physiology. One of the main players is hypoxia-inducible factor (HIF), which initiates a gene transcription program of adaptation. It triggers a complex signaling cascade and thereby activates the expression of a variety of genes linked to such processes as angiogenesis, glycolysis, extracellular matrix remodelling, differentiation, and apoptosis [27]. Many studies in cultured cells suggest that IHT is more potent in activating HIF-1 than sustained hypoxia [12, 17, 57, 65].

Recently, Vogtel and Michels [80] denote the following basic mechanisms of beneficial effects of IHT on patients with BA: (1) HIF-1α induces the expression of erythropoietin (EPO), a glycoprotein hormone that controls erythropoiesis, plays an important role in the brain's response to neuronal injury and is also involved in the wound healing process; (2) HIF-1α provokes expression of the adaptive gene product VEGF, potent mediator of angiogenesis which produces multiple effects in lung development and physiology. Via the target of VEGF pathway – cytokine IL-4, proangiogenic effects in the lung exist under hypoxic conditions; (3) nitric oxide synthase (NOS) and heme oxygenase (HO) are two HIF-1 target genes, both triggering vasodilatation; (4) glucose uptake (glucose transporters) and glycolysis (glycolytic enzymes) are upregulated by HIF-1; (5) various HIFs influence tyrosine hydroxylase, the rate-limiting enzyme for the biosynthesis of dopamine; and (6) HIF transcription factors regulate iron metabolism. Iron is an essential cofactor for oxygen-binding proteins. The links between the cited functions and oxygen homoeostasis show that additional experimental studies are needed to determine the impact of various HIFs upon therapeutic effects of IHT on BA patients.

Numerous studies collectively show that IH (1) increases exercise tolerance, hypoxic ventilatory response, hematocrit, and blood hemoglobin content; (2) stimulates endothelial nitric oxide (NO) production provoking vasodilation, opening of reserve capillaries, and preventing Ca^{2+} overload; (3) stimulates angiogenic growth factor synthesis by endotheliocytes and monocytes; (4) augments the activity of parasympathetic nervous system; (5) enhances antioxidant defense system and increases the resistance of Na^+-K^+ ATPase to oxidative stress; (6) induces changes within mitochondria that increase the O_2 utilization efficiency of ATP production; and (7) mobilizes hematopoietic progenitors and augments cellular and humoral elements of innate immunity, etc. These data served as the basis for IHT in treatment of various diseases including BA.

As previously summarized [38, 69, 75, 76], other basic mechanisms underlying the beneficial effects of IHT were elaborated mainly in three areas: regulation of respiration, free radical production, and mitochondrial respiration. Findings showed that IHT induces increased ventilatory sensitivity to hypoxia and other hypoxia-related physiological changes [32, 72]. A great deal of evidence indicates that the respiratory control system is "plastic," which means that acute hypoxia can trigger a long-term augmentation of respiratory motor output [2, 47]. Following IHT, cellular membranes become more stable and improvement of O_2 transport in tissues is evident. IHT also induces changes in mitochondria, involving NAD-dependent metabolism, which in turn increases the efficiency of oxygen utilization in ATP production [41, 43, 49]. These effects are partly mediated by NO-dependent reactions [40, 51, 52], which are especially important for BA pathogenesis because exhaled NO is related to actual levels of airway inflammation in asthmatic patients [29, 82]. There are pieces of evidence that IHT may actually decrease the pronouncement of tissue hypoxia and intracellular acidosis under acute hypoxic exposure, improve O_2 transport in tissues, increase oxidative metabolism enzyme synthesis and ion-transport systems in cell membranes, and rearrange the cell membrane phospholipid composition. IHT also seems to increase tissue capillary growth. IHT also mobilizes hematopoietic progenitors and augments cellular and humoral elements of innate immunity [74].

The influence of IHT on free radical processes seems of key significance, as these processes are implicated in the pathogenesis of BA. Alveolar macrophages, blood neutrophils, and eosinophils from asthmatic patients have been shown to release more oxygen radicals than healthy subjects do. The mitochondrial damage in asthmatic lung due to reactive oxygen species (ROS) was also described in mice [36]. ROS induce airway hyperreactivity, destruction of lung epithelial cells, mucus hypersecretion, platelet-activating factor synthesis, and other reactions typical for BA in humans and animals [15, 58, 64]. These unwanted changes are often caused by tissue hypoxia and consequent reduction of electron transfer in the respiratory chain, an increase of functional activity of inflammatory cells, and impaired antioxidant defense system. The cyclic hypoxia-reoxygenation episodes in IH also generate ROS. Although high concentrations of these substances are cytotoxic, at physiological concentrations, ROS function as signaling molecules to elicit gene expression and synthesis of cytoprotective proteins. In this manner, ROS may have mediated the induction of cardioprotection [48]. In addition, IHT acts positively on an organism by eliminating tissue hypoxia, normalizing the number and phagocytic activity of white blood cells, and enhancing antioxidant enzymes activity [66]. Interestingly, if the hypoxic periods are much briefer than normoxia, and if this exposure sequence is repeated over a number of days, the antioxidant defenses could be enhanced much more effectively than under sustained hypoxia [50, 53, 72]. Taken together, these data serve as the prerequisite to the use of IHT for treating and correcting various diseases during which the ROS outbreaks are anticipated, in particular, BA.

11.4 Clinical Evidence

All above-mentioned mechanisms may explain positive clinical effects of IHT on BA patients. Many studies showed significant decline in breath shortness and feelings of chest congestion. The cough was diminished or disappeared, and the amount of sputum was reduced and passed more easily. The attacks of asphyxia disappeared or became more occasional. Rebalance of early autonomic dysfunction was also observed [5, 10, 13, 18, 30, 39, 54, 62]. IHT positively affected the psychoemotional state of patients. Most evident positive results were obtained in children (from 4 years) [4, 21, 69, 79].

Anokhin and coauthors [1] performed a normobaric hypoxic stimulation with four sessions of 5 min 12–15% O_2, followed by 5-min normoxic interval (for 10 days) in 200 children aged 4–14 years who suffered from BA. The results were compared with the sham group. A positive effect was seen in 85% of subjects in the group with IH and in 25% of the sham group. In children with mild BA, complete discontinuance of attacks was observed. In patients with middle-severe forms, a significant improvement was registered, namely, the attacks became rare and stopped without medicines. In patients with the severe form, small improvement was noted. As Ehrenburg and Kordykinskaya [20] reported, the lowest efficacy was noted in children with an infection-dependent form of BA. Half of the patients with a severe steroid-dependent form of BA displayed a worsening of the clinical course of the disease. A positive clinical effect in patients with mild and middle atopic BA lasted for an average of 4 months posthypoxic therapy. Hypoxic treatment in children with BA of mild and middle severity can be performed only in between, and not during, the arrest periods. In the hormone-dependent form of BA, IHT was unsatisfactory [30]. These observations have been subsequently confirmed [14, 59, 69].

On the average, a good effect of IHT was noted in 85–95% of BA patients, satisfactory effect in 40–50%, and no effect in only 4–8% of patients who had mostly the hormone-dependent form of BA. The best effect was achieved for atopic form of BA and less pronounced effect was found in the infection-allergic and mixed forms of BA. About 40% of adult patients decreased the dose of constantly taken drugs and almost 90% of children were able to quit the drug treatment. Improvement of the clinical state was retained for 1 year in 40–50% of patients, for 6 months in 20–30%, and for 3–4 months in 15–20%.

Individual differences in respiratory reactions to hypoxia, ranging from ventilatory hypersensitivity to complete absence of reaction, have been described with special approaches suggested for individual dosage of IHT regimen [6, 7, 8, 20, 37, 46, 68, 78].

11.5 Adverse Effects

Meanwhile, a reduction in the partial pressure of inspired oxygen may be a potential risk factor for severe impairment of pulmonary function and even sudden death. It has been postulated that IH-induced oxidative stress may contribute to several chronic diseases associated with obstructive sleep apnea syndrome (OSAS), which has increased predisposition for metabolic dysfunction by impairing insulin sensitivity, glucose effectiveness, etc. [42]. A large number of clinical studies, cell culture and animal models utilizing IH, have demonstrated the central role of oxidative stress in OSAS. Besides, there are some evidences concerning the adverse effect of chronic or intermittent hypoxia on cognition in childhood, more specifically on development, behavior, and academic achievement [3, 35]. Failure to adapt to hypoxia may be a common pathophysiological mediator for a number of other conditions of childhood with cognitive deficit [34]. This should be taken into account in any situation that may expose children to hypoxia. Ability of adaptation to intermittent or sustained hypoxia may determine the type of neurological complications for which patients are at risk when exposed to acute hypoxia [34]. For example, persistently low levels of tissue oxygen in anemia may lead to neuroprotective erythropoietin production, but release of the younger, more adhesive red cells and any associated hemolysis [63] may adversely affect endothelial function [24], eventually leading to irreversible vascular disease. Because the adverse effects have been noted at even mild levels of oxygen desaturation, future research should include precisely defined data on the safety of exposure to all levels of hypoxia.

During the past few years, there are debates about the ethical evaluation of diagnostic and therapeutic use of hypoxia in humans. Although the papers devoted to this problem obtained the approval from the Human Investigation Ethics Committees, there is a lack of evidences about strong evaluation of risk/benefit ratio. The analysis of such ratio and the creation of standardized guidelines for IHT application are complicated due to the differences in criteria for individual dosage and utilized methods. As Vogtel and Michels [80] pointed out, future research examining the potential risks and benefits of IHT could pave the way for the development of new therapeutic approaches for patients suffering from BA. Thereupon, a new mathematical method – "Method of Expert Assessing Scales" (MEAS) – was proposed for estimation of IH application safety in human practice [77]. MEAS expands capabilities of traditional probabilistic safety assessment and allows determining the danger degree at the earliest stage of its development and fulfilling well-timed actions for risk prevention. It includes the description of: (a) hazard causal factors, (b) situations as a set of values of causal factors, (c) influences of separate factors on the origin of basic events, and (d) joint influence of factors on basic events probability. This methodology provides the forming of a system of indexes characterizing the risk of IHT negative effects and determination of legitimate value scopes for basic physiological parameters; creation of a classification system, allowing to set individual cardiorespiratory reactivity; and development of proper IHT regimen for every class of reactivity in humans.

In brief, contraindications to IHT application include acute infectious diseases, exacerbation of chronic inflammatory processes, fever, acute somatic diseases, respiratory insufficiency of II–III stage, pulmonary tuberculosis in active phase, etc. [6, 7, 13, 19, 37, 46, 62, 79].

11.6 Latest Experience in IHT Implementation

After all, we would like to share with readers our latest experience in IHT implementation for treatment of children with BA. Two groups of children aged 9–13 years participated in the study: experimental group (Gr. I) – 16 children (13 boys and 3 girls) who underwent IHT alone with traditional medical treatment – and control group (Gr. II) – 8 children (4 boys and 4 girls) who got received the same medical treatment, but not IHT. All patients had a similar diagnosis: persistent atopic bronchial asthma, moderate form of disease without the signs of respiratory insufficiency.

Before and next day after the 2-week IHT, individual cardiorespiratory reactions to hypoxia were investigated in the morning, 2 h after a light breakfast. With the subject seated, normobaric hypoxia was administered with device "Hypoxotron – Complex," a modified closed spirometer with CO_2 absorption [73]. Initial inspired gas contained atmospheric O_2 (20.9%). The inspired O_2 fell to 12% during the first 60–90 s of rebreathing, and then O_2 was added gradually to the Hypoxotron to maintain inspired O_2 at 12% during the remaining 3.5–4 min. The final arterial O_2 saturation (SaO_2) during first investigation was typically 89–92%. All children easily tolerated the hypoxia periods without any untoward effects. Standard spirometry was performed before and after hypoxic test in accordance with the American Thoracic Society criteria. Between first and second examinations, IHT was conducted bedside using portable device "Hypoxotron-Simplex" [67] during 14 consecutive mornings, after a light breakfast. Every session consisted of four 5–7 min periods, with 5 min interval periods of room air inspiration.

As a result of IHT, a significant decline in breath shortness and feelings of chest congestion were noted in patients of Gr. I. The cough was diminished or disappeared, and the amount of sputum was reduced and passed more easily. The attacks of asphyxia disappeared or became less frequent. Children liked the procedure, and in cases of relapse, they wanted another treatment with IHT. We did not find significant changes in airway conductance before (I) and after (II) IHT (Table 11.1). Significant differences in hypoxic ventilatory sensitivity were found as a result of hypoxic training. Gr. I (in contrast to Gr. II) showed increased hypoxic ventilatory response, which was analyzed by relative minute ventilation (V_E) with respect to $P_{ET}O_2$ and estimated using piecewise linear approximation technique [72]: slope I (S_I) increased by 104% ($p<0.01$); slope II (S_{II}) by 79% ($p<0.05$), maximal lung ventilation by 24% ($p<0.05$; Fig. 11.1). These data suggest that adaptation to IH caused considerable augmentation of ventilatory response to hypoxic stimuli. Several mechanisms are involved in this process, embracing events happening on both central and peripheral levels [31, 71]. At the same time, reaction of heart rate (HR) to increasing hypoxia became less pronounced (Fig. 11.2) and SaO_2 fell less at 12% O_2 (Fig. 11.3). Thus, after IHT, cardiovascular system became more effective to support oxygen supply during hypoxia.

Table 11.1 Lung function parameters before and after IHT

	Before IHT	After IHT
FVC pred (%)	85.51±6.58	91.47±6.97
FEV_1pred (%)	59.7±4.7	64.6±4.5
FEV1/FVC (%)	67.58±3.47	64.18±2.12
PEF pred (%)	61.32±5.25	60.94±5.34

Data are Mean±SD
Abbreviations: *FVC* forced vital capacity, *FEV_1* forced expiratory volume in 1 s, *PEF* peak expiratory flow

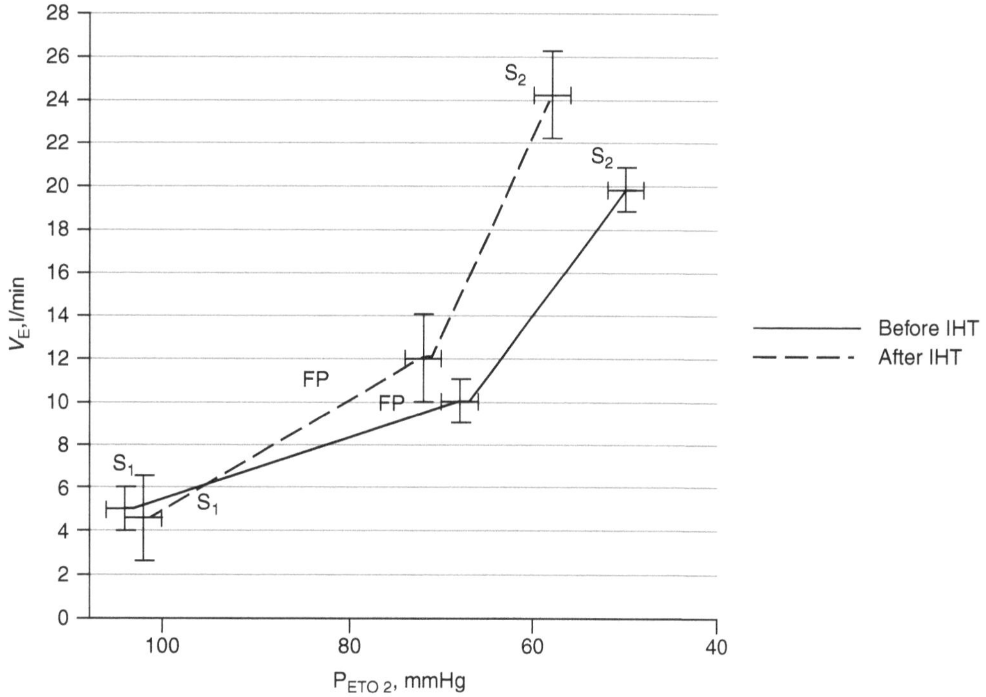

Fig. 11.1 Data plot of hypoxic ventilatory response before and after IHT (Gr. I, Mean±SD). *S_1* slope during the first phase of sharply increasing ventilation, *S_2* slope during the second phase of sharply increasing ventilation, *FP* fracture point co-ordinate

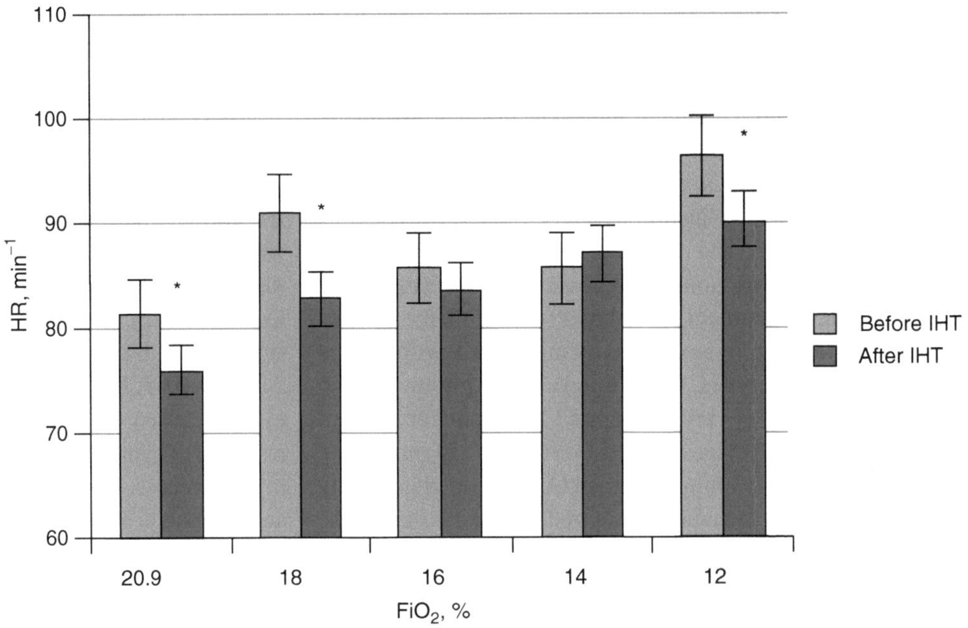

Fig. 11.2 Heart rate during increasing hypoxia test before and after IHT (Gr. I, Mean ± SD; * $p<0.05$)

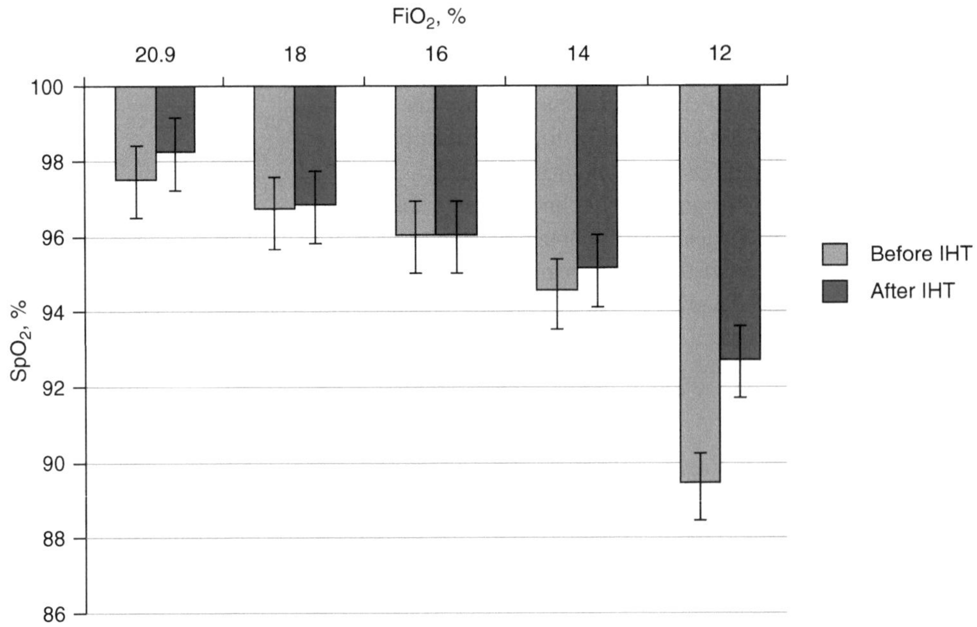

Fig. 11.3 SaO_2 during incremental hypoxia test before and after IHT (Gr. I, Mean ± SD)

Furthermore, IHT influenced mitochondrial enzymes activity of immune cells in asthmatic children, particularly succinate dehydrogenase (SDG) and alpha-glycerophosphate dehydrogenase (GPDG). These enzymes reflect cell energy potential and its reserve mechanisms. Investigation of mitochondrial respiratory chain enzymes is an important step for establishing a diagnosis of mitochondrial dysfunction – one of pathogenetic links of the BA development. Low activity levels of these enzymes suggest cellular metabolic dysfunction that is usually associated with unfavorable clinical signs [22, 33, 36, 55, 61]. Kinetic parameters for mitochondrial enzymes in the substrate region of the respiratory chain correlate with hypoxic resistance [44].

In this investigation, the measurements of SDG and GPDG activities in peripheral lymphocytes were carried out on blood slides cytophotometrically. Both SDG and GPDG activities increased significantly under IHT (by 78% and 42%, respectively, Fig. 11.4). Similar results were obtained in the previous animal investigations [41]. A strong correlation between the individual hypoxic sensitivity and mitochondrial enzymes activities was found by linear regression analysis, mostly expressed according to GPDG: in children

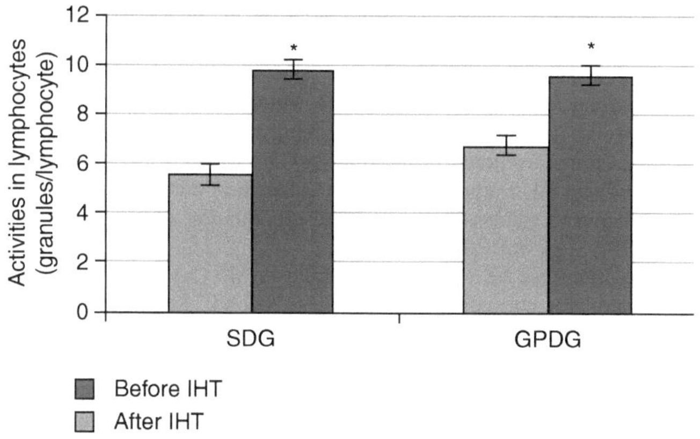

Fig. 11.4 SDG and GPDG activities in lymphocytes under IHT (Gr. I, Mean ± SD; * p<0.05)

with decreased hypoxic ventilatory response (HVR), heightened initial SDG and GPDG activities was observed (for GPDG, $r = -0.64$, $p < 0.05$; for SDG, $r = -0.36$, $p < 0.1$) and greater increase under IHT (for GPDG, $r = -0.58$, $p < 0.05$; for SDG, $r = -0.41$, $p < 0.1$). This reaction was accompanied by more expressed positive clinical effect in children with low hypoxic sensitivity. Reciprocal relationships between hypoxic sensitiveness and enzymatic activity of dehydrogenases indicate an important role of the mitochondrial enzymes in the compensatory reactions of an organism to hypoxia. In addition to their crucial role in energy homeostasis, mitochondria are the main site of ROS generation. When moderately produced, they function as physiological signaling molecules. Thus, mitochondrial ROS trigger hypoxia-dependent gene expression.

On the other hand, the development of inflammatory process in lungs is usually associated with activation of free radical oxidation and decline of antioxidant enzymes activity and intensification of glycolysis in both humans and animals [14, 16, 23, 36]. To elucidate the role of antioxidant enzymes in adaptation to IHT, another investigation was carried out using the same protocol [56]. The effect of 10-day IHT on the mRNA expression and protein content of antioxidant enzymes – Cu,Zn-superoxide dismutase (Cu,Zn-SOD), catalase (CAT), and glutathione-S-transferase (GST) in blood leukocytes of asthmatic children was studied. Level of protein expression of antioxidant enzymes was determined by Western blot analysis [28]. We found that Cu,Zn-SOD protein content did not change significantly, but Cu,Zn-SOD mRNA expression increased by 32.5% ($p < 0.05$). Conversely, GST protein synthesis increased by 90% ($p < 0.05$), but its mRNA gene expression was invariable. CAT protein content and its mRNA gene expression both increased by 37% and 13%, respectively ($p < 0.05$). A previous investigation in animals have also shown a negative correlation between Mn-SOD mRNA expression and its protein content in mitochondria from hypoxic myocardium [25]. It is possible that during hypoxia, the strengthening of translation processes could take place with accelerated protein synthesis without evident activation of mRNA expression at this stage. Nevertheless, analysis of the mRNA expression dynamics may provide additional information of the antioxidant enzymes as the markers of the IHT effectiveness in children with BA.

Conclusion

IHT represents a promising approach in prevention and treatment of BA in childhood. The proper choice of the hypoxic dosage depending on individual's reactivity to hypoxia must be titrated for each patient to avoid negative effects of hypoxia and to augment the favorable ones. Further studies on individual approaches to dosage selection must be performed. The absence of negative side effects, typically observed during drug therapy, and the stimulation of an organism's general resistance to pathological factors of BA would make IHT a beneficial treatment with a bright future.

References

1. Anokhin MI, Geppe NA, Dairova RA. Effects of hypoxic stimulation observed in the animal experiments and in children with bronchial asthma. Fiziol Zh. 1992;38:33–9 [In Russian].
2. Baker TL, Fuller DD, Zabka AGGS, et al. Respiratory plasticity: differential actions of continuous and episodic hypoxia and hypercapnia. Respir Physiol. 2001;129:25–35.
3. Bass JL, Corwin M, Gozal D, et al. The effect of chronic or intermittent hypoxia on cognition in childhood: a review of the evidence. Pediatrics. 2004;114:805–16.
4. Belikova VV. Correlation between clinical and cytochemical changes in bronchial asthma in children. Pediatriia. 1976;11:30–3 [In Russian].
5. Berezovski VA, Levashov MI. Physiological premises and mechanisms of normalizing effect of normobaric hypoxia and inhalation therapy. Fiziol Zh. 1992;38:3–12 [In Russian].
6. Berezovskii VA, Levashov MI. Introduction in orotherapy. Kiev: Academy of Hypoxia Problems of Russian Federation; 2000. p. 75 [In Russian].
7. Berezovskii VA, Levashov MI. The build-up of human reserve potential by exposure to intermittent normobaric hypoxia. Aviakosm Ekolog Med. 2000;34:39–43 [In Russian].
8. Berezovskii VA, Serebrovskaia TV, Lipskii PI. Respiratory function in twins under different gas mixtures. Fiziol Zh. 1981;27:20–5 [In Russian].
9. Bloom B, Cohen RA, Freeman G. Summary health statistics for U.S. children: National Health Interview Survey 2009. Vital Health Stat 10. 2010;1–82.
10. Borukaeva IK. Intermittent hypoxic training in the sanatorium and spa treatment for patients with chronic obstructive pulmonary disease. Vopr Kurortol Fizioter Lech Fiz Kult. 2007;5:21–4 [In Russian].
11. Bousquet J, Mantzouranis E, Cruz AA. Uniform definition of asthma severity, control, and exacerbations: document presented for the World Health Organization Consultation on Severe Asthma. J Allergy Clin Immunol. 2010;126:926–38.

12. Brzecka A. Brain preconditioning and obstructive sleep apnea syndrome. Acta Neurobiol Exp (Wars). 2005;65:213–20.
13. Chizhov AI. Physiologic bases of the method to increase nonspecific resistance of the organism by adaptation to intermittent normobaric hypoxia. Fiziol Zh. 1992;38:13–7 [In Russian].
14. Chizhov AI, Bludov AA. Efficiency of intermittent and resonance intermittent normobaric hypoxia therapy in patients with infection-dependent bronchial asthma. Vestn Ross Akad Med Nauk. 2000;9:48–50 [In Russian].
15. Damon M, Cluzel M, Chanez P, et al. Phagocytosis induction of chemiluminescence and chemoattractant increased superoxide anion release from activated human alveolar macrophages in asthma. J Biolumin Chemilumin. 1989;4:279–86.
16. Daniliak IG, Kogan AK, Bolevich S. The generation of active forms of oxygen by the blood leukocytes, lipid peroxidation and antiperoxide protection in bronchial asthma patients. Ter Arkh. 1992;64:54–7 [In Russian].
17. Dewhirst MW. Intermittent hypoxia furthers the rationale for hypoxia-inducible factor-1 targeting. Cancer Res. 2007;67:854–5.
18. Donenko YI. Comparison of intermittent normobaric hypoxic therapy and hypobaric therapy in treatment of chronic nonspecific lung diseases. In: Intermittent hypoxic training – effectiveness and mechanisms of action. Kiev: Institute of Physical Culture; 1992. p. 65–8 [In Russian].
19. Eckes L. Altitude adaptation. Part III. Altitude acclimatization as a problem of human biology. Gegenbaurs Morphol Jahrb. 1976;122: 535–69 [In German].
20. Ehrenburg IV, Kordykinskaya II. Effectiveness of the use of intermittent normobaric hypoxia in treatment of chronic obstructive lung diseases. In: Intemittent hypoxic training – effectiveness, mechanisms of action. Kiev: Institute of Physical Culture; 1992. p. 96–8 [In Russian].
21. Fesenko ME, Lisyana TO. Approach to employment of hypoxic stimulation for treatment of lingering and relapsing bronchitis in children of early age. Fiziol Zh. 1992;38:31–3 [In Russian].
22. Fursova ZK, Balika IuD, Abubakirova AM. Dynamics of the activity of redox enzymes in peripheral blood lymphocytes of the newborn with a history of chronic intrauterine hypoxia. Akush Ginekol (Mosk). 1995;4:29–31 [In Russian].
23. Gerasimov SV. Lipid peroxidation and antioxidant defense in patients with bronchial asthma. Ukr Med Chasopys. 2000;1:86–94 [In Ukrainian].
24. Gladwin MT, Kato GJ. Cardiopulmonary complications of sickle cell disease: role of nitric oxide and haemolytic anemia. Hematology Am Soc Hematol Educ Program. 2005;51–7.
25. Gonchar OO, Steshenko MM, Mankovska IM, et al. Correction of mitochondrial dysfunction in rat myocardium under hypoxia. Zagalna Patoligia ta Patologichna Phyziologia. 2010;3:44–8 [In Ukrainian].
26. Gordon E, Lazarus SC. Management of chronic obstructive pulmonary disease: moving beyond the asthma algorithm. J Allergy Clin Immunol. 2009;124:873–80.
27. Gordan JD, Simon MC. Hypoxia-inducible factors: central regulators of the tumor phenotype. Curr Opin Genet Dev. 2007;17:71–7.
28. Hanta I, Kocabas A, Canacankatan N, et al. Oxidant–antioxidant balance in patients with COPD. Lung. 2006;184:51–5.
29. Jones SL, Herbison P, Cowan JO, et al. Exhaled NO and assessment of anti-inflammatory effects of inhaled steroid: dose–response relationship. Eur Respir J. 2002;20:601–8.
30. Karash YM, Strelkov RB, Chizhov AY. Normobaric hypoxia in treatment, prophylaxis and rehabilitation. Moscow: Meditsina; 1988 [In Russian].
31. Katayama K. Effect of intermittent hypoxia on hypoxic ventilatory response. In: Xi L, Serebrovskaya TV, editors. Intermittent hypoxia: from molecular mechanisms to clinical applications. New York: Nova; 2009. p. 245–59.
32. Katayama K, Sato Y, Morotome Y, et al. Intermittent hypoxia increases ventilation and SaO_2 during hypoxic exercise and hypoxic chemosensitivity. J Appl Physiol. 2001;90:1431–40.
33. Kiernan MC, Bullpitt P, Chan JH. Mitochondrial dysfunction and rod-like lesions associated with administration of beta2 adrenoceptor agonist formoterol. Neuromuscul Disord. 2004;14:375–7.
34. Kirkham FJ, Datta AK. Hypoxic adaptation during development: relation to pattern of neurological presentation and cognitive disability. Dev Sci. 2006;9:411–27.
35. Kolchinskaya AZ, Hatsukov BH, Zakusilo MP. Oxygen insufficiency: destructive and constructive actions. Nalchik: Kabardino-Balkaria Scientific Center; 1999 [In Russian].
36. Konga DB, Kim Y, Hong SC, et al. Oxidative stress and antioxidant defenses in asthmatic murine model exposed to printer emissions and environmental tobacco smoke. J Environ Pathol Toxicol Oncol. 2009;28:325–40.
37. Korkushko OV, Serebrovskaya TV, Shatilo VB, et al. Selection of the optimal modes for intermittent hypoxia training in medical practice and sports medicine. Methodical recommendations. Kiev Health Ministry; 2010 [In Ukrainian].
38. Kowalski J, Gutkowski P, Serebrovskaya T. Beneficial either detrimental consequences for respiration and hemodynamics. Vestn Hyg Epidemiol. 2007;11:9–13.
39. Kulberg AY. Regulation of the immune response. Moscow: Nauka; 1997. p. 148–57 [In Russian].
40. Kurhalyuk NM, Serebrovskaya TV. Intermittent hypoxic training influences on antioxidant enzymes activity, processes of lipid peroxidation under acute hypoxia and nitric oxide donor treatment. Med Chem. 2001;3:69–71.
41. Kurhalyuk NM, Serebrovskaya TV, Kolesnikova EE, et al. Exogenous L-arginine modulates the effects of acute and intermittent hypoxia on liver mitochondrial and microsomal oxidation. Fiziol Zh. 2002;48:67–73.
42. Louis M, Punjabi NM. Effects of acute intermittent hypoxia on glucose metabolism in awake healthy volunteers. J Appl Physiol. 2009;106:1538–44.
43. Lukyanova LD. Molecular, metabolic and functional mechanisms of individual resistance to hypoxia. In: Sharma BK, Takeda N, Ganguly NK, et al., editors. Adaptation biology and medicine. New Delhi: Narosa Publishing House; 1997. p. 236–50.
44. Lukyanova LD, Dudchenko AM, Tsybina TA, et al. Effect of intermittent normobaric hypoxia on kinetic properties of mitochondrial enzymes. Bull Exp Biol Med. 2007;144:795–801.
45. Lukyanova LD, Germanova EL, Kopaladze RA. Development of resistance of an organism under various conditions of hypoxic preconditioning: role of the hypoxic period and reoxygenation. Bull Exp Biol Med. 2009;147:400–4.
46. Lysenko GI, Serebrovskaya TV, Karaban IN, et al. Use of gradually increasing normobaric hypoxia in medical practice. Methodical recommendations. Kiev: Ukrainian Ministry of Health Care; 1998 [In Russian].
47. Mahamed S, Mitchell G. Is there a link between intermittent hypoxia-induced respiratory plasticity and obstructive sleep apnoea? Exp Physiol. 2007;92:27–37.
48. Mallet RT, Ryou M-G, Manukhina EB, et al. β-Adrenergic signaling and ROS: pivotal roles in intermittent, normobaric hypoxia-induced cardioprotection. In: Xi L, Serebrovskaya TV, editors. Intermittent hypoxia: from molecular mechanisms to clinical applications. New York: Nova; 2009. p. 151–74.
49. Man'kovskaia IN, Vavilova GL, Kharlamova ON, et al. Activity of the cell membrane marker enzymes in rats under adaptation to hypoxia. Ukr Biochem J. 1997;69:79–87 [In Russian].
50. Mankovskaya IN. Peculiarities of lipid peroxidation realization mechanisms in intermittent hypoxic hypoxia. Hypoxia Med J. 1993;4:8–11 [In Russian].

51. Manukhina EB, Downey HF, Mallet RT. Role of nitric oxide in cardiovascular adaptation to intermittent hypoxia. Exp Biol Med. 2006;231:343–65.
52. Manukhina EB, Mashina SY, Smirin BV, et al. Role of nitric oxide in adaptation to hypoxia and adaptive defense. Physiol Res. 2000;49:89–97.
53. Meerson FZ. Adaptation to intermittent hypoxia: mechanisms of protective effects. Hypoxia Med J. 1993;3:2–8 [In Russian].
54. Meerson FZ, Frolov BA, Volianik MN, et al. The effect of adaptation to the periodic action of hypoxia on the indices of the immunity system and on the course of allergic diseases. Patol Fiziol Eksp Ter. 1990;3:16–21 [In Russian].
55. Moroz LA, Sukhorukov VV, Kravchenko LF, et al. Significance of a complex of laboratory methods of study in the differential diagnosis of various forms of bronchial asthma. Med Tr Prom Ekol. 1994;2:32–4 [In Russian].
56. Nesvitalova KV, Gonchar OA, Drevitskaya TI, et al. Changes in mRNA and protein expression of antioxidant enzymes as markers of the interval hypoxic training effectiveness in children with bronchial asthma. Fiziol Zh. 2011;57(6):13–7 [In Ukrainian].
57. Prabhakar NR, Fields RD, Baker T, et al. Intermittent hypoxia: cell to system. Am J Physiol. 2001;281:L524–8.
58. Prasad K, Gupta JB. Relaxant effect of oxygen free radicals on rabbit tracheal smooth muscle. Pulm Pharmacol Ther. 2002;15: 375–84.
59. Ragozin ON. Effectiveness of intermittent normobaric hypoxia in patients with bronchial asthma in various modes of chronotherapy. Vopr Kurortol Fizioter Lech Fiz Kult. 2002;2:8–10 [In Russian].
60. Ragozin ON, Balykin MV, Charikova EI, et al. The analysis of rhythm spectrum of respiratory and cardiovascular parameters in bronchial asthma patients under normobaric hypoxitherapy. Fiziol Zh. 2001;47:36–9 [In Russian].
61. Razumovskiĭ AE, Komissarova IA, Shatalov NN, et al. Effect of atmospheric pressure on leukocyte enzyme activity in bronchial asthma. Sov Med. 1980;12:19–22 [In Russian].
62. Redzhebova OK, Chizhov AI. Results of utilization of intermittent normobaric hypoxia in patients with bronchial asthma and chronic obstructive bronchitis. Fiziol Zh. 1992;38:39–42 [In Russian].
63. Rice L, Alfrey CP. The negative regulation of red cell mass by neocytolysis: physiologic and pathophysiologic manifestations. Cell Physiol Biochem. 2005;15:245–50.
64. Safronova OS, Serebrovskaya TV, Hordiĭ SK. Pro- and antioxidant system during the adaptation to intermittent hypoxia in healthy subjects and patients with bronchial asthma. Exper Clin Physiol Biochem. 1999;4:61–6 [In Russian].
65. Semenza GL. HIF-1: mediator of physiological and pathophysiological responses to hypoxia. J Appl Physiol. 2000;88:1474–80.
66. Serebrovs'ka TV, Safronova OS, Hordiĭ SK. Free-radical processes under different conditions of body oxygen allowance. Fiziol Zh. 1999;45:92–103 [In Ukrainian].
67. Serebrovska TV, Lopata VA, Roy VV, et al. Device for breathing with hypoxic mixtures "Hypoxytron". 2009. Patent 44179, МПК A61M 16/00; Ukraine, 25 Sept 2009, bulletin № 18 [In Ukrainian].
68. Serebrovskaia TV. Hereditary defect of sensitivity to hypoxia in normal sensitivity to hypercapnia. Patol Fiziol Eksp Ter. 1982;4:80–3.
69. Serebrovskaia TV, Man'kovskaia IN, Lysenko GI, et al. A method for intermittent hypoxic exposures in the combined treatment of bronchial asthma patients. Lik Sprava. 1998;6:104–8 [In Ukrainian].
70. Serebrovskaia ZA, Serebrovskaia TV, Afonina GB. Chemiluminescence, blood lipid peroxidation and neutrophil activity during the hypoxic training of persons subjected to ionizing radiation exposure. Radiats Biol Radioecol. 1996;36:394–9.
71. Serebrovskaya TV. Intermittent hypoxia research in the former Soviet Union and the Commonwealth of Independent States (CIS): history and review of the concept and selected applications. High Alt Med Biol. 2002;3:205–21.
72. Serebrovskaya TV, Karaban IN, Kolesnikova EE, et al. Human hypoxic ventilatory response with blood dopamine content under intermittent hypoxic training. Can J Physiol Pharmacol. 1999;77: 967–73.
73. Serebrovskaya TV, Lopata VA. Apparatus for breathing with hypoxic gaseous mixtures. 2010. Patent International Application to all countries of PCT # PCT/UA 2010/000071, 7 Oct 2010.
74. Serebrovskaya TV, Nikolsky IS, Nikolska VV, et al. Intermittent hypoxia mobilizes hematopoietic progenitors and augments cellular and humoral elements of innate immunity in adult men. High Alt Med Biol. 2011;12:243–52.
75. Serebrovskaya TV, Serebrovskaya ZA, Afonina G. Effect of intermittent hypoxic training on human respiration, free radical processes and immune system. In: Ueda G et al., editors. High altitude medicine. Matsumoto: Shinshu University Press; 1992. p. 77–82.
76. Serebrovskaya TV, Swanson RJ, Kolesnikova EE. Intermittent hypoxia: mechanisms of action and some applications to bronchial asthma treatment. J Physiol Pharmacol. 2003;54:35–41.
77. Serebrovsky A, Serebrovska T. Models and algorithms for the assessment of intermittent hypoxia application safety and efficacy in medical practice. In: Hypoxia and consequences: from molecule to malady. 2009. Book of abstracts, Session II, abstract #25, New York, 12–14 Mar 2009.
78. Tsvetkova AM, Tkatchouk EN. "Hypoxia user" – the opportunity of individual programming of interval hypoxic training. In: Hypoxia, mechanisms, adaptation, correction. BEBIM, Moscow; 1999. p. 83–4 [In Russian].
79. Vinnitskaya RS, Davidov EG, Ctruchkov PV. Hypoxic and hypercapnic gas mixtures in complex treatment and rehabilitation of patients with chronic obstructive diseases. In: Intermittent hypoxic training, effectiveness, and mechanisms of action. Kiev: Institute of Physical Culture; 1992. p. 62–4 [In Russian].
80. Vogtel M, Michels A. Role of intermittent hypoxia in the treatment of bronchial asthma and chronic obstructive pulmonary disease. Curr Opin Allergy Clin Immunol. 2010;10:206–13.
81. Zhong H, Belardinelli L, Maa T, et al. Synergy between A2B adenosine receptors and hypoxia in activating human lung fibroblasts. Am J Respir Cell Mol Biol. 2005;32:2–8.
82. Zietkowski Z, Bodzenta-Lukaszyk A. Nitric oxide in bronchial asthma. Pol Merkur Lekarski. 2002;12:519–21 [In Polish].

Part III

Intermittent Hypoxia and Neurological Disorders

Intermittent Hypoxia and Experimental Parkinson's Disease

12

Maria V. Belikova, Evgenia E. Kolesnikova, and Tatiana V. Serebrovskaya

Abstract

Parkinson's disease (PD) is a common neurodegenerative disease which is characterized by a progressive degeneration of dopaminergic neurons in the midbrain. A most reliable mechanism causing the apoptosis in dopaminergic structures of the brain during aging and Parkinson's disease is the activation of oxidative stress. Until now, effective means for the prevention of dopaminergic neurons degeneration and for the retention of damaged neurons functioning is still lacking. A promising way to slacken the pace of degenerative processes during aging and PD could be the adaptation to intermittent hypoxia. Such adaptation strengthens dopamine (DA) synthesis and release at peripheral chemoreceptors in carotid bodies and activates tyrosine hydroxylase – a rate-limiting enzyme for catecholamine synthesis. In this chapter, we examined three groups of rats: adult, old, and old rats with experimental DA deficiency. It was revealed that there was an asymmetry of dopamine distribution between the right and left striatum of adult rats. Prevalent quantity of dopamine was concentrated in right hemisphere. During aging DA, production decreased in the examined structures mainly in right hemisphere of the striatum, so its distribution asymmetry diminished. In PD animals, this decrease was much more expressed and led to practically total abolishment of quantitative difference between right and left hemispheres. Two-week course of intermittent hypoxia training (IHT, five cycles of 15-min exposures to 12% O_2 followed by 15-min room air breathing per day) increased dopamine synthesis in old and experimental PD animals, especially in the right striatum, restored partially the asymmetry of DA distribution between brain hemispheres. IHT also decreased the intensity of lipid peroxidation. Increased plasma antioxidant activity positively correlated with increased DA concentration in the striatum. Therefore, IHT could serve as a good perspective means for the deceleration of aging and prevention/treatment of Parkinson's disease.

M.V. Belikova
Medical Department, Kiev Medical University of Ukrainian Association of Folk Medicine, Academy of Medical Sciences of Ukraine 01004 Kiev, Ukraine

E.E. Kolesnikova (✉) • T.V. Serebrovskaya
Department of Hypoxic States, Bogomoletz Institute of Physiology National Academy of Sciences of Ukraine, 01024 Kiev, Ukraine
e-mail: dr_kolesnikova@ukr.net

L. Xi, T.V. Serebrovskaya (eds.), *Intermittent Hypoxia and Human Diseases*, DOI 10.1007/978-1-4471-2906-6_12, © Springer-Verlag London 2012

Abbreviations

6-OHDA	6-hydroxydopamine
CAT	Catalase
CB	Carotid bodies
DA	Dopamine
EDAD	Experimental DA deficiency
GFAP	Glial fibrillary acid protein
HIF	Hypoxia inducible factor
IHT	Intermittent hypoxia training
MAO	Monoamine oxidase
MDA	Malondialdehyde
PD	Parkinson's disease
ROS	Reactive oxygen species
SN	Substantia nigra
SOD	Superoxide dismutase
TH	Tyrosine hydroxylase

12.1 Introduction

Parkinson's disease (PD) is characterized by a progressive degeneration of dopaminergic neurons in the midbrain. Although there are a number of hypotheses to explain this process, the one on oxidative stress has gained major interest [1, 2]. Experimental studies strongly support the view that the antioxidant system capacity determines life span potential [3]. During many years PD was associated with accelerated aging. The process of aging is accompanied by multiple molecular and cellular changes which promote neurodegeneration. At the same time, it is worthy of notice that regional and subregional pattern of striatal dopamine loss in normal aging differs substantially from the pattern typically observed in PD [4]. The authors consider that the formation of dopamine-derived oxygen radicals in human striatum appears unlikely to be a primary factor responsible for the age-related dopamine loss. It seems that *causa proxima* of PD development is related to the certain specific mechanism of neuronal death different from the reduction of neurocytes quantity in *substantia nigra* (SN) during aging. Until now, an effective means for the prevention of dopaminergic neurons degeneration and for the retention of damaged neurons functioning is still lacking.

One of the more significant symptoms of PD is movement dysfunction (akinesia, rigidity, and tremor). It is known that motor brain sections are characterized by functional asymmetry which shows up in predomination of motive activity of one of the body sides [5, 6]. Motor asymmetry was described in rats, and that typical asymmetric behavior could change under stress stimulus [7]. It is obvious that such asymmetry might cover brain biochemical processes and neurotransmitters secretion, dopamine (DA) in particular [8, 9]. Meanwhile, DA distribution in different hemispheres of striatum during aging and PD development was not carefully investigated. First attempt to elucidate this problem was made by Belikova and Kolesnikova in 2006 [10] using toxin-induced PD rat model. Afterwards, Budilin et al. [11] have shown that DA concentration in the left nucleus accumbens was significantly higher in "left-handed" rats than in "right-handed" animals. Within the group of "right-handers," the DA concentration was significantly higher in the right nucleus accumbens than in the left one. The results confirm in part the experimental data obtained in mice and support the hypothesis that the paw preference is paralleled by elevated tissue DA in the ipsilateral nucleus accumbens of rodents.

Human investigations have shown similar results. Motor deficit asymmetry in individuals with PD correlates with their *substantia nigra* volumes and is associated with poorer spatial memory [5]. DA deficiency in the right hemisphere corresponded mainly to left-side disturbances of motor function and vice versa [12]. Next step was made to test the hypothesis about possible relations between incentive motivation in healthy volunteers and asymmetry of D_2 receptor distribution in striatum [9]. Greater positive incentive motivation was associated with higher receptor availability in the left relative to the right hemisphere.

Vernaleken et al. [13] reported that the asymmetry in dopamine neurotransmission declines during normal aging. Because ventral striatal dopamine neurotransmission is involved in cognitive processes, this loss of physiological asymmetry in caudate nucleus dopamine transmission during aging might be involved in age-related declines of cognitive performance. No such side lateralization or age effects could be found in other brain structures.

The promising way to slacken the pace of degenerative processes during aging could be the adaptation to intermittent hypoxia. It is well established that such adaptation strengthens DA synthesis and release at peripheral chemoreceptors in carotid bodies (CB) [14, 15], activates tyrosine hydroxilase (TH) – rate-limiting enzyme in catecholamine synthesis [16]. At the same time, episodes of hypoxia/reoxygenation during intermittent hypoxia training (IHT) are accompanied by short-time activation of free radical processes which *ultima analysi* serves to the rise of antioxidant defense [17].

In this chapter, we examined DA distribution in nigrostriatal system and the intensity of free radical processes in Wistar male rat under IHT during aging and experimental DA deficiency. We used model of PD with a specific lesion of nigrostriatal dopaminergic pathway which was based on the ability of neurotoxin 6-hydroxydopamine (6-OHDA) to provoke a PD-like prototypic oxidative stress after its injection into the brain [18].

12.2 Materials and Methods

This work was approved and authorized by the Ethics Committee for Animal Experiments of the Bogomoletz Institute of Physiology. Three groups of male Wistar rats participated in the study. Animals of group I (Gr I) were 6-month-old rats ($n=24$). Group II (Gr II) consisted of 22–24-month-old rats ($n=24$). Animals of group III (Gr III) corresponded 22–24-month-old rats with experimental DA deficiency (EDAD). In the age of 4–6 months, they were subjected to surgical lesion of left striatum ($n=12$). The impairment of the striatum was provided stereotaxically by the injection into the left medial bundle of 8 mg 6-OHDA dissolved in 4 ml of saline with 0.1% ascorbic acid [19]. The tip of glass micropipette with diameter about 100 μm was kept in the brain during 5 min for the limitation of neurotoxin diffusion. To ensure the efficacy of 6-OHDA action, the premedication with pargyline (Sigma) in the dose of 40 mg/kg and desipramine (Sigma) in the dose of 25 mg/kg was provided i.p. 25–30 min before 6-OHDA injection. Pargyline inhibits 6-OHDA metabolism by MAO and desipramine blocks 6-OHDA trapping by noradrenergic neurons.

In a week after 6-OHDA injection the rotation movements of animals under dopaminomimetic apomorphine (0.1% solution, 0.5 mg/kg, i.p.) was investigated to indicate the degree of DA-ergic neurons degeneration. The direction of rotation movements was contralateral relatively to surgically impaired hemisphere. Animals which demonstrated more than six full rotation movements on 360° per 1 min during the first 30 min after apomorphine injection were selected for further investigation. Such test indicates significant degree of DA-ergic neurons degeneration (more than 90%) [19].

One half of every animal group underwent sham hypoxic training (control groups) and another half was subjected to IHT (IHT groups). IHT course was provided in flowing chamber five times per day during 2 weeks. Every session consisted of 15 min breathing with hypoxic mixture (12% O_2) and 15 min room air breathing. Next day, after the course of IHT, animals were decapitated. During decapitation, the blood was collected. After that, the striatum was extracted from two brain sides. DA concentration in striatum tissues was studied by fluorescent method [20].

The intensity of lipid peroxidation and antioxidant defense was estimated by measuring of malondialdehyde (MDA) content [21] and the activity of superoxide dismutase (SOD) and catalase (CAT) [22, 23] in blood serum.

Statistical analysis: Data are presented as means ± SD. Probability values of <0.05 was considered statistically significant.

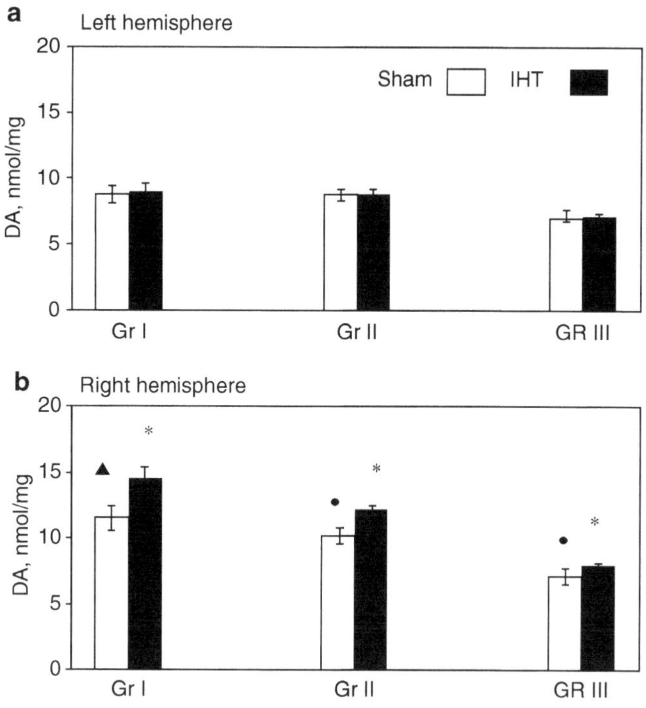

Fig. 12.1 DA distribution in left (**a**) and right (**b**) hemispheres of rat striatum under the adaptation to IHT. *Gr I* – adult (age of 6 months), *Gr II* – old (age of 22–24 months), *Gr III* – experimental DA deficiency (age of 22–24 months). ▲ – $p<0.05$, relatively to left hemisphere; • – $p<0.05$, relatively to Gr.1; * – $p<0.05$ relatively to sham group

12.3 Results and Discussion

12.3.1 DA Distribution in Rat Striatum During Aging

Aging is accompanied by the loss of a part of DA-ergic neuron pool in SN. Every 10-year period of life is accompanied by the loss of about 10% of nigral neurons [24]. Moreover, aging is related to the decrease in TH activity – a rate-limiting enzyme of DA synthesis. It was shown that DA level in one of the areas of the striatum – putamen – began dropping from the first 10-year period of human life and lowered up to nine times from 19 till 72 years [4, 25].

Our study has shown that in adult animals DA level in the striatum of right hemisphere was significantly higher (by 30%, $p<0.05$) than in left one (Fig. 12.1a, b). Results correspond to a notion about functional asymmetry of the brain [5, 6]. During aging, DA production decreased in examined structures mainly in right hemisphere of the striatum, so its distribution asymmetry diminished (Fig. 12.1a, b). In details, no significant differences was found in left hemisphere in Gr II as compared with Gr I, but a decrease by 12% was registered in right hemisphere ($p<0.05$). As a result, in old rats, DA level in right hemisphere of the striatum differed from left side only by 16.6% in comparison with 30% in adult animals ($p<0.05$). This fact demonstrates a decrease in the asymmetry of DA distribution between striatum hemispheres in old animals.

12.3.2 Experimental DA Deficiency

As it was mentioned above, we used a model of PD, which was based on 6-OHDA injection directly into the brain.

6-OHDA shares some structural similarities with DA and norepinephrine (NE), exhibiting a high affinity for several catecholaminergic plasma membrane transporters such as the DA (DAT) and NE (NET) transporters [18, 26]. 6-OHDA destroys catecholaminergic structures by a combined effect of reactive oxygen species (ROS) and quinones, products of this toxin oxidation. 6-OHDA poorly crosses the blood–brain barrier, so to circumvent this problem, 6-OHDA has to be injected directly into the brain. Much more popular and practical model of 6-OHDA is the unilateral intracerebral injection. Maximal reduction of striatal DA level is reached within 3–4 days after lesion, and residual DA content is less than 20% of control [18]. When injected into striatum, 6-OHDA produced more protracted retrograde degeneration of the nigrostriatal system which can last from 1 to 3 week after lesion, and the dying neurons exhibit a varied morphology including some features reminiscent apoptosis. It was shown that 6-OHDA neurotoxicity provoked molecular alteration comparable to those seen in PD [28], thus supporting the meaningfulness of this model to explore the mechanisms of neurodegeneration in PD.

In our own study animals of Gr III with EDAD, it was characterized by the drop of DA level in the striatum relatively to the old control rats and the primary decrease was observed in right hemisphere (by 30% compared to Gr II, Fig. 12.1b). Such drop led to practically total abolishment of quantitative difference between right and left hemispheres. For the assessment of these results, it is necessary to emphasize that EDAD animals had destroyed DA-ergic structures only in left hemisphere. In right hemisphere where the difference between control and EDAD animals was more profound, 6-OHDA was not injected.

Probably, existent cross-communications between right and left hemispheres mediate the decreased DA production in intact structures due to some regulatory mechanisms inflicted by 6-OHDA injection. Such speculative mechanisms inhibiting DA synthesis in the brain of old animals could be due to glutamate-, serotonin-, GABA- and P-ergic systems [27, 28].

It is well known that DA-ergic nigrostriatal system decelerates the activity of cholinergic and glutamatergic systems. In turn, neurons producing acetylcholine, serotonin, GABA, and glutamate inhibit DA release from appropriate neural cells [27, 28]. On the other hand, P-ergic neurons stimulate DA synthesis and release in the striatum. Thus, DA-ergic system functions according to the principle of negative feedback with aforesaid systems and positive feedback with P-ergic system.

Obviously, one-side destruction of DA-ergic brain structures can activate systems that are antagonistic to destroyed neurons [28]. Apparently, the effect of inhibitory mediators manifested preferentially in such hemisphere where nonlesioned target cells persisted after 6-OHDA injection. As a result, DA production and release are depressed in intact hemisphere. As mentioned above, the neurons of P-ergic system and DA-ergic structures collaborate on reciprocal principle. When DA-ergic structures diminish their activating influences on P-ergic neurons, the release of substantial P gradually fades, which in turn abolishes stimulating effect of DA synthesis and release. Thus, in spite of the destruction of DA-synthesized neurons in left hemisphere after toxin injection, relatively more expressed drop of DA content was manifested in right hemisphere.

12.3.3 Adaptation to IHT

Two-week course of IHT practically did not affect DA content in left striatum of all animal groups (Fig. 12.1a). At the same time, significant changes in DA level in right striatum was found (Fig. 12.1b). IHT–group of adult rats (Gr. 1-B) demonstrated significantly heightened DA concentration in right hemisphere by 28% ($p<0.05$) as compared with control (Gr. 1-A). In old rats (Gr. 2-B) DA level increased under IHT by 21% ($p<0.05$) as compared with the control Gr. 2-A but did not restore completely the asymmetry of DA distribution between brain hemispheres. The raise of DA level in right striatum hemisphere of EDAD rats (Gr. 3-B) was modest but statistically significant (by 9.1% as compared with control Gr. 3-A, $p<0.05$).

Mechanism of the above-mentioned shifts in DA distribution in the striatum during adaptation to IHT is rather complicated. It is necessary to take into account that EDAD is a model of hemiparkinsonism when DA neurons are destroyed in strictly certain brain structure that is accompanied by neuronal death and DA deficiency development.

Positive effect of IHT adaptation on DA metabolism could include several molecular and cellular pathways. First of all, IHT influence is probably conditioned by the activation of catecholamine metabolism related to the sensitization of O_2-dependent rate-limiting enzyme, TH. As far as neurons of SN have an embryological affinity with CB chemoreceptor cells (neural crest-derived cells) and similarity in DA synthesis, it is possible to assume that in both structures the adaptive processes during IHT could be similar. So, ROS in SN during IHT may potentiate a periodical cell membrane depolarization, augmentation of cytosolic [Ca^{2+}], activation of cyclic nucleotides in neurons, and the expression of HIF-2α and HIF-3α. This probably can determine an increase in TH gene expression [29–32] and TH promotion at DA synthesis/release in correspondent sites at the striatum.

In the Haavik and Toska's opinion [33], Parkinson's disease can be considered as a TH-deficiency syndrome of the striatum. Similarly, some patients with hereditary L-DOPA-responsive dystonia (neurological disorder with clinical similarities to PD) have mutations in the TH gene and decreased TH activity and/or stability. At the same time, in spite of the decreased TH activity during aging [34] and limited ability to its raise as against young animals [35], our results testify to the presence of certain resource for TH activation in old and EDAD animals.

It is well known that hypoxia is able to change the function of chemosensitive cells. Hence, the cultivation of CB chemoreceptor cells in the medium with lowered PO_2 during 8–10 days showed sixfold increase in DA release from the cells comparing to normoxia [15] that was related to raised spike activity and heightened Ca^{2+} influx facilitating DA release.

Another hypothetical and very attractive mechanism could be related to appearance of new DA-ergic neurons from a certain precursor. Evidently, to initiate this process, it is necessary to have such total toxic damage of nigrostriatum structures as in our PD model. This mechanism was described for CB of adult animals subjected to long-term hypoxic exposure. During hypoxic exposure, the appearance of new neuron-like glomus cells which derived from progenitors (subpopulation of $GFAP^+$ type II cells) was noted [36]. It was identified CB stem cells of glial lineage which can differentiate into functionally normal DA-ergic glomus cells. In fact, this is the first example of neural-crest-derived stem cells with a recognized physiological function identified in adult peripheral nervous system. In our case, such speculation assumes to provide the further detailed morphological research of nigrostriatum.

At the same time, it is necessary to recognize that in the present study, the amount of cells in left hemisphere striatum of EDAD animals which can respond to hypoxic influence was dramatically limited. Obviously, this cause could determine more expressed IHT effect on neurons of right striatum where DA-ergic neurons were not subjected to prior destruction.

Therefore, we conclude that stable increase of nigrostriatum DA level in all groups of the examined animals suggest about real positive IHT effect on DA-ergic neuron pool.

12.3.4 Lipid Peroxidation and Antioxidant Enzymes Activity Under IHT

The level of oxidative stress depends on the intensity of ROS production and the activity of antioxidant system. Aging is accompanied by MDA accumulation and definite changes in antioxidant enzymes activity [37–41]. In our study, old animals had heightened MDA level in blood plasma by 13% ($p<0.05$) relatively to adult rats (Fig. 12.2a). Simultaneously, plasma SOD activity was reduced by 69% ($p<0.05$), and CAT activity was significantly decreased by 28% ($p<0.05$) as compared with adult animals (Fig. 12.2b, c). These results correspond to data of other authors [37–41].

DA-ergic nature of neurons in SN per se promotes high intensity of free radical processes; moreover, the extent of cell surviving is determined by the intensity of DA

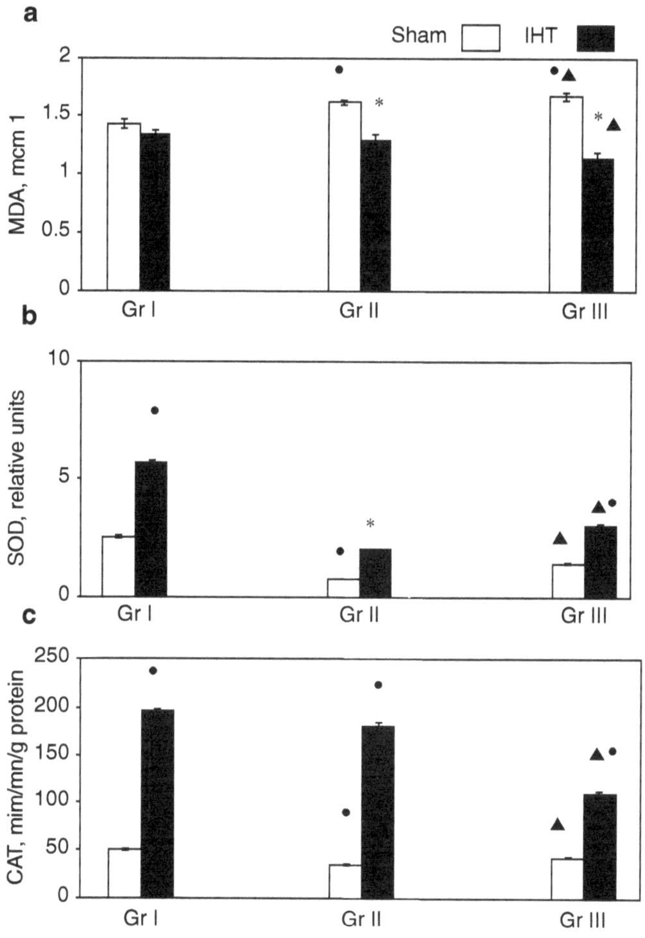

Fig. 12.2 Lipid peroxidation (**a**) and the activities of antioxidant enzymes (**b**, **c**) in rat blood serum under the adaptation to IHT. *Gr I* – adult (age of 6 months), *Gr II* – old (age of 22–24 months), *Gr III* – experimental DA deficiency (age of 22–24 months). (**a**) MDA, (**b**) SOD, (**c**) CAT. • – $p<0.05$, relatively to Gr.1; ▲ – $p<0.05$, relatively to Gr II; * – $p<0.05$ relatively to sham group

metabolism [42]. Toxic products of DA autooxidation – semiquinones – can be polymerized in neuromelatonine. DA oxidation by the MAO-B leads to the formation of H_2O_2 which in normal conditions is inactivated by glutathione/glutathione peroxidase system [42–44].

Thus, shifts in antioxidant enzymes activity are closely related to the disturbances in DA metabolism. This phenomenon is clearly evident in PD patients. It was proved that the neurodegeneration in SN was related to such neurochemical events as increased lipid peroxidation intensity [45–47] and higher activity of antioxidant enzymes [48–50]. For example, it was demonstrated that toxic injury of the striatum in mice was accompanied by three- to fivefold increase in ROS production [51]. Positive correlation between increased MDA accumulation and the severity of PD [45–47] or the degree of striatum damage under toxin injection [52] was also described.

In our study, EDAD animals were characterized by heightened MDA concentration relatively to young ($p<0.01$) and old ($p<0.05$) rats. CAT and SOD activity was also increased as compared with old animals (Fig. 12.2a). These data are compatible with the results of Serra et al. [47].

IHT induced significant decrease in MDA content in old and especially EDAD animals by 32%, ($p<0.05$; Fig. 12.2a). Simultaneously, considerable increase in SOD and CAT activity was registered in all groups (Fig. 12.2b, c). Results were similar to our investigation of PD patients under hypoxic training [37]. Other authors also showed that IHT prevented the activation of free radical oxidation during inflammation and stress [53–55].

Thus, numerous episodes of hypoxia and following reoxygenation which provoke lipid peroxidation are effectively compensated by the rise of antioxidant enzymes activity. Besides, strengthening of the resistance to lipid peroxidation induction can be stipulated by lowered content of fatty acids in cell membranes under IHT [54]. Our results suggest about essential rise in enzymes activity as first line of antioxidant defense in adult, aged, and EDAD animals after the course of IHT.

Investigation of correlations between antioxidant activity and brain dopamine content in all groups of experimental animals revealed a number of statistically meaningful relations between them. DA content in left hemisphere was positively correlated with plasma SOD activity ($r=0.69, p<0.05$). This correlation increased after IHT course ($r=0.74$, $p<0.01$). More significant relations were detected between DA content in right hemisphere and plasma SOD activity: in normoxic group, $r=0.92$ ($p<0.01$); in IHT group, $r=0.80$ ($p<0.01$). Similar relations between CAT activity and DA content were also found: in left hemisphere of control group $r=0.66$ ($p<0.05$), IHT group $r=0.67$ ($p<0.05$); in right hemisphere of control group $r=0.73$ ($p<0.05$), IHT group $r=0.80$ ($p<0.01$).

Thus, the increase in plasma antioxidant activity corresponds to increased DA concentration in the striatum. Present data confirm the significance of antioxidant enzymes in maintenance and renewal of DA synthesis in SN [56, 57].

Conclusion and Perspectives

Our results demonstrate that adaptation to IHT promotes positive influence on DA-ergic neurons in SN and the activity of antioxidant enzymes in adult and old animals as well as in rats with experimental dopamine deficiency. Evidently, major factor caused the increase in DA level could be the activation of DA synthesis enzymes (TH, DOPA decarboxylase) through their gene expression. Besides, the activation of energy metabolism during hypoxic adaptation could promote DA uptake, lower DA autooxidation and prevent further neuron lesion by toxic agents. It was shown that there exists the asymmetry of dopamine distribution between right and left striatum of adult rats. Prevalent quantity of dopamine is concentrated in right hemisphere. Dopamine production in the striatum decreases during aging; at the same time, its distribution asymmetry diminishes. Intermittent hypoxia training increases dopamine synthesis, especially in the right striatum; leads to a decrease in the intensity of lipid peroxidation; and activates antioxidant systems. Increased plasma antioxidant activity positively correlates with increased DA concentration in the striatum. It confirms the hypothesis that the most reliable mechanism causing the apoptosis in dopaminergic structures of the brain during aging and Parkinson's disease is the activation of oxidative stress. Intermittent hypoxia training could serve as good perspective means for the deceleration of aging and prevention/treatment of Parkinson's disease.

References

1. Wei YH, Ma YS, Lee HC, et al. Mitochondrial theory of aging matures-roles of mtDNA mutation and oxidative stress in human aging. Zhonghua Yi Xue Za Zhi (Taipei). 2001;64:259–70.
2. Lee HC, Wei YH. Oxidative stress, mitochondrial DNA mutation, and apoptosis in aging. Exp Biol Med. 2007;232:592–606.
3. Orr WC, Sohal RS. Effects of Cu, Zn superoxide dismutase overexpression on life span and resistance to oxidative stress in transgenic drosophila melanogaster. Arch Biochem Biophys. 1993;301:34–40.
4. Kish SJ, Shannak K, Rajput A, et al. Aging produces a specific pattern of striatal dopamine loss: implications for the etiology of idiopathic Parkinson's disease. J Neurochem. 1992;58:642–8.
5. Foster ER, Black KJ, Antenor-Dorsey JA, et al. Motor asymmetry and substantia nigra volume are related to spatial delayed response performance in Parkinson disease. Brain Cogn. 2008;67:1–10.
6. Hershey T, Wu J, Weaver PM. Unilateral vs. bilateral STN DBS effects on working memory and motor function in Parkinson disease. Exp Neurol. 2008;210:402–8.
7. Chuyan EN. Changes in motor asymmetry of low-intensive high-frequency electromagnetic radiation in normal conditions and under stress. Neurophysiology. 2005;37:164–8 [In Russian].
8. Carlson JN, Stewens KD. Individual differences in ethanol self-administration following withdrawal are associated with asymmetric changes in dopamine and serotonin in the medial prefrontal cortex and amygdale. Alcohol Clin Exp Res. 2006;30:1678–92.
9. Tomer R, Goldshtein RZ, Wang GJ, et al. Incentive motivation is associated with striatal dopamine asymmetry. Biol Psychol. 2008;77:98–101.
10. Belikova MV, Kolesnikova EE. Changes in rat striatum dopamine content under aging and dopamine insufficiency. Probl Aging Longevity. 2006;15:187–91 [In Russian].
11. Budilin S, Midzianovskaia IS, Shchegolevskii NV, et al. Asymmetry in the dopamine content in the nucleus accumbens and the motor preference in rats. Zh Vyssh Nerv Deiat Im I P Pavlova. 2007;57: 598–603 [In Russian].
12. Tomer R, Aharon-Peretz J, Tsitrinbaum Z. Dopamine asymmetry interacts with medication to affect cognition in Parkinson's disease. Neuropsychologia. 2007;45:357–67.
13. Vernaleken I, Weibrich C, Siessmeier T, et al. Asymmetry in dopamine D (2/3) receptors of caudate nucleus is lost with age. Neuroimage. 2007;34:870–8.
14. Bee D, Pallot DJ. Acute hypoxic ventilation, carotid body cell division and dopamine content during early hypoxia in rats. J Appl Physiol. 1995;79:1504–11.
15. Nurse CA, Jackson A, Makintaire F, et al. Adaptation of O_2 chemoreceptors to hypoxia in vitro. In: Women at altitude. Burlingron: Queen City Printers Inc.; 1997. p. 147–53.

16. Vrecko K, Storga D, Bikmayer JG, et al. NADH stimulates endogenous dopamine biosynthesis by enhancing the recycling of tetrahydrobiopterin in rat phaeochromocytoma cells. Biochem Biophys Acta. 1997;1361:59–65.
17. Serebrovskaya TV. Intermittent hypoxia research in the former Soviet Union and the commonwealth of the independent states (CIS): history and review of the concept and selective application. High Alt Med Biol. 2002;3:205–21.
18. Bove J, Prou D, Perier C, et al. Toxin-induced models of Parkinson's disease. NeuroRx. 2005;2:484–94.
19. Oleshko NN. Morphofunctional study of interaction of glutamate-, choline- and dopamine-ergic systems in neostriatum. Ross Fiziol Zh Im I M Sechenova. 1997;1–2:96–101 [In Russian].
20. Jacobowith PM, Richardson JS. Method for the rapid determination of norepinephrine, dopamine, serotonin in the same brain region. Pharmacol Biochem Behav. 1979;8:515–9.
21. Stal'naya ID, Garishvili TG. Method malondialdehyde evaluation with help of tiobarbituric acid. In: Orekhovich VN, editor. Modern methods in biochemistry. Moscow: Medicine; 1977. p. 66–7 [In Russian].
22. Chevari S, Chaba I, Sekei Y. The role of super oxide dismutase in oxidative processes in the cella and the method of its estimation in biological materials. Lab Delo. 1985;11:678–81. [In Russian].
23. Korolyuk MA, Ivanova AI, Majorova IT, et al. Method of catalase activity examination. Lab Delo. 1988;1:16–9 [In Russian].
24. Calne DB, Reppard RF. Aging of nigrostriatal pathway in human. Can J Neurol Sci. 1987;14:424–7.
25. Hornykiewicz O. Neurochimical patology and the ethiology of Parkinson's disease: basic facts and hipotetical possibilities. Mt Sinai J Med. 1988;5:11–20.
26. Betarbet R, Sherer TB, Greenmyre JT. Animal models of Parkinson's disease. Bioessays. 2002;24:308–18.
27. Kryzhanovski GN. Determinant structures in nervous system pathology. In: Generator mechanisms of neuropathological syndromes. Moscow; 1980. p. 360 [In Russian].
28. Kryzhanovski GN. General pathology of nervous system. Moscow; 1997, p. 352. [In Russian].
29. Chen J, Dinger B, Fidone SJ. Second messenger regulation of tyrosine hydroxilase gene expression in rat carotid body. Biol Signals. 1995;4:277–85.
30. Millhorn DE, Conforti L, Beitner-Johnson D, et al. Regulation of ionic conductances and gene expression by hypoxia in an oxygen sensitive cell line. Adv Exp Med Biol. 1996;410:135–42.
31. Raymond R, Millhorn DE. Regulation of tyrosine hydroxylase gene expression during hypoxia: role of Ca^{2+} and PKC. Kidney Int. 1997;51:536–41.
32. Lam SY, Tipoe GL, Long EC, et al. Differential expressions and roles of hypoxia-inducible factor-1alpha, -2alpha and -3alpha in the rat carotid body during chronic and intermittent hypoxia. Histol Histopathol. 2008;23:271–80.
33. Haavik J, Toska K. Tyrosine hydroxilase and Parkinson's disease. Mol Neurobiol. 1998;16:285–309.
34. Ponzio F, Brunello N, Algeri S. Catecholamine synthesis in brain of aging rat. J Neurochem. 1978;30:1617–20.
35. Tumer N, Larochelle JS. Tyrosine hydroxylase expression in rat adrenal medulla: influence of age and cold. Pharmacol Biochem Behav. 1995;51:775–80.
36. Lopez-Barneo J, Ortega-Saenz P, Pardal R, et al. Oxygen sensing in the carotid body. Ann N Y Acad Sci. 2009;1177:119–31.
37. Kolesnikova EE, Safronova OS, Serebrovskaya TV. Age-related peculiarities of breathing regulation and antioxidant enzymes under intermittent hypoxic training. J Physiol Pharmacol. 2003;54:20–4.
38. Rizvi SI, Maurya PK. Alterations in antioxidant enzymes during aging in humans. Mol Biotechnol. 2007;37:58–61.
39. Gomes P, Simão S, Silva E, et al. Aging increases oxidative stress and renal expression of oxidant and antioxidant enzymes that are associated with an increased trend in systolic blood pressure. Oxid Med Cell Longev. 2009;2:138–45.
40. Carvalho C, Santos MS, Baldeiras I, et al. Chronic hypoxia potentiates age-related oxidative imbalance in brain vessels and synaptosomes. Curr Neurovasc Res. 2010;7:288–300.
41. Gautam N, Das S, Mahapatra SK, et al. Age associated oxidative damage in lymphocytes. Oxid Med Cell Longev. 2010;3:275–82.
42. Mann DMA, Yates PO. Possible role of neuromelanin in the pathogenesis of Parkinson's disease. Mech Ageing Dev. 1983;21:193–203.
43. Chiueh CC, Krishna G, Tulsi P, et al. Intracranial microdialysis of salicylic acid to detect hydroxyl radical generation through dopamine autooxidation in the caudate nucleus: effect of MPP^+. Free Radic Biol Med. 1992;13:581–3.
44. Boldyrev AA. Dual role of free radical oxygen forms in ischemic brain. Neirochimiya. 1995;12:3–13 [In Russian].
45. Dexter DT, Holley AE, Flitter WD, et al. Parkinson's disease increased levels of hydroxyperoxides in the Parkinsonian substantia nigra: an HPLC and ESR study. Mov Disord. 1994;9:92–7.
46. Yoritaka A, Hattori N, Uchida K, et al. Immunohistochemucal detection of 4-hydroxynonenal protein adducts in Parkinson's disease. Proc Natl Acad Sci USA. 1996;93:2696–701.
47. Serra JA, Domínguez RO, de Lustig ES, et al. Parkinson's disease is associated with oxidative stress: comparison of peripheral antioxidant profiles in living Parkinson's, Alzheimer's and vascular dementia patients. J Neural Transm. 2001;108:1135–48.
48. Jenner P, Olanow CW. Oxidative stress and the pathogenesis of Parkinson disease. Neurology. 1996;47:S161–70.
49. Martilla RG, Lorentz H, Rinne UK. Oxygen toxicity, protecting enzymes in Parkinson's disease: increase of superoxide dismutase-like activity in the substantia nigra and basal nucleus. J Neurol Sci. 1988;86:321–31.
50. Yoritaka A, Hattori N, Mori H, et al. An immunohostochemical study on manganese superoxide dismutase in Parkinson's disease. J Neurol Sci. 1997;148:181–6.
51. Smith TS, Bennet Jr JP. Mitochondrial toxins in models of neurodegenerative diseases. I. In vivo brain hydroxyl radical production during systemic MPTP treatment or following microialysis infusion of methylpyridinum or azide ions. Brain Res. 1997;765:183–8.
52. Yu YP, Ju WP, Li ZG, et al. Acupuncture inhibits oxidative stress and rotational behavior in 6-hydroxydopamine lesioned rat. Brain Res. 2010;1336:58–65.
53. Gardner HW. Oxygen radical chemistry of polyunsaturated fatty acids. Free Radic Biol Med. 1989;7:65–86.
54. Piretti MV, Pagliuca G. Systematic isolation and identification of membrane lipid oxidation products. Free Radic Biol Med. 1989;7:219–21.
55. Davies KJA. Proteolytic systems as secondary antioxidant defenses. In: Chow CK, editor. Cellular antioxidant defense mechanisms. Boca Raton: CRC; 1988. p. 25–67.
56. Lindgren P, von Campenhausen S, Spottke E, et al. Cost of Parkinson's disease in Europe. Eur J Neurol. 2005;12:68–73.
57. Koutsilieri E, Scheller S, Grunblatt E, et al. Free radicals in Parkinson's disease. J Neurol. 2002;2:II1–5.

Protective Effects of Adaptation to Hypoxia in Experimental Alzheimer's Disease

13

Eugenia B. Manukhina, Anna V. Goryacheva, Maya G. Pshennikova, Igor Yu. Malyshev, Robert T. Mallet, and H. Fred Downey

Abstract

Alzheimer's disease (AD) is characterized by formation of amyloid plaques, intracellular neurofibrillary tangles, and cell death in the brain, resulting in progressive loss of memory and cognitive ability. Efficacy of drugs currently used for prevention and treatment of AD is limited by the fact that each drug influences only a single step of the pathogenesis in AD, and the drugs affect both damaged and normal cells. This is why major attention is now paid to nonpharmacological means that may enhance the adaptive capacity and mobilize the self-defense systems of the body. This chapter focuses on protective effects of adaptation to intermittent hypobaric hypoxia on the memory, brain neurons, and cerebral blood vessels in rats with experimental AD induced by intracerebral injections of beta-amyloid (Aβ) and mechanisms of these protective effects. Special attention is paid to intermittent hypobaric hypoxia's ability to limit early stages in AD pathogenesis, such as nitrosative and oxidative stress in brain tissue. Presented data show that adaptation to hypoxia may be a promising approach to prevention and treatment of AD.

E.B. Manukhina (✉)
Laboratory for Regulatory Mechanisms of Adaptation, Institute of General Pathology and Pathophysiology, Moscow, Russia
e-mail: eugenia.manukhina@unthsc.edu

Department of Integrative Physiology, University of North Texas Health Science Center, Fort Worth, TX, USA

A.V. Goryacheva • M.G. Pshennikova
Laboratory for Regulatory Mechanisms of Adaptation, Institute of General Pathology and Pathophysiology, Moscow, Russia

I.Yu. Malyshev
Laboratory of Stress and Adaptation, Institute of General Pathology and Pathophysiology, Moscow, Russia

Department of Pathophysiology, Moscow State University of Medicine and Dentistry, Moscow, Russia

R.T. Mallet • H.F. Downey
Department of Integrative Physiology, University of North Texas Health Science Center, Fort Worth, TX, USA

Abbreviations

3-NT	3-Nitrotyrosine
Ach	Acetylcholine
AChE	Acetylcholine esterase
AD	Alzheimer's disease
Aβ	β-Amyloid
AMPA	α-Amino-3-hydroxy-5-methyl-4-isoxazolepropionic acid
DNIC	Dinitrosyl iron complex
HIF-1	Hypoxia-inducible factor-1
HRE	Hypoxic response element
HSP	Heat shock protein
LCBF	Local cerebral blood flow
IL	Interleukin
LTP	Long-term potentiation
MPTP	Mitochondrial permeability transition pore
NAC	*N*-Acetylcysteine
NMDA	*N*-Methyl D-aspartate

L. Xi, T.V. Serebrovskaya (eds.), *Intermittent Hypoxia and Human Diseases*,
DOI 10.1007/978-1-4471-2906-6_13, © Springer-Verlag London 2012

L-NNA	N^{ω}-Nitro-*L*-arginine
NO	Nitric oxide
NOS	NO synthase
eNOS	Endothelial NO synthase
iNOS	Inducible NO synthase
nNOS	Neuronal NO synthase
PKC	Protein kinase C
ROS	Reactive oxygen species
TBARS	Thiobarbituric acid-reactive substances
TNFα	Tumor necrosis factor α
VEGF	Vascular endothelial growth factor

13.1 Introduction

Alzheimer's disease (AD) is the most common neurodegenerative disease characterized by death of neurons in the cerebral cortex. AD leads to progressive memory loss and other cognitive disorders, which inevitably progress to total dependence on caregiver care and eventual death. This disease afflicts 5–10% of people older than 65 years [1]. The incidence of AD almost doubles every 5 years for people between 65 and 80 years old [2]. About 25 million people worldwide suffered from AD in 2000, and their number is expected to increase to 114 million by 2050 [3]. Autopsy findings have indicated that the most severe pathology in AD occurs in the hippocampus, temporal cortex, and the basal nucleus [4]. The hippocampus of patients with AD is smaller than in age-matched controls [4].

Histological hallmarks of AD include formation of neurofibrillary tangles and toxic senile plaques in hippocampus and brain cortex. The neurofibrillary tangles are formed inside neurons and consist of hyperphosphorylated tau proteins. The senile plaques are generated by an extra- and intracellular deposition of the β-amyloid peptide (Aβ), a self-aggregating peptide produced by cleavage of a transmembrane glycoprotein, amyloid precursor protein. Aggregated Aβ triggers many neurotoxic mechanisms including oxidative and nitrosative stress, excitotoxicity with Ca^{2+} dysregulation, energy depletion, inflammation, and apoptosis [5].

13.2 Pathogenetic Processes in AD

Excitotoxicity is mediated by excessive activation of the glutamatergic pathway (Fig. 13.1). Glutamate, the major excitatory neurotransmitter in the cerebral cortex, binds to *N*-methyl D-aspartate (NMDA) and α-amino-3-hydroxy-5-methyl-4-isoxazolepropionic acid (AMPA)/kainate receptors. Activation of these receptors induces excessive Ca^{2+} influx. The resulting increase in intraneuronal Ca^{2+} concentration mobilizes a variety of neurotoxic compounds that compromise neuronal viability [6]. Amyloid proteins can directly induce Ca^{2+} influx into neurons, and this Ca^{2+} influx may alter neuronal excitability [7]. In addition, mitochondria take up excessive Ca^{2+} which results in the opening of the mitochondrial permeability transition pore (MPTP), collapse of the mitochondrial membrane potential, generation of reactive oxygen species (ROS), and proapoptotic events [8].

β-Amyloid directly interacts with mitochondria. Aβ traverses both the cell membrane and the mitochondrial membrane and binds to proteins and other molecules. The Aβ targets include β-amyloid binding alcohol dehydrogenase, which functions to detoxify dialdehydes and prevent oxidative stress [9, 10]. It has also been suggested that β-amyloid interacts with protein components of the MPTP, thereby provoking pore opening [11]. Detrimental effects of Aβ in mitochondria also include modification of the membranes, impairment of mitochondrial respiration, activation of free-radical generation, and induction of apoptosis [9].

An important detrimental effect of β-amyloid is inhibition of mitochondrial respiration [12]. By interacting with the α-subunit of ATP synthase [13], Aβ impedes neuronal ATP synthesis [14]. β-amyloid inactivates cytochrome *c* oxidase [15] and conversely increases the activity of respiratory complex III, the cytochrome *c* reductase [16]. These effects combine to inhibit mitochondrial respiration and deplete ATP.

Accumulation of oxidative damage plays a pivotal role in AD pathogenesis [17]. Clinical studies have revealed higher than normal intensity of protein and DNA oxidation in AD patients, which indicates the presence of oxidative stress [18]. Levels of lipid peroxidation measured as thiobarbituric acid-reactive substances were also increased in various brain regions of AD patients [19, 20]. Aβ deposits are considered a major source of reactive oxygen species. Another important source of ROS is activated microglia [21]. Activation of microglia develops early in AD and has been observed in patients with both acute and chronic AD [22]. Aβ-activated microglia, astrocytes, and neurons produce numerous immunoproteins and cytokines in the AD brain. It has been hypothesized that these proteins are responsible for the ongoing chronic inflammation process in the AD brain [21, 23].

Nitric oxide (NO) is involved in both the progression and prevention of AD because NO can both induce and inhibit neuronal death [24]. Normally, NO is produced in brain by neuronal NO synthase (nNOS) in neurons and endothelial NOS (eNOS) of cerebral blood vessels. In AD, NO is overproduced mostly in microglia and astrocytes by inducible NOS (iNOS). Ishii et al. [25] showed that Aβ directly and dose-dependently stimulated NO production by iNOS both in vivo and in vitro. Increased NO production via iNOS has been implicated in impairment of learning behavior and

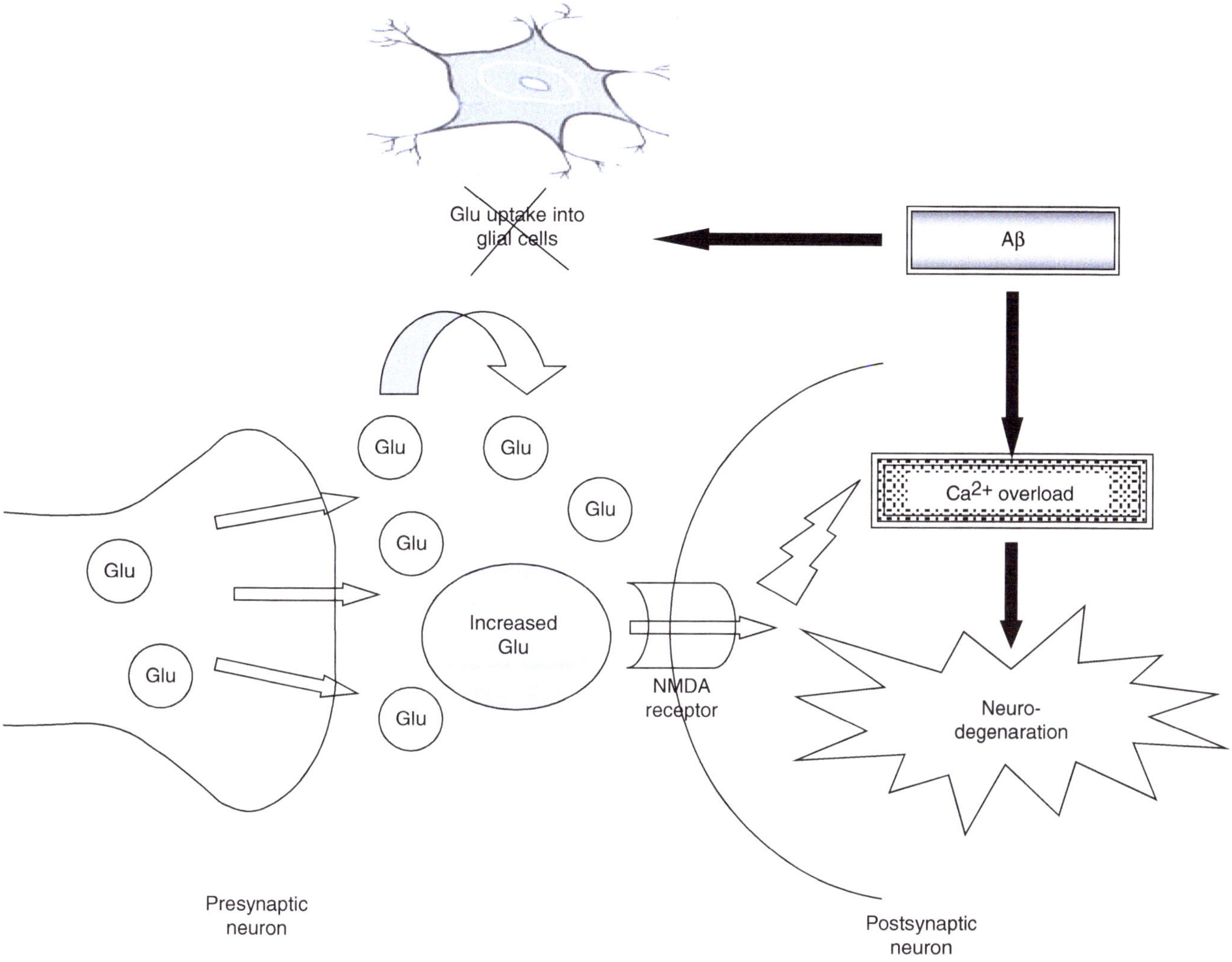

Fig. 13.1 β-Amyoloid (Aβ)-induced excitotoxicity in neurons. *L*-glutamate (*Glu*) binds to NMDA receptors to induce excitation of neurons. Glu uptake into adjacent glial cells terminates the excitation. Aβ inhibits the Glu uptake by glial cells and, thus, increases activation of NMDA receptors. Failure to terminate the NMDA receptor-induced excitation results in neuronal Ca^{2+} overload and neurodegeneration

hippocampal long-term potentiation. Aminoguanidine, a specific iNOS inhibitor, prevented these disorders [26]. Direct neurotoxic effects of excessive NO are mediated by mitochondrial dysfunction and ATP depletion, which lead to the collapse of mitochondrial membrane potential and the release of mitochondrial proteins. These proteins, including cytochrome *c* and Smac [27], in turn, activate the caspase cascade causing apoptotic death of neurons [28].

Nitric oxide condenses with superoxide to form toxic peroxynitrite, a strong oxidant that damages lipids, DNA, carbohydrates, and proteins. Both peroxynitrite decomposition and NO oxidation produce nitrite which is subsequently oxidized to nitrogen dioxide (NO_2) by reactions catalyzed by peroxidases [29, 30]. As potent nitrating species [31], NO_2 readily nitrates tyrosine to form 3-nitrotyrosine (3-NT) [32]. Tyrosine nitration affects many important enzymes and structural proteins, including manganese superoxide dismutase, neurofilament L, actin, and tyrosine hydroxylase [33]. This pathological nitration process is associated with development and progression of several neurodegenerative diseases, including AD, and 3-NT is found in large amounts in affected regions of the brains of patients with AD [34–36]. The nitrative damage occurs early in the progression of AD and may be important for transition from mild cognitive impairment to the severe impairment characteristic of AD [36].

Hence, NO is implicated in AD-related neurodegeneration. At the same time, release of NO from cerebral endothelial cells plays a key role in vascular tone, blood pressure regulation, and vascular homeostasis. NO also acts to inhibit platelet and leukocyte adhesion to the endothelium, a process that may suppress proinflammatory events [37, 38]. Chronic nNOS inhibition may exacerbate inflammatory neurodegeneration [39]. Low concentrations of NO prevent opening of MPTP through the cGMP-PKG pathway and thereby inhibit apoptosis in astrocytes [40, 41]. Another NO-mediated antiapoptotic mechanism is *S*-nitrosylation of caspase-3 [42].

Development of AD is associated with endothelial dysfunction of cerebral blood vessels. Aβ directly induces endothelial dysfunction [43]. In addition, structural microvessel pathology, which is frequently observed in AD [44], results in endothelial dysfunction and dysregulation of NO, primarily in the hippocampus and entorhinal cortex. Constitutively reduced cerebrovascular NO production leads to cerebral hypoperfusion due to impaired vasodilation responses and diminished capacity to remove respiratory waste products and toxins from the extracellular space due to reduced capillary permeability [45]. A study in elderly individuals with mild memory deficits [46], but who had not yet developed AD, showed that AD developed within 2 years only in subjects with significant hypoperfusion of the amygdaloid-hippocampal region. All these vascular effects result in depression of cerebral glucose and oxygen metabolism and correlate with severity of AD [47–49]. Moreover, these metabolic disturbances were shown to precede neurodegeneration in AD [50], and recent data suggest that cerebrovascular disease plays an important role in the pathophysiology of AD [51]. Studies have also shown that optimal use of antihypertensive therapy is associated with a reduction in the incidence of cognitive impairment [52, 53]. A prospective observational study showed that treatment of vascular risk factors in individuals with AD slowed cognitive decline [54]. Collectively, these data prompted de la Torre and Stefano [49] to designate AD as "a vascular disorder with neurodegenerative consequences."

13.3 Pharmacotherapy for AD

Several classes of drugs have been developed and used for therapy of AD, including acetylcholine (ACh) esterase (AChE) inhibitors, drugs influencing NMDA and glutamate receptors, and drugs affecting synthesis of Aβ and formation of neurofibrillary tangles. AChE inhibitors were the first medication developed and approved for the treatment of AD [1]. Since studies showed shortage of ACh in brains of AD patients [55], inhibitors of AChE, the enzyme that degrades ACh, have become a popular medication to combat AD. Later, the NMDA receptor antagonist memantine was approved and introduced to clinical practice [56]. Memantine improves the cognitive function due to prevention of excitotoxicity mediated by overproduction of glutamate [57, 58]. Authors of the Cochrane review evaluating memantine [59] concluded that "memantine has a small beneficial effect at 6 months in moderate to severe AD." At present, AChE inhibitors and/or memantine are considered standard treatments for AD [60, 61].

Development of new therapies for AD is a serious challenge because such drugs must be able to cross the blood–brain barrier to ensure sufficient availability in the brain. All currently available drugs for treatment of AD are symptomatic and they generally have rather modest potential for treatment and prevention of this disease. Some authors concluded that the magnitude of this benefit, though statistically significant, is marginal at best and may even be difficult to detect, measure, and quantify clinically [62, 63]. Other limitations include poor oral bioavailability and common, dose-dependent side effects, such as nausea, diarrhea, and hepatotoxicity [64]. The slowing of cognitive decline by drug therapy is mainly symptomatic and provides only moderate savings of about €1,500 per patient [65]. In addition, development and use of drugs that aim to slow the cognitive decline in patients with AD raise many ethical questions, such as the impact of these drugs for the overall well-being and quality of life of patients [66].

Most pharmacological approaches for AD have been based on simple "compensatory" or "inhibitory" principles. However, many pathogenic mechanisms of this disease have a "dual" nature, i.e., some of them can paradoxically activate neuronal defense. For example, elevated production of neurotoxic Aβ is considered a major event in the development of AD [67]. Under certain conditions, however, Aβ can chelate copper ions and thereby restrict their prooxidant effect on brain neurons [68]. It is well known that the increased production of proinflammatory cytokines (IL-1, IL-6) and tumor necrosis factor α (TNFα) results in neuroinflammation, NO overproduction, and apoptosis in AD. However, the same cytokines activate phagocytosis of Aβ to restrict its proinflammatory and other neurotoxic effects [69]. Another example is that increased glutamate concentrations can provoke excitotoxicity and neuron death [70] but also attenuate the cognitive function decline in AD [71]. Drugs may reduce glutamate receptor sensitivity [72] to enhance neuron resistance, but at the same time, they may impair cognitive functions. Thus, it is difficult to predict which aspect of a pathogenic factor will be more strongly affected by drugs.

Efficacy of available pharmaceutical therapy is limited because each drug influences only a single step of the AD pathogenesis and the drugs affect both damaged and normal cells [1]. To date, only AChE inhibitors and NMDA receptor antagonists have entered clinical practice to treat AD. Cell-selective drug delivery is theoretically possible, but such studies are in their infancy. Promising treatments include controlling vascular risk factors like hypertension and diabetes [73]. New therapeutic agents against AD based on understanding its molecular and biochemical pathogenesis and acting at various steps in the disease mechanism are needed.

Recently, much attention has been paid to therapies that may enhance the adaptive potential and mobilize self-defense systems of the organism, such as natural adaptogens. Many reports suggest that natural products are promising for their anti-AD activity. Among adaptogens, *Ginkgo biloba* is being extensively tested in rodent models of AD and in patients for its efficacy in improving neuropsychological parameters, such as trail-making speed, digit memory span, verbal learning, geriatric symptoms, depressive mood, and memory status [74, 75].

Chauhan showed that garlic extracts effectively reduced levels of Aβ in brains of Alzheimer's Swedish double mutant mice [76]. In these mice, garlic extracts decreased the levels of soluble and fibrillar Aβ and Aβ-immunoreactive plaques by 2.3–3- and 1.67-fold, respectively. Aged garlic extracts prevented early cognitive impairment and improved performance of memory tasks in Tg2576 mice, a strain predisposed to AD [76].

The major phenolic component of green tea, epigallocatechin-3-gallate (EGCG), suppresses Aβ production in APP-transfected cultured murine neuroblastoma cells [77]. EGCG decreased Aβ accumulation and improved memory in mutant AD mice [78]. This effect was further enhanced by addition of fish oil to the treatment [79]. Epidemiological studies have also demonstrated that omega-3 fatty acids, components of fish oil, reduce the risk of AD [80, 81].

13.4 Nonpharmacological Therapy for AD

Multiple studies have suggested that stimulation of self-defense systems of neural cells may attenuate the progression of AD. Even after the disease onset, activation of brain self-defense systems may provide effective protection for a long time. These systems include antioxidants, heat shock proteins (HSPs), NO, and other so-called stress-limiting systems [82, 83]. Nonpharmacological prevention and treatment of AD based on activation of these systems have certain advantages over drug-based therapy. Stress-limiting systems are usually activated by intra- and extracellular adverse factors [82], and these systems respond to changes occurring at the earliest phase of disease. Production of metabolites of stress-limiting systems is generally regulated by the negative feedback mechanism, which prevents overproduction and excessive accumulation of these metabolites. Therefore, activation of self-defense systems appears to be a promising approach to restrict neurodegenerative processes.

Current concepts imply that stimulation of brain metabolic rate and neuronal activity may prevent or delay development of AD [84]. Adequate stimuli for brain neuronal activity include environmental factors, such as education, nutrition, exercise, socialization, and stress. These factors may restore the disturbed balance between neuronal injury and repair and thus prevent or delay progression of brain neurodegeneration [85].

According to the hypothesis of Heininger [86], disorders of memory and other cognitive functions in AD result from exhaustion of adaptive reserves in the brain. The process of brain adaptation to progressive substrate deprivation involves sparing glucose by enhancing the oxidative utilization of ketone bodies. These adaptive metabolic shifts are mediated by Aβ which helps the brain to function in the conditions of substrate deprivation. However, Aβ toxicity increases oxido-nitrosative stress, which in turn suppresses cholinergic neurotransmission and impairs cellular energy metabolism, eventually shifting the brain from a state of resistance to one of exhausted adaptive reserves. This hypothesis suggests a possibility of developing a therapeutic strategy aimed at enhancing the adaptive reserve of the body to prevent or delay the irreversible damage of brain cells in AD. Indeed, available data suggest that adaptation to dietary restriction, physical and mental activity, or mild stress exposure may reduce both the incidence and severity of neurodegenerative disorders in humans [73].

In the triple-transgenic mouse model of AD (3×TgAD mice), 40% calorie restriction and intermittent fasting protected neurons against adverse effects of Aβ. Caloric restriction resulted in lower levels of Aβ1–40, Aβ1–42, and phospho-tau in the hippocampus of AD mice compared to the control diet group and improved their cognitive function [87]. For example, 30% caloric restriction resulted in reduced contents of Aβ1–40 and Aβ1–42 peptides in the temporal cortex of squirrel monkeys, relative to monkeys fed a normal diet [88]. Increased resistance of neurons in the brain to dysfunction and death was also demonstrated in other experimental models of AD where food intake was restricted [89]. Epidemiological studies indicate that caloric intake may influence the relative risk for AD clinical dementia [90, 91]. Clinical observations show that a Mediterranean-style diet is associated with reduced risk of AD and slower decline in Mini-mental State Examination scores [92, 93].

One mechanism potentially underlying the beneficial effects of dietary restriction may involve stimulation of the expression of HSPs and neurotrophic factors. The neurotrophic factors induced by dietary restriction may protect neurons by inducing the production of proteins that suppress oxyradical production, stabilize cellular calcium homeostasis, and inhibit apoptotic biochemical cascades. Interestingly, dietary restriction also increases numbers of newly generated neurons in the adult brain, suggesting that this dietary manipulation increases the brain's capacity for plasticity and self-repair [89].

Low socioeconomic status is detrimental for brain development and raises the risk of developing AD in later life [73]. Moceri et al. [94] studied the relationship between early socioeconomic status and later AD. They found that better socioeconomic environment in childhood and adolescence expands the "brain reserve," i.e., the ability of brain to cope with increasing age- and disease-related changes, and also to decrease the risk of late-life dementia, including AD. Several epidemiological studies have found an association between low educational level or occupations not cognitively demanding and dementia. Intellectual training is considered an effective protection and even therapy for AD. For instance, training in reasoning slows functional decline in AD, and the beneficial effect of such training is sustained for 5 years [95]. The therapeutic benefits of cognitive interventions are associated with substantial biological changes within the brain. Moreover, it was demonstrated that a combination of pharmacological and nonpharmacological interventions more effectively alleviates clinical symptoms in patients with AD than either intervention given alone [96].

The neuroprotective role of intellectual activity training against the development of dementia may have the following explanation. Long-term potentiation (LTP, a biological correlate of learning and memory) increases the sensitivity of hippocampal neurons to synaptically released glutamate while decreasing neuronal responses to glutamate receptor agonists and to hypoxia/ischemia in vitro. The effects of LTP are likely to involve changes in intracellular Ca^{2+} concentration. It was proposed that the LTP-induced neuroprotection may help to explain the epidemiological evidence of a possible neuroprotective role of adaptation to learning against dementia [97].

Exercise training may help decrease the cognitive decline in patients with AD. A comprehensive cognitive-linguistic intervention program for mild to moderate AD, which included physical fitness training and supervised volunteer work, maintained or improved performance on multiple discourse outcome measures, preserving communicative function, slowing of cognitive decline, and improvement of mood [98, 99]. Data from the 1991–1992 Canadian Study of Health and Aging, a prospective cohort study of dementia, showed that compared with no exercise, physical activity was associated with lower risks of cognitive impairment, Alzheimer disease, and dementia of any type [100]. Important additional data were obtained in a recent randomized trial by Lautenschlager et al. [101] who showed that physical exercise was protective against cognitive decline. In the 18-month follow-up of this trial, Lautenschlager et al. used the Alzheimer Disease Assessment Scale–Cognitive Subscale to demonstrate a statistically significant difference between people regularly engaged in physical exercise and a sedentary control group. This effect was more pronounced than the effect of AChE inhibitors [102]. Therefore, regular physical activity can represent an important and potent protective factor for cognitive decline and dementia in the elderly.

An interesting approach to protection of brain against AD and other types of neurodegeneration is increased stimulation of neurons. For instance, the circadian system, which controls the sleep/wake cycle, may be stimulated in AD patients by exposing them to more light or transcutaneous nerve stimulation [103, 104]. Several studies showed that adaptation to hypoxia stimulates proliferation of neural stem cells [105] and neuron growth in hippocampus of adult rats [106]. Based on this evidence, it seems attractive to direct the development of therapeutic strategies toward stimulation of metabolic rate/neuronal activity to improve cognition and other symptoms in AD.

13.5 Neuroprotective Effects of Adaptation to Hypoxia

Protective effects of adaptation to hypoxia have been demonstrated with respect to injuries and diseases of the cardiovascular, immune, and respiratory systems [83]. The ability of this adaptation to prevent or treat disorders of the central nervous system is less studied. In this regard, adaptation to intermittent hypobaric hypoxia in an altitude chamber exerted a protective effect in experimental epilepsy [107], adaptation to high altitude hypoxia in mountains improved formation and retention of conditioned reflex in mice [108], and intermittent hypoxia conditioning during chronic ethanol consumption attenuated oxidative damage to the brain and alleviated behavioral abnormalities during subsequent ethanol withdrawal [109]. In patients, adaptation to hypobaric hypoxia was successfully implemented as a component of multimodal treatment for schizophrenia and alcohol abuse [83]. Hypoxic preconditioning has been demonstrated to prevent ischemic [110–112] and oxidative damage [113] in the mouse brain.

Special attention has been paid by researchers to effects of intermittent hypoxia in Parkinson disease. Adaptation to normobaric hypoxia effectively prevented behavioral disorders associated with experimental Parkinson disease [114]. In patients with Parkinson disease, hypoxia training improved electromyograms, reduced muscle tremor, and facilitated productive motor activity. Importantly, the hypoxia training also improved lung ventilation, which is always impaired in Parkinson patients [115].

One of the possible mechanisms of protective effects of intermittent hypoxia is improved energy production. Hypoxia increases formation of mitochondria in brain of adult mice [116], activates electron flux through respiratory complex I, and increases efficiency of oxidative phosphorylation [117].

Another important mechanism of neuroprotection may be prevention of Ca^{2+} overload in neurons. Studies showed that intermittent hypoxia increases resistance of Na^{+}-K^{+} ATPase to oxidative stress [118, 119]. Thus, the driving force for Ca^{2+} efflux is sustained. In addition, hypoxia-induced protection against Ca^{2+} overload may be mediated by hypoxia-induced activation of NO synthesis, which protects sarcolemmal Na^{+}-K^{+} ATPase function and Na^{+} and K^{+} transport [120, 121].

Induction of hypoxia-inducible factor-1 (HIF-1), a transcription factor that orchestrates expression of myriad genes in response to hypoxia, has been shown to afford neuroprotection in cerebral ischemic stroke and chronic neurodegenerative disorders, such as AD and Parkinson disease [122]. Studies on the effect of adaptation to hypoxia on HIF-1 induction showed that both HIF-1α mRNA [123] and protein [124] increased in rat hippocampus and cortex after each hypoxic session [124, 125]. The increase in HIF-1α took place only in the brain of rats which were able to adapt to hypoxia. In rats with failed adaptation, HIF-1α did not increase [124]. It may be hypothesized that the adaptive resistance of nerve cells to Aβ toxicity may partially be due to an enhanced flux of glucose through both the energy-yielding glycolytic pathway and the hexose monophosphate shunt, which maintains endogenous antioxidant defenses, secondary to HIF-1-driven expression of the enzymes of these pathways [126].

Lower levels of constitutive heat shock protein 70 (HSP70) mRNA are considered important for development of AD [127]. HSP70 is a well-recognized neuroprotective factor [37, 128]. Prior increase in HSP70 expression decreases apoptosis in hippocampal neurons [129] and prevents death and injury of neurons both in vitro and in vivo [130]. Multiple mechanisms may underlie this neuroprotection, including suppression of apoptosis, restriction of NO production, dissolution of extracellular Aβ aggregates, enhancement of Aβ elimination from extracellular spaces, restriction of tau-protein hyperphosphorylation, protection of neurons from glutamate toxicity, and restriction of intracellular Aβ cytotoxicity [131, 132].

In our experiments, adaptation to hypobaric hypoxia (5,000 m; 10–30 min daily for 8 days) induced pronounced HSP70 accumulation in rat brain and increased the survival time of rats during subsequent, more severe hypoxia at a simulated altitude of 11,000 m. The NO synthase inhibitor, *L*-NNA, completely abolished both the accumulation of HSP70 and the development of hypoxia resistance. These results suggested that the activation of HSP70 synthesis is mediated by NO-dependent mechanisms [82, 133].

We obtained direct evidence of the hypoxia-induced neuroprotection by histopathological analysis of rat brain [134]. To visualize degenerating neurons, 10-μm sections of parietotemporal cortex were Nissl-stained with hematoxylin-eosin, acid vanadium fuchsin, and cresyl violet. Degenerating neurons were not found in rats which did not receive Aβ-injections (Fig. 13.2). Multiple shrunken, hyperchromic degenerating neurons were present in the parietotemporal cortex of rats

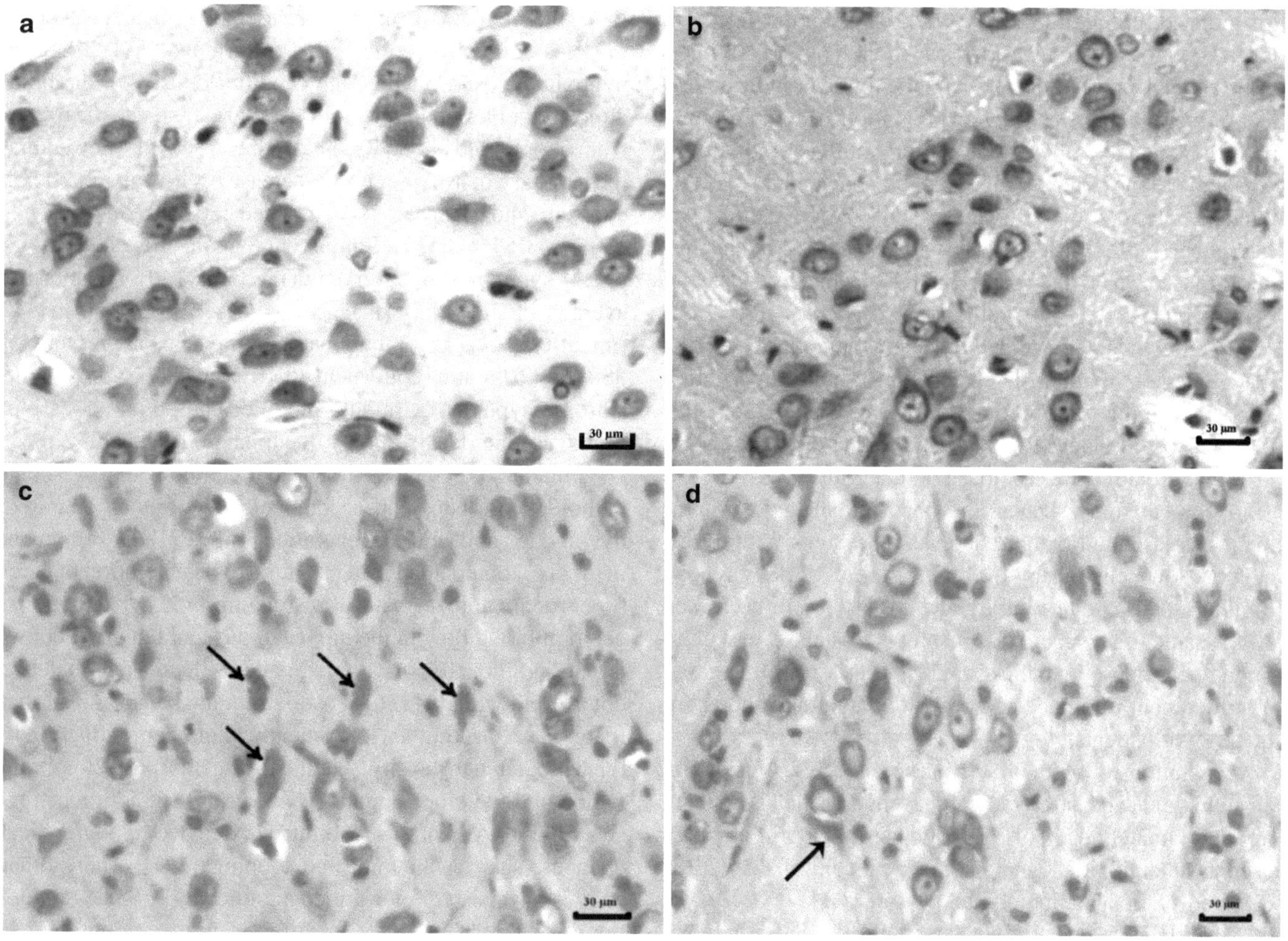

Fig. 13.2 Representative sections of Nissl-stained rat parietotemporal cortex. (**a**) Naïve control; (**b**) adaptation to hypoxia; (**c**) effect of Aβ; (**d**) adaptation to hypoxia + Aβ (From [134] and presented with the kind permission of Elsevier) (*arrows* indicate shrunken and hyperchromic, degenerating neurons)

injected with Aβ. Neurons with these pathomorphological signs were essentially absent in the brains of rats injected with Aβ after adaptation to hypoxia. Therefore, AIH prevented Aβ toxicity-induced neurodegeneration in the brain.

13.6 Alleviation of Oxidative Stress by Adaptation to Hypoxia: Role in Neuroprotection

Experiments on rats showed that a 7-h exposure to 10% O_2 left unaffected the Fe^{2+}-induced chemiluminescence and rate of accumulation of thiobarbituric acid-reactive substances (TBARS) in plasma and brain [135]. Two-week adaptation to intermittent hypoxia induced some activation of free-radical oxidation and a pronounced potentiation of the endogenous antioxidant system.

In our experiments, Alzheimer's disease was modeled by bilateral administration of Aβ into the basal magnocellular nucleus of rats [136, 137]. Experiments were started 30 days after Aβ administration. Adaptation of rats to intermittent hypobaric hypoxia was performed in an altitude chamber at a simulated altitude of 4,000 m, 4 h daily for 14 days. The last adaptation session was performed 24 h before Aβ injection. The Aβ-induced damage and the hypoxia-induced protection were evaluated by memory retention in the conditioned passive avoidance reflex 14 days after administration of Aβ. Adaptation to hypoxia significantly prevented the Aβ-induced deterioration of memory. This protective effect was associated with restriction of oxidative stress in the hippocampus of rats with experimental AD, which was detected by respective changes in brain tissue TBARS.

Direct evidence demonstrates that adaptation to hypoxia potentiates antioxidant defense. High altitude intermittent hypoxia training (30 min/day for 15 days) increased activities of the antioxidant enzymes superoxide dismutase, catalase, and glutathione peroxidase in rat erythrocytes [138].

A clinical study showed that intermittent hypoxia treatment increased antioxidant defense in patients with dyscirculatory encephalopathy [139]. After a 10-day hypoxic training, total oxidant activity and TBARS were decreased. At the same time, superoxide dismutase, catalase, and glutathione peroxidase activities in erythrocytes were increased. The treatment improved cerebral circulation and short-term memory of patients.

Adaptation to hypoxia activates synthesis of melatonin, an antioxidant and a free-radical scavenger, which is deficient in approximately 45% of AD patients. Melatonin is widely used as an antioxidant and also for treatment of sleep disorders and sundown agitation in AD [140, 141].

Melatonin has been shown to be highly effective in reducing oxidative damage in the central nervous system. In addition, melatonin can stimulate other antioxidant enzymes including superoxide dismutase, glutathione peroxidase, and glutathione reductase [142]. Importantly, melatonin also possesses antiamyloidogenic properties [143]. Recently, it was found that melatonin inhibits apoptotic pathways in neurodegenerative diseases [144]. A single, 2-h hypoxia exposure at 8,000-m simulated altitude sharply increased plasma melatonin level, which peaked at 7 days after hypoxia and returned to baseline after another 7 days [145]. Collectively, there is much evidence that adaptation to hypoxia may be beneficial for prevention of AD-related disorders due to restriction of free-radical processes.

13.7 Role of Brain Angiogenesis in the Neuroprotective Effect of Intermittent Hypoxia

Adaptive structural changes in response to prolonged hypoxia include increased capillary density. This mechanism decreases intercapillary diffusion distance [146]. Vascular capacity was increased in both left and right ventricles of rats adapted to intermittent high altitude hypoxia [147]. Intermittent hypoxia increased vascularity also in skeletal muscles and enhanced exercise performance [148]. During hypoxia exposure of rats, the capillary density in the brain almost doubles, and the intercapillary distance decreases from about 50 to about 40 μm [149]. Harik et al. showed that the capillary density begins to increase by 1 week of hypoxic exposure and the process is completed between 2 and 3 weeks of exposure [150, 151]. Similar angiogenic effects of adaptation to hypoxia were observed in rat brain [149], in which the average intercapillary distance decreased from ~50 to ~40 μm after 3 weeks of hypobaric hypoxia at a pressure of 380 Torr (0.5 atm, equivalent to 10% normobaric oxygen). Chronic hypoxia in 2-month-old mice caused an increase in brain vascular density, likely due to angiogenesis [152].

Clinical studies have shown that cerebral microvascular pathology precedes and accompanies age-related cognitive dysfunction and neurodegeneration [153, 154]. Development of AD is accompanied by a progressive degeneration of cerebrocortical capillary wall ultrastructure [155]. The regional cerebral blood flow in the hippocampus and temporal cortex is also significantly lower in AD patients than in age-matched control individuals [156]. Postmortem analysis showed that there was a striking and statistically significant reduction in the vascular net density specifically in the basal forebrain region and the hippocampus of AD brains. In addition, vessels in the AD brains exhibited extensive topographical changes, such as kinking and looping [157]. Many other studies have also demonstrated significant (16–38%) reductions in capillary density in different brain regions of AD patients [57, 64, 83, 105, 106, 112]. The decline in vascular density correlated with increasing Clinical Dementia Rating

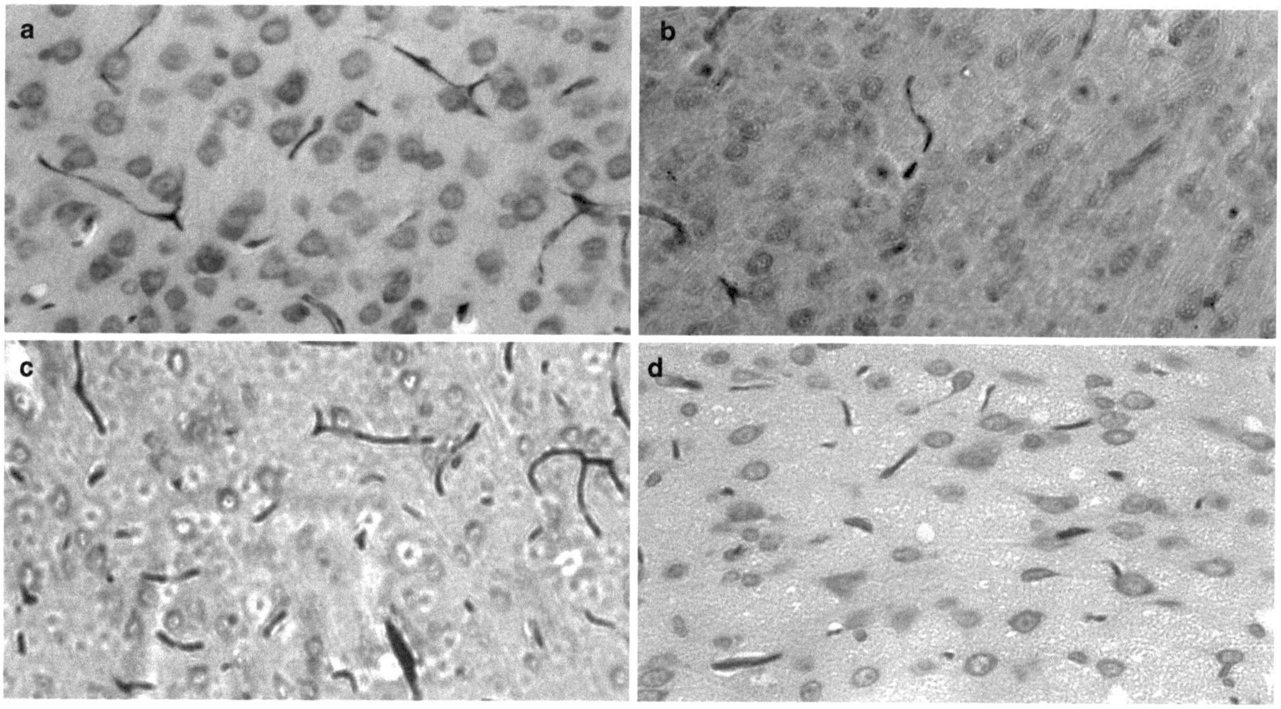

Fig. 13.3 Prevention of vascular rarefaction in the cortex of rats with experimental AD by adaptation to hypoxia. (**a**) Naïve control; (**b**) effect of Aβ; (**c**) adaptation to hypoxia; (**d**) adaptation to hypoxia + Aβ

score [113]. Similar microvascular changes were found in animal models of AD [113, 115, 116].

Cerebral angiogenesis is initiated in hypoxia by HIF-1 through activation of downstream genes containing hypoxic response elements (HRE), including vascular endothelial growth factor (VEGF) [158, 159]. VEGF is upregulated primarily in the glial end feet of the astrocytes surrounding the capillaries [146]. The capacity for cerebral angiogenesis declines with age and in AD [160–162] apparently due to decreased responsiveness of HIF-1 to hypoxia, which reduces VEGF expression [163]. This HIF-1 decline is associated with neuronal loss [164]. The failure of vascular recovery and other cerebrovascular changes represent a loss of brain vascular reserve and functional reserve [162].

Angiogenesis produced by intermittent hypoxia may be protective. In spontaneously hypertensive rats, adaptation to intermittent hypobaric hypoxia prevented the functional rarefaction of arterioles and capillaries in brains of spontaneously hypertensive rats [165, 166]. Chronic (3 weeks) hypobaric hypoxia decreased the average intercapillary distance [149] and improved O_2 availability to the brain parenchyma [167]. Increased vascular density in brain is a possible mechanism for the antihypertensive effect of adaptation to hypoxia [165, 166].

Recently, we tested if adaptation to hypoxia might prevent the vascular rarefaction in rats with experimental AD induced by bilateral injection of Aβ (unpublished data). Brain blood vessels were stained by transcardiac injection of Indian ink. Brain sections of 10 μm were stained with cresyl violet, and blood vessels were counted. In rats with experimental AD, vascular density was significantly decreased in both hippocampus and cortex by 22–25% (Fig. 13.3). Adaptation to intermittent hypobaric hypoxia increased vascular density so that it did not significantly differ from the vascular density in respective brain areas of control rats. Therefore, prevention of brain vascular rarefaction may be a protective mechanism of adaptation to hypoxia in experimental AD.

13.8 Role of NO in the Neuroprotective Effect of Adaptation to Hypoxia in AD

Whereas excessive NO is neurotoxic and contributes to development and progression of AD, NO shortage or reduced availability also aggravates AD-related disorders. Inadequate NO production may mediate cerebral hypoperfusion and insufficiency of NO-inducible protective mechanisms including synthesis of HSP70 and HSP32 [168–170]. Studies showed that promotion of endothelial NO formation may decrease the risk of age-related neurodegeneration [171]. Accordingly, NO-based strategies to prevent or delay AD may seek to establish a moderate rate of NO production.

Chronic, nonpharmacological enhancement of endogenous NO production can be produced most efficiently by special diets [172, 173] or adaptation to environmental stresses such as hypoxia, exercise, mental stress, cold, or heat [174]. Among nonpharmacological treatments, adaptations to hypoxia and exercise are the strategies most commonly used in experimental and clinical settings for disease prevention and therapy [120, 175].

After finding that adaptation to intermittent hypoxia can prevent cognitive disorders and cortical neurodegeneration in rats [131], we focused on the possible role of NO in this protection [136]. The study showed that the development of experimental AD induced by Aβ injection was associated with decreased plasma nitrite + nitrate (NO_x). Prior adaptation to hypoxia moderately stimulated NO synthesis and alleviated the decrease in plasma NO_x after β-amyloid injection. Daily administration of the NOS inhibitor, *L*-NNA, to rats for 14 days aggravated the loss of memory induced by Aβ. When *L*-NNA was injected during adaptation to hypoxia, it abolished the protective effect of adaptation to hypoxia and, moreover, induced memory disorders in rats similar to those observed in experimental AD. In contrast, the increase in plasma NO level by administration of NO donor, dinitrosyl iron complex (DNIC), like adaptation to hypoxia, prevented the Aβ-induced memory impairment (Fig. 13.4).

NO is commonly regarded as not only a detrimental factor in AD, but it is also a protective factor in AD [176]. Astrocytes and epithelial cells which intensively produce NO are better protected against toxic effects of NO overproduction than are neuronal cell lines characterized by weak NO production [177]. iNOS knockout mice develop more severe cognitive decline and dramatic neuron loss in AD-relevant brain regions in response to Aβ compared to control [178]. NO_x concentration in the cerebrospinal fluid negatively correlates with the degree of mental disorders in AD patients [179].

These literature reports and our results [136] are consistent with our observations that rats of the August strain, which have constitutively elevated NO production, are better protected against neurodegenerative damage than Wistar rats [180, 181]. Indeed, NO production is significantly higher in August than in Wistar rats [182, 183], so content of nNOS protein was 67% higher in brains of August vs. Wistar rats [182]. Aβ injections induced only a slight decrease in plasma NO_x in August rats and did not induce any significant impairment of memory in these rats vs. Wistar rats [181, 182]. Histopathological analysis showed that the number of dead neurons per high-power field in cerebral cortex was significantly less in August (26.4±4.2) than in Wistar rats (48.4±6.0) with experimental AD ($P<0.05$) [182]. Therefore, reduced NO production plays an important role in cognitive disorders and neuronal death induced by Aβ, and prevention of NO deficiency is protective in experimental AD.

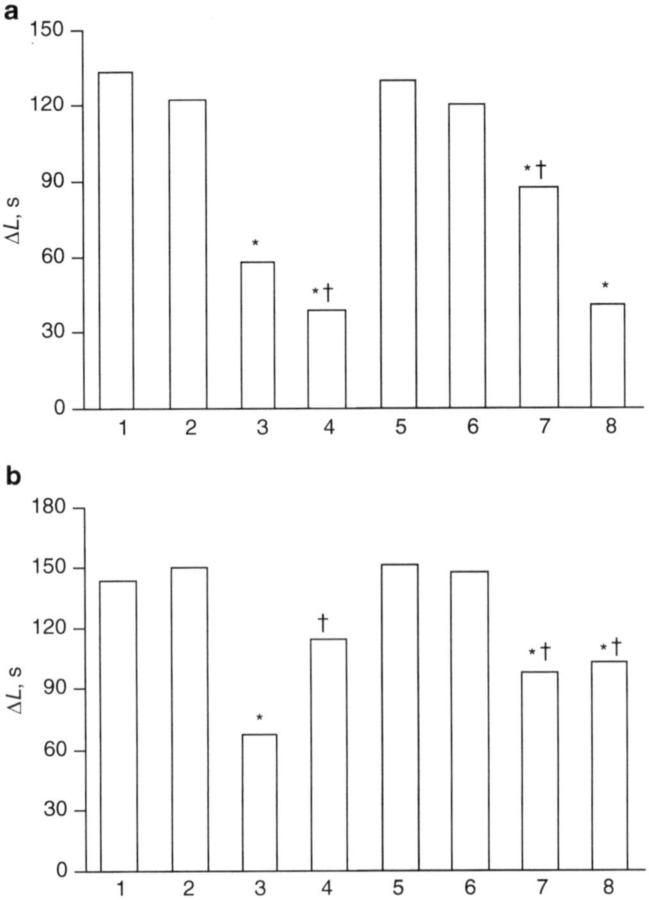

Fig. 13.4 Effects of adaptation to hypoxia, NOS inhibitor L-NNA (**a**) and NO-donor DNIC (**b**) on Aβ-induced memory disorders in rats. (*Panel* **a**) *1* control; *2* L-NNA; *3* Aβ; *4* L-NNA+Aβ; *5* adaptation; *6* adaptation+L-NNA; *7* adaptation+β-amyloid; *8* adaptation+L-NNA+Aβ. (*Panel* **b**) *1* control; *2* DNIC; *3* β-amyloid; *4* DNIC+Aβ; *5* adaptation; *6* adaptation+DNIC; *7* adaptation+β-amyloid; *8* adaptation+DNIC+Aβ. $^*P<0.05$ vs. control; $^\dagger P<0.05$ vs. Aβ (From [136] and presented with the kind permission of Russian Academy of Medical Sciences)

Endothelial dysfunction of cerebral vessels considerably impairs autoregulation of local cerebral blood flow (LCBF) in Aβ-treated animals and transgenic animals with Aβ overexpression. Furthermore, the severity of endothelial dysfunction positively correlates with Aβ concentration in the brain [184]. The reduction in temporoparietal LCBF correlates positively with cognitive decline in patients diagnosed with AD [185].

Attenuated endothelium-dependent dilation impairs the vasodilatory response of cerebral blood vessels to decreases in transmural pressure, which makes the brain highly susceptible to blood pressure variations even within the normal range and aggravates damage induced by ischemia and occlusion of cerebral vessels [186]. Importantly, the Aβ-induced endothelial dysfunction precedes neurodegenerative changes in the brain [184] and, therefore, constitutes an important pathophysiological mechanism of AD.

We studied endothelium-dependent dilation of blood vessels in the parietal cortex using continuous recording of LCBF by a laser Doppler flowmeter [187]. Endothelium-dependent dilation was evaluated by response to injection of ACh into the carotid artery. Aβ reduced the endothelium-dependent dilation of cerebral vessels by 75–80% [187]. Adaptation had no effect on endothelium-dependent dilation at the basal condition but completely prevented the Aβ-induced endothelial dysfunction.

Recent reports suggest that development of AD is associated with endothelial dysfunction of not only cerebral but also peripheral blood vessels. Gentile et al. [43] showed that Aβ induced endothelial dysfunction of skin vessels. Dede et al. [188] observed attenuated flow-dependent vasodilation in patients with AD. In our experiments, rats with experimental AD had pronounced endothelial dysfunction of the aorta (unpublished data). Maximum endothelium-dependent relaxation of isolated aorta in response to ACh was $52.2 \pm 3.5\%$ in control rats vs. $39.8 \pm 5.2\%$ in Aβ-injected rats ($P < 0.05$). Adaptation to hypoxia itself did not significantly influence the endothelium-dependent relaxation, but this adaptation did prevent Aβ-induced endothelial dysfunction ($51.9 \pm 2.9\%$, $P < 0.05$). These data suggest that AD may contribute to development and progression of cardiovascular disease associated with endothelial dysfunction such as hypertension and heart failure.

Nitric oxide is a highly reactive substance which can be bound into complexes used for transport and intracellular storage of NO, mainly *S*-nitrosothiols and dinitrosyl iron complexes [189]. These NO stores are formed after any increase in NO, irrespective of the cause. NO stores can provide protection from NO overproduction by sequestering excess free NO. On the other hand, NO stores can be an additional NO source when NO is deficient [189].

Important evidence for the protective role of NO stores against NO overproduction was obtained in rats with experimental AD induced by Aβ injections [187]. NO stores were estimated by a method based on the ability of *N*-acetylcysteine (NAC) to interact with intracellular NO stores and release vasoactive products, which increased LCBF [190]. NO stores were estimated in the presence of the NO synthase inhibitor, *L*-NNA, which prevented any contribution of de novo synthesized NO to the vasodilatory response. To reveal NO stores, NAC was injected into the carotid artery. The increase in LCBF reflected dilation of cerebral blood vessels. The magnitude of changes in LCBF corresponded to the size of NO stores and was expressed as a percent of resting LCBF. Since the size of NO stores correlated significantly with NO production [191], increased NO stores may be regarded as an indirect marker of NO overproduction. NO stores were absent in cerebral blood vessels of control rats [187], but in both hypoxia-adapted and Aβ-treated rats, NAC administration revealed NO stores. In rats injected with Aβ after adaptation, NO stores were increased compared to nonadapted rats treated with Aβ. It had been previously shown that adaptation to hypoxia moderately increased NO synthesis with formation of NO stores in the aorta [189, 191]. Adaptation to hypoxia also enhances the NO-storage capacity of blood vessels [192]. This mechanism may underlie the protection of blood vessels against subsequent NO overproduction in rats with experimental AD, as reported by Mashina et al. [187].

Injections of Aβ resulted in large increases in expression of all three NOS isoforms, nNOS, iNOS, and eNOS, in both cortex and hippocampus [134]. Adaptation to hypoxia did not significantly influence NOS expression in the cortex. However, the expression of all three NOS isoforms was increased in the hippocampus of hypoxia-adapted rats, although these increases were considerably smaller than the increases in NOS isoform expression induced by Aβ. The most important result of these experiments was that adaptation to hypoxia significantly blunted the increases in NOS isoform expression induced by Aβ in both cortex and hippocampus. We found stronger induction of eNOS than of iNOS by Aβ, although a prior report indicated that the iNOS isoform, which is induced in astrocytes associated with amyloid plaques, is a major source of NO in AD [193]. More recent evidence, however, has demonstrated also a significant role for eNOS [194, 195]. While eNOS is found in endothelial cells, this NOS isoform had been also detected in neurons and glial cells [195, 196].

Astrocytes with elevated levels of iNOS or eNOS are found in direct association with Aβ-deposits, and experimental AD is associated with astrocytosis accompanied by significant increases of both iNOS and eNOS [195]. Thus, increased expression of these NOS isoforms contributes to the maintenance and progression of the neurodegenerative process. Contrary to iNOS, the eNOS and nNOS isoforms are constitutively expressed, and their activation does not require new enzyme protein synthesis. However, these constitutive forms of NOS are also inducible, since synthesis of new enzyme protein is stimulated by pathological conditions [197, 198].

All three NOS isoforms, as well as 3-NT, a product of nitrosation of tyrosyl residues in proteins, are found in sections of temporal cortex taken from postmortem brains of patients with AD [199]. Aberrant expression of nNOS in cortical pyramidal cells and of iNOS and eNOS in glial cells is highly colocalized with 3-NT. Therefore, it is likely that increased expression of all NOS isoforms in astrocytes and neurons contributes to formation of reactive nitrogen intermediates that attack proteins, leading to severe damage to brain neurons [200]. Our measurements of the stable NO metabolites, nitrite and nitrate, directly demonstrated that Aβ induced pronounced NO overproduction resulting from excessive expression of all three NOS isoforms [134]. Adaptation to hypoxia completely prevented NO overproduction in Aβ-injected rats [134].

β-Amyloid injections were associated with increased 3-NT in cortex and in hippocampus [134]. The increase in 3-NT was greater in hippocampus than in cortex following injection of Aβ, consistent with the suggestion that the hippocampus is the region more vulnerable to AD [36, 201]. Adaptation to hypoxia did not significantly influence tissue 3-NT in the hippocampus, but moderately increased 3-NT in the cortex by 42% compared to the naïve control ($P<0.05$). However, adaptation to hypoxia significantly restricted the increases in 3-NT in both the cortex and hippocampus of rats injected with Aβ. Therefore, although adaptation to hypoxia per se moderately increases NO production [120, 189], it prevents fulminate NO overproduction in experimental AD and alleviates adverse effects of AD [134].

Conclusion

Literature reports and the results of our experiments substantiate the hypothesis that adaptive medicine can be used as a strategy to improve neuronal self-defense mechanisms which suppress progression toward AD. The diagram on Fig. 13.5 shows the effect of adaptation to hypoxia on major pathogenetic processes in brain neurodegeneration during development of AD. Briefly, Aβ induces increased generation of reactive oxygen species, particularly superoxide, and activates expression of all NOS isoforms. Excessive NO reacts with superoxide to form toxic peroxynitrite. Together with excessive NO, peroxynitrite damages DNA and proteins including mitochondrial enzymes, which disrupts energy supply and cell structure and function. These processes harm brain neurons and blood vessels. The loss of cerebral blood vessels, with ensuing rarefaction of the vasculature together with endothelial dysfunction, facilitates progression of neurodegeneration. Death of neurons results in cognitive decline and progression of AD.

Adaptation to hypoxia blocks all steps of this pathological process, primarily by prevention of ROS generation and restriction of increased NOS expression. Moderate stimulation of NO synthesis by adaptation to hypoxia provides restriction of subsequent NO overproduction by a negative feedback mechanism. In addition, adaptation to hypoxia substantially enhances binding of excessive NO to NO stores and thus restricts the interaction of NO with superoxide and formation of peroxynitrite. Adaptation to hypoxia almost completely prevents endothelial dysfunction of both cerebral and extracerebral blood vessels, rarefaction of brain vascular net, and the loss of neurons in the brain cortex. Due to all these protective effects, adaptation to hypoxia eventually prevents the impairment of memory and development of experimental AD.

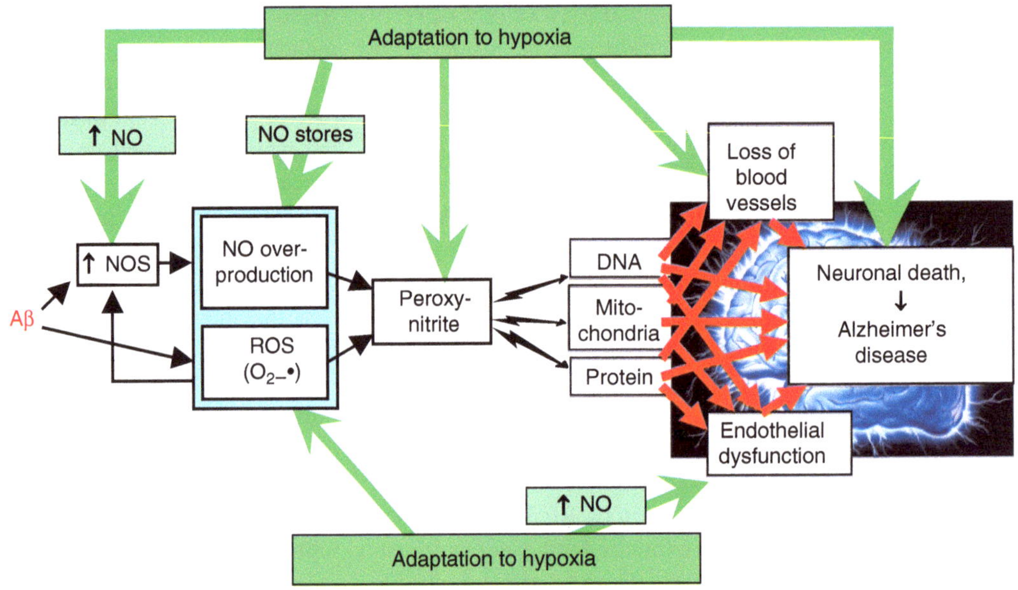

Fig. 13.5 The role of NO in neuroprotective mechanisms against AD-mediated neurodegeneration activated by adaptation to hypoxia. *Green arrows* show protective effects of adaptation to hypoxia; *black* and *red arrows* show progressive detrimental effects leading to AD. For explanation, see the text

Acknowledgments This work was supported by the Russian Foundation for Basic Research (grant 07–04–00650).

References

1. Park SY. Potential therapeutic agents against Alzheimer's disease from natural sources. Arch Pharm Res. 2010;33:1589–609.
2. Katzman R, Kawas C. Epidemiology of dementia and Alzheimer disease. In: Terry RD, Katzman R, Bick KL, editors. Alzheimer disease. New York: Raven; 1994. p. 105–22.
3. Wimo A, Winblad B, Aguero-Torres H, et al. The magnitude of dementia occurrence in the world. Alzheimer Dis Assoc Disord. 2003;17:63–7.
4. Cummings JL, Vinters HV, Cole GM, et al. Alzheimer's disease: etiologies, pathophysiology, cognitive reserve, and treatment opportunities. Neurology. 1998;51:S2–17.
5. LaFerla FM. Pathways linking Abeta and tau pathologies. Biochem Soc Trans. 2010;38:993–5.
6. Green KN, Smith IF, Laferla FM. Role of calcium in the pathogenesis of Alzheimer's disease and transgenic models. Subcell Biochem. 2007;45:507–21.
7. Small DH. Dysregulation of calcium homeostasis in Alzheimer's disease. Neurochem Res. 2009;34:1824–9.
8. Ferreiro E, Oliveira CR, Pereira CM. The release of calcium from the endoplasmic reticulum induced by amyloid-beta and prion peptides activates the mitochondrial apoptotic pathway. Neurobiol Dis. 2008;30:331–42.
9. Mancuso M, Orsucci D, LoGerfo A, et al. Clinical features and pathogenesis of Alzheimer's disease: involvement of mitochondria and mitochondrial DNA. Adv Exp Med Biol. 2010;685:34–44.
10. Murakami Y, Ohsawa I, Kasahara T, et al. Cytoprotective role of mitochondrial amyloid beta peptide-binding alcohol dehydrogenase against a cytotoxic aldehyde. Neurobiol Aging. 2009;30: 325–9.
11. Singh S, Suman S, Chandra S, et al. Possible role of amyloid-beta, adenine nucleotide translocase and cyclophilin-D interaction in mitochondrial dysfunction of Alzheimer's disease. Bioinformation. 2009;3:440–5.
12. Tillement L, Lecanu L, Papadopoulos V. Alzheimer's disease: effects of β-amyloid on mitochondria. Mitochondrion. 2011;11: 13–21.
13. Sergeant N, Wattez A, Galvan-Valencia M, et al. Association of ATP synthase alpha-chain with neurofibrillary degeneration in Alzheimer's disease. Neuroscience. 2003;117:293–303.
14. Schmidt C, Lepsverdize E, Chi SL, et al. Amyloid precursor protein and amyloid beta-peptide bind to ATP synthase and regulate its activity at the surface of neural cells. Mol Psychiatry. 2008; 13:953–69.
15. Hauptmann S, Scherping I, Dröse SU, et al. Mitochondrial dysfunction: an early event in Alzheimer pathology accumulates withy age in AD transgenic mice. Neurobiol Aging. 2009;30:1575–86.
16. Rhein V, Baysang G, Rao S, et al. Amyloid-beta leads to impaired cellular respiration, energy production and mitochondrial electron chain complex activities in human neuroblastoma cells. Cell Mol Neurobiol. 2009;29:1063–71.
17. Aslan M, Özben T. Reactive oxygen and nitrogen species in Alzheimer's disease. Curr Alzheimer Res. 2004;1:111–9.
18. Mecocci P, MacGarvey U, Beal MF. Oxidative damage to mitochondrial DNA is increased in Alzheimer's disease. Ann Neurol. 1994;36:747–51.
19. Lovell MA, Ehmann WD, Butler SM, et al. Elevated thiobarbituric acid-reactive substances and antioxidant enzyme activity in the brain in Alzheimer's disease. Neurology. 1995;45:1594–601.
20. Sayre LM, Zelasko DA, Harris PL, et al. 4-Hydroxynonenal-derived advanced lipid peroxidation end products are increased in Alzheimer's disease. J Neurochem. 1997;68:2092–7.
21. Agostinho P, Cunha RA, Oliveira C. Neuroinflammation, oxidative stress and the pathogenesis of Alzheimer's disease. Curr Pharm Des. 2010;16:2766–78.
22. Cagnin A, Brooks DJ, Kennedy AM, et al. In-vivo measurement of activated microglia in dementia. Lancet. 2001;358:461–7.
23. Di Bona D, Scapagnini G, Candore G, et al. Immune-inflammatory responses and oxidative stress in Alzheimer's disease: therapeutic implications. Curr Pharm Des. 2010;16:684–91.
24. Brown GC. Nitric oxide and neuronal death. Nitric Oxide. 2010;23:153–65.
25. Ishii K, Muelhauser F, Liebl U, et al. Subacute NO generation induced by Alzheimer's β-amyloid in the living brain: reversal by inhibition of the inducible NO synthase. FASEB J. 2000;14:1485–9.
26. Mori K, Togashi H, Ueno KI, et al. Aminoguanidine prevented the impairment of learning behavior and hippocampal long-term potentiation following transient cerebral ischemia. Behav Brain Res. 2001;120:159–68.
27. Hsu MJ, Sheu JR, Lin CH, et al. Mitochondrial mechanisms in amyloid beta peptide-induced cerebrovascular degeneration. Biochim Biophys Acta. 2010;1800:290–6.
28. Bertoni-Freddari C, Fattoretti P, Casoli T, et al. Neuronal apoptosis in Alzheimer's disease: the role of age-related mitochondrial metabolic competence. Ann N Y Acad Sci. 2009;1171:18–24.
29. Kirsch M, Korth HG, Sustmann R, et al. The pathobiochemistry of nitrogen dioxide. Biol Chem. 2002;383:389–99.
30. Augusto O, Bonini MG, Amanso AM, et al. Nitrogen dioxide and carbonate radical anion: two emerging radicals in biology. Free Radic Biol Med. 2002;32:841–59.
31. Brennan ML, Wu W, Fu X, et al. A tale of two controversies: defining both the role of peroxidases in nitrotyrosine formation in vivo using eosinophil peroxidase and myeloperoxidase-deficient mice, and the nature of peroxidase-generated reactive nitrogen species. J Biol Chem. 2002;277:17415–27.
32. Souza JM, Daikhin E, Yudkoff M, et al. Factors determining the selectivity of protein tyrosine nitration. Arch Biochem Biophys. 1999;371:169–78.
33. Gow AJ, Duran D, Malcolm S, et al. Effects of peroxynitrite-induced protein modifications on tyrosine phosphorylation and degradation. FEBS Lett. 1996;385:63–5.
34. Castegna A, Thongboonkerd V, Klein JB, et al. Proteomic identification of nitrated proteins in Alzheimer's disease brain. J Neurochem. 2003;85:1394–401.
35. Cenini G, Sultana R, Memo M, et al. Elevated levels of pro-apoptotic p53 and its oxidative modification by the lipid peroxidation product, HNE, in brain from subjects with amnestic mild cognitive impairment and Alzheimer's disease. J Cell Mol Med. 2008; 12:987–94.
36. Butterfield DA, Reed TT, Perluigi M, et al. Elevated levels of 3-nitrotyrosine in brain from subjects with amnestic mild cognitive impairment: implications for the role of nitration in the progression of Alzheimer's disease. Brain Res. 2007;1148:243–8.
37. Ohtsuka K, Suzuki T. Roles of molecular chaperones in the nervous system. Brain Res Bull. 2000;53:141–6.
38. Kubes P, Kanwar S, Niu XF. Nitric oxide synthesis inhibition induces leukocyte adhesion via superoxide and mast cells. FASEB J. 1993;7:1293–9.

39. Harry GJ, Sills R, Schlosser MJ, et al. Neurodegeneration and glia response in rat hippocampus following nitro-L-arginine methyl ester (LNAME). Neurotox Res. 2001;3:307–19.
40. Takuma K, Phuagphong P, Lee E, et al. Anti-apoptotic effect of cGMP in cultured astrocytes: inhibition by cGMP-dependent protein kinase of mitochondrial permeable transition pore. J Biol Chem. 2001;276:48093–9.
41. Bonthius DJ, Luong T, Bonthius NE, et al. Nitric oxide utilizes NF-kappaB to signal its neuroprotective effect against alcohol toxicity. Neuropharmacology. 2009;56:716–31.
42. Na HJ, Chung HT, Ha KS, et al. Detection and measurement for the modification and inactivation of caspase by nitrosative stress in vitro and in vivo. Methods Enzymol. 2008;441:317–27.
43. Gentile MT, Vecchione C, Maffei A, et al. Mechanisms of soluble beta-amyloid impairment of endothelial function. J Biol Chem. 2004;279:48135–42.
44. Kalaria RN, Hedera P. Differential degeneration of the cerebral microvasculature in Alzheimer's disease. Neuroreport. 1995;6:477–80.
45. Mueller XM, Tevaearai H, Chaubert P, et al. Mechanism of action of transmyocardial revascularization. Schweiz Med Wochenschr. 1999;129:1889–92 [In French].
46. Johnson KA, Jones K, Holman BL, et al. Preclinical prediction of Alzheimer's disease using SPECT. Neurology. 1998;50: 1563–71.
47. Meier-Ruge W, Bertoni-Freddari C. The significance of glucose turnover in the brain in the pathogenic mechanisms of Alzheimer's disease. Rev Neurosci. 1996;7:1–19.
48. Ferreira IL, Resende R, Ferreiro E, et al. Multiple defects in energy metabolism in Alzheimer's disease. Curr Drug Targets. 2010;11: 1193–206.
49. de la Torre JC, Stefano GB. Evidence that Alzheimer's disease is a microvascular disorder: the role of constitutive nitric oxide. Brain Res Rev. 2000;34:119–36.
50. Duara R, Barker WW, Chang J, et al. Viability of neocortical function shown in behavioral activation state PET studies in Alzheimer disease. J Cereb Blood Flow Metab. 1992;12:927–34.
51. Massoud F, Gauthier S. Update on the pharmacological treatment of Alzheimer's disease. Curr Neuropharmacol. 2010;8:69–80.
52. Tzourio C, Anderson C, Chapman N, et al. Effects of blood pressure lowering with perindopril and indapamide therapy on dementia and cognitive decline in patients with cerebrovascular disease. Arch Intern Med. 2003;163:1069–75.
53. Forette F, Seux ML, Staessen JA, et al. Systolic hypertension in Europe investigators. The prevention of dementia with antihypertensive treatment: new evidence from the systolic hypertension in Europe (Syst-Eur) study. Arch Intern Med. 2002;162: 2046–52.
54. Deschaintre Y, Richard F, Leys D, et al. Treatment of vascular risk factors is associated with slower decline in Alzheimer disease. Neurology. 2009;73:674–80.
55. Francis PT, Palmer AM, Snape M, et al. The cholinergic hypothesis of Alzheimer's disease: a review of progress. J Neurol Neurosurg Psychiatry. 1999;66:137–47.
56. Lipton SA. Pathologically-activated therapeutics for neuroprotection: mechanism of NMDA receptor block by memantine and S-nitrosylation. Curr Drug Targets. 2007;8:621–32.
57. Ferris S, Ihl R, Robert P, et al. Treatment effects of memantine on language in moderate to severe Alzheimer's disease patients. Alzheimers Demen. 2009;5:369–74.
58. Mecocci P, Bladstrom A, Stender K. Effects of memantine on cognition in patients with moderate to severe Alzheimer's disease: post-hoc analyses of ADAScog and SIB total and single-item scores from six randomized, double-blind, placebo-controlled studies. Int J Geriatr Psychiatry. 2009;24:532–8.
59. McShane R, Areosa Sastre A, Minakaran N. Memantine for dementia. Cochrane Database Syst Rev. 2009;2:CD003154. doi:10.1002/14651858.CD003154.pub5.
60. Doody RS, Stevens JC, Beck C, et al. Practice parameter: management of dementia (an evidence-based review). report of the quality standards subcommittee of the American Academy of Neurology. Neurology. 2001;56:1154–66.
61. Lyketsos CG, Colenda CC, Beck C, et al. Position statement of the American Association for Geriatric Psychiatry regarding principles of care for patients with dementia resulting from Alzheimer disease. Am J Geriatr Psychiatry. 2006;14:561–72.
62. Kaduszkiewicz H, Zimmermann T, Beck-Bornholdt HP, et al. Cholinesterase inhibitors for patients with Alzheimer's disease: systematic review of randomised clinical trials. BMJ. 2005;331:321–7.
63. Raina P, Santaguida P, Ismaila A, et al. Effectiveness of cholinesterase inhibitors and memantine for treating dementia: evidence review for a clinical practice guideline. Ann Intern Med. 2008;148:379–97.
64. Lleo A, Greenberg SM, Growdon JH. Current pharmacotherapy for Alzheimer's disease. Annu Rev Med. 2006;57:513–33.
65. McDonnell J, Redekop WK, van der Roer N, et al. The cost of treatment of Alzheimer's disease in the Netherlands: a regression-based simulation model. Pharmacoeconomics. 2001;19:379–90.
66. Berghmans RL. Anti-Alzheimer drugs: ethical aspects of research and practice. Tijdschr Gerontol Geriatr. 2000;31:100–6 [In Dutch].
67. Clippingdale AB, Wade JD, Barrow CJ. The amyloid-beta peptide and its role in Alzheimer's disease. J Pept Sci. 2001;7:227–9.
68. Kontush A. Amyloid-beta: an antioxidant that becomes a pro-oxidant and critically contributes to Alzheimer's disease. Free Radic Biol Med. 2001;31:1120–31.
69. Kakimura J, Kitamura Y, Takata K, et al. Microglial activation and amyloid-beta clearance induced by exogenous heat-shock proteins. FASEB J. 2002;16:601–3.
70. Dodd PR. Excited to death: different ways to lose your neurons. Biogerontology. 2002;3:51–6.
71. Penner J, Rupsingh R, Smith M, et al. Increased glutamate in the hippocampus after galantamine treatment for Alzheimer disease. Prog Neuropsychopharmacol Biol Psychiatry. 2010;34:104–10.
72. Wild-Bode C, Yamazaki T, Capell A, et al. Intracellular generation and accumulation of amyloid beta-peptide terminating at amino acid 42. J Biol Chem. 1997;272:16085–8.
73. Larson EB. Prospects for delaying the rising tide of worldwide, late-life dementias. Int Psychogeriatr. 2010;22:1196–202.
74. Ahlemeyer B, Krieglstein J. Pharmacological studies supporting the therapeutic use of Ginkgo biloba extract for Alzheimer's disease. Pharmacopsychiatry. 2003;36 Suppl 1:S8–14.
75. Shi C, Liu J, Wu F, et al. Ginkgo biloba extract in Alzheimer's disease: from action mechanisms to medical practice. Int J Mol Sci. 2010;11:107–23.
76. Chauhan NB, Sandoval J. Amelioration of early cognitive deficits by aged garlic extract in Alzheimer's transgenic mice. Phytother Res. 2007;21:629–40.
77. Rezai-Zadeh K, Shytle D, Sun N, et al. Green tea epigallocatechin-3-gallate (EGCG) modulates amyloid precursor protein cleavage and reduces cerebral amyloidosis in Alzheimer transgenic mice. J Neurosci. 2005;25:8807–14.
78. Lee JW, Lee YK, Ban JO, et al. Green tea (-)-epigallocatechin-3-gallate inhibits beta-amyloid-induced cognitive dysfunction through modification of secretase activity via inhibition of ERK and NF-kappaB pathways in mice. J Nutr. 2009;139:1987–93.
79. Giunta B, Hou H, Zhu Y, et al. Fish oil enhances anti-amyloidogenic properties of green tea EGCG in Tg2576 mice. Neurosci Lett. 2010;471:134–8.
80. Kalmijn S, van Boxtel MP, Ocke M, et al. Dietary intake of fatty acids and fish in relation to cognitive performance at middle age. Neurology. 2004;62:275–80.
81. Morris MC, Evans DA, Bienias JL, et al. Consumption of fish and $n-3$ fatty acids and risk of incident Alzheimer disease. Arch Neurol. 2003;60:940–6.
82. Malyshev IYu, Manukhina EB. Stress, adaptation and nitric oxide. In: Pandolf BB, Takeda N, Singal PK, editors. Adaptation biology and medicine. New Delhi: Narosa Publ House; 1999. p. 375–92.

83. Meerson FZ. Essentials of adaptive medicine: protective effects of adaptation. Moscow: Hypoxia Medical Ltd.; 1994.
84. Esposito E, Cuzzocrea S. New therapeutic strategy for Parkinson's and Alzheimer's disease. Curr Med Chem. 2010;17:2764–74.
85. Ball LJ, Birge SJ. Prevention of brain aging and dementia. Clin Geriatr Med. 2002;18:485–503.
86. Heininger K. A unifying hypothesis of Alzheimer's disease. IV. Causation and sequence of events. Rev Neurosci. 2000;11:213–328.
87. Halagappa VK, Guo Z, Pearson M, et al. Intermittent fasting and caloric restriction ameliorate age-related behavioral deficits in the triple-transgenic mouse model of Alzheimer's disease. Neurobiol Dis. 2007;26:212–20.
88. Qin W, Chachich M, Lane M, et al. Calorie restriction attenuates Alzheimer's disease type brain amyloidosis in Squirrel monkeys (*Saimiri sciureus*). J Alzheimers Dis. 2006;10:417–22.
89. Mattson MP. Neuroprotective signaling and the aging brain: take away my food and let me run. Brain Res. 2000;886:47–53.
90. Hendrie HC, Ogunniyi A, Hall KS, et al. Incidence of dementia and Alzheimer disease in 2 communities – Yoruba residing in Ibadan, Nigeria, and African Americans residing in Indianapolis, Indiana. JAMA. 2001;285:739–74.
91. Luchsinger JA, Tang MX, Shea S, et al. Caloric intake and the risk of Alzheimer disease. Arch Neurol. 2002;59:1258–63.
92. Féart C, Samieri C, Rondeau V, et al. Adherence to a Mediterranean diet, cognitive decline, and risk of dementia. JAMA. 2009; 302:638–48.
93. Scarmeas N, Luchsinger JA, Schupf N, et al. Physical activity, diet, and risk of Alzheimer disease. JAMA. 2009;302:627–37.
94. Moceri VM, Kukull WA, Emanuel I, et al. Early-life risk factors and the development of Alzheimer's disease. Neurology. 2000; 554:415–20.
95. Willis SL, Tennstedt SL, Marsiske M, et al. Long-term effects of cognitive training on everyday functional outcomes in older adults. JAMA. 2006;296:2805–14.
96. Buschert V, Bokde AL, Hampel H. Cognitive intervention in Alzheimer disease. Nat Rev Neurol. 2010;6:508–17.
97. Addae JI, Youssef FF, Stone TW. Neuroprotective role of learning in dementia: a biological explanation. J Alzheimers Dis. 2003; 5:91–104.
98. Mahendra N, Arkin S. Effects of four years of exercise, language, and social interventions on Alzheimer discourse. J Commun Disord. 2003;36:395–422.
99. Teri L, Gibbons LE, McCurry SM, et al. Exercise plus behavioral management in patients with Alzheimer disease: a randomized controlled trial. JAMA. 2003;290:2015–22.
100. Laurin D, Verreault R, Lindsay J, et al. Physical activity and risk of cognitive impairment and dementia in elderly persons. Arch Neurol. 2001;58:498–504.
101. Lautenschlager NT, Cox KL, Flicker L, et al. Effect of physical activity on cognitive function in older adults at risk for Alzheimer disease: a randomized trial. JAMA. 2008;300:1027–37.
102. Malouf R, Birks J. Donepezil for vascular cognitive impairment. Cochrane Database Syst Rev. 2004;1:CD004395.
103. Swaab DF, Dubelaar EJ, Scherder EJ, et al. Therapeutic strategies for Alzheimer disease: focus on neuronal reactivation of metabolically impaired neurons. Alzheimer Dis Assoc Disord. 2003; 17:S114–22.
104. Song Y, Dowling GA, Wallhagen MI, et al. Sleep in older adults with Alzheimer's disease. J Neurosci Nurs. 2010;42:190–8.
105. Zhu LL, Wang X, Wang X-M, et al. Effects of intermittent hypoxia on neurogenesis in the adult and parkinsonian rat. In: Xi L, Serebrovskaya TV, editors. Intermittent hypoxia: from molecular mechanisms to clinical applications. New York: Nova Science Publ., Inc.; 2009. p. 329–43.
106. Zhu XH, Yan HC, Zhang J, et al. Intermittent hypoxia promotes hippocampal neurogenesis and produces antidepressant-like effects in adult rats. J Neurosci. 2010;30:12653–63.
107. Meerson FZ, Pinelis VG, Koshelev VB, et al. Adaptation to periodic hypoxia restricts subdural hemorrhages in audiogenic epileptiform convulsions in rats. Biull Eksp Biol Med. 1993;116:572–4 [In Russian].
108. Meerson FZ. Adaptation, stress and prophylaxis. Berlin: Springer; 1984.
109. Jung ME, Simpkins JW, Wilson AM, et al. Intermittent hypoxia conditioning prevents behavioral deficit and brain oxidative stress in ethanol-withdrawn rats. J Appl Physiol. 2008;105:510–7.
110. Bernaudin M, Nedelec AS, Divoux D, et al. Normobaric hypoxia induces tolerance to focal permanent cerebral ischemia in association with an increased expression of hypoxia-inducible factor-1 and its target genes, erythropoietin and VEGF, in the adult mouse brain. J Cereb Blood Flow Metab. 2002;22:393–403.
111. Prass K, Scharff A, Ruscher K, et al. Hypoxia-induced stroke tolerance in the mouse is mediated by erythropoietin. Stroke. 2003;34:1981–6.
112. Sharp FR, Ran R, Lu A, et al. Hypoxic preconditioning protects against ischemic brain injury. NeuroRx. 2004;1:26–35.
113. Lin AMY. Hypoxic preconditioning protects against oxidative injury in the central nervous system. In: Xi L, Serebrovskaya TV, editors. Intermittent hypoxia: from molecular mechanisms to clinical applications. New York: Nova Science Publ., Inc.; 2009. p. 313–27.
114. Gulyaeva NV, Stepanichev MV, Onifriev MV, et al. Interval hypoxia training prevents oxidative stress in striatum and locomotor disturbances in a rat model of Parkinsonism. In: Fisher A, Hanln I, Yoshida M, editors. Progress in Alzheimer's and Parkinson's diseases. New York: Plenum Press; 1998. p. 717–23.
115. Kolesnikova EE, Serebrovskaya TV. Parkinson's disease and intermittent hypoxia training. In: Xi L, Serebrovskaya TV, editors. Intermittent hypoxia: from molecular mechanisms to clinical applications. New York: Nova Science Publ., Inc.; 2009. p. 549–60.
116. Gutsaeva DR, Carraway MS, Suliman HB, et al. Transient hypoxia stimulates mitochondrial biogenesis in brain subcortex by a neuronal nitric oxide synthase-dependent mechanism. J Neurosci. 2008;28:2015–24.
117. Lukyanova LD. Novel approach to the understanding of molecular mechanisms of adaptation to hypoxia. In: Hargens A, Takeda N, Singal PK, editors. Adaptation biology and medicine. New Delhi: Narosa Publ.; 2005. p. 1–19.
118. Sazontova TG, Arkhipenko YuV. Membranoprotective effects of adaptation in the heart and skeletal muscles. In: Hargens A, Takeda N, Signal PK, editors. Adaptation biology and medicine. New Delhi: Narosa Publ.; 2005. p. 112–23.
119. Arkhipenko IuV, Sazontova TG, Rozhitskaia II, et al. Effects of adaptation to periodic hypoxia on Ca^{2+} pump of the cardiac sarcoplasmic reticulum and its resistance to endogenous damaging factors. Kardiologiia. 1992;32:57–61 [In Russian].
120. Manukhina EB, Downey HF, Mallet RT. Role of nitric oxide in cardiovascular adaptation to intermittent hypoxia. Exp Biol Med. 2006;231:343–65.
121. Xu KY, Kuppusamy SP, Wang JQ, et al. Nitric oxide protects cardiac sarcolemmal membrane enzyme function and ion active transport against ischemia-induced inactivation. J Biol Chem. 2003;278:41798–803.
122. Correia SC, Moreira PI. Hypoxia-inducible factor 1: a new hope to counteract neurodegeneration? J Neurochem. 2010;112:1–12.
123. Lukyanova LD, Dudchenko AV, Germanova EL, et al. Mitochondrial signaling in formation of body resistance to hypoxia. In: Xi L, Serebrovskaya TV, editors. Intermittent hypoxia: from molecular mechanisms to clinical applications. New York: Nova Science Publ., Inc.; 2009. p. 391–417.
124. Heidbreder M, Frolich F, Johren O, et al. Hypoxia rapidly activates HIF-3α mRNA expression. FASEB J. 2003;10:1096–115.

125. Sazontova TG, Arkhipenko YuV. Intermittent hypoxia in resistance of cardiac membrane structures: role of reactive oxygen species and redox signaling. In: Xi L, Serebrovskaya TV, editors. Intermittent hypoxia: from molecular mechanisms to clinical applications. New York: Nova Science Publ., Inc.; 2009. p. 113–50.
126. Soucek T, Cumming R, Dargusch R, et al. The regulation of glucose metabolism by HIF-1 mediates a neuroprotective response to amyloid beta peptide. Neuron. 2003;39:43–56.
127. Wakutani Y, Urakami K, Shimomura T, et al. Heat shock protein 70 mRNA levels in mononuclear blood cells from patients with dementia of the Alzheimer type. Dementia. 1995;6:301–5.
128. Behl C, Schubert D. Heat shock partially protects rat pheochromocytoma PC12 cells from amyloid beta peptide toxicity. Neurosci Lett. 1993;154:1–4.
129. Yao S, Peng M, Zhu X, et al. Heat shock protein 72 protects hippocampal neurons from apoptosis induced by chronic psychological stress. Int J Neurosci. 2007;117:1551–64.
130. Brown IR. Heat shock proteins and protection of the nervous system. Ann N Y Acad Sci. 2007;1113:147–58.
131. Malyshev IY, Wiegant FA, Mashina SY, et al. Possible use of adaptation to hypoxia in Alzheimer's disease: a hypothesis. Med Sci Monit. 2005;11:HY31–8.
132. Malyshev IYu, Manukhina EB. Stress proteins in Alzheimer's disease. Vestn Ross Akad Med Nauk. 2005;7:40–6 [In Russian].
133. Malyshev IY, Zenina TA, Golubeva LY, et al. NO-dependent mechanisms of adaptation to hypoxia. Nitric Oxide. 1999; 3:105–13.
134. Goryacheva AV, Kruglov SV, Pshennikova MG, et al. Adaptation to intermittent hypoxia restricts nitric oxide overproduction and prevents beta-amyloid toxicity in rat brain. Nitric Oxide. 2010;23:289–99.
135. Belykh AG, Gukasov VM, Chukaev SA. State of the free-radical oxidation system in normobaric hypoxia. Fiziol Zhurnal. 1992; 38:73–6 [In Russian].
136. Manukhina EB, Pshennikova MG, Goryacheva AV, et al. Role of nitric oxide in prevention of cognitive disorders in neurodegenerative brain injuries in rats. Bull Exp Biol Med. 2008;146:391–5.
137. Manukhina EB, Goryacheva AV, Barskov IV, et al. Prevention of neurodegenerative damage to the brain in rats in experimental Alzheimer's disease by adaptation to hypoxia. Neurosci Behav Physiol. 2010;40:737–43.
138. Asha Devi S, Subramanyam MV, Vani R, et al. Adaptations of the antioxidant system in erythrocytes of trained adult rats: impact of intermittent hypobaric-hypoxia at two altitudes. Comp Biochem Physiol C Toxicol Pharmacol. 2005;140:59–67.
139. El'chaninova SA, Koreniak NA, Smagina IV, et al. Intermittent hypoxia in the treatment of dyscirculatory encephalopathy. Zh Nevrol Psikhiatr Im SS Korsakova. 2002;102:29–32 [In Russian].
140. Cardinali DP, Brusco LI, Liberczuk C, et al. The use of melatonin in Alzheimer's disease. Neuro Endocrinol Lett. 2002;1(suppl):20–3.
141. Sánchez-Barceló EJ, Mediavilla MD, Tan DX, et al. Clinical uses of melatonin: evaluation of human trials. Curr Med Chem. 2010;17:2070–95.
142. Reiter RJ, Cabrera J, Sainz RM, et al. Melatonin as a pharmacological agent against neuronal loss in experimental models of Huntington's disease, Alzheimer's disease and Parkinsonism. Ann N Y Acad Sci. 1999;890:471–85.
143. Pappolla MA, Sos M, Omar RA, et al. The heat shock/oxidative stress connection. Relevance to Alzheimer disease. Mol Chem Neuropathol. 1996;28:21–34.
144. Wang X. The antiapoptotic activity of melatonin in neurodegenerative diseases. CNS Neurosci Ther. 2009;15:345–57.
145. Kaur C, Srinivasan KN, Singh J, et al. Plasma melatonin, pinealocyte morphology, and surface receptors/antigen expression on macrophages/microglia in the pineal gland following a high-altitude exposure. J Neurosci Res. 2002;67:533–43.
146. LaManna JC, Chavez JC, Pichiule P. Structural and functional adaptation to hypoxia in the rat brain. J Exp Biol. 2004;207:3163–9.
147. Turek Z, Hoofd L, Rakusan K. Myocardial capillaries and tissue oxygenation. Can J Cardiol. 1986;2:98–103.
148. Wagner PD. Skeletal muscle angiogenesis. A possible role for hypoxia. Adv Exp Med Biol. 2001;502:21–38.
149. Lauro KL, LaManna JC. Adequacy of cerebral vascular remodeling following three weeks of hypobaric hypoxia. Examined by an integrated composite analytical model. Adv Exp Med Biol. 1997;411:369–76.
150. Harik N, Harik SI, Kuo N-T, et al. Time course and reversibility of the hypoxia-induced alterations in cerebral vascularity and cerebral capillary glucose transporter density. Brain Res. 1996;737: 335–8.
151. Harik SI, Hritz MA, LaManna JC. Hypoxia-induced brain angiogenesis in the adult rat. J Physiol (Lond). 1995;485:525–30.
152. Boero JA, Ascher J, Arregui A, et al. Increased brain capillaries in chronic hypoxia. J Appl Physiol. 1999;86:1211–9.
153. Bell RD, Zlokovic BV. Neurovascular mechanisms and blood-brain barrier disorder in Alzheimer's disease. Acta Neuropathol. 2009;118:103–13.
154. Brown WR, Moody DM, Thore CR, et al. Microvascular changes in the white mater in dementia. J Neurol Sci. 2009;283:28–31.
155. Farkas E, De Jong GI, Apró E, et al. Similar ultrastructural breakdown of cerebrocortical capillaries in Alzheimer's disease, Parkinson's disease, and experimental hypertension. Ann N Y Acad Sci. 2000;903:72–82.
156. Hanyu H, Sato T, Hirao K, et al. The progression of cognitive deterioration and region al cerebral blood flow patterns in Alzheimer's disease: a longitudinal SPECT study. J Neurol Sci. 2010;290:96–101.
157. Fischer VW, Siddiqi A, Yusufaly Y. Altered angioarchitecture in selected areas of brains with Alzheimer's disease. Acta Neuropathol. 1990;79:672–9.
158. Chávez JC, Agani F, Pichiule P, et al. Expression of hypoxic inducible factor 1alpha in the brain of rats during chronic hypoxia. J Appl Physiol. 2000;89:1937–42.
159. Pichiule P, LaManna JC. Angiopoietin-2 and rat brain capillary remodeling during adaptation and deadaptation to prolonged mild hypoxia. J Appl Physiol. 2002;93:1131–9.
160. Black JE, Polinsky M, Greenough WT. Progressive failure of cerebral angiogenesis supporting neural plasticity in aging rats. Neurobiol Aging. 1989;10:353–8.
161. Rivard A, Fabre JE, Silver M, et al. Age-dependent impairment of angiogenesis. Circulation. 1999;99:111–20.
162. Brown WR, Thore CR. Review: cerebral microvascular pathology in aging and neurodegeneration. Neuropathol Appl Neurobiol. 2011;37:56–74.
163. Rivard A, Berthou-Soulie L, Principe N, et al. Age-dependent defect in vascular endothelial growth factor expression is associated with reduced hypoxia-inducible factor 1 activity. J Biol Chem. 2000;275:29643–7.
164. Rapino C, Bianchi G, Di Giulio GC, et al. HIF-1alpha cytoplasmic accumulation is associated with cell death in old rat cerebral cortex exposed to intermittent hypoxia. Aging Cell. 2005;4:177–85.
165. Manukhina EB, Sokolova IA, Rodionov IM. Changes in density of the vascular network on brain surface in rats in experiments hypertension and adaptation to high altitude. Kardiologiya. 1982;10:1982 [In Russian].
166. Prewitt RL, Cardoso SS, Wood WB. Prevention of arteriolar rarefaction in the spontaneously hypertensive rat by exposure to simulated high altitude. J Hypertens. 1986;4:735–40.
167. LaManna JC, Vendel LM, Farrell RM. Brain adaptation to chronic hypobaric hypoxia in rats. J Appl Physiol. 1992;72:2238–43.
168. Calabrese V, Boyd-Kimball D, Scapagnini G, et al. Nitric oxide and cellular stress response in brain aging and neurodegenerative disorders: the role of vitagenes. In Vivo. 2004;18:245–67.

169. Takahashi K, Hara E, Suzuki H, et al. Expression of heme oxygenase isozyme mRNAs in the human brains and induction of heme oxygenase-1 by nitric oxide donors. J Neurochem. 1996;67:482–9.
170. Kurauchi Y, Hisatsune A, Isohama Y, et al. Nitric oxide-cyclic GMP signaling pathway limits inflammatory degeneration of midbrain dopaminergic neurons: cell type-specific regulation of heme oxygenase-1 expression. Neuroscience. 2009;158:856–66.
171. McCarty MF. Vascular nitric oxide may lessen Alzheimer's risk. Med Hypotheses. 1998;51:465–76.
172. Cellermajer DS. Endothelial dysfunction: does it matter? Is it reversible? J Am Coll Cardiol. 1997;30:325–53.
173. Pedrazachaverri J, Tapia E, Medinacampos ON, et al. Garlic prevents hypertension induced by chronic inhibition of nitric oxide synthesis. Life Sci. 1998;62:PL71–7.
174. Manukhina EB, Malyshev IYu. Role of nitric oxide in protective effects of adaptation. In: Moravec J, Takeda N, Singal PK, editors. Adaptation biology and medicine. New Delhi: Narosa Publishing House; 2002. p. 312–27.
175. Lange-Asschenfeldt C, Kojda G. Alzheimer's disease, cerebrovascular dysfunction and the benefits of exercise: from vessels to neurons. Exp Gerontol. 2008;43:499–504.
176. Chung KKK, David KK. Emerging roles of nitric oxide in neurodegeneration. Nitric Oxide. 2010;22:290–5.
177. Ghosh C, Lahiri DK. Increased vulnerability of neuronal cell lines to sodium nitroprusside-mediated toxicity is caused by the decreased level of nitric oxide metabolites. J Mol Neurosci. 1999;13:77–92.
178. Wilcock DM, Lewis MR, Van Nostrand WE, et al. Progression of amyloid pathology to Alzheimer's disease pathology in an amyloid precursor protein transgenic mouse model by removal of nitric oxide synthase 2. J Neurosci. 2008;28:1537–45.
179. Tarkowski E, Ringqvist A, Blennow K, et al. Intrathecal release of nitric oxide in Alzheimer's disease and vascular dementia. Dement Geriatr Cogn Disord. 2000;11:322–6.
180. Pshennikova MG, Popkova EV, Khomenko IP, et al. Resistance to neurodegenerative brain damage in August and Wistar rats. Bull Exp Biol Med. 2005;139:540–2.
181. Pshennikova MG, Popkova EV, Pokidyshev DA, et al. The effects of adaptation to hypoxia on the resistance to neurodegenerative disorders in the brain of rats of different genetic strains. Vestn Ross Akad Med Nauk. 2007;2:50–5 [In Russian].
182. Manukhina EB, Goryacheva AV, Barskov IV, et al. Nitric oxide prevents cognitive disorders and neurodegeneration in rats with experimental Alzheimer's disease. FASEB J. 2010;24:568.4.
183. Mikoyan VD, Kubrina LN, Manukhina EB, et al. Differential stimulation of NO synthesis by heat shock in rats of genetically different populations. Bull Exp Biol Med. 1996;6:634–7 [In Russian].
184. Niwa K, Kazama K, Younkin L, et al. Cerebrovascular autoregulation is profoundly impaired in mice overexpressing amyloid precursor protein. Am J Physiol. 2002;283:H315–23.
185. Bartenstein P, Minoshima S, Hirsch C, et al. Quantitative assessment of cerebral blood flow in patients with Alzheimer's disease by SPECT. J Nucl Med. 1997;38:1095–101.
186. Zhang F, Eckman C, Younkin S, et al. Increased susceptibility to ischemic brain damage in transgenic mice overexpressing the amyloid precursor protein. J Neurosci. 1997;17:7655–61.
187. Mashina SY, Aleksandrin VV, Goryacheva AV, et al. Adaptation to hypoxia prevents disturbances in cerebral blood flow during neurodegenerative process. Bull Exp Biol Med. 2006;142:169–72.
188. Dede DS, Yavuz B, Yavuz BB, et al. Assessment of endothelial function in Alzheimer's disease: is Alzheimer's disease a vascular disease? J Am Geriatr Soc. 2007;55:1613–7.
189. Manukhina EB, Vanin AF, Malyshev IYu, et al. Intermittent hypoxia-induced cardio- and vasoprotection: role of NO stores. In: Xi L, Serebrovskaya TV, editors. Intermittent hypoxia: from molecular mechanisms to clinical applications. New York: Nova Science Publ., Inc.; 2009. p. 113–46.
190. Vlasova MA, Vanin AF, Muller B, et al. Detection and description of various stores of nitric oxide store in vascular wall. Bull Exp Biol Med. 2003;136:226–30.
191. Manukhina EB, Malyshev IYu, Smirin BV, et al. Production and storage of nitric oxide in adaptation to hypoxia. Nitric Oxide. 1999;3:393–401.
192. Vlasova MA, Smirin BV, Pokidyshev DA, et al. Mechanism of adaptation of the vascular system to chronic changes in nitric oxide level in the organism. Bull Exp Biol Med. 2006;142:670–4.
193. Wallace MN, Geddes JG, Farquhar DA, et al. Nitric oxide synthase in reactive astrocytes adjacent to β-amyloid plaques. Exp Neurol. 1997;144:266–72.
194. de la Monte SM, Lu BX, Sohn YK, et al. Aberrant expression of nitric oxide synthase III in Alzheimer's disease: relevance to cerebral vasculopathy and neurodegeneration. Neurobiol Aging. 2000;21:309–19.
195. Lüth HJ, Holzer M, Gärtner U, et al. Expression of endothelial and inducible NOS-isoforms is increased in Alzheimer's disease, in APP23 transgenic mice and after experimental brain lesion in rat: evidence for an induction by amyloid pathology. Brain Res. 2001;913:57–67.
196. Gabbott PL, Bacon SJ. Localisation of NADPH diaphorase activity and NOS immunoreactivity in astroglia in normal adult rat brain. Brain Res. 1996;714:135–44.
197. Förstermann U, Kleinert H. Nitric oxide synthase expression and expressional control of the three isoforms. Naunyn Schmiedebergs Arch Pharmacol. 1995;352:351–64.
198. Aguilera P, Chánez-Cárdenas ME, Floriano-Sánchez E, et al. Time-related changes in constitutive and inducible nitric oxide synthases in the rat striatum in a model of Huntington's disease. Neurotoxicology. 2007;28:1200–7.
199. Fernández-Vizarra P, Fernández AP, Castro-Blanco S, et al. Expression of nitric oxide system in clinically evaluated cases of Alzheimer's disease. Neurobiol Dis. 2004;15:287–305.
200. Lüth HJ, Münch G, Arendt T. Aberrant expression of NOS isoforms in Alzheimer's disease is structurally related to nitrotyrosine formation. Brain Res. 2002;953:135–43.
201. Smith MA, Richey Harris PL, Sayre LM, et al. Widespread peroxynitrite-mediated damage in Alzheimer's disease. J Neurosci. 1997;17:2653–7.

Neuroprotective Mechanisms of Intermittent Hypoxia: An In Vitro Study

14

Galina Skibo, Maxim Orlovsky, Anastasiia Maistrenko, Victor Dosenko, and Iryna Lushnikova

Abstract
It is well known that brief sublethal anoxia episodes can render neurons resistant against subsequent longer or more severe anoxia and ischemia. The progress in applications of hypoxia in medicine is largely dependent on availability of appropriate experimental models. In this chapter, we describe an in vitro model for anoxia investigations using organotypic-cultured hippocampal slices. We investigate the efficiency of different regimes of anoxia preconditioning. We also describe a new single-cell real-time RT-PCR method for analyzing individual neurons within cultured hippocampal slices. This approach allows investigation of short-term neuronal reactions on anoxia preconditioning and oxygen-glucose deprivation – an experimental model of ischemic brain damage. Using these methods, we demonstrated that hypoxia-inducible factors (HIF), a family of transcription regulators, are involved in the mechanisms of anoxia-induced neuroprotection in hippocampus. In particular, brief intermittent anoxia prevented the decrease in HIF-1 mRNA expression caused by severe oxygen-glucose deprivation, which is closely correlated with its neuroprotective action. Possible mechanisms of such endogenous neuroprotective effect are discussed.

Abbreviations

APC	Anoxia preconditioning
HBSS	Hanks' balanced salt solution
HIF	Hypoxia-inducible factor
OGD	Oxygen-glucose deprivation
PI	Propidium iodide

G. Skibo (✉) • M. Orlovsky • A. Maistrenko • I. Lushnikova
Department of Cytology,
State Key Laboratory of Molecular and Cellular Biology,
Bogomoletz Institute of Physiology,
National Academy of Sciences, Kiev,
Ukraine
e-mail: skibo@biph.kiev.ua

V. Dosenko
Department of General Pathophysiology,
State Key Laboratory of Molecular and Cellular Biology,
Bogomoletz Institute of Physiology,
National Academy of Sciences,
Kiev, Ukraine

14.1 Introduction

The protective action of mild hypoxia environments was shown for the first time in 1950s by a famous Russian physiologist and pathologist Felix Meerson (see [1] for review). His observations were lately confirmed by Kitagawa in 1990, who had described increased resistance to the prolonged ischemia induced in hippocampus by exposition to a short-term hypoxia [2]. Furthermore, potentiation of this effect was observed if the applied hypoxia was intermittent. Later on, the adaptive action of hypoxic preconditioning is proved in clinical observations [3, 4] as well as in vitro experiments [5].

In the present time, intermittent hypoxia and anoxia in the forms of ischemic preconditioning and postconditioning are known and proven to increase neuronal resistance to ischemia (see [6–8] for reviews). Hypoxic preconditioning with brief exposures to hypoxia environment is able to significantly decrease brain damage following ischemic stroke, as well as improve resistance to transient ischemic attacks. Research on

L. Xi, T.V. Serebrovskaya (eds.), *Intermittent Hypoxia and Human Diseases*,
DOI 10.1007/978-1-4471-2906-6_14, © Springer-Verlag London 2012

preconditioning has resulted in various promising strategies for the treatment of patients with acute brain injury [7].

14.2 An In Vitro Model of Anoxia Preconditioning

Notwithstanding the vast amount of evidence for the neuroprotective action of hypoxic environments, the mechanisms of such neuroprotection are still not clear. The progress on applications of hypoxic environments in medicine is largely dependent on availability of appropriate experimental models to delineate the mechanisms of action. There are several in vitro systems to study brain cell damage resulting from various pathologic conditions, including acute brain slices, dissociated cell cultures, and organotypic slice cultures. The latter offers several advantages since it allows preservation of the native hippocampal organization, neuronal networks, and synaptic contacts [9–11]. This makes slice culture an appropriate model for studies on brain ischemic damage and mechanisms of hypoxia/anoxia preconditioning.

14.2.1 Model of Organotypic Hippocampal Slices

In our work, organotypic hippocampal slice cultures were prepared according to Stoppini et al. [10]. Seven-day-old Wistar rat pups were decapitated, and brains were quickly removed into ice-cold dissection medium (50% of minimal essential medium (MEM), 5 mM Tris, 2 mM $NaHCO_3$, 12.5 mM HEPES, 15 mM glucose, 25% Hanks' balanced salt solution (HBSS), 100 units/ml penicillin, and 100 mg/ml streptomycin, pH 7.3). Then, 350–400-μm-thick transversal slices were prepared from the middle third of isolated hippocampi using tissue chopper (McIllwain, UK). Slices were put on porous Millicell membrane inserts (Millicell, Bedford, USA) and placed in plates (Nunc, Denmark) with 1 ml culture medium per well (50% of MEM, 25% horse serum, 2.5 mM Tris, 2 mM $NaHCO_3$, 12.5 mM HEPES, 15 mM glucose, 25% HBSS, 100 units/ml penicillin, and 100 mg/ml streptomycin, pH 7.2). Slices were kept at 35°C in 5% CO_2 atm. Medium was changed twice a week starting from the next day of the slices preparation. All experiments were performed on 12-day-old cultures.

14.2.2 Modeling Anoxia Preconditioning and Ischemia

To model intermittent hypoxia, we have used repeated brief exposures of cultured hippocampal slices to anoxic environment. This procedure is well known from the literature as anoxia preconditioning (APC). APC was carried out in a thermostatically controlled chamber (35°C) that was filled with 95% N_2 and 5% CO_2. The slices were placed into Petri dish with 1 ml culture medium and put into chamber. Slices were exposed to APC from 1 to 3 times for 2 or 5 min (depending on the experimental group) with 12-h intervals between exposures and returned to normal incubating conditions thereafter. The optimal protocol of APC was selected empirically by observing the results of PI staining in different time series. Oxygen-glucose deprivation (OGD) in APC + OGD experiments was carried out 12 h following the last APC exposure.

As a model of ischemic neuronal damage, we have used OGD for 30 min. OGD is one of the most common approaches to produce the ischemic damage in experimental conditions [12–14]. OGD is also a well established in vitro model for investigating molecular and cellular events in ischemic damage. At least 30-min long, OGD was shown to be sufficient for ischemia-like neuronal death in cultured hippocampal slices [15]. It is generally assumed that long-term OGD induces significant neuronal damage while brief OGD episodes are less destructive.

The OGD procedure was described in details in our previous works [12–14]. Briefly, hippocampal slices were washed three times with deoxygenated glucose- and serum-free artificial cerebrospinal fluid medium (ACSF, pH 7.4, containing NaCl 124 mM, KCl 1.6 mM, $NaHCO_3$ 24 mM, KH_2PO_4 1.2 mM, ascorbic acid 2 mM, $CaCl_2$ 2.5 mM, $MgCl_2$ 1.5 mM, sucrose 10 mM instead of glucose). Then, the slices were placed into a thermostatically controlled chamber (35°C) and exposed to 95% N_2 and 5% CO_2 for 30 min. The slices thereafter were returned to the normal incubating conditions. Control slices were incubated by the same procedure using glucose-containing ACSF in the same incubating environment.

14.3 Comparing the Efficiency of Different Anoxia Preconditioning Regimes

14.3.1 Design of the Experiments

To find out the most efficient regime of intermittent anoxia in terms of minimal of neuronal damage and maximal effect of preconditioned neuroprotection by APC, we have used two durations of anoxia exposure: 2 and 5 min. Anoxia was applied in a consequent manner from 1 to 3 times with 12-h interval between the exposures (for details, please refer to the previous section). Neuronal damage was analyzed 4 h after the last APC or OGD episode using propidium iodide (PI) cellular uptake according to the established procedure [12–14]. PI is a stable nontoxic fluorescent dye entering cells through the damaged plasma membrane that interacts with DNA yielding a bright red fluorescence [14, 16, 17].

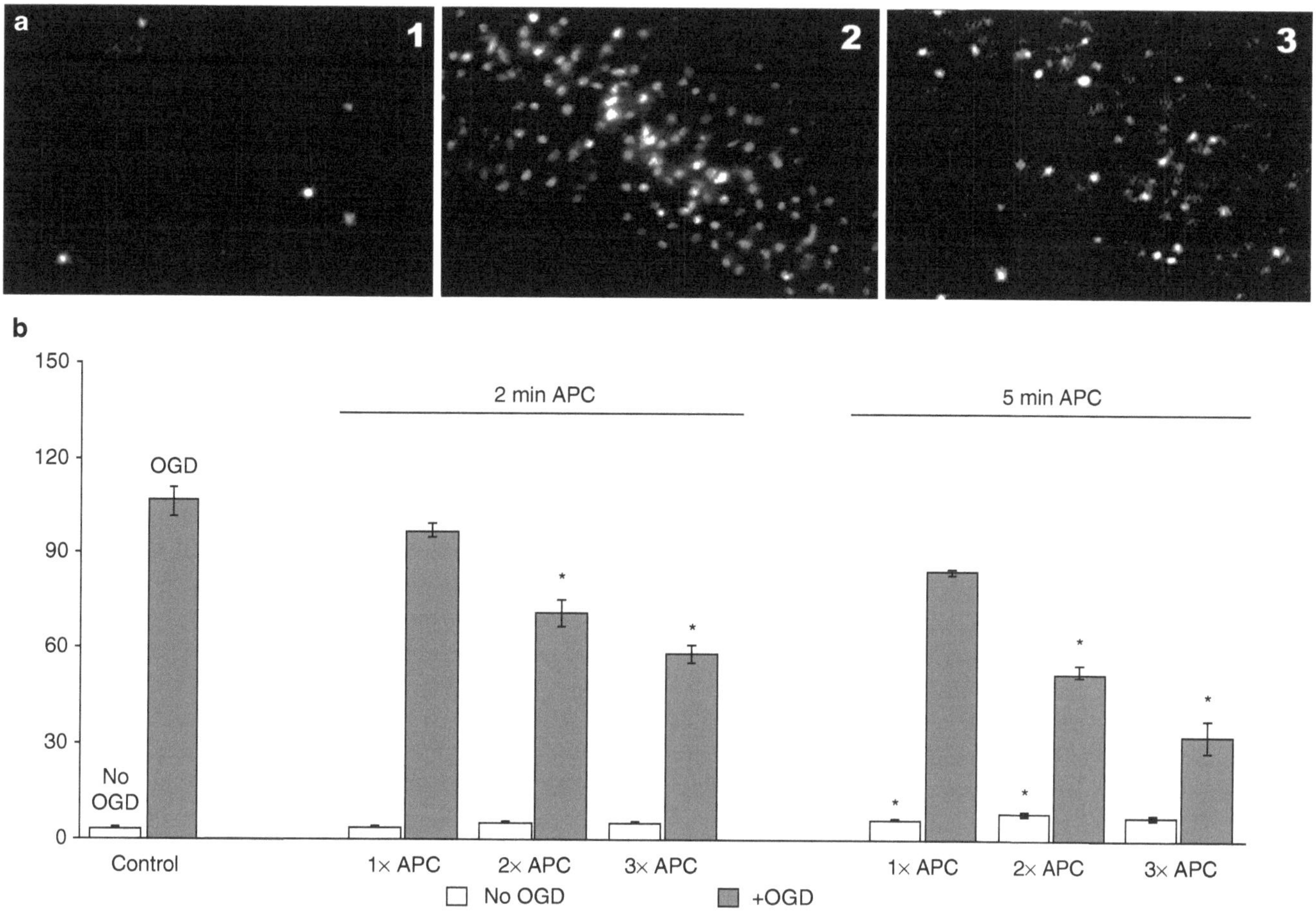

Fig. 14.1 Neuronal damage (indicated by the amount of propidium iodide-positive cells per mm²) in CA1 area of hippocampus following different regimes of anoxia preconditioning and subsequent test oxygen-glucose deprivation (OGD) exposure: (**a**) Images of PI-labeled slices: 1 – Control untreated slices; 2 – OGD applied alone without anoxia preconditioning; 3 – OGD applied following triple 5-min anoxia preconditioning; (**b**) Data on the amount of PI+ cells in experimental series

Two micrometer of PI was added to the culture medium after the experimental treatment for 15–20 min in compliance with the protocol (Fig. 14.1). Samples were analyzed on fluorescent microscope XSP-139A-TP equipped with digital camera Cannon Power Short G-6 (NNJOI Co. Ltd., Japan-China) using excitation wavelength 530 nm. The amount of PI-positive (PI+) cells per 1 μm^2 was calculated in stratum pyramidale of CA1 and CA3 regions.

14.3.2 Neuronal Survival Following Different Regimes of APC

A few sparse cells in CA1 and CA3 cells were found to be PI+ under the control conditions (see Fig. 14.1). OGD applied without preconditioning had dramatically increased this amount; the neuronal damage was significantly more prominent in CA1 (25-fold increase) than in CA3 (12-fold increase). This goes in accord with other findings showing higher ischemia sensitivity of CA1 neurons [18, 19].

APC does not produce significant neuronal loss neither in a single, double, or triple 2-min exposure. At the same time, 5-min single, double, and triple exposure resulted in a slight increase in the amount of PI-positive cells in CA1 area to the level of 6.3 ± 0.7, 8.4 ± 0.9, and 7.4 ± 0.9 per μm^2 correspondingly as compared to 3.1 ± 0.6 per μm^2 in the untreated control group (see Fig. 14.1). However, APC led to a significant and prominent decrease in the number of damaged cells following OGD exposure. This effect linearly increases with each additional anoxia exposure – from a nonsignificant effect for a single exposure to the most prominent effect for the triple exposure. Furthermore, repeated 5-min exposures appeared to be relatively more efficient than the corresponding repeated 2-min exposures. The highest efficiency was demonstrated by triple 5-min APC exposure, as it did not lead to a significant neuronal loss under control conditions and decreased neuronal damage 3-fold followed by OGD. This effect was 1.7 times better than those of triple 2-min APC and 1.5 times better than double 5-min APC. Thus, triple 5-min APC exposure was selected as the best model for further studies of the mechanisms of endogenous neuroprotection.

14.4 Role of Hypoxia-Inducible Factors in Mechanisms of Endogenous Neuroprotection

Generally, data concerning the time frame between application of APC and subsequent formation of ischemic resistance are sparse. Existing reports in this area primarily focused on the facts of inhibition of neuron apoptosis, neurogenesis, or the survival rate of neurons induced by such preconditioning [20]. A number of studies had shown that in many tissues, including brain, the effects of APC are related to the activation of hypoxia-inducible factors (HIF) – the heterodymeric transcription regulators [21–23]. HIF-1, the first investigated member of the family, was shown to increase cell survival by inducing expression of endothelial growth factors, glucose transporters, antioxidant enzymes, heat shock proteins, antiapoptotic genes, and many other [21, 24, 25]. HIF-1 also participates in early brain development and proliferation of neuronal precursor cells [22]. Intracellular quantity of active HIF-1 α/β dimer is dependent on HIF prolyl-hydroxylase activity. This enzyme catalyzes HIF-1α subunit hydroxylation leading to ubiquitin-depending proteasome degradation [26–28]. However, it is still unknown how brain HIF-1 expression reacts on APC and ischemia and whether that changes are important for neuroprotection.

Another member of the HIF family, HIF-3, in cerebellum, corneal epithelium, kidney tissue, and some cell lines can suppress HIF-mediated gene expression and inhibits HIF-1 action by binding its β subunit [25, 29, 30]. Generally, HIF-3 expression is rapidly activated following hypoxia [31], and while this factor is expressed in some brain regions [30, 31], there is no clear indication on its role and possible interference with HIF-1 in hippocampus following hypoxia exposure.

In the present work, we have examined effects of APC, OGD, and their combination on neuronal viability and HIF-1α and HIF-3α mRNA expression, measured using single-cell reverse transcription real-time PCR in CA1 and CA3 neurons. These two regions of hippocampus are known to have difference in ischemia sensitivity [15, 19], which can be partially related to the difference in HIF expression.

14.4.1 Single-Cell qRT-PCR

In order to achieve high data precision on the timeframe following anoxia exposures, we developed a method of CA1 and CA3 stratum pyramidale single-cell microsampling from the cultured hippocampus slices. The samples were subsequently analyzed using quantitative real-time RT-PCR. Since CA1 and CA3 regions are known to have different anoxia sensitivity [18, 19], HIF mRNA expression in the individual neurons was compared between these regions. The single-cell was extracted by micropipette (hole size 10–20 μm) using micromanipulator under light microscope (×200). Then, microprobes were placed into separate vials containing reverse transcription buffer. The buffer was prepared ex tempore by mixing 50 mmol of Tris–HCl (pH 8.3), 50 mmol of KCl, 4 mmil of $MgCl_2$, 40 mmol of ditiotreitol, 40 U of RiboLock, 0.2 μg of random hexamer primer, and 1 mmol each of dNTP. All chemicals were purchased from Fermentas, Lithuania. Samples were kept in the buffer at 4°C for 3–4 h. Subsequently, samples were incubated at 37°C for 2 h with 20 U of M-MuLV reverse transcriptase. The resulting cDNAs was amplified in two rounds in a total volume of 25 μl of a buffer containing 5 μl of 5× buffer with NH3Cl, 2.5 mM $MgSO_4$, 0.5 U Taq polymerase, 200 μM of dNTP mixture (5 pM of each for the first amplification cycle and 20 pM for the second), and a pair of specific primers (Table 14.1).

The first amplification round included 15 cycles and was performed using termocycler GeneAmp System 2700 (Applied Biosystems, USA). The product of the first round was used for quantitative measurements of corresponding mRNA using 7500 Fast Real-time PCR System (Applied Biosystems, USA). Amplification mixture was composed of 10 μl SYBR Green PCR Master Mix (Applied Biosystems, USA) and 30 pM of corresponding specific primers. Before the amplification, DNA-polymerase was preactivated using AmpliTaq applied at 94°C for 10 min. A separate dissociation phase was used to control reaction specificity at the end of the round. Product purity was checked by dissociation curve analysis and confirmed afterward using agarose gel electrophoresis.

Sample mRNA levels were normalized to glyceraldehyde-3-phosphate dehydrogenase (GADPH) mRNA level [31]. No differences between the experimental series in GADPG mRNA expression were found. All samples were analyzed for neuronal-specific enolase (NSE, neuron-specific marker) mRNA expression; samples without NSE (originating from non-neuronal cells) were excluded from the experiments.

14.4.2 Effects of OGD and APC on HIF mRNA Expression

The existing data on HIF mRNA and protein expression under hypoxia and glucose deprivation are controversial. While it was found that ischemia inhibits HIF prolyl-hydroxylase leading to HIF accumulation [28], Ndubuizu et al. recently showed that HIF-1 responses to ischemia are subjected to an age-dependent decline [32]. This effect is caused by an increase in HIF prolyl-hydroxylase activity and is not associated with a changed HIF-1 mRNA expression [32].

Table 14.1 Primer sequences used for single-cell qRT-PCR

Gene	Sequence	PCR product size	Gene bank accession no.
HIF-1α	5′– AGA AAC CGC CTA TGA CGT G –3′ 5′– CCA CCT CTT TTT GCA AGC AT –3′	301	AF057308
HIF-3α	5′– AGA GAA CGG AGT GGT GCT GT –3′ 5′– ATC AGC CGG AAG AGG ACT TT –3′	301	NM022528
β-actin	5′– AAC CCT AAG GCC AAC CGT GAA A –3′ 5′– TCA TGA GGT AGT CTG TCA GGT C –3′	300	81822
Neuron-specific enolase (NSE)	5′– TGT GGT GGA GCA GGA GAA GC –3′ 5′– GAT GCA TCG GGA AGG GTC AG –3′	564	AF019973

It was also established that ischemia leads to the increase in HIF-1α protein levels following hypoxia-ischemia in vivo and in vitro in brain [33, 34]. Regarding hippocampus, it was previously reported that moderate hypoxia in vivo did not affect HIF-1α mRNA levels, but increased HIF-3α mRNA expression in the whole hippocampus at 2 h after exposure [31]. However, no specific studies on HIF mRNA expression in CA1 and CA3 neurons were made under anoxia conditions so far. In our present study, accomplished using single-neuron sampling technology, we observed that OGD decreases HIF-1α mRNA expression only in CA1 but not in CA3 neurons, which suggests the difference in mechanisms of neuroprotection in these two regions.

Our data showed that CA1 neurons had higher HIF-1α mRNA expression than CA3 neurons. We also found that HIF-3α expression was significantly weaker comparing to HIF-1α and did not demonstrate any difference between the areas (0.196 ± 0.009 in CA1 and 0.194 ± 0.005 in CA3; P_{HSD} = 0.842). This is consistent with other studies confirming that HIF-1α mRNA is expressed under normoxic conditions in mouse brain [33] and rat hippocampus [31]. Also, small amount of HIF-1α protein, detectable with Western blotting was constantly presented in rat brain cortex [35]. Heidbreder et al. reported detectable HIF-3α mRNA expression in whole rat hippocampus under normoxic conditions; however, they did not detect any difference between HIF-1α and HIF-3α mRNA amounts [31]. It is established that HIF is expressed not only by in neurons but also by astrocytes, ependymal cells, and endothelium [35]. Thus, the difference between HIF-1α and HIF-3α mRNA expression observed by us can be explained by the neuron-specific single-cell sampling technology used in our work in combination with highly sensitive quantitative real-time PCR.

Neuronal damage produced by OGD (Fig. 14.1) was accompanied by a significant decrease in HIF-1α and HIF-3α mRNA expression in CA1 neurons (Fig. 14.2). HIF-1α mRNA expression in the CA1 area was decreased to 0.237 ± 0.007 per cell (P_{HSD} < 0.001). The OGD action was more prominent for HIF-3α. Following OGD, the level of HIF-3α was reduced from the control 0.196 ± 0.009 down to 0.143 ± 0.010 per cell (P_{HSD} < 0.05). We did not observe any significant changes in HIF-1α and HIF-3α mRNA levels in CA3 neurons.

Triple short-term (5-min) APC did not affect neuronal viability. The amount of PI-positive cells was not significantly increased as compared to control (Fig. 14.3). APC did not produce any significant changes neither in HIF-1α nor HIF-3α mRNA expression in both CA1 and CA3 areas. If APC was followed by OGD, it led to prevention of OGD-induced neuronal death both in CA1 and CA3 regions as compared with those observed after OGD alone (Fig. 14.3). We also found that in CA1 region APC + OGD did not affect intracellular HIF-1α and HIF-3α mRNA, which remained at the comparable levels to the control, although it underwent significant decrease following OGD treatment (Fig. 14.2). In fact, APC followed by OGD did not lead to HIF-1α expression decrease in the CA1 (control 0.268 ± 0.002 vs. 0.255 ± 0.002 per cell; P_{HSD} = 0.423) and the CA3 areas (control 0.196 ± 0.008 vs. 0.183 ± 0.010 per cell; P_{HSD} = 0.082) as well. However, there was an important difference between the groups exposed to OGD with or without APC, i.e., OGD-treated slices had significantly lower HIF-1α expression level than the slices pre-treated with APC (0.237 ± 0.007 vs. 0.255 ± 0.002 per cell; P_{HSD} < 0.01). Similar significant difference was observed between slices exposed to OGD and APC alone, i.e., the former ones had significantly higher HIF-1α expression (0.237 ± 0.007 vs. 0.262 ± 0.008 per cell; P_{HSD} = 0.001).

To a lesser extent, such effects were observed for HIF-3α mRNA expression, which was not affected by APC (P_{HSD} = 0.920) or APC + OGD (P_{HSD} = 0.677), but for anoxia-treated slices, it was significantly higher than for those exposed to OGD (0.214 ± 0.014 vs. 0.143 ± 0.010 per cell; P_{HSD} = 0.025). Thus, we can conclude that APC action to a certain degree could prevent OGD-induced *HIF1A* and *HIF3A* genes suppression.

Li have recently reported that APC comparing to ischemia presents a stronger stimulus for HIF-1α protein expression in brain [36]. However, we did not detect any significant

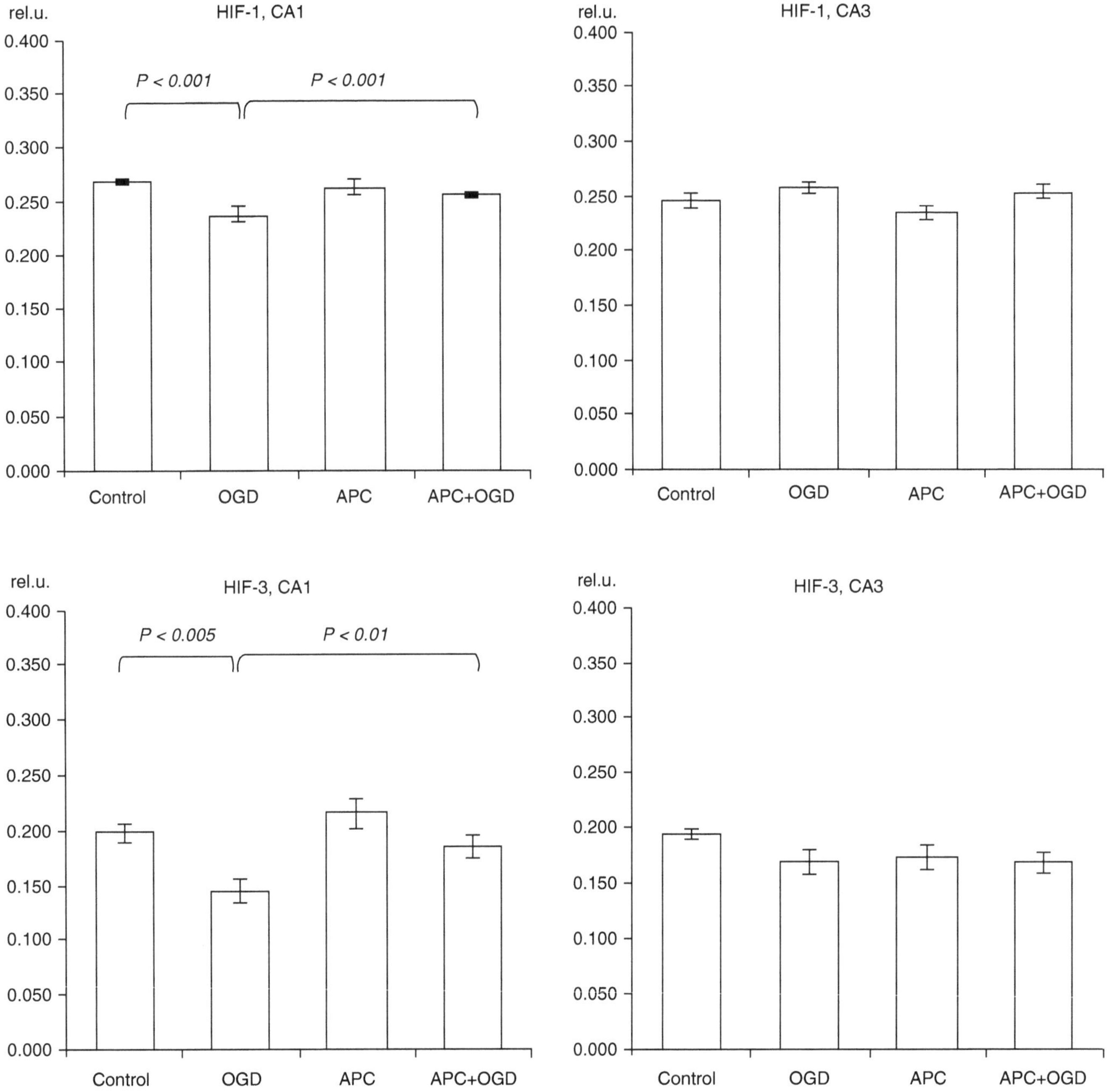

Fig. 14.2 HIF-1α and HIF-3α mRNA transcript expression in individual neurons from CA1 and CA3 areas of cultured hippocampal slices following different experimental procedures

changes in the level of HIF-1α and HIF-3α mRNA transcripts after APC in our experiments. Thus, we can conclude that neuroprotective effect of APC can be, at least in part, explained by the prevention of HIF mRNA suppression. Apparently, mechanisms of APC-induced neuroprotection are rather related to the inhibited HIF protein degradation than increased HIF mRNA expression. One of such mechanisms can be related to HIF prolyl-hydroxylase – an enzyme that is responsible for HIF degeneration under normoxic conditions. It was previously found that HIF prolyl-4-hydroxylase olygopeptide inhibitor given prior to ischemia protects embryonic rat cortical neurons from oxidative stress [28]. The authors had shown that HIF prolyl-hydroxylase inhibitors and RNA interference both protect neurons from normoxic oxidative damage. So while it is clear that prevention of HIF-1α mRNA expression by a triple APC has a strong neuroprotective action, further studies are required to elucidate the exact mechanisms of such action.

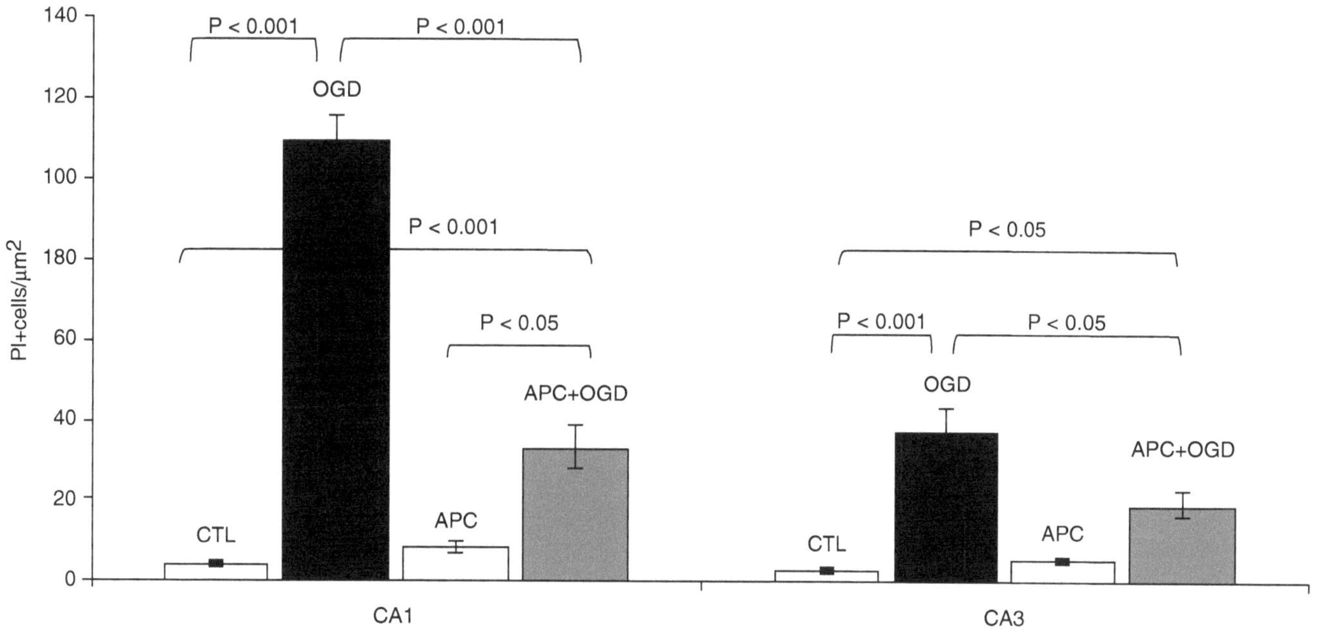

Fig. 14.3 Amount of PI+ cells in CA1 and CA3 areas of cultured hippocampal slices following different experimental exposures

Conclusion

Organotypic hippocampal cultured slices represent a useful model for complex in vitro studies of endogenous neuroprotective mechanisms. Using this model, we have established that triple 5-min intermittent anoxia exposure has a strong neuroprotection action, preventing CA1 and CA3 hippocampal neurons from ischemic death caused by a subsequent oxygen-glucose deprivation. This variant of anoxia preconditioning appears more efficient than single or double anoxia, as well as repeated 2-min intermittent anoxia exposures.

In general, neuronal damage occurring after OGD is more prominent in CA1 region, where it is also accompanied by a significant decrease in HIF-1α and HIF-3α mRNA expression. Intermittent anoxia preconditioning is shown to reduce neuronal damage caused by a subsequent oxygen-glucose deprivation in CA1 and CA3 area and prevent decrease in HIF-1α and HIF-3α mRNA levels in CA1, but not in CA3 area. Thus, HIF-1α and HIF-3α are important factors of anti-ischemic neuroprotection at least in the CA1 area of hippocampus.

Acknowledgment This work was funded by the grant of SFFD 46.2/001.

References

1. Viru A. Early contributions of Russian stress and exercise physiologists. J Appl Physiol. 2002;92:1378–82.
2. Kitagawa K, Matsumoto M, Tagaya M, et al. "Ischemic tolerance" phenomenon found in the brain. Brain Res. 1990;528:21–4.
3. Moncayo J, de Freitas GR, Bogousslavsky J, et al. Do transient ischemic attacks have a neuroprotective effect? Neurology. 2000;54:2089–94.
4. Weih M, Kallenberg K, Bergk A, et al. Attenuated stroke severity after prodromal TIA: a role for ischemic tolerance in the brain? Stroke. 1999;30:1851–4.
5. Sakaki T, Yamada K, Otsuki H, et al. Brief exposure to hypoxia induces bFGF mRNA and protein and protects rat cortical neurons from prolonged hypoxic stress. Neurosci Res. 1995;23:289–96.
6. Schaller B. Endogenous neuroprotection. New York: Nova Publishers; 2008.
7. Dirnagl U, Becker K, Meisel A. Preconditioning and tolerance against cerebral ischaemia: from experimental strategies to clinical use. Lancet Neurol. 2009;8:398–412.
8. Pignataro G, Scorziello A, Di Renzo G, et al. Post-ischemic brain damage: effect of ischemic preconditioning and postconditioning and identification of potential candidates for stroke therapy. FEBS J. 2009; 276:46–57.
9. Lipton P. Ischemic cell death in brain neurons. Physiol Rev. 1999;79:1431–568.
10. Stoppini L, Buchs PA, Muller D. A simple method for organotypic cultures of nervous tissue. J Neurosci Methods. 1991;37:173–82.
11. Buddle M, Eberhardt E, Ciminello LH, et al. Microtubule-associated protein 2 (MAP2) associates with the NMDA receptor and is spatially redistributed within rat hippocampal neurons after oxygen-glucose deprivation. Brain Res. 2003;978:38–50.
12. Lushnikova IV, Voronin KY, Malyarevskyy PY, et al. Morphological and functional changes in rat hippocampal slice cultures after short-term oxygen-glucose deprivation. J Cell Mol Med. 2004;8:241–8.
13. Skibo GG, Lushnikova IV, Voronin KY, et al. A synthetic NCAM-derived peptide, FGL, protects hippocampal neurons from ischemic insult both in vitro and in vivo. Eur J Neurosci. 2005;22:1589–96.
14. Laake JH, Haug FM, Wieloch T. A simple in vitro model of ischemia based on hippocampal slice cultures and propidium iodide fluorescence. Brain Res Brain Res Protoc. 1999;4:173–84.
15. Wilde GJ, Pringle AK, Wright P, et al. Differential vulnerability of the CA1 and CA3 subfields of the hippocampus to superoxide and hydroxyl radicals in vitro. J Neurochem. 1997;69:883–6.

16. Hassen GW, Tian D, Ding D, et al. A new model of ischemic preconditioning using young adult hippocampal slice cultures. Brain Res Brain Res Protoc. 2004;13:135–43.
17. Raval AP, Bramlett H, Perez-Pinzon MA. Estrogen preconditioning protects the hippocampal CA1 against ischemia. Neuroscience. 2006;141:1721–30.
18. Griesemer D, Mautes AM. Closed head injury causes hyperexcitability in rat hippocampal CA1 but not in CA3 pyramidal cells. J Neurotrauma. 2007;24:1823–32.
19. Newrzella D, Pahlavan PS, Kruger C, et al. The functional genome of CA1 and CA3 neurons under native conditions and in response to ischemia. BMC Genomics. 2007;8:370.
20. Zhao T, Zhang CP, Liu ZH, et al. Hypoxia-driven proliferation of embryonic neural stem/progenitor cells–role of hypoxia-inducible transcription factor-1alpha. FEBS J. 2008;275:1824–34.
21. Chang AY, Chan JY, Cheng HL, et al. Hypoxia-inducible factor 1/heme oxygenase 1 cascade as upstream signals in the prolife role of heat shock protein 70 at rostral ventrolateral medulla during experimental brain stem death. Shock. 2009;32:651–8.
22. Fan X, Heijnen CJ, van der Kooij MA, et al. The role and regulation of hypoxia-inducible factor-1alpha expression in brain development and neonatal hypoxic-ischemic brain injury. Brain Res Rev. 2009;62:99–108.
23. Sorond FA, Shaffer ML, Kung AL, et al. Desferroxamine infusion increases cerebral blood flow: a potential association with hypoxia-inducible factor-1. Clin Sci. 2009;116:771–9.
24. Dawn B, Bolli R. HO-1 induction by HIF-1: a new mechanism for delayed cardioprotection? Am J Physiol Heart Circ Physiol. 2005; 289:H522–4.
25. Grimm C, Hermann DM, Bogdanova A, et al. Neuroprotection by hypoxic preconditioning: HIF-1 and erythropoietin protect from retinal degeneration. Semin Cell Dev Biol. 2005;16:531–8.
26. Maxwell PH, Wiesener MS, Chang GW, et al. The tumour suppressor protein VHL targets hypoxia-inducible factors for oxygen-dependent proteolysis. Nature. 1999;399:271–5.
27. Kamura T, Maenaka K, Kotoshiba S, et al. VHL-box and SOCS-box domains determine binding specificity for Cul2-Rbx1 and Cul5-Rbx2 modules of ubiquitin ligases. Genes Dev. 2004;18:3055–65.
28. Siddiq A, Aminova LR, Troy CM, et al. Selective inhibition of hypoxia-inducible factor (HIF) prolyl-hydroxylase 1 mediates neuroprotection against normoxic oxidative death via HIF- and CREB-independent pathways. J Neurosci. 2009;29:8828–38.
29. Hara S, Hamada J, Kobayashi C, et al. Expression and characterization of hypoxia-inducible factor (HIF)-3alpha in human kidney: suppression of HIF-mediated gene expression by HIF-3alpha. Biochem Biophys Res Commun. 2001;287:808–13.
30. Makino Y, Cao R, Svensson K, et al. Inhibitory PAS domain protein is a negative regulator of hypoxia-inducible gene expression. Nature. 2001;414:550–4.
31. Heidbreder M, Frohlich F, Johren O, et al. Hypoxia rapidly activates HIF-3alpha mRNA expression. FASEB J. 2003;17:1541–3.
32. Ndubuizu OI, Chavez JC, LaManna JC. Increased prolyl 4-hydroxylase expression and differential regulation of hypoxia-inducible factors in the aged rat brain. Am J Physiol Regul Integr Comp Physiol. 2009;297:R158–65.
33. Stroka DM, Burkhardt T, Desaillets I, et al. HIF-1 is expressed in normoxic tissue and displays an organ-specific regulation under systemic hypoxia. FASEB J. 2001;15:2445–53.
34. van den Tweel ER, Kavelaars A, Lombardi MS, et al. Bilateral molecular changes in a neonatal rat model of unilateral hypoxic-ischemic brain damage. Pediatr Res. 2006;59:434–9.
35. Chavez JC, Agani F, Pichiule P, et al. Expression of hypoxia-inducible factor-1alpha in the brain of rats during chronic hypoxia. J Appl Physiol. 2000;89:1937–42.
36. Li L, Qu Y, Li J, et al. Relationship between HIF-1alpha expression and neuronal apoptosis in neonatal rats with hypoxia-ischemia brain injury. Brain Res. 2007;1180:133–9.

Part IV

Intermittent Hypoxia and Occupational, Environmental, and Other Disorders

Intermittent Hypoxic Training to Enhance Endurance in Elite Swimmers

15

Nikolai I. Volkov

Abstract

Intermittent hypoxic training (IHT) with normobaric hypoxia has been used as an adjunct method to enhance performance of endurance athletes. Twelve swimmers of high qualification were divided into two groups: control and experimental. The control group was trained with usual capacity using traditional techniques. The experimental group of swimmers underwent the same traditional methods of training combined with different variants of IHT during the recovery periods followed the main physical training loads. "Hypoxicator Everest" (a device jointly developed by the Climbi Ltd. of Russia and the Praxsep Inc. of Canada) was used for generating hypoxic atmosphere with hypoxic gas mixtures (10% or 12% O_2). Each hypoxic exposure was 3–10 min followed by 3–10 min of normoxia period when the athletes breathed regular air. The combined exposure to hypoxia did not exceed 1.5–2 h/day. The adjunct IHT training continued for a period of 3 months. Before and immediately after the end of experiments, the athletes of both groups were tested in standard ergonomic procedures for the maximum of aerobic and anaerobic work capacity. IHT resulted in significant increase in parameters of maximum aerobic capacity for the experimental group: VO_2max increased on average 11% from its pretraining baseline; V_E, 6.4%; W_{cr}, 10.8%; ΔpH, 44.6%; ExcCO_2, 23%, and W_{max}, 9.8%. Results for the control group were significantly lower. According to these findings, the greater improvement in swimming performance was to be expected for athletes in the IHT group in middle distances such as 200, 400, and 800 m. In conclusion, the use of IHT as additional training method for elite swimmers has considerably improved their performance results during a relatively short period of training.

Abbreviation

IHT Interval hypoxic training

15.1 Introduction

The improvement of sports achievements reflects the process of adaptation under the influence of divergent tools and methods used in athletic training. Means and methods used in training of swimmers are differentiated by the direction of physiological influence. Depending upon the chosen characteristics of physical loads, such as type of exercise, its intensity, and duration, recovery breaks, number of repetitions, and all training loads used in swimmers can be divided into the following groups: (1) loads of aerobic effect, (2) loads of combined aerobic-anaerobic effect, (3) loads of glycolytic anaerobic effect, and (4) loads of alactate anaerobic effect. In quantification of the effectiveness of a training plan, the volume

N.I. Volkov
Russian State University of Physical Education, Sport and Tourism, Moscow, Russia
e-mail: olegpo57@gmail.com

L. Xi, T.V. Serebrovskaya (eds.), *Intermittent Hypoxia and Human Diseases*,
DOI 10.1007/978-1-4471-2906-6_15, © Springer-Verlag London 2012

of training is usually regarded as a separate variable of the general "dose"-dependent effect, which reflects the regularity of training adaptation [1, 2].

The characteristic feature of the training process of skilled athletes is the application of heavy volume and intensity. However, the further increase of volume and intensity of exercise is limited. There is a necessity to find out additional means, which will enable to significantly reduce the time for achieving certain training effect and considerably increase performance results. One of such means is the method of intermittent (or interval) hypoxia training (IHT), which is based on the reaction of athletes organism to the decrease of partial O_2 pressure in inhaled air. In this case, the total dose of hypoxia influence is divided into several periods of hypoxic exposition performed repeatedly in certain periods of normobaric respiration [3, 4].

The aim of present chapter is to report the results of our study on the functional parameters and physical exercise capacity of the elite swimmers following regular training loads and in combination with IHT.

15.2 Theoretical and Experimental Premises

The condition of hypoxia at the cellular level is determined by the status of O_2-limited cytochrome metabolism [5, 6]. The speed of turnover of cytochromes depends on the concentration of O_2 and pO_2 on the mitochondrial membrane. Nevertheless, because of the influence of homeostatic mechanisms tending to minimize sharp changes in intracellular pO_2 and also because of the great reserves of convection and diffusion transport, considerable deviations from the standards of PiO_2 and PaO_2 are not necessarily accompanied by similar changes in intracellular pO_2 to become limiting factor for oxidative phosphorylation in mitochondria.

The development of tissue hypoxia in connection with the change in intracellular pO_2 takes place in several stages, and each of these stages of hypoxia may be identified by change in pO_2 in a particular area [5]. According to L. D. Lukyanova [7], the first stage of latent hypoxia (with normal O_2 saturation) is connected with the activation of NAD-independent pathway in mitochondria. The second stage of metabolic adaptation in which the speed of turnover of ATP in the cell remains unchanged is marked by inactivation of the NAD-dependent pathway and intensification of succinate dehydrogenase oxidation. The third stage of hypoxia with the appearance of decompensation is marked by inhibition of the electron transport function of the respiratory chain. Only at the fourth stage of marked hypoxia, a reduction in the activity of cytochrome oxidase occurs and cause reduction in the turnover of ATP that is linear to the drop in intracellular pO_2. The metabolic shifts associated with hypoxia may influence change both in membrane transport [13] and in blood flow velocity [14, 15]. The *Threshold 3* marked in Fig. 15.1 corresponds to the pO_2 value, below which cell functions and their integration may be considerably impaired.

The system of intracellular regulation ensures balance between the speed of uptake and consumption of ATP depends on pH and Pi as the main feedback signals [8]. The dynamics of pO_2, the condition of hypoxia in working muscles, can be established on the basis of studying the metabolic shifts directly linked to the occurrence of a hypoxic condition in cells. Such metabolic measurements include the concentration of phosphate, formation of lactate as a result of glycolytic activity, and changes in the indicators of acid–base balance in the tissues and cardiorespiratory parameters. Measurement of all these indicators as a set can be used to establish the severity of hypoxic conditions and establish common physiological criteria for diagnosis of such conditions [10–12, 16, 17].

The typical signs of workload (exercise)-induced hypoxia are formation of oxygen deficit and oxygen debt, reduction in tension of oxygen in muscular tissue and mixed venous blood, accumulation of incompletely oxidized products of metabolism in the blood, shift of pH, disturbance of acid–base balance, excessive production of CO_2, along with accelerated O_2 utilization and transfer [18–22]. Four degrees of load hypoxia are distinguished, i.e., (1) latent, (2) compensated, (3) marked hypoxia with beginning of decompensation, and (4) uncompensated hypoxia [17, 23].

In the first degree of hypoxia, when it appears in limited parts of the muscle fibers, positive oxygen supply at rest could eliminate local hypoxia using the oxygen resources within the fiber itself without involving the systemic compensatory mechanisms [9, 24–26]. In the second degree of hypoxia, which is the most common in normal humans who are performing muscular activities of moderate intensity, the whole respiratory system becomes involved in compensating the local hypoxia. Pulmonary ventilation, blood flow, and speed of oxygen delivery increase. With the increasing demand for O_2 by working muscles, oxygen deficit forms, and a certain number of acidic products are released into the blood and rapidly neutralized, leading to no substantial shifts of pH. This small (3–5%) oxygen debt may accumulate and cause a tendency to shift pH to more acidic range. This degree of load hypoxia is characterized by the most economical external respiration, where the ventilation equivalent is minimal and the rate of O_2 utilization is maximal [27].

The third degree of marked hypoxia with the beginning of decompensation is usually developed in the workload with 75–85% of the maximal oxygen consumption. As the speed of delivery of oxygen does not match with the tissue demand for O_2, oxygen debt forms, and excess exhaled CO_2 can be observed. Not only severe venous hypoxemia but also arterial hypoxemia can be observed. With high levels of ventilation (up to 90–110 l/min) and blood flow volume (up to 25–28 l/min in sportsmen), there is a rise in oxygen delivery

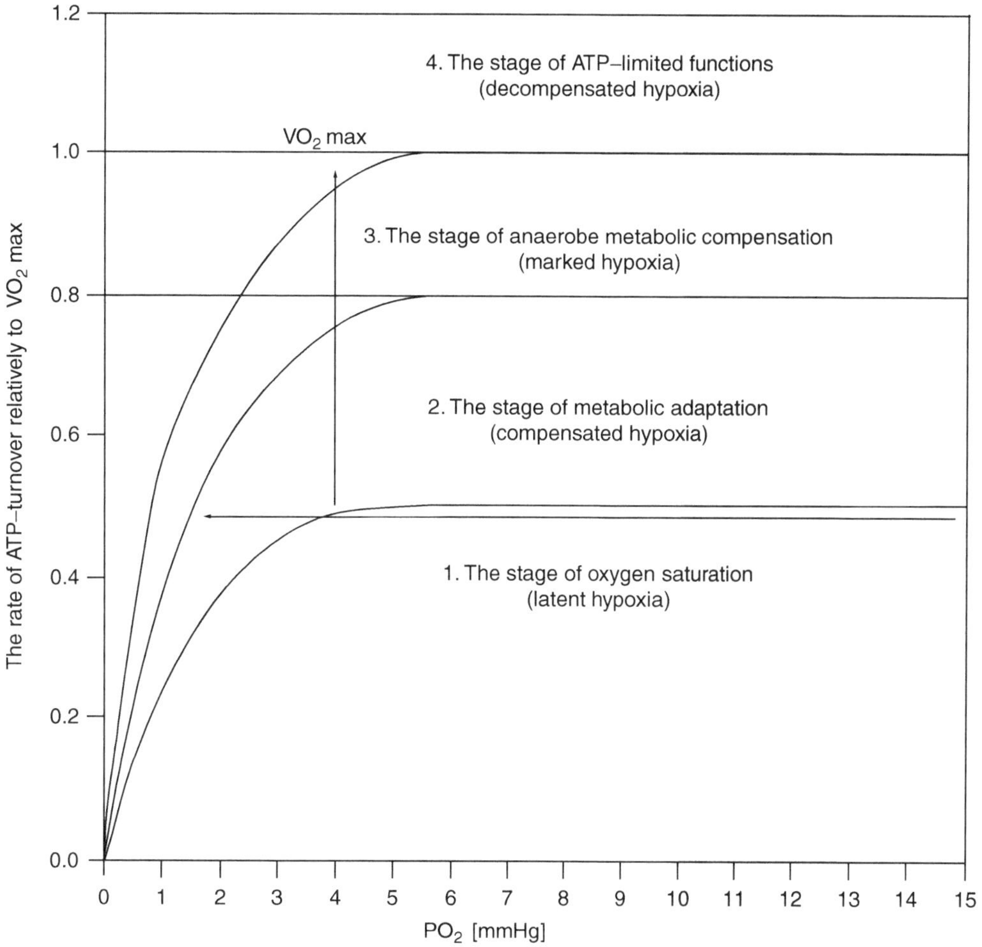

Fig. 15.1 Change in the speed of ATP turnover and its dependence on intracellular oxygen pressure. Ordinate: the rate of resynthesis of ATP, in relation to V_{max}. Abscissa: the intracellular oxygen pressure, torr

and consumption, but further increase in the oxygen utilization from arterial blood becomes impossible [28]. This type of hypoxia may serve as a triggering mechanism for the development of muscle fatigue. The enhanced respiration and blood circulation aimed at maintaining oxygen uptake and transport are parts of the compensatory mechanisms for overcoming fatigue.

In uncompensated load hypoxia (the fourth degree), the exacerbated imbalance between oxygen delivery and demand can be observed. Although the oxygen debt is increasing, oxygen consumption has reached its maximal level as plateau even with further increase in workload. Oxygen saturation of arterial blood drops to 83–85% and oxygen tension drops to 8–10 torr [28]. Ventilation increases to a considerably greater degree than oxygen consumption, and further intensification is not effective, as a considerable part of oxygen uptake is used by the respiratory muscles themselves. The work of the heart also becomes less effective with decline of stroke volume and the high blood flow is maintained largely by increasing heart rate. The development of marked tissue hypoxia leads to impairment of the compensatory systems, and their operation eventually ceases. The duration of exercise under this form of hypoxic condition is counted in tens of seconds, and only a few highly trained athletes can perform it for a few minutes.

The degrees of workload hypoxia which may appear during muscular work with either incremental or constant intensity. The exercise-induced hypoxia may be combined with other types of hypoxia, for example, with hypoxic hypoxia and, in a sick individual, with respiratory, circulatory, or anemic hypoxia [17, 28–32]. The effects of crossover adaptation induced by various combinations of different types of hypoxia and the potentiating action of additionally superimposed factors have a substantial effect on the development of adaptation to hypoxic stimulus caused by exercise. Many types of professions, such as military service and sports, involve the performance of intense muscular work with sharply raising oxygen demand and leading to the occurrence of tissue hypoxia in a reversible nature. This is followed by a considerable intensification of aerobic metabolism on the cessation or reduction of the work intensity.

In order to ensure successful activities in such challenging conditions and to maintain high physical fitness, special hypoxic training has been investigated for decades. The majority of such hypoxic training are carried out with artificially induced hypoxia, such as living in hypobaric chambers, respiration in enclosed space, or simply holding breath and inhalation of hypoxic gas mixtures, varying in their duration and degree of low pO_2 [33–36]. The effect of hypoxic treatment is determined by the total duration of the session of hypoxia and the degree of reduction of partial oxygen pressure in inhaled air [28, 36]. With a sharp drop in pO_2 accompanied by the abrupt development of severe hypoxic conditions, maintenance of the baseline functional levels can only last for some seconds or minutes. With a moderate drop in pO_2, the normal functional activities will continue over a time period of many minutes or even hours. Therefore, when setting optimal conditions of IHT, one general principle should be followed: the strength and duration of hypoxic treatment should be limited by the physiological norm at which effective compensation of the functional shifts taking place and rapid restoration after the end of hypoxia are still possible [32, 37, 38]. It has been established that the development of adaptation to hypoxia and of the general nonspecific resistance in an organism are considerably accelerated if the total dose of hypoxic treatment is divided into several separate periods of hypoxia with certain periods of normoxic interval [36–38]. One should consider that it takes certain time for the body to react to acute hypoxia [39]. The necessary duration of individual hypoxic treatment ranges from 3 to 10 min. The total duration of the daily session of IHT should be sufficient for the development of the organism's adaptive reaction to the hypoxic treatment. The total dose of hypoxia will depend on its degree and the general nonspecific resistance of the organism. As a rule, the total duration of sessions of hypoxia during 1 day should not exceed 1.5–2 h.

15.3 Methods

Twelve swimmers of high qualification using the training programs of the same type were randomly divided into two groups: control and experimental. The control group was trained with usual capacity using the traditional means and methods. The experimental group of swimmers underwent the traditional methods of training in combination with IHT during the recovery period following the main workload.

The following three protocols of IHT were applied: (1) 60 repetitions of 30-s hypoxia (inhalation of gas mixture with 10% O_2) that were divided by equally duration of normoxic breathing, (2) 30 repetitions of 1-min hypoxia (10% O_2) with 1 min normoxia intervals, (3) six repetitions of 5-min hypoxia (12% O_2) with 5 min normoxia intervals. To create the hypoxia conditions, "Hypoxicator Everest-l" (a device jointly developed by the Climbi Ltd. of Russia and the Praxsep Inc. of Canada) was applied.

The period of experimental training lasted 3 months. Before the beginning of training and immediately after the end of the experiment, the athletes of both control and experimental groups were tested in the progressive examination on Monark cycle ergometer to determine the maximum of aerobic and anaerobic work capacity and in repeated swimming 5×100 m freestyle and in hypoxia test to the moment of the decrease of blood oxygenation degree to 85% SO_2. Heart rate and blood oxygenation degree were continuously registered in the swimming and hypoxic tests. All gasometrical indexes by laboratory and swimming pool assessment were determined by Metalayser monitor system (Cortex, Germany). The indexes of acid–base equilibrium and blood lactate concentration were measured with the microanalisator ABL Radiometer (Denmark). Pulseoxymeter NQNIN-8000 (USA) was used to register blood oxygenation degree and heart rate. In quantification of performed training loads, diaries arid fixed planning tasks for each swimmer of both control and experimental groups were evaluated.

15.4 Results and Discussion

The summary of data on the executed training loads of various effect and increase in indexes of working capacity is shown in Table 15.1. Table 15.2 demonstrates the specific effects of IHT as compared with the traditional methods of training. IHT resulted in a significant increment in the maximum aerobic capacity. A greater increment in swimming performance was found in the middle distances, such as 200, 400, and 800 m.

An example of the functional improvement in the test of repeated swimming 5×100 m freestyle swimming (for the

Table 15.1 Volume of the executed training loads and increase in indexes of various working capacity of swimmers in the period of experimental training

Group	Control $n=6$	IHT $n=6$	Statistical significance
Total volume of executed work (min)	4,450±312	4,024±273	$P>0.05$
Loads of aerobic effect (min)	1,234±202	1,137±174	$P>0.05$
Loads of combined aerobic anaerobic effect (min)	2,341±256	2,049±264	$P<0.05$
Loads of glycolytic anaerobic effect (min)	594±102	557±86	$P<0.05$
Loads of alactate anaerobic effect (min)	280±58	279±47	$P>0.05$
Result increase in test 5×100 m freestyle (s)	10.2±1.0	15.6±1.0	$P<0.01$
T-85% increase (min)	0.5±0.2	4.5±1.6	$P<0.01$
T-kt increase (min)	0.15±0.02	3.1±0.3	$P<0.01$
T-ad increase (min)	0.35±0.09	1.4±0.1	$P<0.01$

Table 15.2 Alterations in the pattern of swimmers training of 4 weeks with intermittent hypoxia

		VO_2max (l/min)	V_E (l/min)	W_{cr} (kpm/min)	ΔpH	$ExcCO_2$ (l/min)	W_{max} (kpm/min)
Pre	Mean	3.80	161.1	1,989	−0.130	1.71	4,052
	SD	±0.137	±18.6	±189	±0.061	±0.24	±284
Post	Mean	4.23	171.1	2,205	−0.188	2.12	4,453
	SD	±0.11	±20.6	±207	±0.043	±0.31	±231
Change	%	11.1	6.4	10.8	44.6	23.1	9.8

*Significant at the $P<0.05$ level

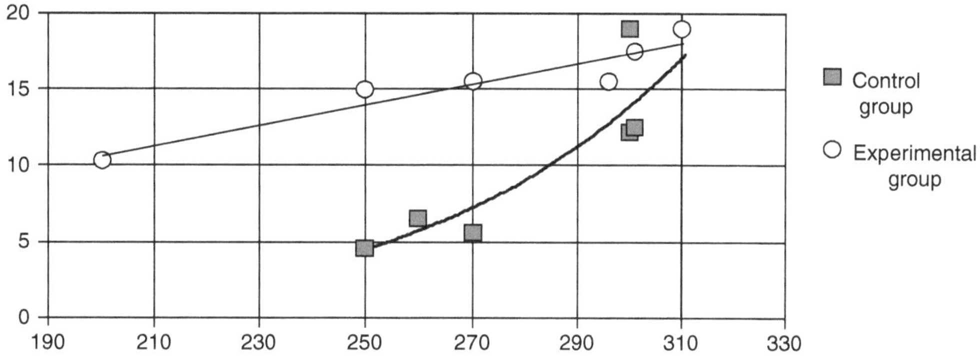

Fig. 15.2 Relationship of increase results in test 5 × 100 m freestyle from volume of alactic anaerobic loads

alactate-anaerobic effect) is shown in Fig. 15.2. As Fig. 15.2 indicates, the use of IHT as an additional training tool significantly modifies the dose-dependent effect by anaerobic alactate loads. Similar changes are noted in other types of physical loads.

Training under hypoxic conditions has been widely used among swimming coaches. Swimming with breath holding, breathing through dead space, and training in high mountains or in the hypobaric chamber have been successfully used to maintain the reduced contents of O_2 in tissues [40–42]. Our present study has employed an inexpensive system with simple design for breathing through a sealed space with absorption of CO_2 and reduced O_2 contents in the inhaled air. In different kinds of repeated and interval exercises, the application of such IHT enabled us to achieve significant effects on the function of aerobic and anaerobic metabolism. Figure 15.3 illustrates the dependence of hypoxia index on relative power of exercise. The hypoxia index is a ratio of oxygen requirement rate to the actual level of oxygen consumption during a performance of exercise. A greater degree of tissue hypoxia (indicated by deviation of the curve to the left) is achieved by hypoxic conditions in a dose-dependent manner. Thus, the combination of two types of hypoxic stimulus alters considerably the training effect of any kind of studied workload. The intensification of anaerobic glycolysis under the influence of hypoxic hypoxia shifts training loads to the type of mixed aerobic-anaerobic regime of work. Repeated performance of 30 s exercises with a rest of 30 s is closer to the loads of glycolytic character in respect of its effect. Under the conditions of hypoxia, the glycolytic source of energy plays more important role in energy supply of alactic-anaerobic exercises of 10 s duration with a rest period of 1 min.

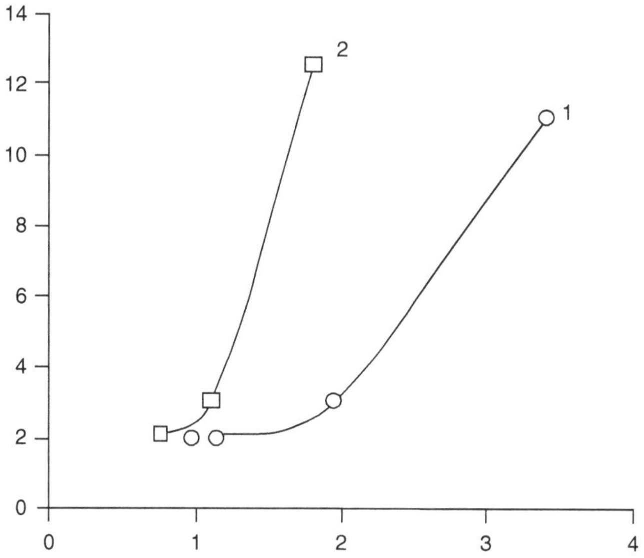

Fig. 15.3 Relationship of hypoxia index (ordinate) on relative power of exercise as a ratio the rate of oxygen requirement to a level of individual maximum of oxygen consumption, MMR units (abscissa). Before (1) and after (2) intermittent hypoxia training

Our current study in elite swimmers proved that IHT intensified the effect of exercise training. The IHT during the period of 3 months enhanced the absolute level of adaptation in anaerobic alactate loads, but it decreased the rate of adaptation changes in this type of training loads. Conversely, the 3-month duration of the trainings was insufficient to obtain any significant changes in other types of training loads. An advantage of IHT is the fact that it does not break the regular exercise training schedule. Overall, the adjunct use of IHT for high-level swimmers has considerably improved their performance results after the 3-month period of training.

Conclusion and Prospects

The physiological changes observed in the human organism under the action of various modes of intermittent hypoxia depend on the strength of the hypoxic stimulus used, i.e., the percentage of oxygen in inhaled air, the duration of individual exposures to hypoxia, the duration of periods of normoxic respiration, the total number of repeated exposures to hypoxia, or the total duration of hypoxia treatment during the day [32]. By varying the selected parameters of hypoxic load, it is possible to achieve the required degree of effect on particular physiological functions and to act directly on the key reactions of the body's metabolism. This opens wide possibilities for using IHT in the prophylaxis and treatment of various types of diseases [28, 32, 35, 37, 43] and to improve human health and increase the work productivity [44, 45]. By analogy with the process of sports training in which the training effect to be achieved arises as a result of a combination of effects caused by change in particular parameters of physical load in the use of artificially caused intermittent hypoxia, there exists the same possibility of constructing various modes of physiological effects [30, 37].

Our results indicate that systematic use of IHT in the training of elite swimmers can achieve a noticeable improvement in the indicators of functional condition and physical fitness. The most marked physiological changes could be observed following the IHT conducted after a mixed aerobic-anaerobic and anaerobic-glycolytic workloads. In highly skilled sportsmen, the regular use of IHT over a 5-week period of training led to a substantial improvement in the indicators of aerobic fitness as well as speed and strength. This new method of sports training can be successfully used in combination with the main types of physical load. In this case, IHT acts as a potentiating agent for improving the development of adaptation to the primary physical training. The hypoxic treatments are mainly applied during the recovery periods between the training loads when this method is used as an additional means, making it possible to load leading functions to the necessary degree and to accelerate their recovery from preceding training loads.

From the standpoint of the general theory of adaptation [1, 32, 37], the call to seek new combinations of the method of IHT with other modalities appears perfectly appropriate. The exhaustion of the organism's adaptation reserves during the maximal physical loads can be replaced by a new "splash" of adaptation changes in the organism only in response to a new, unusual, and stronger stimulus or a new combination of known stimuli. Based on the results reported in this chapter, we can assume that a number of possibilities in the development of new methodologies of sports training are opened up in practice by the use of combined treatment with interval physical training and IHT [38] and also pharmaceutical preparations with adaptogenic and antihypoxic effects [2]. The combined efforts of scientists and people practically involved in sport (athletes, coaches, and trainers) in the development and introduction of this advanced training modality will undoubtedly give positive results in the effort to further enhance athletic performance.

References

1. Viru A. Adaptation in sports training. Boca Raton: CRL Press; 1995.
2. Volkov NI. Bioenergetics of sport activities. In: Theory and practice of physical culture and sports. Moscow; 2010 [In Russian]
3. Kolchinskaya AZ. Hypoxic training in sport. Hypoxia Med J. 1993; 1:30–6 [In Russian].
4. Wolkov NI. Trening hypoxemiczny – skuteczny srodec zwickezania widolnosci fizycznej sportowcow. Sport Wyczynowy. 1994;XXXII (11–12):53–5 [In Polish].
5. Connett RJ, Gayeski TE, Honig CR. Defining hypoxia: a system view of VO_2, glycolysis, energetic and intracellular pO_2. J Appl Physiol. 1990;68:833–42.
6. Kondrashova MN. Functional hypoxia as factor of enhancing power in working act. In: Hypoxia load: mathematical modeling, prognosis and correction. Kiev: Acad Sci UkrSSR Publ; 1991 [In Russian].
7. Lukyanova LD. Bioenergetical hypoxia: definition, mechanisms and means of correction. Bull Exp Biol Med. 1997;124:244–53.
8. Roos A, Boron WF. Intracellular pH. Physiol Rev. 1981;61:296–434.
9. Drake-Holland AJ, Laird JD, Noble MI, et al. Oxygen and coronary vascular resistance during autoregulation and metabolic vasodilatation in the dog. J Physiol. 1984;348:285–99.
10. Wilson DF, Erecinska M, Drown C. The oxygen dependence of cellular energy metabolism. Arch Biochem Biophys. 1979;195:485–93.
11. Kolchinskaya AZ. Oxygen: physical states. In: Work capacity. Kiev: Naukova Dumka; 1991 [In Russian].
12. Volkov NI. The energy continuum and metabolic states of athletes in strenuous muscular activities. In: Biochemistry of sport. Materials of the international symposium. Leningrad; 1990 [In Russian].
13. Hollmann W. Hochst und dankerleistagsfahigkeit des sportlers. J A Barth (Munchen). 1983:344 [In German].
14. Kovalenko EA. The question of theory for gases dynamics in organism. Sechenovs Physiol J USSR. 1973;2:45–6 [In Russian].
15. Marshak ME. About the regional oxygen insufficiency. In: Oxygen insufficiency. Kiev: Acad Sci UkrSSR Publ; 1963 [In Russian].
16. Piiper J. Factors limiting the O_2 transporting capacity in exercise by hypoxia. In: Margaria R, editor. Exercise at altitude. Milan: Exepta Medica; 1967.
17. Volkov NI. Energy metabolism and human work capacity in strenuous muscular activity. Ph.D. thesis, Institute of Med Biol Problems, Acad Med Sci USSR, Moscow; 1969 [In Russian].
18. Armstrong Y. Aviation medicine. Moscow: Foreign Literature Publ; 1934. p. 522.
19. Foster RE. Oxygenation of muscle cell. Circ Res. 1967;20:1.
20. Gayeski TE, Honig CR. Intracellular pO_2 in long axis of individual fibers in working dog gracilis muscle. Am J Physiol. 1988;254: H1179–86.
21. Federspiel WJ, Popel AS. A theoretical analysis of the effect of the particulate nature of blood on oxygen release in capillaries. Microvasc Res. 1986;32:164–89.
22. Kolchinskaya AZ. Oxygen insufficiency: about the classification of hypoxic states. In: Kolchinskaya AZ, editor. Special and clinical physiology of hypoxic states. Kiev: Naukova Dumka; 1979 [In Russian].

23. Kolchinskaya AZ. Combined interval hypoxic and sportive training effectiveness. Hypoxia Med J. 1993;3:28–32 [In Russian].
24. Bulgakova NG, Volkov NI, Kovalenko EA. Adaptation of athletes to combined action of interval training and hypoxical hypoxia. In: Hypoxia of load: mathematical modeling, forecasting and correction. Kiev; 1990 [In Russian].
25. Karash YM, Strelkov RB, Chijov AY. In: Strelkov RB, editor. Normobaric hypoxia in therapy, prophylactic and rehabilitation. Moscow: Meditsina; 1988 [In Russian].
26. Sirotinin NN. Hypoxia and its signification for pathology. In: Hypoxia. Kiev: Acad Sci Ukr SSR Publ; 1949 [In Russian].
27. Volkov NI. Hypoxic training for rehabilitation and prophylactics of pathogenesis states. In: Rehabilitation and therapy in health resort conditions. 1983 [In Russian].
28. Brovko AP, Fefilatjev LP, Volkov NJ. Intermittent hypoxia as a method of enhancing adaptation to high mountains. Bishkek: MUK; 1996. p. 410 [In Russian].
29. Kovaenko EA, Volkov NI, Erinburg IV. Activation of adaptation processes in organism by therapy of patients with different diseases. Hypoxia Med J. 1993;1:8–9 [In Russian].
30. Meerson FS, Tverdokhlib VP. Adaptation to intermittent hypoxia in therapy and prophylactics. Moscow: Nauka; 1989 [In Russian].
31. Volkov NI, Bulgakova NJ, Kovalenko EA. Impulsive hypoxia and interval training. Hypoxia Med J. 1994;2:64–5 [In Russian].
32. Volkov NI, Damarchi A, Darduri U. Physiological characteristics of different regimes of interval hypoxic training. In: Hypoxia: mechanisms, adaptation, correction. In: Proceedings of all Russian science conference, Moscow; 1997 [In Russian].
33. Volkov NI, Smirnov VV, Dardouri U. Hipoxia e treio intervalado. Treinamento Desportivo (Brasil). 1957;2:23–30.
34. Volkov NI, Smirnov VV. Intermittent hypoxia as new method in the enhancing of sportsmen's endurance. In: Book of abstracts II. Copenhagen; 1997, p. 1032–3.
35. Iordinskaja FA, Arharov CI, Dmitriev ET, et al. About the using hypoxia in sport training. Theor Pract Phys Cult. 1967;2:32–5 [In Russian].
36. Krijstev K. Hypoxic training of sportsmen. Quest of Phys Cult (Bulgaria). 1962;7:426–31.
37. Wolkow NI, Szmatlan-Gabrys U, Gabrys T. Hipoksja w treningu sportowym: interwalowy trening hipoksyczny. In: AWF Jozefa Pilsudskiego, Warszawa; 2003 [In Polish].
38. Strelkov RB. Normobaric hypoxic therapy. Moscow: Ministry of Healthcare, Russian Federation; 1994 [In Russian].
39. Bruner H, Jovy D, Zhein HE. Hypoxia as a stressor. Aerospace Med. 1961;32:1009.
40. Butterfield YE. Elements of energy balance at altitude. In: Sutton JR, Coates Y, Remmers JE, editors. Hypoxia: the adaptation. Philadelphia: Deeber; 1990.
41. Platonov VN, Bulatova MM. Hypoxic training in sport. Hypoxia Med J. 1994;4:17–23 [In Russian].
42. Volkov NI, Karasev AB, Smetanin VY, et al. Interval hypoxic training. Moscow: Great Peter's Military Acad; 1990 [In Russian].
43. Volkov NI, Darduri U, Smetanin VY. Interval hypoxic training – new method to enhanced work capacity of athletes. In: Materials of all Russian scientific practical conference, development of top-performance sport and strategy of preparation of top-class athletes by 1997–2000. Moscow; 1997 p. 124–32.
44. Bobkov YG, Vinogradov VM, Katkov VF. Pharmacological correction of fatigue. Moscow: Medicine Publ; 1964 [In Russian].
45. Stegeman J. Exercise physiology: physiological bases of work and spirit. Chicago: Year Book Med Publ; 1981.

Adaptation to Intermittent Hypoxia/Hyperoxia Enhances Efficiency of Exercise Training

16

Tatyana G. Sazontova, Antonina V. Bolotova, Irina V. Bedareva, Nadezhda V. Kostina, and Yuriy V. Arkhipenko

Abstract

This chapter provides an overview of the current concepts on redox signaling pathways, particularly, under hypoxic conditions. The principle of intermittent adaptation effects of variable oxygen levels (short-term hypoxia and hyperoxia) was substantiated and confirmed experimentally in vivo for the first time. The goal of our experiments in rats was to estimate (1) efficiency of physical training conducted separately and in combination with adaptation to intermittent hypoxia/hyperoxia, (2) changes in the rates of free radical processes, and (3) concentration of heat shock proteins (HSP). We found that short-term physical training increased the duration of swimming in acute exhaustive exercise. Combination of physical training with adaptation to hypoxia–normoxia had no effect on this parameter, while adaptation to physical load combined with adaptation to hypoxia–hyperoxia increased the duration of the active swimming phase and, as a consequence, the efficiency of adaptation. Adaptation to physical load and its combination with adaptation to variable oxygen levels increased the resistance of membrane structures to free radical oxidation at the expense of excessive activation of antioxidant defense enzymes in the course of physical training, which was partly compensated for by adaptation to hypoxia/normoxia and was fully prevented by adaptation to hypoxia/hyperoxia. Combination of two forms of adaptation to physical load and to variable oxygen levels markedly compensated/reversed the elevated content of HSP in the course of physical training, which is especially well pronounced during adaptation to hypoxia/hyperoxia. The novel technique is biologically less expensive and more beneficial for the organism.

Abbreviations

AEE	Acute exhaustive exercise
AP-1	Activator protein 1
ClO^-	Hypochlorite
H_2O_2	Hydrogen peroxide
H/H	Hypoxia/hyperoxia
H/N	Hypoxia/normoxia
HIF	Hypoxia-inducible factor
$HO_2^{\bullet}$	Hydroperoxyl radical
HSP	Heat shock protein
IH	Intermittent hypoxia
IRP	Iron-regulatory protein
$LOO^{\bullet}$	Peroxy radicals
LOOH	Lipid hydroperoxides
NF-κB	Nuclear factor kappa B
NO	Nitric oxide
$O_2^{-\bullet}$	Superoxide anion radical
$OH^{\bullet}$	Hydroxyl radical
ROS	Reactive oxygen species
SOD	Superoxide dismutase

T.G. Sazontova (✉) • A.V. Bolotova • I.V. Bedareva •
N.V. Kostina • Y.V. Arkhipenko
Faculty of Fundamental Medicine,
M.V. Lomonosov Moscow State University,
Lomonosovsky pr., 31/5, Moscow 119192, Russia
e-mail: yva1950@gmail.com

L. Xi, T.V. Serebrovskaya (eds.), *Intermittent Hypoxia and Human Diseases*,
DOI 10.1007/978-1-4471-2906-6_16, © Springer-Verlag London 2012

16.1 Introduction

Increasing attention has been given to the nonmedicamentous approach to improving the resistance of the organism to environmental factors. These approaches consist of, in particular, the use of different forms of adaptation to stress, physical load, hypoxia, changes in ambient temperature, etc. A search for novel adaptation technologies with the ultimate goal to increase the efficiency of adaptation, to reduce the time required for the formation of adequate adaptive responses, to minimize negative side effects, and to elaborate mild stress or hypoxic conditions is currently under way. Much attention is given to cross effects of adaptation and simultaneous adaptation to several factors.

In particular, adaptation to intermittent hypoxia (IH) that is able to increase the resistance of an organism to damaging factors has been studied extensively in the past two decades. Its mechanism combines adaptation to hypoxia and reoxygenation after inhalation of air with normal oxygen content. As it is known, reoxygenation is concomitant with generation of reactive oxygen species (ROS); their induction exerts a damaging effect and/or triggers an intracellular redox signaling cascade resulting in the formation of an adaptive response, which manifests itself in increased resistance of the organism [1].

It was found that in addition to the well-established role of excessive ROS in the pathogenesis of various pathological states, generation of ROS and initiation of free radical reactions represent naturally and continuously occurring physiological processes. The main physiological functions of ROS include oxidation of damaged molecules and their further metabolism [2–4], synthesis of messenger molecules (e.g., eicosanoids) in the course of free radical oxidation of polyunsaturated fatty acids [5, 6], and extra-/intracellular signaling functions. The role of redox signaling and the ROS-dependent intracellular system effecting the transmission of external signals to the cell nucleus with subsequent initiation of protein synthesis was the subject of in-depth studies in the past decade [7, 8]. By initiating redox signaling in the absence of specific receptors, ROS triggers a series of cell responses to hypoxia and oxidizing or reducing agents. Besides, the agents whose effects are mediated by specific (hormonal, cytokine) receptors stimulate the activity of the nonspecific redox signaling system and thus participate in cross activation and interaction between specific receptors underlying cross effects of adaptation, where training to one damaging factor increases the resistance of the organism to other factors.

Activation of the transcription factors nuclear factor kappa B (NF-κB) [9], activator protein 1 (AP-1) [10], hypoxia-inducible factor 1α and 3α (HIF-1α and HIF-3α) [7], which augments the activity of defense proteins and thus promotes adaptation and survival, is among the most crucial events in redox signaling activation. The major proteins responsible for initiating responses to ROS signals under stress, hypoxia, and ischemia include antioxidant defense enzymes, HSP proteins, iron-regulating proteins, repair enzymes and peroxyredoxins [10–14]. As a result of redox signaling, the cells become saturated with the aforementioned and other molecules responsible for improved cell resistance to damaging factors. Noteworthy, intracellular protection [15] is much more effective than external (i.e., based on the use of exogenous additives) protection.

The free radical signals generated in the course of adaptation to IH increase the resistance of body cells to a vast variety of damaging factors including ROS-mediated ones. This was established under stress and cold adaptation conditions, after the use of food-borne adaptogens [16–18] and in the course of hypobaric training, a yet another type of interval hypoxic training, which has a membrane-stabilizing effect and increases the general resistance of the organism [19]. It was established that long-term adaptation to intermittent normobaric hypoxia increases the resistance of heart, liver, and brain membranes to ROS. This phenomenon most likely underlies the cross effect of adaptation to IH under the conditions of physical load, based on the results of its application in sports medicine [20]. However, the procedure of adaptation to intermittent hypoxia/normoxia takes a lot of time for its development, whereas its short duration may be achieved with more severe hypoxia and enhancement of the ROS signal [21]. In order to enhance the ROS signal without inducing hypoxic side effects, we hypothesized that normoxia as a constituent element of adaptation to hypoxia/normoxia should be replaced by moderate hyperoxia. Compared to hypoxia–normoxia, the novel type of adaptation to hypoxia and moderate hyperoxia (Russian Federation Patent No. 2289432 of 20.12.2006) affords a faster increase in the resistance of membrane structures [22]. The efficiency of the novel adaptation procedure in protecting membrane structures against in vitro ROS-induced injuries was previously demonstrated [14]; however, little is known about its effects at the whole-body level. The first examples of the defense potential of the novel adaptation procedure to variable oxygen level (hypoxia and hyperoxia) under conditions of sharply decreased (hypokinesia) or increased (acute exhaustive physical training) physical activity are described in our recent publication [23].

The mechanism of the damaging effect of exhaustive physical load on body cells is based on excessive activation of ROS-associated processes. The exhaustive physical load has both hypoxic and stress components. Interestingly, simultaneous adaptation to several external factors (hypoxia + cold, hypoxia + immobilization, cold + physical training, etc.) often gives more impressive results than adaptation to each individual factor. It was also suggested that training to physical load combined with adaptation to hypoxia and/or hyperoxia is much more effective with regard to the ultimate effect of physical training. At the same time, information on adaptation to hypoxia/hyperoxia is very scarce; therefore, the efficiency of combined adaptation requires further experimental verification.

A search for a clue to this enigma made the subject of the present study. Our experimental goal was to estimate (1) efficiency of physical training used separately and in combination with adaptation to intermittent hypoxia/hyperoxia, (2) changes in the rates of free radical processes, and (3) concentration of heat shock proteins (HSP).

The following experimental tasks were performed: (1) estimation of efficiency of physical training alone and in combination with two types of adaptation to intermittent hypoxia/normoxia or hypoxia/hyperoxia, (2) estimation of effects of a combination of two modes of adaptation to physical training and variable oxygen levels on the rate of free radical oxidation and activity of antioxidant defense enzymes, and (3) comparison of efficiency of adaptation to hypoxia/normoxia and hypoxia/hyperoxia combined with physical training in normalization of concentrations of HSPs induced during the course of acute exhaustive exercise (AEE). The scientific and practical significance of this study is in demonstration of protective effects of adaptation to hypoxia/hyperoxia combined with short-term physical training against AEE-induced injuries and rationalization of broadening the range of applications of adaptation to transient changes in O_2 content.

16.2 Role of Free Radical Processes in the Organism: Reactive Oxygen Species

The bulk (95–98%) of molecular oxygen consumed by the organism is utilized for generating energy and oxidative catabolism of reaction substrates. The four-electron reduction of O_2 in different components of the mitochondrial respiratory chain of aerobic cells is accompanied by incomplete (1–3-electron) reduction of ROS, namely, the superoxide anion radical ($O_2^{-\bullet}$), hydrogen peroxide (H_2O_2), and the hydroxyl radical ($OH^\bullet$). In other words, primary ROS are generated in response to stepwise single-electron reduction of molecular oxygen.

The most characteristic features of ROS, which make them a "local action tool," include short life cycle, low concentration in tissues, and high reactivity. Recent studies established that free radicals are key regulatory elements of many physiological processes occurring in the cell at different levels. The involvement of the same molecules in cell and tissue injuries, protection against external damaging factors, and intra- and intercellular regulation strongly suggests that ROS generation is a typical physiological process and a result of evolutional selection [24].

The $O_2^{-\bullet}$ is formed upon binding of one electron to the molecule of O_2. Since $O_2^{-\bullet}$ anion carries an electric charge hindering its transmembrane transport and is able to withdraw and accept electrons, it can act both as a reducing agent and an oxidant. Its biological targets include small organic molecules (catecholamines, low-molecular thiols, ascorbate, tetrahydropterins, etc.). In acid media, $O_2^\bullet$ generates a hydroperoxyl radical ($HO_2^\bullet$), which is a much more potent oxidant than the superoxide anion radical.

Under normal conditions, $O_2^{-\bullet}$ is converted into H_2O_2 under the action of superoxide dismutase (SOD) involved in the synthesis of hypochlorite (ClO^-) or undergoes nonradical decomposition in the presence of antioxidant enzymes, for example, peroxidases, among which catalase and glutathione peroxidase manifest the highest activity.

Nitric oxide (NO) is another highly reactive free radical, which controls an immense diversity of physiological and pathological processes occurring in the organism. The biological role of NO is determined by the small size of its molecule, its high reactivity, and the ability to diffuse into tissues [25].

Secondary free radicals are generated from H_2O_2, lipoperoxides, and hypochlorite in the presence of Fe(II) ions. They include the hydroxyl radical and some lipid radicals involved in oxidative reactions of unsaturated fatty acid chains of membrane lipids and blood plasma lipoproteins.

Further single-electron reduction of H_2O_2 in the presence of free Fe^{2+} or Cu^+ ions (Fenton reaction) gives $OH^\bullet$, which is a strong oxidant endowed with an ability to attack nucleic acids, proteins and phospholipids:

$$H_2O_2 + Fe^{2+} \rightarrow OH^- + OH^\bullet + Fe^{3+} \quad (16.1)$$

Besides, $OH^\bullet$ is known for its ability to induce effective cleavage of C–H and C–C bonds. The rate of its interaction with the majority of organic molecules reaches a level commensurate with its diffusion rate [23]. Under normal conditions, $OH^\bullet$ generation proceeds at a slow rate, but is activated in the presence of transition metal ions.

The $OH^\bullet$ attacks at the side chains of unsaturated fatty acids are accompanied by detachment of H_2 and generation of the lipid radical ($L^\bullet$) (Reaction 16.2). In the presence of oxygen, the latter is converted into organic radicals of O_2 ($LOO^\bullet$) (so-called peroxy radicals), which, in their turn, withdraw hydrogen from fatty acid chains of phospholipids to give lipid hydroperoxides (LOOH). This reaction is accompanied by generation of additional lipid radicals able to reenter the reaction cycle.

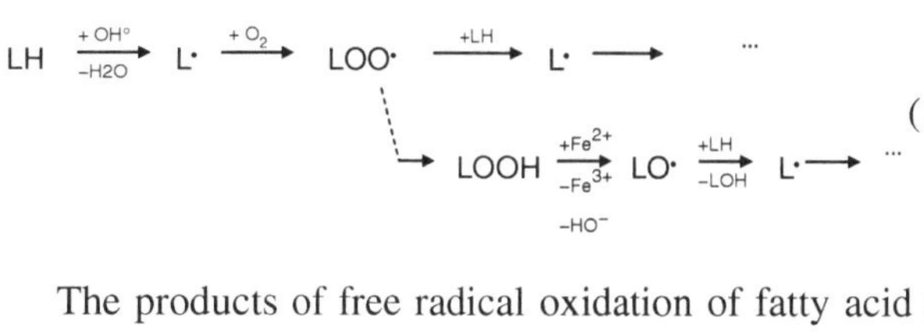

(16.2)

The products of free radical oxidation of fatty acid residues of phospholipids serve as a source of many biologically active substances. Before free radical oxidation takes place, polyenic fatty acyls can be withdrawn from phospholipids by hydrolysis with phospholipase A_2. Under these conditions, oxidation of fatty acids in the presence of lipoxygenase yields leukotrienes, while oxidation in the presence of cyclic oxygenase gives prostaglandins, thromboxanes, and prostacyclins. Oxidation of fatty acid acyls without cleavage from phospholipids yields dienoic conjugates and lipid hydroperoxides with subsequent formation of gaseous products, aldehyde-like carbonyl compounds, and last but not least, Schiff bases. All of them represent primary, secondary, or final lipid peroxidation products.

16.3 Sources of ROS in the Organism

In living organisms, free radicals are formed in miscellaneous reactions occurring both inside and outside the cell. In cells, $O_2^{-\bullet}$ is formed as an intermediate product of many biochemical reactions, such as oxidation of thiols, flavins, quinones, and catecholamines or metabolic conversions of xenobiotics [26]. However, the main sources of $O_2^{-\bullet}$ are enzymatic systems, namely, mitochondrial cytochrome-*c*-oxidase, NADPH oxidase, phagocytic cells, xanthine oxidase, and microsomal monooxygenases [27]. Studies in human and animal cardiomyocytes established that mitochondria are the main intracellular sources of ROS ($O_2^{-\bullet}$, H_2O_2, $OH^{\bullet}$) in myocardial cells. Under normal conditions, less than 5% of molecular oxygen is converted into ROS in the course of oxidative phosphorylation in mitochondria [28]. The main sites of ROS generation in the mitochondrial respiratory chain are NADH-dependent dehydrogenase and NADH-dependent ubiquinone reductase [29]. $O_2^{-\bullet}$ and H_2O_2 are metabolized in mitochondria by Mn-SOD and glutathione peroxidase; as a result, the concentration of these ROS is maintained at a relatively low level. However, the rate of ROS generation in mitochondria increases in various pathological states, for example, ischemia/reperfusion of internal organs, such as heart and kidney, hypoxia/reoxygenation of cardiomyocytes [30] and upon aging [31, 32]. A crucial role in ROS generation is played by changes in the membrane potential of mitochondria. It was found that inhibition of oxidative phosphorylation in mitochondria increases the membrane potential and the rate of ROS generation [27].

Under physiological conditions, the rate of ROS production by the microsomal monooxygenase system is controlled by a vast variety of antioxidant enzymes and substances, such as SOD, catalase, glutathione peroxidase, α-tocopherol, glutathione, and so on [33]. The highly ordered structure of the monooxygenase ensemble can be impaired as a result of disturbances in the coordination between the systems responsible for generation and inactivation of ROS; in the absence of their substrates, one of its components can attack polyunsaturated fatty acids of the neighboring membranes. A similar situation is observed under the influence of stress factors, for example, during excessive production of catecholamines in the adrenal gland medulla. In this case, autoxidation of adrenaline in liver microsomes is concomitant with excessive production of $O_2^{-\bullet}$ and free radical oxidation of polyunsaturated fatty acids of the microsomal membrane. As a result, the membrane structure and function become impaired [34]. Thus, 6-h emotional–pain stress and excessive physical load stimulate lipid peroxidation in liver microsomes and reduce the activity and concentration of cytochrome P-450 [35]. Considering that microsomal oxidation is especially intense in the liver, it was suggested that liver microsomes are the main sources of ROS (of $O_2^{-\bullet}$, in particular) [36].

Apart from the enzymatic mechanisms of ROS formation considered above, intracellular single-electron reduction of oxygen takes place in reactions of readily oxidized compounds, for example, during oxidation of catecholamines in the presence of Fe ions, oxidation of semireduced flavins, semiquinones, and heme iron, etc. by molecular oxygen. The role of reducing agents for O_2 is played by transition metal ions, NADPH, etc. For example, $O_2^{-\bullet}$ is produced upon oxidation of arachidonic acid via the cyclooxygenase and lipoxygenase routes, where NADH and NADPH are used as cofactors.

ROS can also be generated in the cell as a result of antioxidants oxidation. A salient feature of naturally occurring low-molecular antioxidants is their ability to fulfill a prooxidant function in certain situations. This capability was first demonstrated for ascorbate oxidase under conditions where this typical antioxidant initiated lipid peroxidation in the presence of iron ions by virtue of its ability to reduce trivalent iron to bivalent iron. Under these conditions, the ascorbate molecule passed into the oxidized form. This reaction is reversible and its direction is controlled by the general redox potential of the cell [37]. A similar dual role was established for glutathione and lipoic acid. Autoxidation of glutathione used at physiological concentrations is concomitant with generation of ROS and damage of DNA [26].

16.4 Role of Free Radical Oxidation in the Cell

As it is known, enhanced production of ROS and excessive activation of intracellular free radical oxidation processes play the role of damaging factors impairing the structure and function of intracellular components, which contributes to the development of various pathological states.

The mechanism of ROS generation is common for all pathologies. Some of its distinctive features can be detected only in the very earliest stages of the disease. Thus, free radical processes can be triggered by oxidative burst as a result of abnormally high activity of phagocytic cells in inflammation, by disturbances in the electron-transport function of the mitochondrial respiratory chain in hypoxia or ischemia or by activation of the microsomal oxidation system in chemical injuries. The factors stimulating excessive production of ROS and, as a consequence, oxidative stress are schematically presented in Fig. 16.1 (partially adopted from [38, 39]). It may be inferred from these data that the reasons for excessive activation of free radical processes are different, but the changes at the molecular level are similar and so are the results [40, 41].

There is no universally accepted opinion in the current literature concerning the role of ROS in cell metabolism. Until recently, this role was confined to the beneficial bactericidal effect of $O_2^{-\bullet}$ generated by macrophagal plasma membrane NADPH oxidase. In actual practice, the biological role of ROS is much more diverse.

In addition to the aforesaid bactericidal function, two more activities of ROS deserve special mention. In all body cells and tissues irrespective of their origin and specific function, ROS mediate two differently directed physiological processes, namely, catabolism of old and synthesis of new molecules. In the cell, ROS induce oxidation of depleted protein and lipid molecules and, in so doing, stimulate the activity of degradation enzymes (phospholipases and proteases) whose affinity for the oxidized substrate is much higher [2–4]. Simultaneously, ROS participate in continuous synthesis of new molecules. By illustration, free radical oxidation of polyunsaturated fatty acids of biomembrane phospholipids initiates the synthesis of many physiologically active lipids including leukotrienes, thromboxanes, and prostaglandins [5, 6, 42]. Being active participants of many catabolic and synthetic processes, ROS maintain the functional status of the cell and provide its adaptation to variable conditions of the environment by changing the composition of cellular membrane lipids and broadening the range of their intrinsic proteins. ROS play an essential role in early steps of intracellular signaling by virtue of their ability to stimulate the activity of the multicomponent redox signaling system affecting the transmission of external signals to the cell nucleus. This system owes its name to its initial component, which is extremely sensitive to free radical oxidation [7, 8, 27, 43].

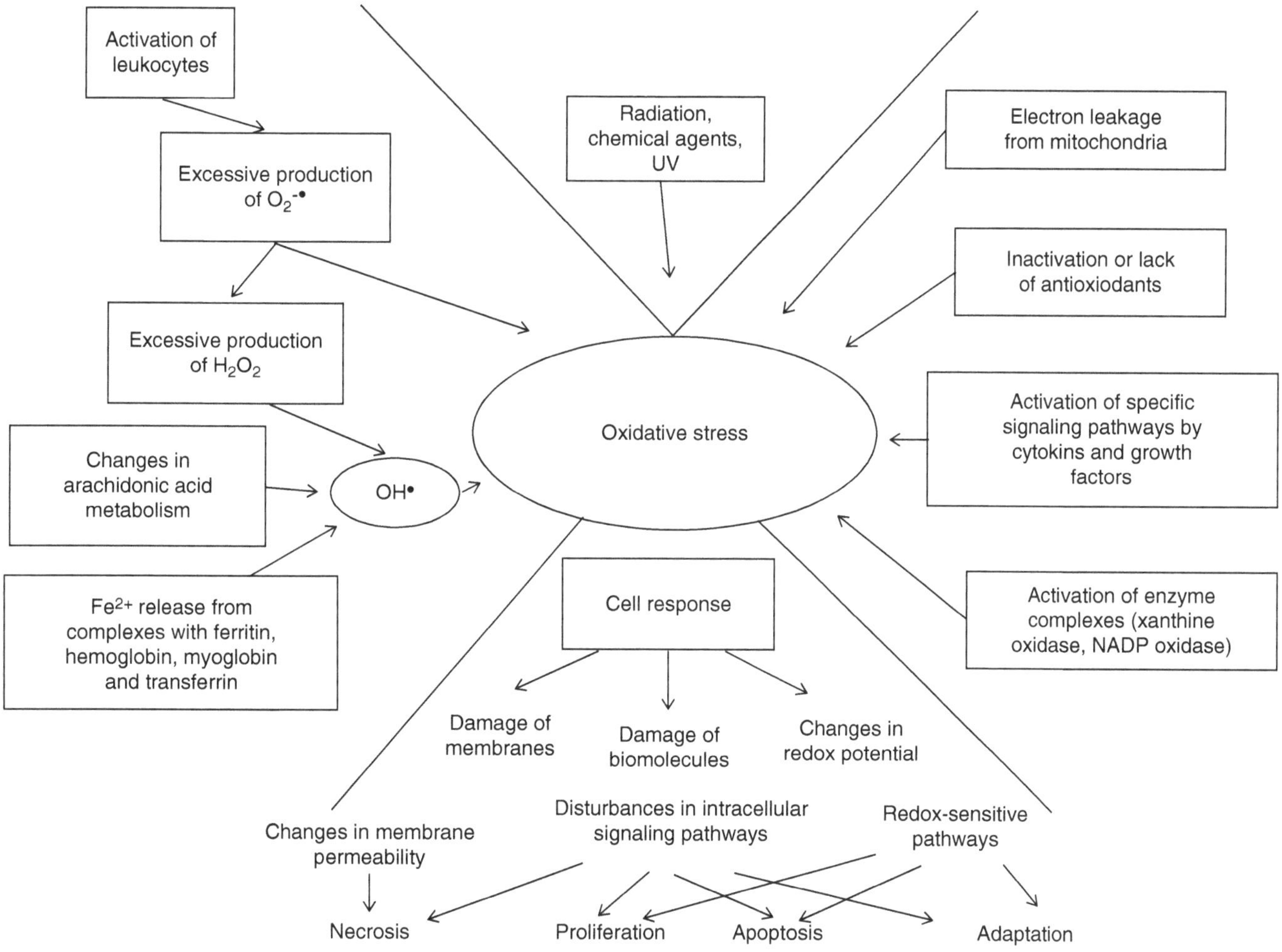

Fig. 16.1 The main factors responsible for oxidative stress and various types of the cell response

16.5 The Antioxidant Defense System of the Cell

The antioxidant system is one of the most potent mechanisms, whereby body cells maintain ROS at the physiological level and protect the organism against cell and tissue injuries. The biochemical mechanisms of the complex antioxidant defense system consist of four main components: (1) antioxidant defense enzymes; (2) endogenous (intrinsic) low-molecular antioxidants synthesized by body cells; (3) exogenous (naturally occurring) antioxidants used as supplements to diets and entering the organism with food (so-called dietary adaptogens) (these include ascorbic acid (vitamin C), α-tocopherol (vitamin E), rutin (vitamin P), flavonoids, β-carotene and other carotenoids, and vitamin A precursors; chemical substances localized in active centers of antioxidant enzymes (e.g., selenium) can also be related to this group); and (4) specific proteins and peptides able to binding to transition metal ions catalyzing free radical oxidation processes. This category includes the cell-specific protein ferritin, the plasma-specific proteins transferrin and ceruloplasmin, the muscle-specific protein carnosine, etc. The coordinated functioning of these ensembles maintains, at the constant level, the formation and subsequent transformations of free radicals and other potentially hazardous substances.

In the course of their evolution, body cells synthesize special substances (called antioxidant defense systems) that protect them against ROS. These include SOD catalyzing the conversion of $O_2^{-\bullet}$ into H_2O_2, catalase responsible for degradation of H_2O_2, glutathione-dependent peroxidases, and transferases for specifically scavenging organic peroxides. SOD and catalase do not need cofactors for their activity, which makes their functioning independent of other cellular structures. At the same time, normal functioning of glutathione-dependent enzymes is provided by reduced glutathione synthesized in the liver under the action of glutathione synthase or formed in glutathione reductase-catalyzed reactions. Antioxidant defense enzymes are distinguished for high specificity against definite forms of ROS and specific localization in body cells and tissues [44].

SOD is a primary source of ROS scavenger and one of the key mechanisms of body cell protection [45]. In human and animal cells, this enzyme is represented by three main isoforms, i.e., the cytosolic isoform (Cu,Zn-SOD), the mitochondrial isoform (Mn-SOD), and the extracellular high-molecular isoform Cu,Zn-SOD. Each of them is coded by a specific gene localized in human chromosomes 21q21, 6q27, and 4p, respectively [46]. Cu,Zn-SOD is found in the nucleus, cytoplasmic matrix, peroxisomes, and the intermembrane space of mitochondria [47]. This isozyme has a molecular mass of 31 kDa; its molecule consists of two identical subunits linked together through a disulfide bridge. Each subunit contains one copper and one zinc atom. It is assumed that Zn^{2+} is responsible for stabilization of the SOD molecule, whereas Cu^{2+} is directly involved in dismutation of $O_2^{-\bullet}$ [24]. Mn-SOD is localized in mitochondria, has a molecular mass of about 40 kDa, and is made up of four subunits, which contain a Mn^{2+} atom in their active center. The most distinctive features of Mn-SOD include high resistance to hydrogen peroxide and high inducibility. In human fibroblasts, ionizing radiation increases the rate of transcription and stability of Mn-SOD mRNA (2- and 3-fold, respectively) [48].

Another important feature of SOD is its ability to generate hydroxyl radicals in the presence of excess H_2O_2 [45]. Their attacks at the SOD molecule are terminated by its fragmentation and inactivation. From the above-said, it follows that SOD needs low-molecular antioxidants or coordination of its functional activity with that of peroxidases.

Catalase is one of the key regulators of H_2O_2 metabolism. This Fe-containing protoporphyrin (MW ~250 kDa) fulfills a dual function by acting as catalase and peroxidase. At high intracellular concentrations of H_2O_2, it is the catalase activity that is predominant, whereas at low concentrations of H_2O_2, the peroxidase pathway is triggered on. Inside the cell, catalase is predominantly localized in peroxisomes, but its low concentrations can also be detected in the cytosol and mitochondria [49, 50]. Catalase can retain high activity for sufficiently long periods of time; the rates of catalase-mediated reactions depend exclusively on the rate of substrate diffusion to the active center of the enzyme [51]. At the same time, in intracellular fluids, catalase rapidly loses its activity under the action of proteolytic enzymes.

16.6 Interval Hypoxic Training in Sports Medicine

It is well known that acute physical load is concomitant with excessive production of ROS, which exert strong damaging effects on body cells. This, in turn, stimulates the activity of antioxidant defense systems and general resistance of the body to exhaustive physical exercise [52]. Regular training is accompanied by generation of a series of weak repetitive ROS signals resulting in the formation of defense systems in various body cells and tissues. This phenomenon underlies the cross effect of hypoxic training on physical endurance of the organism and is corroborated by the beneficial effects of intermittent normobaric hypoxia on athletes.

The use of interval hypoxic training as a tool for improving sports achievements has been practiced for decades [20]. For example, a study showed that the total amount of work and the total number of strokes performed by boat racers in the terminal steps increased from 500 to 780 after preliminary hypoxic training. Adaptation to IH reduced the time required for holding up the race (both up- and downstream); the rate of respiration and cardiac rhythm also returned to the normal level. The combined training protocol was also effective in training highway bicyclists and volleyball players [53].

A series of questions arise. What is the cost of increasing the resistance of the human organism? What are the mechanisms underlying its resistance to acute physical load? How can the beneficial effects of adaptation be enhanced without deleterious side effects?

One of the ways to minimize adverse side effects in different forms of adaptation is to reduce the intensity of the active factor. However, formation of long-lasting adaptive responses using the stressor with moderate or low intensity would take a lot of time (no less than 3–5 weeks), which may not be very practical for both clinical medicine (i.e., therapeutic management of patients, implementation of preoperative procedures, preventive measures during remission, etc.), and sports (training of athletes). The main challenge is to reduce the time required for long-lasting adaptation with preservation or improvement of its efficiency at the organ level. This issue can be solved through increasing the intensity of the adaptive signal at the expense of excessive production of ROS and the degree or duration of hypoxia, while eliminating the negative side effects [19]. A clue to the practical solution of this problem is to develop an approach to increase the intensity of the adaptive signal without affecting the hypoxic component. A positive cross effect can be attained, for example, through combination of two different adaptation regimens or the use of a novel technique combining interval hypoxia with hyperoxia. Analysis of the efficiency of these approaches has made the subject of the present work.

16.7 Materials and Methods

16.7.1 Experimental Design

The experiments were performed on 40 male Wistar rats weighing 200–230 g. The animals were kept under standard vivarium conditions (School of Fundamental Medicine, Moscow State University, Moscow, Russia). The animals were divided into five groups, eight animals in each group. The experimental protocol included three steps.

In the first step, we evaluated the efficiency of short-term physical exercise using two regimens of adaptation to variable oxygen levels. To this end, we estimated the total time of staying on water surface during swimming test to exhaustion for the rats and also evaluated the share of the active swimming phase in the total time of staying on water surface.

In the second step, we evaluated the damaging effect of AEE and protective effect of adaptation to hypoxia/normoxia (H/N) or hypoxia/hyperoxia (H/H) combined with physical load by measuring the rate of free radical oxidation and activity of antioxidant defense enzymes.

In the third step, we examined the changes in the concentration of constitutive and inducible urgent response proteins and the iron-regulatory protein (IRP) after short-term physical training combined with adaptation to variable oxygen levels. In a special series of our experiments, we performed a comparative analysis of the "cost" of adaptation in the H/N and H/H regimens.

The following physiological models were used: (1) damaging model, physical training by forced swimming to exhaustion with additional load (5% of body mass); (2) adaptation models, *direct model* – physical training by swimming in a moderate mode, and *cross model* – adaptation to variable oxygen levels was implemented in two variants, i.e., classical intermittent normobaric hypoxia (hypoxia + normoxia, H/N) and a novel type of adaptation to intermittent hypoxia and moderate hyperoxia (hypoxia + hyperoxia, H/H).

The experimental and control animals were kept under standard vivarium conditions (25–26°C, eight animals in a cage) and on a standard diet. Twenty-four hours before acute exposure to physical load (multiple swimming sessions), the animals were deprived of food. Tissue fragments were collected 2 h after acute exposure.

16.7.2 Physiological Models

Acute Physical Load by Swimming to Exhaustion with Additional 5% Load (AEE): AEE included manifold exhaustive swimming sessions ($t_{H_2O}+21^{\circ}C$) with additional load (5% of body mass) implemented 3 h after the last adaptation to variable oxygen levels. The total time of staying on water surface and duration of passive and active training were determined individually for each animal. Tissue samples were collected 2 h after cessation of AEE. The physical status of experimental animals was characterized by low mobility, which correlated with that observed in acute stress (anxiety neurosis).

Adaptation to Moderate Physical Load by Swimming (8Swim): The adaptation protocol included 30-min manifold ($n=8$) swimming sessions at 24°C, daily for 8 days; their duration was gradually increased from 10 to 20 and 30 min on the 1st, 2nd, and subsequent days, respectively. Adaptation of control and experimental animals was implemented in a moderate regime on the same day (2 h after adaptation to H/N or H/H).

Adaptation to Variable Oxygen Levels (Hypoxia and/or Hyperoxia): Preconditioning to interval normobaric hypoxia was performed using two regimens:

1. H/N – classical training, which combined alternating H/N exposures (5-min 10% O_2 + 3-min normoxia; 64 min daily for 15 days).
2. H/H – a novel regime (RF Patent No. 2289432 of 20.12.2006), which combined hypoxia and hyperoxia (5-min 10% O_2 + 3-min moderate hyperoxia (30% O_2); 64 min daily for 15 days). The novel adaptation protocol was introduced progressively (20 min on day 1, 40 min on day 2, and 64 min on day 3 and subsequent days).

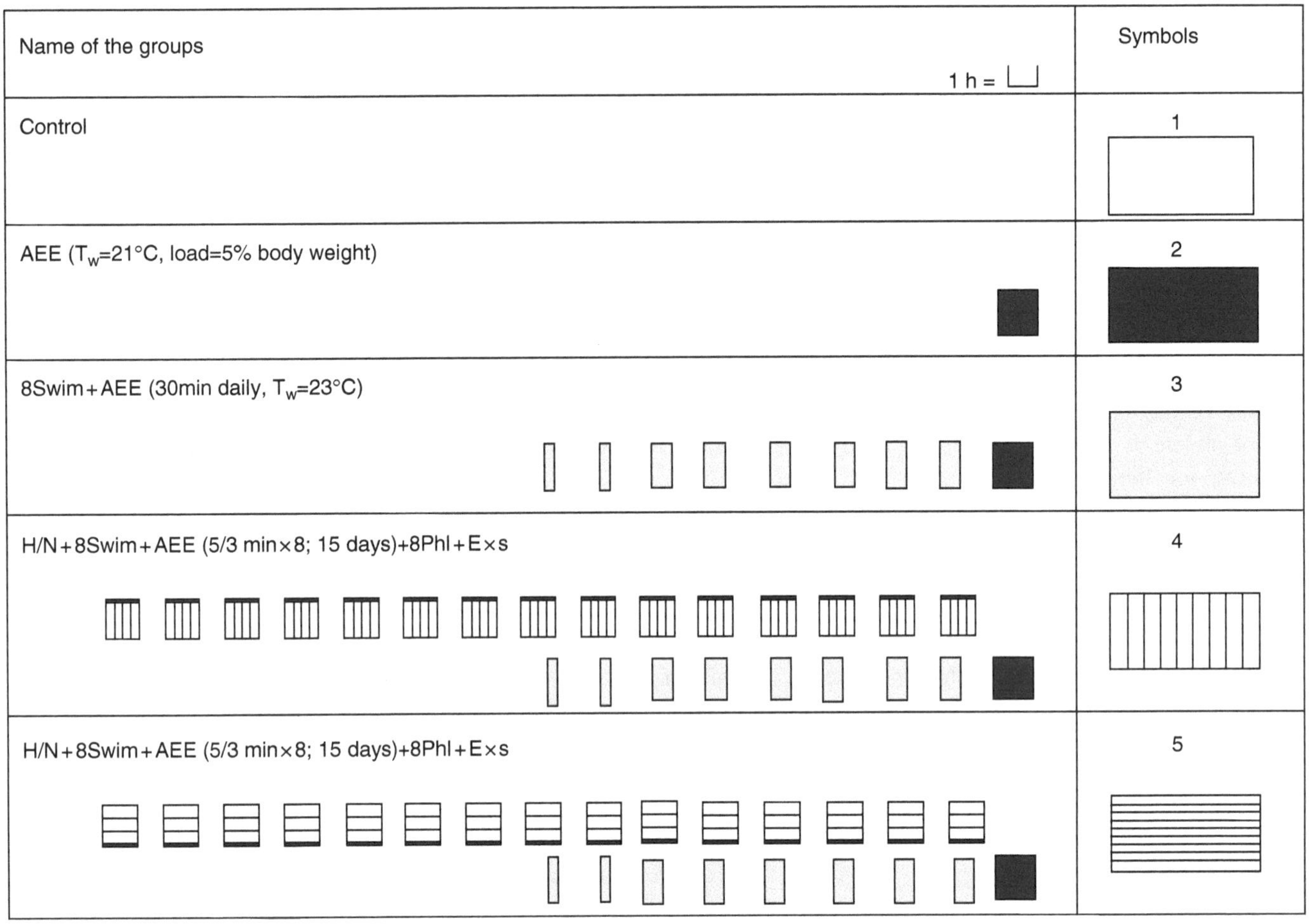

Fig. 16.2 Experimental design and abbreviations

Figure 16.2 shows the experimental design and abbreviations. The following five animal groups were investigated: (1) C – control; (2) AEE – acute physical load by swimming to exhaustion with additional weight (5% of body mass); (3) 8Swim + AEE – AEE performed after 30-min daily physical training, eight exposures; (4) H/N + 8Swim + AEE – AEE performed after physical training combined with adaptation to hypoxia/normoxia; and (5) H/H + 8Swim + AEE – AEE performed after physical training combined with adaptation to hypoxia/hyperoxia.

16.7.3 Biochemical Methods

Preparation of Tissue Samples: Fragmented tissue samples were collected after decapitation of animals under urethane anesthesia (40 g/100 ml of solution, 0.5 ml/100 g of body mass). Fragments of heart, left lobe of liver, and skeletal muscle (quadriceps muscle of thigh) were stripped of connective tissue, washed carefully with ice-cold saline, and frozen in liquid nitrogen until use.

Homogenate Preparation: The tissue samples were homogenized in knife- (heart) or Teflon-glass homogenizer (liver) in 12 volumes of a medium containing 30 mM Trizma@ and 100 mM NaCl pH 7.4. Protein concentration was determined by the method of Lowry et al.

Lipid Peroxidation: The resistance of myocardial and liver tissues to free radical oxidation was studied in vitro by oxidation in ROS-inducing systems. Freshly prepared diluted (1:5) homogenates (3 mg protein) were incubated at 37°C in 20 mM Trizma@ (pH 7.0), 100 mM NaCl, $FeSO_4^{2+}$ (10–50 nmol/mg of protein), and 0.3 mM sodium ascorbate. The concentrations of ROS-induced oxidation products were determined by following characteristic absorption using the method of Ohkawa et al. [54] in the modification of Kikugawa et al. [55].

Antioxidant Enzymes Assays: Catalase activity was determined by the method of Luck [56] at 240 nm. SOD activity was measured by the rate of inhibition of superoxide radical formation in the xanthine-xanthine oxidase system [57] at 560 nm by formazan formation from tetranitrotetrazolium blue.

Western Blot Analysis: HSP72, HSP32, and HSC73 were determined in the cytoplasmic fractions of heart and liver.

The tissues were homogenized in a Teflon-glass homogenizer (4°C) in a lyzing buffer containing 50 mM Tris–HCl, 5 mM EDTA, 1 mM DTT, and 1% Triton X-100 pH 7.5 (buffer: tissue ratio=6:1, by weight). The homogenate was filtered through six layers of gauze and centrifuged for 30 min at 12,000 g (4°C). The proteins were separated in 10% polyacrylamide gel and transferred to a PVDF membrane by electroelution (overnight). Preincubation of Western blots was carried out in TBST supplemented with 1% Tween-20 containing 5% (w/v) defatted milk (1 h). The positive controls prepared from rat thymuses and H35 hepatoma cells were subjected to heat shock (41.5°C, 30 min). The Western blots were incubated in the presence of primary monoclonal antibodies against HSP72, HSP32 (Stressgen, Canada; Santa Cruz, USA) (1:1,000), and primary polyclonal antibodies against (Stressgen) used in the same dilution for 1 h, washed and incubated in the presence of secondary antibodies (Jackson Immuno Research) conjugated with horseradish peroxidase (1:2,000) for 1 h. Detection of HSP72, HSP32, and HSC73 was performed in a reaction with ECL reagents (Kodak film).

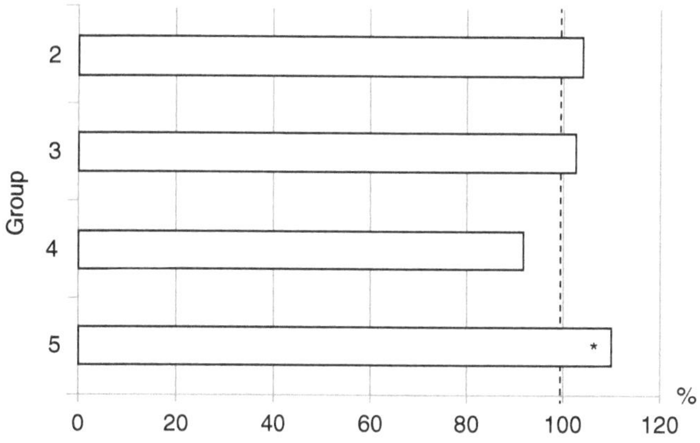

Fig. 16.3 The body mass of rats determined after cessation of swimming sessions (% of control – 100% – *dotted line*). *Experimental groups*: *2* – AEE (acute physical load by swimming to exhaustion with additional weight (5% of body mass)); *3* – 8Swim+AEE (AEE performed after 30 min daily physical training, 8 exposures); *4* – H/N+8Swim+AEE (AEE performed after physical training combined with adaptation to hypoxia/normoxia); *5* – H/H+8Swim+AEE (AEE performed after physical training combined with adaptation to hypoxia/hyperoxia). *Note*: * significance of differences ($P \leq 0.05$) compared to H/N+8Swim+AEE (Mann–Whitney *U* Test)

16.8 Results and Discussion

16.8.1 Changes in the Duration of Test Swimming After Adaptation to Physical Load Combined with Adaptation to Variable Oxygen Levels

A comparison of changes in body mass of experimental rats measured before and after cessation of training sessions indicated a lack of notable changes in comparison with the control group. This lack of significant decrement of body mass in both control and experimental groups suggests that the given training mode has a moderate stressor effect on the organism.

At the same time, we observed a significant difference between the effects of two forms of adaptation to variable oxygen levels combined with physical exercise (Fig. 16.3). After cessation of swimming sessions, the body mass in the group where adaptation to physical load was combined with 2-week adaptation to hypoxia–hyperoxia (H/H+8Swim+AEE) significantly exceeded that in the group where physical exercise was implemented together with adaptation to hypoxia–normoxia (H/N+8Swim+AEE). The general increment of body mass in the (H/H+8Swim+AEE) group was 19.4 g.

It may be inferred from these data that combination of AEE performed after adaptation of experimental animals to hypoxia/hyperoxia with physical load training by forced swimming is not accompanied by decreased body mass, but rather stimulates the synthesis of structural proteins.

16.8.2 Changes in the Duration of Physical Load (Swimming)

After short-term adaptation to physical load combined with adaptation to variable oxygen levels or without it, the duration of forced swimming to exhaustion increased appreciably (Fig. 16.4). When physical training (8Swim+AEE) was used alone, i.e., without hypoxic exposure, the average duration of AEE increased by 54%. After combining physical training with adaptation to hypoxia/normoxia (H/N+8Swim+AEE) or hypoxia/hyperoxia (H/H+8Swim+AEE), this parameter increased 2.3 and 2.0 fold, respectively.

Very impressive results were obtained in the duration of active swimming phase. In the control group, the share of active swimming relative to the total time of staying on water surface was not very large (16%), suggesting that most of the time the animals hovered in water in the upright position since the passive phase was preferable.

Eight-day physical training (8Swim+AEE) markedly increased the duration of the active swimming phase in comparison with control group AEE, while the share of active swimming in the total time of staying on water surface increased by 34% (i.e., 52% of total time of staying on the water surface) (Fig. 16.4).

Although combination of adaptation to hypoxia–normoxia with training to physical load (H/N+8Swim+AEE) increased the duration of staying on water surface, the duration of the active swimming phase did not increase in comparison with the 8Swim+AEE group. Moreover, the share of active

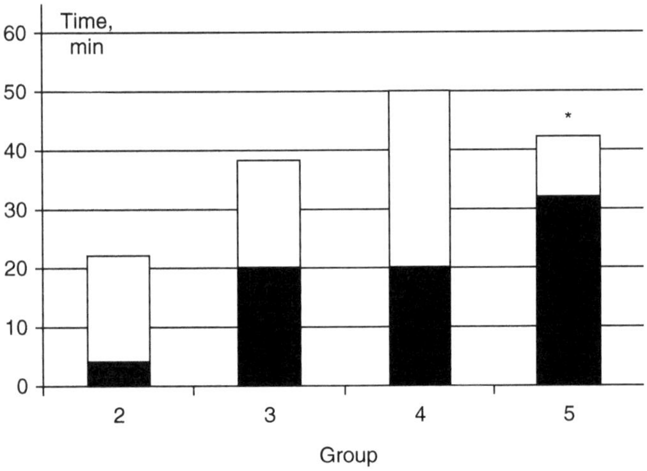

Fig. 16.4 The total time of staying on water surface and duration of the active swimming phase. *Experimental groups*: *2* – AEE (acute physical load by swimming to exhaustion with additional weight (5% of body mass)); *3* – 8Swim+AEE (AEE performed after 30 min daily physical training, 8 exposures); *4* – H/N+8Swim+AEE (AEE performed after physical training combined with adaptation to hypoxia/normoxia); *5* – H/H+8Swim+AEE (AEE performed after physical training combined with adaptation to hypoxia/hyperoxia). *Note*: *dark-colored areas* active swimming phase

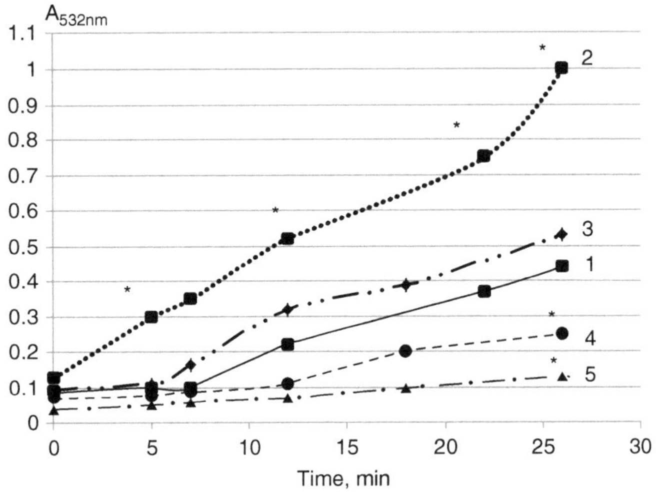

Fig. 16.5 Effect of adaptation to hypoxia/normoxia and hypoxia/hyperoxia combined with adaptation to physical load on the level of TBA-active lipid peroxidation products during LPO induction in the liver in vitro. *Experimental groups*: *1* – *C* (control); *2* – AEE (acute physical load by swimming to exhaustion with additional weight (5% of body mass)); *3* – 8Swim+AEE (AEE performed after 30 min daily physical training, 8 exposures); *4* – H/N+8Swim+AEE (AEE performed after physical training combined with adaptation to hypoxia/normoxia; *5* – H/H+8Swim+AEE (AEE performed after physical training combined with adaptation to hypoxia/hyperoxia). *Note*: A_{532} optical density at 532 nm

swimming showed a tendency to decrease from 52% to 40% of the total time of staying on water surface.

Conversely, combination of adaptation to physical load with adaptation to hypoxia/hyperoxia (H/H+8Swim+AEE) prolonged the active phase by 24% in comparison with the (8Swim+AEE) group, while combined adaptation to physical load with intermittent hypoxia–hyperoxia changed the active swimming phase from minor in the control group to dominant in the experimental group. This finding provides additional support in favor of the hypothesis on beneficial effect of adaptation to hypoxia/hyperoxia on the synthesis of structural proteins.

Thus, the time of staying on water surface in the course of exhaustive AEE after combined adaptation to physical load and variable oxygen levels increases, but the duration of the active swimming phase increases appreciably; however, only after the addition of adaptation to hypoxia/hyperoxia to the protocol.

16.8.3 Changes in the Intensity of Free Radical Oxidation and Activity of Antioxidant Defense Enzymes in AEE After Different Adaptation Regimens

We examined the changes in the rates of free radical processes in the most ROS-sensitive organ, i.e., the liver, during AEE in control rats as well as after adaptation to physical load with or without combined adaptation to variable oxygen levels.

In AEE group, the rate of lipid peroxidation products accumulation during in vitro initiation of free radical oxidation increased more than twofold versus the control group (Fig. 16.5), suggesting a drastic decrease in the resistance of animal tissues to ROS-dependent processes. Adaptation to physical load used alone (8Swim+AEE) or in combination with adaptation to variable oxygen levels (H/N+8Swim+AEE and H/H+8Swim+AEE) diminished the rate of free radical oxidation induced by AEE. After implementation of direct adaptation (short-term physical training, 8Swim+AEE), the rate of accumulation of lipid peroxidation products did not differ essentially from control, being time-dependent and 1.6–2.7 times lower than in the AEE group.

Addition of cross adaptation to physical load to adaptation to variable oxygen levels further increased the resistance of animal tissues to free radical oxidation. After adaptation to hypoxia/normoxia (H/N+8Swim+AEE), the concentration of TBA-active metabolites diminished 1.4- to 2.9-fold, whereas after adaptation to hypoxia/hyperoxia (H/H+8Swim+AEE), it decreased for 2.2- to 4.6-fold.

Measurement of activities of the major antioxidant defense enzymes, i.e., SOD and catalase (Fig. 16.6), established that AEE-induced activation of free radical oxidation was accompanied by inhibition of antioxidant defense enzymes (21% significant decrease of SOD activity as compared with the control).

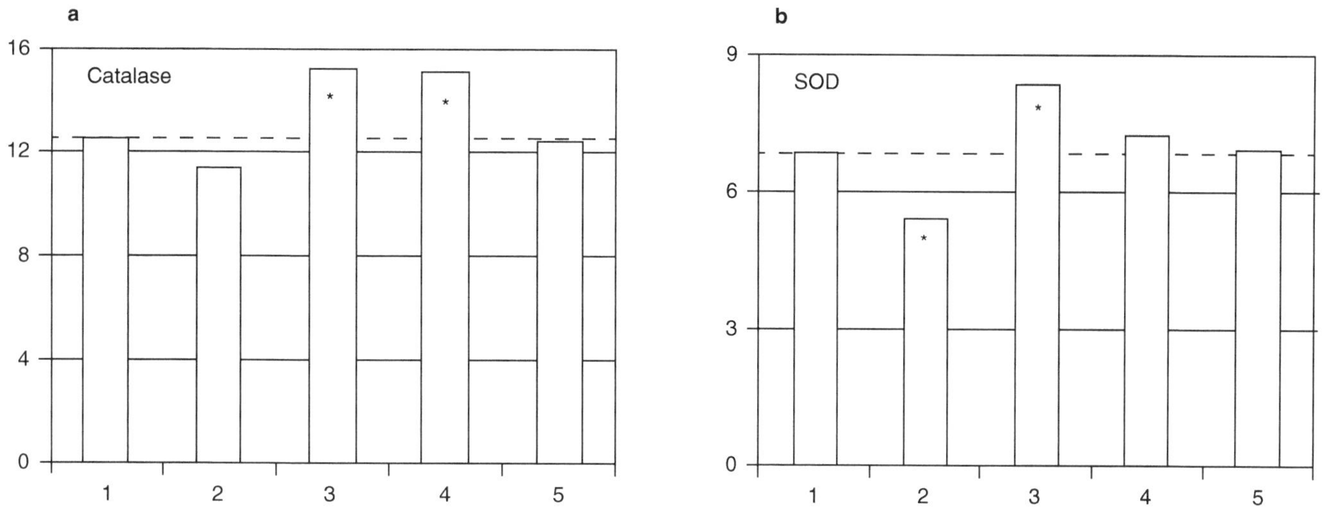

Fig. 16.6 Activities of catalase (**a**) and superoxide dismutase (**b**) in the liver of Wistar rats after a single session of swimming to exhaustion with additional load (5% of body mass). *Experimental groups*: *1* – *C* (control); *2* – AEE (acute physical load by swimming to exhaustion with additional weight (5% of body mass)); *3* – 8Swim+AEE (AEE performed after 30 min daily physical training, 8 exposures); *4* – H/N+8Swim+AEE (AEE performed after physical training combined with adaptation to hypoxia/normoxia); *5* – H/H+8Swim+AEE (AEE performed after physical training combined with adaptation to hypoxia/hyperoxia). Note: the dotted lines indicate the enzyme activity levels found in Group 1 (control)

Compensation of free radical processes after 8-day training (8Swim+AEE) was possible due to significant increases in the activities of both enzymes in comparison with AEE and control groups: the activity of SOD exceeded the control level by 24%, while that of catalase surpassed it by 35%. In addition, AEE changed the ratio of pro- and antioxidant enzymes in both control group and after short-term preconditioning to physical load (8Swim+AEE).

Combination of adaptation to physical load with adaptation to variable oxygen levels not only initiated a significant decrease in the rate of lipid peroxidation but also failed to induce significant activation of antioxidant defense systems at the end of the 2-week adaptation period characteristic of physical training in the absence of adaptation to variable oxygen levels (8Swim+AEE). When adaptation to physical load was combined with adaptation to hypoxia/normoxia (H/N+8Swim+AEE), this regularity was only partly realized, which manifested itself in a drastic decrease of the elevated content of SOD to nearly control values, while the activity of catalase remained at a sufficiently high level. This finding can be interpreted by the fact that 2-week adaptation to hypoxia/normoxia is insufficient for eliciting a stable adaptive response and elevated activity of one of antioxidant defense enzymes can be regarded as a "cost" of adaptation.

Noteworthy, the hypoxia/hyperoxia mode ensures eliciting of long-lasting adaptive responses within the same time period as the new form of adaptation to variable oxygen levels. When physical training is combined with adaptation to hypoxia/hyperoxia (H/H+8Swim+AEE), the decrease in the intensity of AEE-induced lipid peroxidation is concomitant with a return of the elevated content of antioxidant defense systems to the control level as is the case with SOD and catalase.

It seems probable that augmented synthesis of antioxidant defense enzymes is a peculiar kind of a "cost" of improved resistance following short-term adaptation to physical load. If such training is combined with adaptation to hypoxia/hyperoxia, we may deal with a more efficient defense mechanism affording potent protection against ROS-induced injuries. It should be remembered that it is the restoration of the balance between pro- and antioxidants that is a reason for high efficiency of adaptation to physical training.

In other words, combination of two adaptation protocols, namely, adaptation to variable oxygen levels and adaptation to physical load, effectively prevents inhibition of antioxidant defense systems in AEE and their excessive activation during adaptation to physical load. This, in turn, may influence the efficiency of physical training.

16.8.4 Determination of Levels of HSP Proteins (HSP72, HSP32, HSC73) in AEE After Adaptation in Different Regimes

The regularities characteristic of changing levels of antioxidant defense enzymes were also established for other defense proteins. In this study, we examined the levels of three HSP proteins, namely, two inducible forms (HSP72 and HSP32) and the constitutive form (HSC73).

Protein HSP72 is characterized by enhanced expression in response to different stress factors which increase the denaturation of intracellular proteins. HSP72 expression proceeds at a much faster rate than activation of proteins acting as cell protectors and diminishes when normal cell activity is resumed.

HSP32 (HOx-1) is an inducible isoform of the protein, usually referred to as heme oxygenase. The rate of its synthesis provides information about the activity of its stressor and hypoxic components. It is important to note that the HSP32 level must be considered in the paradigm of variable levels of other ROS-induced proteins. Indeed, HSP32 induction may be suggestive of simultaneous presence of the ROS signal and the hypoxic component, while elevated content of HSP72 is characteristic of ROS-induced stress, but not hypoxia. In this context, HSP32 elevation against the background of HSP72 induction may testify, with a high degree of probability, to the presence of a ROS signal and the lack of changes in the HSP72 level, while HSP32 induction suggests the predominance of the hypoxic signal.

Continuous expression of HSC73 is characteristic of physiological conditions. In the absence of stress, the constitutive protein HSC73 plays the role of a molecular chaperone for newly synthesized proteins and controls their transport into cell organelles. In addition, HSC73 is engaged in targeted delivery of irreversibly damaged proteins and polypeptides to proteasomes where the latter undergo degradation under the action of Bag-1, CHIP, and ubiquitin.

Some papers describe differently directed changes in HSC73 content after thermal and hypoxic exposures. Among the most recent findings, the results obtained by Andreeva et al. [58] present particular interest. These authors succeeded in demonstrating that under conditions of thermal stress, the level of the constitutive protein HSC73 does not change, but increases in the subsequent period, most probably due to augmented synthesis of intracellular proteins during adaptation to the stress factor [58]. It was suggested that HSC73 accumulation in mononuclear cells in response to thermal stress is prerequisite to chaperoning and folding of newly synthesized functional proteins, adaptive changes in the cell, formation of adaptive responses, and improvement of cell resistance to damaging factors.

At the same time, a single course of normobaric hypoxic training from manifold 30-min continuous inhalation of 10% oxygen failed to elicit stress responses at the body level, suggesting a lack of inducible HSP72 elevation in mononuclear cells [59]. However, the nonspecific resistance increased in parallel with a simultaneous increase in the content of the constitutive protein HSC73. Apparently, the presence of the hypoxic component of adaptation can be inferred from the level of HSC73.

The contribution of the stress and hypoxic components to adaptation can adequately be evaluated only on the basis of in-depth analysis of complex changes in the three HSP proteins.

Our study established the following changes in stressory and hypoxic proteins. AEE initiates significant (by 61% in comparison with control) accumulation of the inducible form of the stress protein HSP72. Adaptation to physical load (8Swim + AEE) and its combination with adaptation to variable oxygen levels (H/N + 8Swim + AEE and H/H + 8Swim + AEE) compensates for the stress component, while the HSP72 content drops down to a level characteristic of the control group (Fig. 16.7). This indicates that training to physical load combined with adaptation to variable oxygen levels and without it prevents the enhancement of ROS-induced processes. These findings are consistent with the results described in the foregoing section.

Quite different regularities were established for urgent response proteins characteristic of hypoxia. Figure 16.8a, b shows that AEE implemented after short-term training (8Swim + AEE) increases the level of both HSP32 (by 34% in comparison with control and by 43% in comparison with AEE) and HSC73 (by 24% in comparison with control), being suggestive of the hypoxic effect. In other words, direct adaptation as a short-lasting mode of adaptation to physical load has a "cost" of its own manifested in a noncompensated hypoxic (as opposed to compensated) stress signal as can be judged from continuous synthesis of hypoxic proteins even at the end of the 2nd adaptation week.

Such high cost can be reduced through combination of adaptation to physical load (8Swim + AEE) with adaptation to variable oxygen levels. If adaptation to physical load is combined with adaptation to hypoxia/normoxia (H/N + 8Swim + AEE), its effect is only partly apparent as in the case with antioxidant defense enzymes, and it is the level of only one protein, namely, the rapidly synthesized low-molecular protein HSP32 that is decreased. The novel procedure for short-term adaptation to variable oxygen levels, namely, hypoxia/hyperoxia combined with physical training (H/H + 8Swim + AEE), is sufficient for complete compensation of the "cost" of physical training, namely, a return to the content of all intrinsic proteins of the hypoxic component to the control level.

These data altogether suggest that adaptation to physical load alone compensates for the stress component of acute exhaustive exercise. Notwithstanding, after such adaptation, the hypoxic component is obviously apparent. Combination of physical training with adaptation to hypoxia–normoxia partly eliminates the hypoxic component, while combination of adaptation to physical load with adaptation to hypoxia/hyperoxia fully normalizes the level of rapidly and slowly synthesized proteins characteristic of the hypoxic component of adaptation.

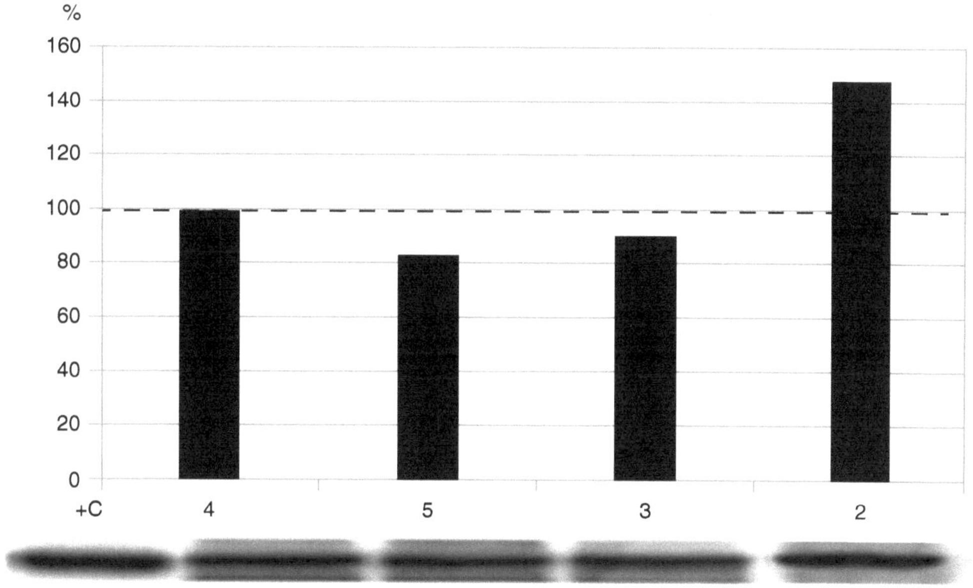

Fig. 16.7 Effect of adaptation to variable oxygen levels combined with adaptation to physical load on the content of the inducible form of the stress protein HSP72 in the heart of Wistar rats after AEE. *C* control (100%) (*dotted line*), +*C* positive control. Fragments of rat thymus tissue and H35 cells were subjected to 30-min thermal treatment at 41.5°C. *Experimental groups*: *2* – AEE (acute physical load by swimming to exhaustion with additional weight (5% of body mass)); *3* – 8Swim + AEE (AEE performed after 30 min daily physical training, 8 exposures); *4* – H/N + 8Swim + AEE (AEE performed after physical training combined with adaptation to hypoxia/normoxia); *5* – H/H + 8Swim + AEE (AEE performed after physical training combined with adaptation to hypoxia/hyperoxia)

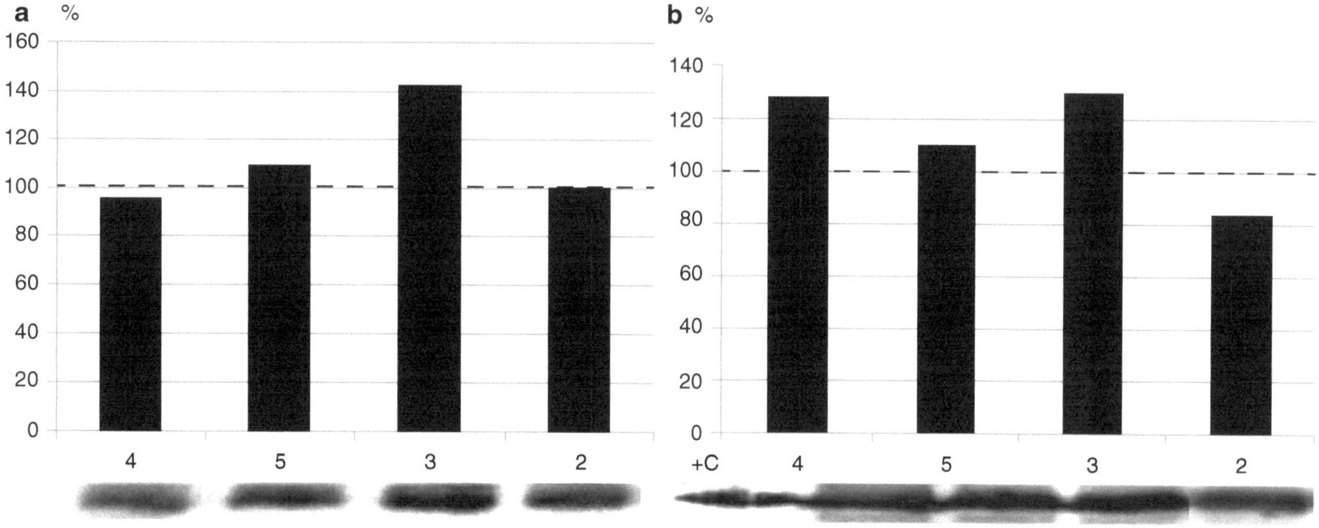

Fig. 16.8 Effect of adaptation to variable oxygen levels combined with adaptation to physical load (physical training) on the content of the inducible protein HSP32 (**a**) and the constitutive protein HSP73 (**b**) in the heart of Wistar rats under AEE. *C* control (100%) (*dotted line*), +*C* positive control: fragments of rat thymus tissue and H35 cells were subjected to 30-min thermal treatment at 41.5°C. *Experimental groups*: *2* – AEE (acute physical load by swimming to exhaustion with additional weight (5% of body mass)); *3* – 8Swim + AEE (AEE performed after 30 min daily physical training, 8 exposures); *4* – H/N + 8Swim + AEE (AEE performed after physical training combined with adaptation to hypoxia/normoxia); *5* – H/H + 8Swim + AEE (AEE performed after physical training combined with adaptation to hypoxia/hyperoxia)

Conclusions

Short-term physical training increases the duration of swimming in AEE. Its combination with adaptation to variable oxygen levels has no effect on this parameter, while adaptation to physical load combined with adaptation to hypoxia–hyperoxia increases the duration of the active swimming phase and, as a consequence, the efficiency of adaptation. Adaptation to physical load and its combination with adaptation to IH increase the resistance of membrane structures to free radical oxidation at the expense of excessive activation of antioxidant defense enzymes in the course of physical training, which is partly compensated by adaptation to hypoxia/normoxia and is fully prevented by adaptation to hypoxia/hyperoxia. The combination of two forms of adaptation (i.e., direct adaptation to physical load and cross adaptation to variable oxygen levels) compensates for the markedly elevated content of HSP proteins in the course of physical training, which is especially well pronounced during adaptation to hypoxia/hyperoxia. This novel technique is apparently less expensive and more beneficial for the organism.

References

1. Das DK. Redox regulation of cardiomyocyte survival and death. Antioxid Redox Signal. 2001;3:23–37.
2. Ungemach FR. Plasma membrane damage of hepatocytes following lipid peroxidation: involvement of phospholipase A2. In: Free radicals liver injury. Washington, D.C.: Oxford; 1985. p. 127–34. Proc. Int. Meet., Turin.
3. Sazontova TG. Stress-induced moderation of heart Ca-transporting system SR function and its resistance to endogenous damaging factors. Bull Exp Biol Med. 1989;108:271–4 [In Russian].
4. Zolotarjova N, Ho C, Mellgren RL, et al. Different sensitivities of native and oxidized forms of Na^+/K^+-ATPase to intracellular proteinases. Biochim Biophys Acta. 1994;1192:125–31.
5. Hemler ME, Cook HW, Lands WE. Prostaglandin biosynthesis can be triggered by lipid peroxides. Arch Biochem Biophys. 1979;193:340–5.
6. Roberts AM, Messina EJ, Kaley G. Prostacyclin (PGI_2) mediates hypoxic relaxation of bovine coronary artery strips. Prostaglandins. 1981;21:555–69.
7. Semenza GL. Perspectives on oxygen sensing. Cell. 1999;98:281–4.
8. Chandel NS, Schumacker PT. Cellular oxygen sensing by mitochondria: old questions, new insight. J Appl Physiol. 2000;88:1880–9.
9. Flohe L, Brigelius-Flohe R, Salion C, et al. Redox regulation of NF-kappa B activation. Free Radic Biol Med. 1997;22:1115–26.
10. Maulik N, Yoshida T, Das DK. Regulation of cardiomyocyte apoptosis in ischemic reperfused mouse heart by glutathione peroxidase. Mol Cell Biochem. 1999;196:13–21.
11. Graven KK, Zimmerman LH, Dickson EW, et al. Endothelial cell hypoxia associated proteins are cell and stress specific. J Cell Physiol. 1993;157:544–54.
12. Peng J, Jones GL, Watson K. Stress proteins as biomarkers of oxidative stress: effects of antioxidant supplements. Free Radic Biol Med. 2000;28:1598–606.
13. Ryter SW, Tyrrell RM. The heme synthesis and degradation pathway: role in oxidant sensitivity. Free Radic Biol Med. 2000;28:289–309.
14. Zhukova AG, Sazontova TG. Heme oxygenase: function, regulation, biological role. Hypoxia Med J. 2004;3–4:30–43.
15. Hu ML, Frankel EN, Leibowitz BE, et al. Effect of dietary lipids and vitamin E on in vitro lipid peroxidation in rat liver and kidney homogenates. J Nutr. 1989;119:1574–82.
16. Sanz MJ, Ferrndiz ML, Cejudo M, et al. Influence of a series of natural flavonoids on free radical generating systems and oxidative stress. Xenobiotica. 1994;24:689–99.
17. Singh B, Sharma SP, Goyal R. Evaluation of Geriforte, an herbal geriatric tonic, on antioxidant defense system in Wistar rats. Ann N Y Acad Sci. 1994;717:170–3.
18. Cai YN, Appelkvist EL, Deplerre JW. Hepatic oxidative stress and related defenses during treatment of mice with acetylsalicylic acid and other peroxisome proliferators. J Biochem Toxicol. 1995;10:87–94.
19. Arkhipenko YuV, Sazontova TG, Rice-Evans C. Hypertrophy and regression of rat heart: free radical related metabolic systems. Pathophysiology. 1997;4:241–8.
20. Kolchinskaya AZ. Intermittent hypoxic training in sports of highest achievements. Sports Med. 2008;1:9–25 [In Russian].
21. Sazontova TG, Tkatchouk EN, Kolmykova SN, et al. Comparative analysis of peroxidation and antioxidant enzyme activities in rats adapted to different regimes of normobaric hypoxia. Hypoxia Med J. 1994;2:4–7.
22. Sazontova TG, Arkhipenko YuV. The role of free-radical processes in adaptation of the organism to variable oxygen levels. In: Lukyanova LD, Ushakov IB, editors. Problems of hypoxia: molecular, physiological and medical aspects. Moscow: Publ. Istoki; 2004. p. 112–38 [In Russian].
23. Sazontova TG, Arkhipenko YuV. Intermittent hypoxia in resistance of cardiac membrane structures: role of reactive oxygen species and redox signaling. In: Xi L, Serebrovskaya TV, editors. Intermittent hypoxia: from molecular mechanisms to clinical applications. New York: Nova Science Publishers, Inc.; 2009. p. 147–87.
24. Zenkov NK, Lankin VZ, Menschikova EB. Oxidative stress. Moscow: MAIK Science/Interperiodica; 2001 [in Russian].
25. Moncada S, Palmer RMJ, Higgs EA. Nitric oxide: physiology, pathophysiology and pharmacology. Pharmacol Rev. 1991;43:109–40.
26. Thomas S, Lowe JE, Hadjivassiliou V, et al. Use of the comet assay to investigate the role of superoxide in glutathione-induced DNA damage. Biochem Biophys Res Commun. 1998;243:241–5.
27. Skulachev VP. Mitochondrial in the programmed death phenomena; a principle of biology: "It's better to die than to be wrong". IUBMB Life. 2000;49:365–77.
28. Sohal RS, Svensson I, Brunk UT. Hydrogen peroxide production by liver mitochondria in different species. Mech Ageing Dev. 1990; 53:209–15.
29. Beyer RE. The analysis of the role of coenzyme Q in free radical generation and as an antioxidant. Biochem Cell Biol. 1992;70:390–403.
30. Zorov DB. Mechanisms of cardioprotection in hypoxia/reoxygenation. In: Reception and intracellular signaling. Puschino: Nauka; 2003. p. 160–2 [in Russian].
31. Sohal RS. Ageing, cytochrome oxidase activity, and hydrogen peroxide release by mitochondria. Free Radic Biol Med. 1993;14:583–8.
32. Richter C. Role of mitochondrial DNA modifications in degenerative diseases and aging. Curr Top Bioenerg. 1994;17:1–19.
33. Nikonorov AA, Tverdokhlib VP, Krasikov SI. Correction of biotransformation of xenobiotics in extreme states. In: Biochemistry: from molecular mechanisms investigation to implementation in clinical practice. Orenburg: OGMA; 2003. p. 305–11 [in Russian].
34. Deev LI, Ahalaya MYa, Illarionova EA, et al. Relation of changes in the content and activity of rat liver microsomal cytochrome P-450 to the intensification of lipid peroxidation under stress. Biull Eksp Biol Med. 1983;95:51–3 [In Russian].
35. Nikonorov AA. Application of adaptation to interval hypobaric hypoxia for increase of sportsmen' organism resistance to competition load. Thesis for MD. Siberian State Medical University, Tomsk; 2002 [In Russian].
36. Bondy SC, Naderi S. Contribution of hepatic cytochrome P450 systems to the generation of reactive oxygen species. Biochem Pharmacol. 1994;48:155–9.
37. Podmore I, Griffiths H, Herbert K. Vitamin C exhibits pro-oxidant properties. Nature. 1998;392:559.
38. Droge W. Free radicals in the physiological control of cell function. Physiol Rev. 2002;82:47–95.
39. Saenko YuV, Shutov AM. Role of oxidative stress in pathology of cardiovascular system in nephrologic patients. II. Clinical aspects of oxidative stress. Nephrol Dial. 2004;6:138–44.

40. Dubinina EE. Role of reactive oxygen species as signal molecules in tissue metabolism under oxidative stress. Vopr Med Khim. 2001;47:561–81 [In Russian].
41. Sergienko VI, Panasenko OM. Reactive oxygen species in disease pathogenesis. Technol Living Syst. 2004;1:37–46 [In Russian].
42. Moldovan NI, Moldovan L. Oxygen free radicals and redox biology of organelles. Histochem Cell Biol. 2004;122:395–412.
43. Valko M, Leibfritz D, Moncol J, et al. Free radicals and antioxidants in normal physiological functions and human disease. Int J Biochem Cell Biol. 2007;39:44–84.
44. Sies H. Oxidative stress – from basic research to clinical application. Am J Med. 1991;91:S31–8.
45. Fridovich I. Fundamental aspects of reactive oxygen species, or what's the matter with oxygen? Ann N Y Acad Sci. 1999;893:13–8.
46. Zakharova MN, Zavalishin IA, Boldyrev AA. Role of SOD in pathogenesis of amyotrophic lateral sclerosis. Bull Exp Biol Med. 1999;127:460–2 [In Russian].
47. Wanders RJA, Denis S. Identification of superoxide dismutase in rat liver peroxisomes. Biochem Biophys Acta. 1992;1115:259–62.
48. Akashi M, Hachiya M, Paquette RL. Irradiation increases manganese superoxide dismutase mRNA levels in human fibroblasts – possible mechanisms for its accumulation. J Biol Chem. 1995;270:15864–9.
49. Radi R, Turrens JF, Chang LY. Detection of catalase in rat heart mitochondria. J Biol Chem. 1991;266:22028–34.
50. Eriksson AM, Lundgren B, Andersson K, et al. Is the cytosolic catalase induced by peroxisome proliferators in mouse liver on its way to the peroxisomes? FEBS Lett. 1992;308:211–4.
51. Antunes F, Han D, Cadenas E. Relative contributions of heart mitochondria glutathione peroxidase and catalase to H_2O_2 detoxification in in vivo conditions. Free Radic Biol Med. 2002;33:1260–7.
52. Finaud J, Lac G, Filaire E. Oxidative stress: relationship with exercise and training. Sports Med. 2006;36:327–58.
53. Khotochkina LV, Statsenko NI. Intermittent hypoxic training as a method of physical state improvement and increase of efficiency in highly qualified oarsmen. Hypoxia Med J. 1993;2:38–40 [In Russian].
54. Ohkawa H, Ohishi N, Yagi K. Assay for lipid peroxides in animal tissues by thiobarbituric acid reaction. Anal Biochem. 1979;95: 351–8.
55. Kikugawa K, Kojima T, Yamaki S, et al. Interpretation of the thiobarbituric acid reactivity of rat liver and brain homogenates in the presence of ferric ion and ethylenediaminetetraacetic acid. Anal Biochem. 1992;202:249–55.
56. Luck H. Catalase. In: Bergmeyer HU, editor. Methods of enzymatic analysis. New York: Verlag-Chemie, Academic; 1963. p. 885–8.
57. Beauchamp C, Fridovich I. Superoxide dismutase: improved assay and an assay applicable to acrylamide gels. Anal Biochem. 1971;44: 276–87.
58. Andreeva LI, Goranchuk VV, Shustov EB, et al. Human adaptation to hypothermia and changes in leucocytes of peripheral blood. Sechenov Ross Physiol J. 2001;87:1208–16 [In Russian].
59. Boykova AA, Andreeva LI, Margulis BA, et al. Constitutive isoform of heat shock protein 70 in human blood mononuclears as marker of adaptation during normobaric hypoxia training. Sechenov Ross Physiol J. 2006;92:835–42 [In Russian].

Hypobaric Interval Hypoxia as a Nonmedication Method for Improving the Functional State of Aerospace Pilots and Astronauts

17

Igor B. Ushakov, Anatoli A. Shishov, Vladimir N. Komarevtsev, and Vladimir N. Filatov

Abstract

Maintenance of health of risky profession workers (such as aerospace pilots and astronauts) and rendering them rehabilitative procedures remains to be one of the major medical issues. There is an apparent necessity to seek and adopt effective methods of rehabilitating the workers of risky professions who usually suffer with fatigue, impairment of body tolerance to negative factors, deadaptation, and asthenization (a condition experienced by astronauts with symptoms such as fatigue, irritability, lack of appetite, and sleep disorders) following stressful situations of aerospace flights. These adverse effects could potentially lead to functional and organic diseases in the pilots and astronauts. A method of hypobaric interval hypoxia (HIH) was devised and test validated for the needs of aviation, space, military, preventive, and rehabilitation medicine. The course of HIH treatment consists of ten 1-h daily sessions of exposure to HIH in a hypobaric chamber simulating high altitude of 3,000–5,000 m. In each of the 10-min periods, 7-min hypoxic air breathing alternates with 3-min hyperoxic air mixture breathing with air pressure simulating same altitude. In the first session, the subjects "climb" to 3,000 m; in sessions 2–4, the altitude increases in 500 m steps; and finally the sessions 5–10 are performed at the altitude of 5,000 m. HIH has showed high effectiveness in improving human organism functionality and tolerance to the environmental adverse factors, that is, hypoxia, flight accelerations, and motion sickness, as well as in preventing and correcting the impaired functional states.

Abbreviations

BP	Blood pressure
CCCA	Continuous cumulation of Coriolis accelerations
FR	Physiological reserve
HIH	Hypobaric interval hypoxia
ICCA	Intermittent cumulation of Coriolis accelerations
MS	Motion sickness
SET	Statoergometric test
SV	Systolic volume
TPR	Total peripheral resistance
VBV	Volumetric blood flow velocity
VVR	Vestibulovegetative reactions

I.B. Ushakov (✉) • A.A. Shishov • V.N. Komarevtsev • V.N. Filatov
Russian Federation State Scientific Center, Institute of Biomedical Problems of the Russian Academy of Sciences,
Moscow, Russia
e-mail: ibushakov@gmail.com

17.1 Introduction

Duties of workers of risky professions (such as aerospace pilots and astronauts) are challenged by exposure to extreme conditions, severe psychoemotional stresses, and utmost mobilization of the functional reserve of the body. Reequipment of the armed forces with new aviation materials usually increases the roughness of extreme flight conditions. These changes would intensify the demands and requirements for personal protection of the aircrew and for the pilot's basic functional state and level of physiological reserve (FR) [1, 2]. In this context, there are still most critical and urgent needs to search for new strategy and ways to strengthen tolerance of hostile environmental factors

L. Xi, T.V. Serebrovskaya (eds.), *Intermittent Hypoxia and Human Diseases*,
DOI 10.1007/978-1-4471-2906-6_17, © Springer-Verlag London 2012

and maintenance of health of these risky profession workers and to render them rehabilitative therapy after exhaustive flight stresses [3–5].

Broadened application of nonmedicament methods of correcting changed functional states in risky professional workers is an emerging domain of the supportive and rehabilitative therapy. As one of the nonmedicament methods that have successfully treated detriments in the functional state caused by stress factors and diseases, the method of adaptation to hypoxia has been well recognized in aviation, sport, clinical, and military medicine [6–11]. Adaptation to hypoxia not only increases tolerance to hypoxia itself, producing the direct protective effect, but also strengthens resistance of organism to other stress factors, particularly with a hypoxic component providing the cross protective effect [12–14].

Animal experiments demonstrated substantial changes in the brain induced by exposure to the extreme factors of aviation and space flight, such as accelerations, vibration, microgravity, ionizing radiation, etc. These changes were associated primarily with disorders in structural organization and permeability of the hematoencephalic barrier [15, 16]. Adaptation to any stress factor produces resistance to the particular factor and also develops cross protective effects by activation of stress-limiting systems that control stress reactions and moderate damaging effects of stress hormones on target organs, as well as of local cytoprotective mechanisms [17].

17.2 Basic Concepts of Adaptation to Intermittent Hypoxia: Normobaric Versus Hypobaric

17.2.1 Concept of the Five Complexes of Adaptation to Intermittent Hypoxia

The mechanism of gaining stable adaptation to intermittent hypoxia includes the following five main distinguishable complexes [18, 19].

The first complex (early adaptation stage) is characterized by mobilization of the systems responsible for oxygen uptake and transport. Activation of ribonucleic acids and protein synthesis in the lung, heart, bone marrow, and blood has already been observed in the initial days of hypoxia. Consequently, respiratory surface of the lungs expands and functionality of the cardiovascular system and coronary blood flow increases, proliferation of erythrocytes becomes more intensive, and oxygenation capacity of blood increases [20, 21].

The distinguishing feature of the second complex is extensive synthesis of protein and ribonucleic acids in the brain in parallel with accumulation of serotonin and dopamine and a slight reduction in noradrenaline. Reductions in serotonin and histamine occur in blood. The protective reaction of organism leads to complete or partial prevention of stress-induced fermentemia through control of cytosolic and lysosomal enzymes excretion typically induced by severely stressful conditions [22].

The third complex is described as stable shifts in regulation of water-electrolyte metabolism and myogenic tone of resistive vessels. Incomplete atrophy of the supraoptical nucleus in the hypothalamus and zona glomerulosa, limited secretion of aldosterone, and antidiuretic hormone could cause excessive loss of sodium chloride and water, which in turn, together with degradation of arterial and arteriole stiffness, weakens the pressor reflexes and reduces the probability of hypertension development [13].

Changes in the immune system are directed toward prevalence of B lymphocytes over T lymphocytes in lymphoid organs (such as the spleen) constitute the forth complex. The principal consequence of this shift is partial suppression of immune reactions and decreases in the number of antibody-forming cells and antibodies in blood [13].

The fifth adaptation complex is recognized by activation of the antioxidant system and elevated concentration of cytochrome P-450 enzymes in hepatocytes that could be advantageous for the detoxication ability of the liver. Together, these changes fortify organism against atherogenic factors and toxic agents [23–25].

17.2.2 Adaptation to Hypobaric Versus Normobaric Intermittent Hypoxia

Previous publications have demonstrated that enhancement of the adaptive processes in living organism can be achieved by exposure to hypoxia in high mountains, during artificial "ascents" in hypobaric chamber, and through breathing of hypoxic gas mixtures at normal pressure [26–28]. The increased tolerance to altitude hypoxia and other extreme factors (including accelerations, vestibular stimulation, low and high ambient temperatures) by mountain acclimation has been established in numerous scientific expeditions to mountains [29]. Yet, the known methods of altitude training are counterweighed by several drawbacks, that is, long distraction from professional activity, heavy financial expenses, organization difficulties, unfeasibility of prescribing individual dose of hypoxic exposure and reoxygenation therapy, and the risk of deadaptation syndrome after an extended period of living in mountains [13]. Conversely, the programs of hypobaric chamber training offer a more convenient approach to formation of adaptation to hypoxia as they permit to vary hypoxia dose and duration [30]. Significant improvement of altitude tolerance in a number of investigations using various hypobaric chamber training regimes provided strong evidence for the development of a specific antihypoxia effect in humans and animals [31].

The key factors in formation of the adaptation during mountain or hypobaric chamber training are oxygen deficit and reduced air density, which trigger profound physiological reactions including a more effective alveolar ventilation, accelerated mass transfer of biologically active gases, and stimulation of energy and plasticity processes in cells. The morphological data from hypoxia-adapted rats demonstrated more dense vascularity in the brain and increased number of capillaries [32]. Importantly, intermittent (interval) hypoxia has some advantages over stationary (constant) hypoxia due to the presence of reoxygenation intermissions in the normoxia intervals that are favorable to synthesis of nucleic acids and proteins [33]. Altitude tolerance was enhanced in the animals subjected to 13 days of interval hypobaric chamber training as compared with their counterparts continuously exposed to the same altitudes [34]. It was shown that formation of the adaptation is dependent on the final altitude achieved, duration of exposure, and altitude rise gradient. Rapid "ascent" to the final altitude and/or extended duration of exposure to hypobaric hypoxia may impact or even cause failure of a stable adaptation to intermittent hypoxia [18].

Credible improvement of altitude tolerance as well as of tolerance for high and low temperatures (cross adaptation effect) can be reached in healthy men by 4 weeks of daily 30-min chamber "ascents" to 6,000 m. Besides, it was found that development of the adaptation effect correlated with concentration of free corticosteroids [35].

In aerospace medicine, hypobaric chamber "ascents" were used to improve pilots' tolerance of altitude for more than five decades [36]. This method is also used as a functional loading test (5,000 m for 20 min) for the applicants to aviation schools and cosmonauts' detachment, and medical certification of flying personnel [37]. The regular decreases of partial pressure of oxygen inside space vehicles were also applied for the purpose of preventing cosmonauts' deadaptation in the long duration of space missions [38]. In addition, the course of hypobaric hypoxia consisting of 15 sessions of chamber "ascents" to 1,500–3,000 m augmented human tolerance to breathing under a positive pressure of 2,000 mmHg, improved the quality of operator's performance by 8–15%, extended the period of tolerance for statokinetic stimulation 1.6–2.8 times, and also increased resistance to orthostatic effects [39]. This method also gave good results in increasing tolerance to accelerations and its associated hypoxia [40].

Methods of hypoxic adaptation have also been used for prophylaxis and treatment of hypertension-type cardiopsychoneurosis, essential hypertension stages 1–2, bronchial asthma, asiderotic anemia, consequences of irradiation, etc. [41, 42]. "Ascents" of animals over 20-day periods made them more resistant to influenza virus [43]. To prolong the adaptation effect, some special training regimes were proposed such as chamber "ascents" once or twice a week with altitude exposure from one to several hours [44]. It was also stated that short hypoxia prevents the possibility of exhaustive effect of low oxygen partial pressure, while reproducible, close to natural rhythm, and discreteness of tissue and cell oxygen tension activate the compensatory reactions and lead to stable adaptation to hypoxia [6]. A similar phenomenon of organism reaction to intermittent stimulation revealed itself by a more effective increase of tolerance for heat and cold stresses as a result of intermittent but not continuous thermal training [45].

Interval hypoxic exposure can be provided by repeated "ascents" and "descents" in pressurized chamber [46]. Conversely, normobaric hypoxic training/therapy, which usually involves breathing with hypoxic gas mixtures (10–12% of oxygen) [1], has been widely used in clinical medicine and its experimental and theoretical basis has been actively investigated in the recent decades [47–49]. In comparison with normobaric training, hypobaric chamber training possesses the following advantages: (1) more accurate "dosage" of hypoxia due to exclusion of air inflow in the mask dead space while breathing the rarified air without mask; (2) low-pressure rarified air is less resistant to respiration and favorable to functioning of the cardiovascular system; (3) although the initial cost for building a pressure chamber facility is quite high, its service life can last over 50 years; and (4) hypoxic training can utilize the capabilities of existing pressure chambers intended for psychophysiological training, health examination and certification, and other purposes. On the other hand, the relative shortcoming of hypobaric chamber training is the possibility of barocavepathy that can be provoked by pressure changes due to repeated "ascents" and "descents."

17.3 Methodological Evolution and Application in Aerospace Medicine

17.3.1 Theoretical Assumption, Justification, and Premises of Adaptation to Hypoxia

Assumption that altitude flight factors have the potential to help correcting the changes in functional states of human bodies is based on the well-known principle of physiology and medicine – use of a damaging pathogenic agent as an effective homeostatic means. There are examples of how some flight-related stress factors (such as hypoxia, hyperoxia, hypobaria, breathing positive pressure oxygen) can be beneficially applied in sport, clinical, and aviation medicine [2, 50].

A new method of adaptation to hypoxia was developed on the basis of knowledge obtained in previous investigations with due account of the merits and faults of the existing mountain, hypobaric chamber, and normobaric interval hypoxic training regimes. Consideration was given to the following fundamental propositions: (1) methods of adaptation to hypoxia have been widely used for nonmedication treatment of diseases and correction of the functional state [51, 52]; (2) extended hypoxia of stationary continuous methods may result in exhaustive effect on human organism [53]; (3) frequent repeated changes in barometric pressure due to "ascents" and "descents" create potential danger of barocavepathy [54]; (4) reaction of human organism to intermittent stimulation is manifested by a much higher rise of resistance to stress factors as compared with permanent training regimes [45]; and (5) breathing with pure oxygen arrests effectively functional disorders provoked by hypoxic conditions [55].

Theoretical justification of the nonmedication method of adaptation relied, first and foremost, on hypoxia as one of the key potential factors of high-altitude flight. The choice of hypoxia was guided by the following processes and changes associated with evolution of life on Earth and ontogenesis of humans: (1) growth of oxygen partial pressure in atmosphere from 0.15 to 159 mmHg [56]; (2) development by living organisms of the aerobic energy supply system over a long historical period; (3) retention of the ability to activate anaerobic glycolysis as a backup energy production mechanism; (4) intrauterine germination in the hypoxic medium and ensuing formation of aerobic glycolysis; (5) high resistance to hypoxia in newborns and resistance declines in the course of human life; and (6) the noted longer life span and lower morbidity of mountain dwellers. Hence, the centuries-long maturation of the processes of adjusting to atmospheric changes and the genetic memory of ancient energy production mechanisms were the premises for considering hypoxic hypoxia as a basic genetic factor in the development of specific and nonspecific physiological adaptation.

17.3.2 Methodological Development of Adaptation to Intermittent Hypobaric Hypoxia

Of theoretical and practical interests, there was an issue of whether such permanent stress factor during high-altitude flight as hypobaria can also be used to elicit adaptation effects. It can be assumed that low-density atmosphere facilitates gas exchange in the lung and positively influences the function of respiratory and closely associated cardiovascular systems.

It was shown that the adaptation effect established by different types of training is particularly strong after the intermittent, interval discrete exposures to certain stimulus rather than the continuous (or chronic, stationary) regimes [57]. With this in view, the adaptation procedure was devised on the principle of interval action of hypoxia and hyperoxia as a possible concomitant high-altitude factor in human body with the goal to activate compensatory reactions of homeostasis-maintaining systems on the one hand, and prevention of the damaging effect of chronic oxygen deficit on the other. Additionally, alternation of hypoxia and hyperoxia periods without barometric pressure change could minimize the risk of altitude decompression disorders and contributed also to the gaining of positive adaptive effect.

17.4 Experimental Protocols, Results, and Discussion

17.4.1 Effect of HIH on Tolerance to High Altitude

The course of hypobaric interval hypoxia (HIH) consisted of 10 virtually daily hour-long sessions of interval hypoxic exposure during "ascents" to incrementally growing altitude from 3,000 to 5,000 m. "Ascent" to 3,000–5,000 m was made at the rate of 10–15 m/s; "descent" rate was 5–10 m/s. During session 1, altitude of ascent was 3,000 m; in sessions 2–4, "ascent" altitude grew in 500 m increments; in sessions 5–10, altitude was 5,000 m. The HIH session continued 60 min and included six 10-min steps: "ascent" (1), staging point (2–5), and "descent" (6). Each step consisted of 7 min of unmasked breathing with rarified air (hypoxic exposure) and 3 min of masked breathing with 100% oxygen (hyperoxic exposure).

The investigation (647 experiments with participation of 34 volunteers with informed consent) was aimed at HIH evaluation as a method of improving human tolerance of high-altitude flight stress factors including hypoxia, longitudinal accelerations, motion sickness, and also rapid elimination of the motion sickness syndrome.

The first part of the investigation was designed to study effectiveness of HIH for development of specific adaptation to altitude hypoxia. Seven volunteers performed 91 experiments; 70 experiments were HIH sessions and 21 chamber "ascents" in order to test altitude tolerance of the volunteers. The procedure was divided into the next stages: testing baseline altitude tolerance, 10-day HIH training, and altitude tolerance testing in a day and 1–2 months after the HIH training to assess adaptation effect of the chamber training and length of its retention. Altitude tolerance (expert "ascents") was determined by the time of retaining the ability to do mental work or exhibiting apparent signs of changes in volunteer's functional state during incremental "ascent" to 8,000 m without mask with 5-min "staging points" at the altitudes higher than 5,000 m. Quantitatively, altitude tolerance was assessed by "high-altitude ceiling" – maximal "ascent" height and "reserve time" (T_R) – total time at altitudes higher than 5,000 m including 5 min at 5,000, 6,000, and 7,000 m "staging points," and time of climbing (1 min) to the next "staging point."

While at a "staging point," volunteers were given 1 min to do a written digital test, that is, sequential subtraction 17 from 3 figures. In the remaining time, the volunteers were asked to calculate from a multiplication table. The first wrong answer, late or incorrect solution of simple sums, and full

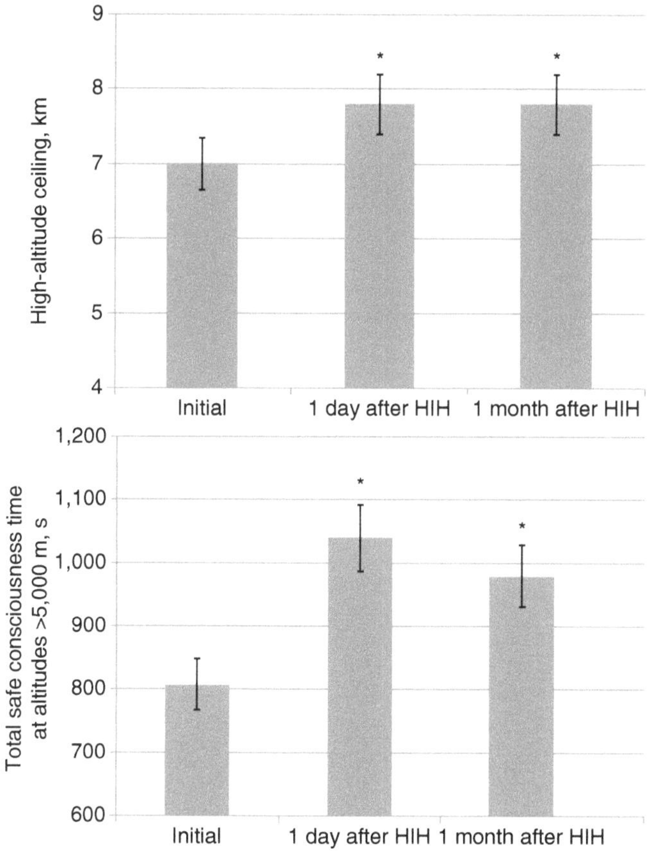

Fig. 17.1 Human hypoxia tolerance dynamics following the HIH training. *Top graph*: High-altitude ceiling indicates maximal "ascent" height or maximal tolerable altitude. *Bottom graph*: Total safe consciousness time ("reserve time") measures the total time at altitudes higher than 5,000 m, including 5 min at the "staging points" of 5,000, 6,000, and 7,000 m, and time of climbing (1 min) to the next "staging point." * Indicates $p<0.05$ as compared with the initial values

failure were qualified as an ambiguous sign of deteriorated mental ability and impairment of long-term memory, which indicated the necessity to terminate the hypoxic exposure with supplementation of oxygen. In several cases, degradation of long-term memory was preceded by distinct subjective symptoms of hypoxic condition and cardiovascular and respiratory functional disorders, which required reoxygenation and "descent." Hemodynamic reactions to altitude hypoxia were studied using records of ECG and tetrapolar rheography, BP measurements, calculated values of systolic volume (SV), cardiac output, volumetric blood flow velocity (VBV), and total peripheral resistance (TPR) of vessels. Reserve capacity of the external respiration apparatus was studied prior to and after the HIH sessions.

As summarized in Fig. 17.1, the baseline altitude tolerance of the volunteers was characterized by "high-altitude ceiling" $=7{,}000\pm0.2$ m and $T_R=808\pm62$ s. The HIH training significantly increased the tolerance by increasing the "high-altitude ceiling" for 800 ± 0.2 m immediately after HIH training and keeping it high even 1 month later. Increase in T_R averaged 232 ± 50 s in a day after HIH training, and this adaptation effect was maintained in the next 30 days (ΔPB – 172 ± 41 s). The HIH effect of specific adaptation showed itself also by a reliable gain in static muscular tolerance by 40–50%: 76 s ± 10 prior to the initial "ascent," 112 s ± 13, and 120 s ± 15 1 day and 1 month after the HIH training, respectively.

Following the hypoxic training, mental performance during the written digital test at the critical altitude of 7,000 m was better. Whereas during the initial "ascent" to 7,000 m the volunteers were able to perform 6.8 ± 0.6 sums in a minute with 3.5 ± 1.0 errors, 1 day after HIH the number of successful sums increased to 8.5 ± 1.0 and the number of errors dropped to 1.6 ± 0.7. A month later, the numbers of right sums and errors were 7.5 ± 0.7 and 0.5 ± 0.2, respectively.

17.4.2 Effect of HIH on the Parameters of Cardiorespiratory Function

Changes in the hemodynamic parameters and respiration rate during repeated expert "ascents" to the altitudes of 5,000–7,000 m are shown in Table 17.1. The effects of HIH training on hypoxic reactions of the cardiorespiratory system were revealed by less intensive response in heart rate, BP, and respiration parameters; increase in systolic output; and TPR reduction at the altitudes of 5,000–7,000 m, particularly 1 month after HIH training. All these facts indicated a more economical functioning of the cardiorespiratory system in the conditions of hypobaric hypoxia following the HIH training. Spirometry of the external respiration function showed a reliable gain in maximal lung ventilation and extension of the length of arbitrary eupnoea averaging 30% and 25%, respectively (Table 17.2). These data also pointed to the HIH positive adaptation effect on the reserve capacity of external respiration and oxygen demands of human organism.

This increase may have practical implications as redeployment in high-altitude region affects implementation of expert tests with chamber "ascents" to 5,000 m with a 20-min staging point and to 5,000–6,000 m with 5-min staging points as well as of short flights in an open-air aircraft to altitudes above 4,000 m. These results suggested that hypobaric interval hypoxia produces a distinct effect of specific adaptation manifested by increased altitude tolerance for up to a month.

17.4.3 HIH-Induced Cross-Tolerance to G-force During Head-to-Pelvis Accelerations

We also evaluated the effectiveness of HIH training for development of the cross (nonspecific) adaptation. The objective was to study the effects of HIH on tolerance of head-to-pelvis accelerations (+*Gz*) created on centrifuge as well as the effect

Table 17.1 Hemodynamics and respiration parameters during "ascents" to 5,000, 6,000, and 7,000 m before and after HIH training ($n=7$)

						Period after HIH							
		Pre-HUH "ascent"				One day				One month			
Altitude, m		0	5	6	7	0	5	6	7	0	5	6	7
HR, beats/min		73±5.3	90±3.2*	94±3.8*	102±3.3*	73±6.8*	90±5.1	92±2.8*	100±8.4*	73±6.2	87±8.1	90±2.9*	91±8.1
BP, mmHg	Max	129±3.2	131±3.4	133±4.9	139±4.0	124±4.0	128±4.2	131±4.5	139±5.4*	129±5.4	129±4.4	129±3.9	128±3.7
	Mean	90±4.8	91±6.0	95±5.6	89±6.0	89±4.1	94±3.2	92±4.1	89±4.2	89±4.0	92±3.6	93±4.1	86±3.1
	Minimal	63±4.1	59±4.9	59±3.9	46±6.8	61±3.7	63±2.6	63±4.6	58±6.1	64±3.4	68±3.1	69±3.9	59±4.0
CO, ml		61±5.0	58±5.2	59±3.5	72±6.0	60±2.8	55±3.1	58±3.2	72±7.6	57±4.6	58±3.5	65±4.6	68±4.5
MV, l/min		4.4±0.2	5.2±0.1*	5.5±0.5	7.3±0.4*	4.4±0.3	5.0±0.4	5.7±0.4*	7.2±0.6*	4.2±0.3	5.0±0.4	6.2±0.6*	6.2±1.0
VBV, ml/s		240±14	250±9.9	256±14	326±25*	234±8.4	239±13	244±10	274±17	227±13	243±11	254±23	296±30
TPR, dyn/cm·s^{-5}		755±111	1,409±93	1,409±129	1,012±96*	1,717±132	1,563±153	1,408±116	1,242±181	1,788±127	1,625±155	1,449±166	1,205±189*
RR, breaths/min		15±1.2	15±1.2	19±1.5	16±1.1	15±1.0	15±0.9	14±1.4	17±1.7	15±0.8	13±0.6	14±1.9	16±1.2

*Indicates significant difference from the baseline value ($p<0.05$)

Table 17.2 External respiration parameters before and after HIH training ($n=7$)

Parameters	Post-HIH training period		
	Baseline	One day	One month
RR, breaths/min	17±1.8	16±1.7	13±1.4
RV, l	0.8±0.1	0.8±0.1	0.9±0.1
MRV, l/min	13.6±1.5	12.8±0.9	11.7±1.3
BC, l	4.6±0.2	4.7±0.2	4.7±0.2
FEV, l/s	3.7±0.1	3.8±0.1	3.8±0.1
Tifno index, %	82±2.1	80±2.0	80±2.2
MPV, l/min	101±8.1	130±5.5*	133±8.1*
Apnea, s	69±5.7	87±4.9*	84±3.4*

*Indicates significant difference from the baseline value ($p<0.05$)

Table 17.3 HIH effectiveness (Δ points) in improving tolerance of static muscular effort during statoergometric test (SET)

Stage of post-HIH testing	Number of subjects, n	Character of static effort tolerance change (Δ point)			
		Distribution of subjects			% of positive shifts
		+0.5 ÷ +1.5	0	−0.5 ÷ −1.2	
In 5 days	8	5	0	3	63
In 1–2 months	8	6	1	1	88

Δ points – difference in scoring three-step statoergometry test; the SET scoring: excellent (% points), good (4 points), satisfactory (3 points), unsatisfactory (2 points), very bad (1 points)

Table 17.4 Comparison of shifts in SET tolerance and CVS reactivity following the HIH training

Effect	n	SET tolerance shift, Δ points	Δ MV l/min	TPR Δ dyn/cm·s^{-5}	Δ %
+	11	+0.81±0.11*	−0.11±0.22	−80±70	−4.6±4.3
−	4	−0.88±0.1*	−0.14±0.14	+160±13*	+12.1±1.2*

*Indicates significant difference from the pre-HIH training data ($p<0.05$)

of HIH training on tolerance of static muscular effort during statoergometry.

Fourteen subjects volunteered for a 2-week training period of ten sessions of HIH. The total number of experiments was 180 including 24 statoergometry, 16 centrifuge, and 140 HIH sessions. The subjects were tested for tolerance of static muscular effort and accelerations before, 5 days, and 1–2 months after the HIH training. Level of static muscular tolerance was determined using the statoergometric test (SET) that predicts individual tolerance of flight accelerations in 75% cases. The SET procedure did not differ from standard [58], that is, human subject produced progressive static muscular efforts of 120, 160, 200, 240, and 280 kg during 30 s increments until the limit of individual tolerance. The regimes of accelerations were 2–6 units with an elevation gradient of 0.5 unit/s. The subjects were centrifuged without wearing antiacceleration suit and there were 5–10 min intervals between runs.

To study the central hemodynamic responses of seating subject during statoergometry, BP was measured according to Korotkov method and ECG recorded in the second standard lead of mingograph. Data of systolic and diastolic BP and heart rate measurements were used to calculate the following hemodynamic indices: mean BP, systolic output, minute volume, and TPR [58].

Characteristic of the HIH training effectiveness in improving tolerance of static muscular effort is presented in Table 17.3. The HIH training triggered multidirectional shifts in the level of static muscular tolerance, that is, from ±0.5 to −1.2 and +1.5 points. Five days after the training, positive shifts scored 63% of the subjects, whereas in 1–2 months, the percent of positive shifts went up to 88%. It is noteworthy that a downward trend in occurrence of negative shifts in static muscular tolerance was found at 1–2 months after HIH in two of three subjects who exhibited decline in SET tolerance immediately after HIH. This normalization at 1–2 months later suggested a delayed positive effect of HIH. To interpret the diversity of shifts in SET tolerance, individual hemodynamic reactivity was analyzed based on the SET data obtained before and after the HIH training. Dynamics of minute volume and TPR of vessels was correlated with changes in SET tolerance.

As shown in Table 17.4, the results display different trends in SET tolerance irrespective of the post-HIH duration. The positive adaptation effects of HIH training include a considerable improvement of static muscular tolerance in the majority of subjects (88%), which was associated with hypotensive neutral reaction and other favorable alteration of cardiac regulation. At the same time, several cases of degraded SET tolerance were marked by elevation of vascular tone, that is, the hypertensive reaction. Taken together, HIH training may optimize hemodynamic reactions to static physical loads and improve myocardial functional capacity.

It is known that SET reproduces only part of acceleration impacts, that is, static straining of leg and abdominal muscles and hemodynamic shifts caused by sharp TPR increase along with reduction of systolic blood volume. The drop of hydrostatic pressure in the head region and hypoxic changes in cerebral and retinal neurons cannot be provoked by SET because of small gradient of hydrostatic pressure which rises sharply during head-to-pelvic acceleration [59]. We believe that the shifts in SET tolerance following HIH reflect some but not all processes underlying adaptation to flight accelerations.

Figure 17.2 illustrates our results showing that HIH training increased tolerance of head-to-pelvis accelerations in all six subjects, that is, from the baseline value of 4.5±0.1 units to 5.3±0.2 units immediately after HIH and 5.9±0.1 units 1–1.5 months later ($p<0.05$). Conversely, there was no significant shift in hemodynamic parameters in the resting subjects right after the HIH training. However, 1–1.5 months later there was a reliable gain in minute volume ($p<0.05$, +1.2±0.3 l/min) because of increase in both heart rate

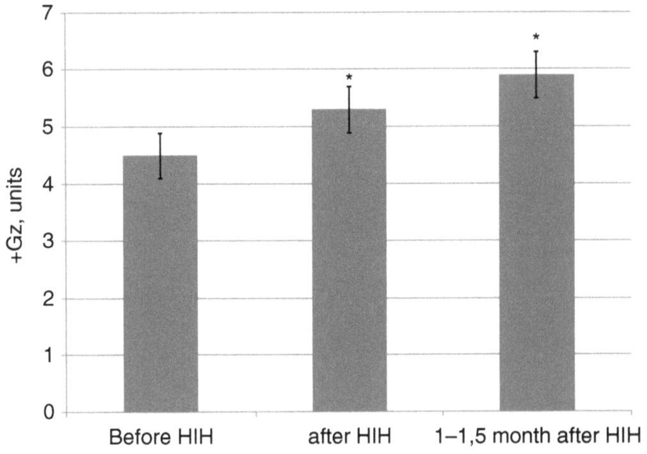

Fig. 17.2 Human tolerance to G-force (generated by head-to-pelvis accelerations in centrifuge) following the HIH training. * Indicates statistical significance ($p<0.05$) as compared with the initial values

(+9 ± 3.6 beats/min) and systolic output (+4.5 ± 0.3 ml), and substantial reduction of TPR of vessels (−138 ± 13 dyn/s·cm^{-5}). The TPR changes match well with the alterations in cardiac regulation of hemodynamics that has been previously shown to be favorable to adaptation to static muscular effort on statoergometer [58].

In summary, HIH training is an effective nonspecific method of increasing tolerance of static muscular effort and +*Gz* accelerations of 5–6 units without antiacceleration suit. Gain in SET tolerance immediately and 1–1.5 months after HIH averaged 0.81 ± 0.11 points in 63% and 88% cases, respectively. Improvement of acceleration tolerance in 100% cases made up +0.8 ± 0.2 units and +1.4 ± 0.1 units, respectively. The primary mechanism of nonspecific adaptation to accelerations can be rearrangement of the central hemodynamics regulation on the cardiac pattern.

17.4.4 HIH Improved the Training Benefits of Continuous Cumulation of Coriolis Accelerations (CCCA) Against Motion Sickness

We further studied the potentiality of HIH in improving human statokinetic tolerance and rapid elimination of the motion sickness syndrome. Motion sickness (MS) has been a major issue in aerospace medicine [60]. Approximately 60% of aviation school students develop MS symptoms in various degrees of severity at the beginning of the first airfield training, and the student dropout rate due to MS may reach 5%. Among flying personnel, MS is often associated with different partial health insufficiency; it can be a problem for nonpiloting navigators, operators, and some other personnel [61]. MS may also be a possible cause for flight accidents, particularly among the student pilots. The dynamic flight factors provoke development of the MS syndrome, which is associated with not only discomfort but also difficulties in acquiring proficiency and fulfillment of the flight plan, and ultimately jeopardizes flight safety [60]. Therefore, it is necessary to enhance not only the special selection procedure of pilots/astronauts but also the program for strengthening flying personnel tolerance to the dynamic flight factors through search for new and upgrade of existing methods of increasing statokinetic tolerance and rapid elimination of the MS syndrome.

The methods of vestibular training constitute an important component in such a program. Vestibular training employs the procedures of intermittent and continuous cumulation of Coriolis accelerations (ICCA and CCCA, respectively) performed on a revolving chair in absence of visual stimulation. The adaptation effect of this training is especially high if visual (optokinetic) stimulation is added to the procedure and the training program is extended. In addition, the elements of active training, e.g., repeated tonic head movements, are also advantageous [60].

Therefore, the third part of our present investigation focused on evaluation of the CCCA and HIH training, especially the combined specific (vestibular, CCCA) and nonspecific (hypoxic, HIH) methods to improve statokinetic tolerance of humans. We further collected experimental evidence of HIH utility as a method of rapid elimination of the MS syndrome. The theoretical basis for our investigation was that the specific and cross adaptation resulted from the combined vestibular and hypoxic training would potentiate an increasing statokinetic tolerance. The anticipated MS-reducing effect of HIH may originate from factors such as hypobaria, hypoxia, and hyperoxia that could assist circulation, oxygenation of vital organs, and equilibration of excitation and inhibition processes in the cerebral cortex due to stimulation of baroreceptors in the middle ear, gastrointestinal tract, and other receptor zones.

A total of 24 subjects performed 376 experiments including 88 vestibulometric CCCA tests, 160 HIH sessions, 8 single HIH session for MS reduction, and 120 CCCA training sessions. Effectiveness of the statokinetic tolerance improvement methods was evaluated by provoking MS by exposure of the subjects to the open-eye CCCA test either prior to or in 1 day and 1 month after the training. The vestibular test was performed on the Polyet-M stand simulating the joint vestibular-ocular effect. Chair and optokinetic drum rotated clockwise at the speed of 90°/s and 120°/s, respectively. Before rotation, the volunteered subject was fastened to the chair and briefed on the character and order of actions. During rotation, the subject followed the physician's instructions to open eyes and make head turns from one shoulder to the other and the reverse in 2 s with vertical deviation of about 30°. Turns were made continuously and smoothly; no other head movements about the vertical axis were allowed.

The registered test parameters included the onset time and severity of vestibulovegetative reactions (VVR) and the latent time of illusions as reported by the subjects. Tests had been terminated with appearance of distinct VVR symptoms (dramatic paleness, profuse hyperhidrosis, vomiting, retching) or following the subjects' request or complaints of sharp discomfort. Heart rate and BP were measured before and after the test. Statokinetic tolerance was assessed by tolerance time, latency and amplitude of illusion of rocking, and VVR severity in each of the time points.

The nonspecific (vestibular) training was conducted using a modified vestibulometric CCCA procedure, that is, combined exposure to CCCA and optokinetic stimulation of peripheral fields of vision. Electrorotating chair Polyet-M was used for the procedure. In brief, the subject seated on the chair with open eyes and the control console was then turned on and in 10 min after chair stabilization at 180°/s, human subject was instructed to start head turns in the frontal plane at 30°. Deviation angle was adjusted with headstops mounted on the chair. Movements were made smoothly and continuously with a 2-s half-period. Optokinetic stimulation involved alternation of dark and light strips on the internal surface of the stationary drum.

During training, the subject reported regularly about his condition. In the event of mild vestibulovegetative disorders (slight paleness and hyperhidrosis, light nausea) or on expiration of 5 min, doctor instructed to quit head turns and stopped chair rotation. The vestibular training was conducted once a day no earlier than in 1.5–2 h after meal. The training program according to only the CCCA or HIH procedure took 10 days. The combined program started with 2 HIH sessions; sessions 3–7 were preceded by 5 sessions of the modified CCCA vestibular training till the development of mild motion sickness symptomatology.

The HIH training alone had a positive effect on statokinetic tolerance, as all eight subjects had significantly increased CCCA tolerance time from averaged baseline 276 ± 14 to 402 ± 17 s 1 day after HIH ($p<0.05$). This effect was persistent over a month period maintaining the tolerance time at 348 ±9 s ($p<0.05$).

In the CCCA test, latency of illusion of rocking increased considerably from 30 ±1.9 s of the pretraining control level to 37 ± 1.5 and 35.1 ± 1.8 s immediately after HIH training and a month later, respectively. Similarly, the amplitude of rocking illusion declined from 25 ± 3° to 15 ± 2 and 20 ± 3°, respectively. VVR severity also reduced from 8.4 ± 0.7 to 4.2 ± 0.4 and 4.8 ± 0.9 points.

Results of modified vestibulometric CCCA training show close values of increases in resistance to motion sickness in comparison with hypoxic training. On the average, time of CCCA test tolerance increased from 252 ± 12.4 (baseline) to 330 ± 13.7 and 295 ± 8.9 immediately after CCCA training and a month later, respectively.

Our next objective was to evaluate effectiveness and utility of combining the specific vestibular training as one of the methods of improving statokinetic tolerance of flying personnel with the method of hypobaric interval hypoxia.

Table 17.5 CCCA tolerance time after combined CCCA-HIH training ($n=8$)

Time point of testing	Tolerance time, s
Pretraining baseline	243 ± 16
One day after training	486 ± 16*
One month after training	315 ± 8*

*Indicates significant difference in comparison with pretraining baseline ($p<0.05$)

Table 17.6 Comparative effectiveness of modified CCCA, HIH, and combined CCCA-HIH training

	Extension of CCCA vestibular tolerance time by different methods (Δ % of baseline value)		
	CCCA ($n=8$)	HIH ($n=8$)	CCCA-HIH ($n=8$)
Period of testing	1	2	3
One day after training	31 ± 9*	46 ± 6*	100 ± 6
One month after training	17 ± 6*	26 ± 1	30 ± 3

*Indicates significantly different versus CCCA-HIH group ($p<0.05$)

The time of vestibular CCCA test tolerance prior to the program of combined CCCA-HIH training, in 1 day and 1 month after the training completion, is summarized in Table 17.5. Parameters in the table evidence for the fiducial increase of vestibular tolerance of the subjects owing to the program of combined specific (i.e., CCCA) and nonspecific (i.e., HIH) training with an apparent delayed effect persisting 30 days as a minimum. Data on effectiveness of the combined CCCA-HIH training in the context of improvement of vestibular tolerance in comparison with the results of either CCCA or HIH training alone are presented in Table 17.6 and Fig. 17.3.

Comparative analysis of the results of effectiveness evaluation of the combined, modified CCCA vestibular and HIH training programs showed that the greatest gain and longest effect on human vestibular tolerance is achieved with the combined CCCA-HIH training.

Improvement of vestibular stimulation tolerance after the combined specific-nonspecific training was witnessed also by the subjects' statements about general health in the SAN questionnaire. It was shown that upon completion of the training program, the average assessment of general health, activity, and mood in the SAN questionnaire was 17%, 15%, and 28% higher even after prolonged vestibular tests. Furthermore, the trained subjects had markedly reduced severity of vestibulovegetative disorders, that is, from 9.7 ± 0.9 points at baseline to 6.6 ± 1.7 points after the training, which also suggests a very positive effect of the combined training on the vestibular apparatus.

Therefore, implementation of specific vestibular CCCA training together with HIH training led to significant gain

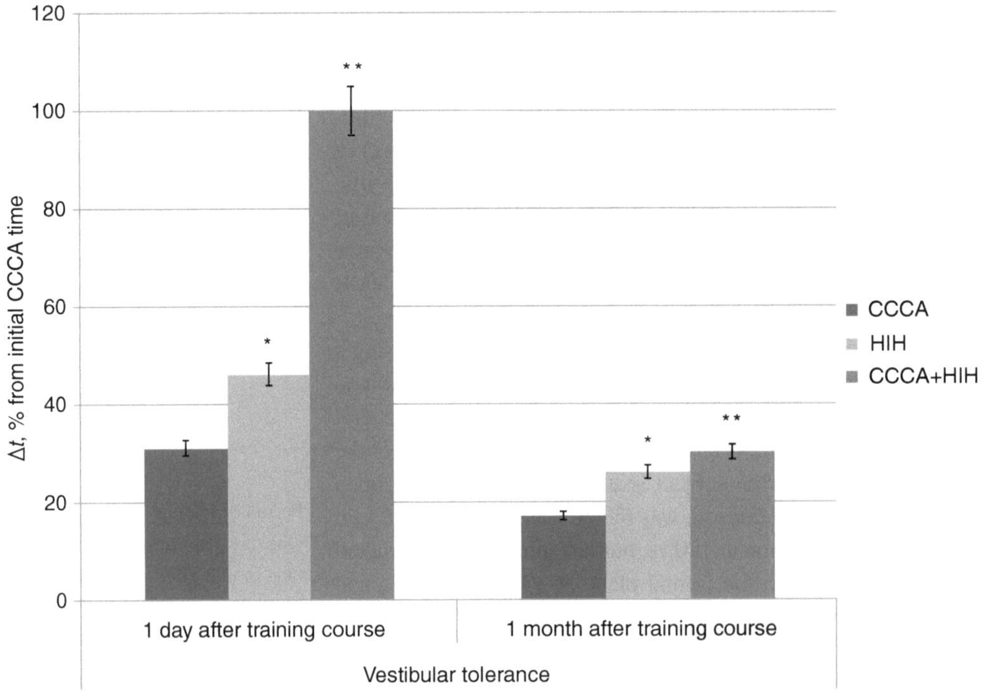

Fig. 17.3 Effectiveness of the combined CCCA-HIH training in the context of improvement of vestibular tolerance to CCCA (continuous cumulation of Coriolis accelerations) in comparison with the results of either CCCA or HIH training alone. * Indicates statistical significance ($p<0.05$) as compared with the CCCA alone group; ** Indicates statistical significance ($p<0.05$) versus the HIH alone group

(nearly double) in vestibular tolerance, which remained fairly high over the period of time more than 30 days. The positive effect of combined CCCA-HIH training relative to statokinetic tolerance is achieved largely through the use of specific vestibular training. The positive effect on statokinetic tolerance is possibly associated with formation of nonspecific cross adaptation to hypoxic hypoxia, which in turn could increase tolerance to circulatory hypoxia that attends motion sickness and, consequently, improving tolerance of vestibular stimulation.

In addition, implementation of the HIH sessions immediately after CCCA within the combined training program had an accelerated moderation effect on the negative vestibulo-vegetative reactions (see the following section), mitigated their severity, improved general health of the subjects and, consequently, facilitated adaptation to MS as well as increased statokinetic tolerance.

17.4.5 HIH Accelerated the Recovery from Motion Sickness and Normalization of General Functional State of Human Bodies

To study HIH effectiveness in reducing the motions sickness syndrome during the CCCA test with vestibular and optokinetic stimulation, each subject was provoked into motion sickness until development of severe symptoms scored 8–10 points according the Galle scale [60]. The control group ($n=8$) was not rendered rehabilitation treatment from motion sickness and recovered spontaneously; the experimental group ($n=8$) was given 1-h HIH session within 15–20 min after the CCCA test. The HIH sessions included "ascent" to 3,000 m (step 1) and subsequent climbing to the altitude of 5,000 m in increments of 500 m (steps 2–5). During each step, 7 min of unmasked breathing with rarified air alternated with 3 min of oxygen breathing in mask. Step 6 was "descent" to sea level.

The subjects were required to strictly follow the sequence of participation in the control and experimental investigations. Some subjects entered the investigation doing the control test first and then experimental test, whereas the others had a reversed test arrangement. The interval between the CCCA tests was at least 14 days long. Both groups of subjects had a period of full elimination of the MS syndrome after the investigation. In the subjective reports, they scored high (5-point rating scale) in general functional state; stated the absence of nausea, vertigo, headache, general ill at ease, drowsiness, and discomfort; and had no changes in hemodynamic parameters.

As shown in Fig. 17.4, a single HIH training reduced the time for MS elimination three times on the average. The averaged time for the spontaneous full disappearance of MS symptoms and normalization of general state in the control group was 222 ± 12 min from the end of CCCA test. One-hour HIH session in the experimental group significantly reduced the time for MS elimination to 72 ± 12 min (Fig. 17.4). In the majority of cases, disappearance of the MS syndrome produced by the CCCA test could already be seen during the course of chamber "ascent" or immediately after the end of test.

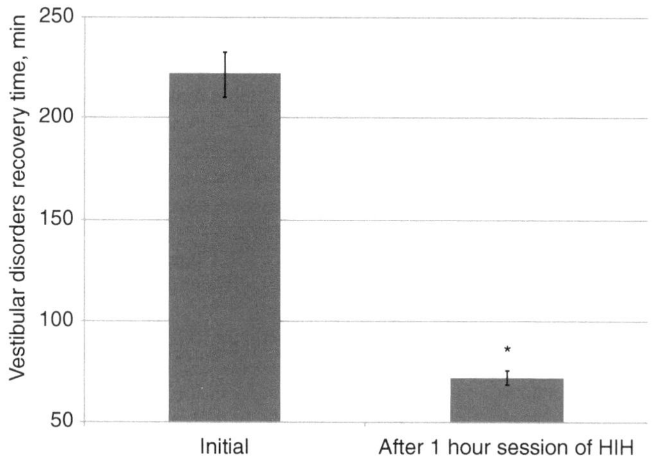

Fig. 17.4 Time of full disappearance of motion sickness symptoms and normalization of general state in nontrained subjects and 1 h after the HIH session. * Indicates statistical significance ($p<0.05$) compared with initial values

Rating of general functional state (points) by the subjects changed with the following patterns: the control group ($p<0.05$): baseline – 5.0 ± 0, after MS development – 2.3 ± 0.6, in 15 min – 2.7 ± 0.8, 30 min – 3.1 ± 0.6, and 60 min – 3.3 ± 0.7; and the experimental group with HIH session: baseline – 4.9 ± 0.1, after MS development – 2.3 ± 0.8, in 15 min – 4.1 ± 0.4, in 30 min – 4.4 ± 0.4, and virtually full recovery to 4.9 ± 0.1 in 60 min ($p<0.05$). The hemodynamic parameters measured during the HIH session after the CCCA test did not show noteworthy differences. In contrast, during the time period of 15–60 min, the control group displayed statistically significant reductions (as compared with the baseline values) in systolic pressure, 12–14 mmHg; mean pressure, 7–11 mmHg; diastolic pressure, 5–10 mmHg; and TPR 123–457 dyn/s·cm^{-5}, which served as an objective criterion of incomplete recovery of subjects' general state.

Hence, these results demonstrate high effectiveness of single HIH session in accelerating MS elimination. Considering one of the major mechanisms of MS syndrome development, that is, sharp blood redistribution and pooling in abdominal organs leading to disorders in cerebral circulation, the positive effect of HIH on the MS syndrome can be explained by blood flow centralization and intensification of oxygen supply to the brain and other vital organs. Additionally, it can be presumed that the MS-eliminating effect of hypobaria as one of the HIH factors is stipulated by stimulation of baroreceptors in the middle ear, gastrointestinal tract, lung, diaphragm, and other receptor zones, which, being an external inhibitor, blocks the constant excitation focus and assists to equilibration of inhibition and excitation processes in the cerebral cortex impaired by statokinetic overstress.

Conclusion

The results of our investigations demonstrate that hypobaric chamber training with the proposed HIH procedure is safe for human health and significantly enhances human tolerance for environmental stress factors. This beneficial effect is achieved via formation of the specific and nonspecific (cross) adaptation to intermittent hypoxic exposures alternating with short hyperoxic periods under hypobaric condition. These protective-adaptive reactions lead to activation of oxidative phosphorylation and intensification of anaerobic and aerobic energy production in tissues and organs across the central nervous, cardiorespiratory, and hormonal systems.

The HIH effect was the strongest on altitude tolerance, as multiple hypoxic intervals develop the specific adaptation to oxygen deficiency first. The subsequent gain in tolerance to other adverse factors and improvement of physiological capacity of human bodies following the HIH training reflect the formation of nonspecific cross adaptation. The immediate adaptation to a single HIH session also had motion sickness–eliminating effects, such as triple reduction of time for VVR disappearance as compared with passive rest and normalization of general health and condition after the CCCA stress test.

The high effectiveness of the nonmedication method of HIH combining the factors of high-altitude flight, that is, hypoxia, hyperoxia and low barometric pressure, can remarkably improve the functional condition and body's tolerance to adverse environmental stress factors that endanger the aerospace pilots and astronauts.

Special Note

The theoretically justified and experimentally verified method of hypobaric interval hypoxia has been covered by Russian Federation patent No. 2098867 "Method of improving human organism tolerance of exposure to flight stress-factors" [62].

References

1. Ushakov IB, Cherniakov IN, Shishov AA. Physiology of high-altitude flight. Moscow: Istoki; 2007 [In Russian].
2. Shishov AA, Cherniakov IN, Nizky AM. Hyperbaric oxygenation as a method of normalizing reduced functional state of human operator. Problems of prophylaxis and rehabilitation in aviation and space medicine. 1994;3:19–20 [In Russian].
3. Bodrov VA. On the problem of performance rehabilitation in flying personnel. Voenno-Med J. 1982;8:46–8 [In Russian].
4. Ponomarenko VA, Belinsky AV. Substantiation of differential assessment of mental health of flying personnel. Aviakosmich Ekologich Med. 1995;4:67c [In Russian].
5. Stupakov GP, Ushakov IB, Lapa VV. Aviation medicine to military science and practice. Voenno-Med J. 1995;7:76–9 [In Russian].

6. Kovalenko EA. Hypoxic training in medicine. Hypoxia Med J. 1993; 1:3–5 [In Russian].
7. Kovalenko EA. Problems of hypoxia in space medicine. Hypoxia Med J. 1994;2:53–4 [In Russian].
8. Kolchinskaya AZ, Tkachuk EN, Tsyganova TN. Interval hypoxic training of sportsmen. In: Interval hypoxic training. Kiev; 1992 [In Russian].
9. Mirrakhimov MM. Treatment of internal diseases with mountain climate. Moscow: Meditsina; 1977 [In Russian].
10. Truijens MJ, Rodríguez FA, Townsend NE, et al. The effect of intermittent low-pressure hypoxic exposure and sea level training on submaximal economy in well-trained swimmers and runners. J Appl Physiol. 2008;104:328–37.
11. Rodríguez FA, Truijens MJ, Townsend NE, et al. Performance of runners and swimmers after four weeks of intermittent low-pressure hypoxic exposure plus sea level training. J Appl Physiol. 2007;103: 1523–35.
12. Barbashova ZI. Acclimation to hypoxia and its physiological mechanisms. Moscow: AN SSSR; 1960 [In Russian].
13. Meerson FZ, Tverdokhlib VP, Boev VM, et al. Adaptation to periodic hypoxia in therapy and prophylaxis. Moscow: Nauka; 1989 [In Russian].
14. Pshennikova MG, Meerson FZ. Mechanisms of protective effects of adaptation to hypoxia. In: Hypoxia: mechanisms, adaptation, correction. Moscow; 1997 [In Russian].
15. Kovalenko EA, Cherniakov IN. Tissue oxygen and extreme flight factors. Probl Space Biol. 1972;21:263 [In Russian].
16. Fedorov VP, Ushakov IB, Saurina OS. Hypoxia as a type neuropathological process under the action of flight factors. In: Hypoxia: mechanisms, adaptation, correction. Moscow; 2002 [In Russian].
17. Meerson FZ. Adaptation, stress and prophylaxis. Moscow: Meditsina; 1981 [In Russian].
18. Meerson FZ. Adaptation medicine: concept of long-term adaptation. Moscow: Meditsina; 1993 [In Russian].
19. Meerson FZ, Malyshev IYu. Phenomenon of adaptive stabilization of the heart structures and protection. Moscow: Meditsina; 1993 [In Russian].
20. Burton RR, Smith AH. Induction of cardiac hypertrophy and polycythemia in the developing chick at high altitude. Fed Proc. 1969;28: 1170–7.
21. Hurtado A. Studies of myohemoglobin at high altitudes. Am J Med Sci. 1937;194:708.
22. Meerson FZ. General mechanisms of adaptation and prophylaxis. Moscow: Meditsina; 1973 [In Russian].
23. Fradette C, Du Souich P. Effect of hypoxia on cytochrome P450 activity and expression. Curr Drug Metab. 2004;5:257–71.
24. Grek OP, Sharapov VI, Grek OO. Effect of hypoxic stress on xenobiotic metabolism and activities of various isoforms of cytochrome P-450. Eksp Klin Farmakol. 2001;64:42–4 [In Russian].
25. Bayanov AA, Brunt AR. Role of hypoxia and constitutionally different resistance to hypoxia/stress as the determiners of individual profile of cytochrome P450 isozyme activity. Gen Pharmacol. 1999; 33:355–61.
26. Agadzhanyan NA. Organism and gas environment. Moscow: Meditsina; 1972 [In Russian].
27. Agadzhanian NA, Gnevushev VV, Katkov AYu. Adaptation to hypoxia and bioeconomy of external respiration. Moscow: UDN; 1987 [In Russian].
28. Goranchuk VV, Novikov LA, Kalinina SN. Methodological aspects of hypoxic therapy. In: Barotherapy in complex treatment and rehabilitation of the wounded, sick, and damaged. 1997 [In Russian].
29. Vasiliev PV, Uglova NN. Effects of adaptation to reduced partial pressure of oxygen on g-tolerance. Probl Space Biol. 1967;6:215c [In Russian].
30. Haldane JS. Acclimatization to high altitudes. Physiol Rev. 1927; 7:363.
31. Voitkevich VI. Chronic hypoxia: adaptive reactions of organism. Leningrad: Nauka; 1973.
32. Domontovich EN. Material on the problem of organism adjustment to hypoxic form of oxygen deficiency. Dissertation, Moscow; 1957 [In Russian].
33. Kolchinskaya AZ. Peculiarities of the mechanisms of effectiveness of using hypoxia adaptation in interval hypoxic training in medicine and sport. In: Hypoxia: mechanisms, adaptation, correction. Moscow; 2002. p. 63–4 [In Russian].
34. Vasiliev PV, Malkin VB, Babchinsky FV. Comparative evaluation of effectiveness of different regimes of adaptation to hypoxia. Probl Space Biol. 1968;8:122–9 [In Russian].
35. Bruner H, Klein KE. Hypoxia as stressor. Aerosp Med. 1960;1: 1009–19.
36. Vasilenko ME, Gazenko OG, Gramenitsky PM, et al. Changes in altitude tolerance during chamber training. In: Functions of organism in the conditions of altered gas environment. Moscow: AN SSSR; 1958. p. 137–52 [In Russian].
37. Malkin VB, Cherniakov IN. Altitude hypoxia. In: Aviation Med. 1986:25–42 [In Russian].
38. Malkin VB. Barometric pressure and gas composition. Found Space Biol Med. 1975;2:11–73 [In Russian].
39. Lustin S.I. Physiological substantiation of increasing tolerance to hypoxia for correction of the functional state of organism. Dissertation, St. Petersburg; 1994.
40. Vasiliev PV, Kotovskaya AR. Long-term linear and radial accelerations. Found Space Biol Med. 1975;2:177–231 [In Russian].
41. Aliev MA. Adaptation to mountain climate in the event of arterial hypertension. Frunze: Ilim; 1978 [In Russian].
42. Bannikov VK. Application of low-pressure hypoxia to treatment and rehabilitation of patients with atopic neurodermatitis. Hypoxia Med J. 1994;2:74–5 [In Russian].
43. Berry LJ, Mitchell RB, Rubenstein D. Effect of acclimatization to altitude on susceptibility of mice to influenza virus infection. Proc Soc Exp Biol Med. 1957;96:501–6.
44. Malkin VB, Guippenreiter EB. Acute and chronic hypoxia. Probl Kosm Biol. 1977;35:320S [In Russian].
45. Lukyanova LD, Kharadurov SV, Romanova VE. Physiological and clinical issues of adaptation of human and animal organism to hypoxia, hyperthermia, hypodynamia and nonspecific methods of recovery. Moscow; 1978 [In Russian].
46. Katkov AYu, Kovalenko EA, Davydov GA, et al. Antihypoxic effectiveness of the "impulse" regime of chamber training of human. Kosmicheskaia Biologiya i Meditsina. 1981;5:56–8 [In Russian].
47. Tverdokhlib VP, Tkachuk EN. Organization of adaptation therapy in patient care institutions of the Russian Federation. Hypoxia in medicine; 1996. p. 110–1 [In Russian].
48. Tsyganova TN. Interval hypoxic training during sanatorium-and-spa treatment. Yalta. 1993;6:90 [In Russian].
49. Ushakov IB, Usov VM, Dvornikov MV et al. Modern aspects of the problem of hypoxia in theory and practice of altitude physiology and aviation medicine. In: Lukyanova LD, Ushakov IB, editors. Problems of hypoxia. Moscow; 2004. p. 170–200 [In Russian].
50. Cherniakov IN. Stress-factors in altitude flight and homeostasis. In: Humanization and humanization of education. Pikalevo. 2002:40–7 [In Russian].
51. Tkachuk EN. Prevention of post-operation complications in gynaecological patients as a result of interval hypoxic training. Hypoxia Med. 1994;26:50–1 [In Russian].
52. Chizhov AYa, Strelkov RB, Potievskaya VI, et al. Normobaric hypoxic therapy. Moscow: RUDN; 1994 [In Russian].
53. Kolchinskaya AZ. Interval hypoxic training. effectiveness, action mechanisms. Kiev; 1992 [In Russian].
54. Ushakov IB, Cherniakov IN, Shishov AA. Low-pressure modification of interval hypoxic training in aerospace medicine. Voenno-Med J. 2003;2:54–7 [In Russian].

55. Belyi YuN, Kazennyi YuB. Methods of increasing work ability of operator profile ship specialists. Voenno-Med J. 1987;11:52–3 [In Russian].
56. Zakoshchikov KF. Adaptation, hypoxia, and health. Moscow; 1996 [In Russian].
57. Marianovich AT. Comparative characteristics of the regimes of smooth and fractional adaptation. Dissertation, Leningrad; 1981 [In Russian].
58. Ushakov IB. Special psychophysiological and physical training of flying personnel for increasing tolerance of flight g-loads and hypoxia. Moscow; 2006 [In Russian].
59. Glod GD, Migachev SD, Plakhotnyuk LS, et al. Reactions of the cardiovascular system to graded static and dynamic physical tests. Space Biol Aerosp Med. 1982;1:234S [In Russian].
60. Krylov YuV, Lapaev EV, Kuznetsov VS. Function of the auditory and vestibular analyzers under the action of aerospace flight factors. Probl Space Biol. 1983;47:241S [In Russian].
61. Sidelnikov IA, Pavlov GI. Methodical guidelines on determination of vestibular tolerance and vestibular training of aviation schools students for use by LAM, KAM doctors. Moscow; 1976 [In Russian].
62. Ushakov IB, Cherniakov IN, Shishov AA et al. Russian patent #2098867 for invention "Method of improving human organism tolerance of exposure to flight stress-factors". 1997 [In Russian].

18 Intermittent Hypoxia Remedies Male Subfertility

R. James Swanson and Zoya Serebrovska

Abstract

Progressive motility with high velocity that exhibits normal lateral head displacement is one of the most important characteristics of spermatozoa directly influencing their fertilizing capacity. A subfertile condition often depends more on sperm motility than count. Application of noninvasive methods of motility stimulation is an important treatment modality for male infertility. In this chapter, we demonstrate the efficacy of an intermittent hypoxic training (IHT) regimen on improving sperm motility in humans. The IHT consisted of 14 consecutive days having four repetitions of 5–7 min each of induced hypoxia interspersed with 5 min periods of ambient inspiration. Initial inspiration began with atmospheric air (20.9%) O_2. During the procedure, inspired O_2 fell to a value of 5–7%, with the final arterial O_2 saturation typically at 84–85%. This IHT regimen produced a stimulatory effect on male reproductive function in the gametes, and this significant increase in the number of spermatozoa with high motility was coupled with a decrease of seminal plasma chemiluminescence (ChL), while sperm count and morphology did not change. Motility and free radical status are some of the most labile parameters when compared to other characteristics of male reproductive function, and their response to external influences is very rapid. Sperm count is more inert. Of course, sperm count also depends on spermatozoal survival. Lack of mitochondrial enzyme activity, high-energy phosphates, oxidative stress, or other stress factors can lead to decreased motility and eventually to apoptosis or necrosis. The increase we have found in motility after 2 weeks of IHT implies that experimenting with the parameters and regimens of the IHT might produce an increase in sperm count along with the motility increase. Our future investigations will include prolonged IHT duration in multiple protocols. We propose that the mechanism of sperm motility augmentation that occurred in our study is due to inhibition of free radical processes. Positive changes in free radical processes should lead to membrane stabilization and improvement of spermatozoal function. Decrease of free radical levels in blood and increase of erythrocyte superoxide dismutase activity could be two likely causes of decreased free radical oxidation in sperm leading to our improved motility results.

R.J. Swanson (✉)
Biological Sciences Department,
Old Dominion University,
Norfolk, VA 23529, USA
e-mail: jswanson@odu.edu

Z. Serebrovska
Bogomoletz Institute of Physiology,
Kiev 01601, Ukraine

L. Xi, T.V. Serebrovskaya (eds.), *Intermittent Hypoxia and Human Diseases*,
DOI 10.1007/978-1-4471-2906-6_18, © Springer-Verlag London 2012

Abbreviations

ChL	Chemiluminescence
DNA	Deoxyribonucleic acid
HE	High energy
iChL	Initiated chemiluminescence
IHT	Intermittent hypoxic training
MEA	Mitochondrial enzyme activity
NADP	Nicotinamide adenine dinucleotide phosphate
pChL	Peak chemiluminescence
ROS	Reactive oxygen species
sChL	Spontaneous chemiluminescence
SOD	Superoxide dismutase

18.1 Introduction

According to most published data, the influence of a chronic or intermittent hypoxic treatment or experience on spermatogenesis and spermatozoal fertilizing capacity is always negative. Chronic or intermittent hypoxia would generally never be considered as a cure for sterility but quite the reverse; completely normal males of any species, including humans, become infertile or subfertile after exposure to certain doses of hypoxia [1]. Spanish emigrants who moved to Latin America in the sixteenth century experienced this high-altitude problem when they could not conceive for decades [2]. The same problem occurred in domestic animals brought from Europe; they could not produce offspring at altitudes higher than 3,500–4,000 m [3]. Nevertheless, a reduction in oxygen partial pressure has not caused fertility problems for the plateau aborigines or their animals, a privilege achieved by centuries of adaptation [4].

Present day investigations would indicate that no significant changes have taken place in the male response to hypoxia over the last four centuries. Present day investigations on mountaineers [1, 2, 5] found considerable inhibition of spermatogenesis in long-term sojourns at high altitude, both in permanent and intermittent regimes. In 1968, Donayre et al. reported [2] a significant decrease in sperm count and motility with marked and sustained increases in abnormal forms in semen samples from nine volunteers who lived at 14,000 ft (about 4,000 m) for 28 days. The men's levels of testosterone decreased, while fructose concentrations rose. Decreases in motility did not parallel the increase in abnormal forms. Similarly, there was no clear relationship between decreased motility and increased fructose. The loss of motility without a significant change in the percentage of live spermatozoa could have been due to a toxic, but nonlethal effect of hypoxia on the energy-utilizing mechanism of the spermatozoa or on reduced resources.

Verratti et al. reported [5] results of a study on six mountaineers who spent 26 days at altitudes of 2,000–5,600 m. Their sperm count was cut in half with a 20% drop in motility and a 20% increase in abnormal or immature forms after this high-altitude exposure. A complete recovery of sperm parameters occurred only after 6 month at sea level. According to the authors, the main mechanism of sperm damage was thought to be an increased generation of reactive oxygen species (ROS). Much reproductive pathology pathogenesis is based on the excess of ROS [6–8]. At an altitude of 4,000 m, oxygen is only 63% of sea level air. Tissue hypoxia leads to mitochondrial respiratory chain overloading and ROS accumulation with consequent augmentation of membrane fluidity and DNA damage. This damage, if it occurs during spermatogenesis, before the final nuclear compaction, cannot be repaired in the mature spermatozoon because of the chromatin's six-fold increase in condensation.

Similar results have been obtained in studies on animals (monkeys and rats) [9–14]. Acclimation to altitudes of 3,500–4,000 m leads to decreased sperm count and motility and increased abnormal forms. The main pathogenic ways are decrease in mitochondrial enzyme activity (MEA) and high-energy (HE) phosphates, ROS accumulation, and increased temperature in the testes due to vessel growth.

Saxena [9] observed the following in the rhesus monkey after 21 days at 4,411 m: nonreversible reduction of sperm count and motility, sperm epithelium degeneration, arrest of spermatogenesis, and both increased pH and fructose concentration.

Cikutovic et al. [10] studied the adaptation of rats to high altitude in an intermittent regime: 7 days at 3,400 m followed by 7 days at sea level, repeated cyclically seven times. A significant decrease was found in epididymal spermatozoal concentration, seminiferous tubule diameter, and height of spermatogenic epithelium. These changes were proportional to the hypoxia exposure. In addition to tissue hypoxia, the authors considered the increase of testicular temperature as a possible pathogenic way for the spermatogenic damage seen in these animals.

In a study by Gasco et al. [11], rats resided at 4,340 m for 42 days. In just 7 days, a significant decrease in epididymal spermatozoal concentration occurred in the II–III and IX–XII spermatogenic stages.

Farias et al. [12] studied rats at 4,600 m ($PO_2 = 89.6$ mmHg) for 60 days. Significant changes in testis morphology, metabolism of round spermatids, and death of spermatogenic cells of all stages of spermatogenesis were observed. Similar data were obtained by Shevantaeva and Kosyuga [13] as well as Liao et al. [14].

In all the studies we have cited, humans and animals were exposed to hypoxia of about 4,000 m for weeks. Such dosages clearly negatively influence spermatogenesis and spermatozoal function. Similar phenomenon of decompensation in circulatory and immune systems appear after long-term exposure to altitudes between 4,000 and 5,000 m [15].

In this chapter, we propose that a mild hypoxic dosing, maintained below the threshold of maladaptation, would produce a stimulatory effect on male reproductive function in the gametes, not inhibitory. Physiological correction within several major body systems has been attained by intermittent hypoxic therapy in a number of different laboratories [16–18]. Therefore, we are confident that an effective regimen of training can be experimentally defined for improving all areas of male reproductive function.

Another reason for our optimism is the proven positive influence of intermittent hypoxia on antioxidants [19–21]. Free radical oxidation in controlled amounts is necessary for proper preparation of spermatozoa for the final fertilization phases of capacitation and hyperactivation [22, 23]. A special membrane enzyme, NADP oxidase, is responsible for producing this limited superoxide synthesis in spermatozoa. However, excesses of free radicals cause damage of sperm membranes, and higher levels of ROS can lead to DNA damage, apoptosis or necrosis, inhibition of spermatogenesis, increases in abnormal forms, and decreased motility [24, 25]. Free radical damage is especially dangerous for haploid cells because no repair mechanisms for DNA exist at this developmental stage. Moreover, human spermatozoa are very sensitive to free radical damage because of high concentrations of nonsaturating acids [26]. The extent of damage depends on the level of oxidative stress, which in turn depends on the balance between pro- and antioxidant processes. The latter is a good predictor of fertility [27].

Intermittent hypoxia stimulates both ROS production and antioxidant synthesis [28–31]. During 5-min periods of hypoxia, lack of oxygen causes electron-transport-chain overloading with the resultant accumulation of reduced mitochondrial products. When the subject returns to normoxic breathing, oxygen concentration increases rapidly, thereby increasing the probability of superoxide formation. An increase in free radicals stimulates antioxidant formation and thus becomes a nonpharmaceutical antioxidant therapy for spermatozoa.

Another reason to presume a positive influence of intermittent hypoxia on spermatogenesis and sperm function is that hypoxic training increases vascular endothelial growth factor (VEGF), which plays an important role in spermatozoon formation and survival. Caires et al. [32] have shown that VEGF increases proliferation and survival of spermatozoa in bovine testis. In the testicular Sertoli and Leydig cells, VEGF is produced and carried to the germinal cell receptors. The number of germinal cells significantly increases in culture when VEGF has been added [33]. Hwang et al. [34] reports a dose-dependent stimulation of Leydig cell proliferation with testosterone secretion under VEGF influence.

Thus, intermittent hypoxia produced during a training regimen causes antioxidant stimulation and VEGF secretion. These factors will positively influence sperm parameters. In our research, we therefore investigated the influence of hypoxic training on human sperm function and morphology, and on free radical processes in semen and blood.

18.2 Methods

This work was approved and authorized by the Ethics Committee for Human Experiments at the Bogomoletz Institute of Physiology. All subjects gave their informed consent at the time of enrollment.

18.2.1 Design of Study

Our study consisted of two sets of experiments: (1) a comparative retrospective investigation of sperm count and motility in two groups of men from environmentally diverse regions of Ukraine and (2) a prospective study to determine the effect of hypoxic training on improving male reproductive parameters.

1. The L'viv Group (800 km from Chernobyl; $n=37$; mean age $=21\pm1$ year, SEM) was comprised of healthy male volunteers. These males were students attending the L'viv Military Academy. L'viv is considered to be a "radiation clean" region when compared to Chernobyl and Kiev. Investigation of sperm parameters were done one time in the morning after an overnight fast.
2. The Kiev Group ($n=22$; mean age $=25\pm1$ year, SEM) was also comprised of healthy male volunteers. These males were students attending the Kiev Military Academy. Although Kiev is approximately 90 km from Chernobyl, its residents have been exposed to varying amounts of radiation since the nuclear reactor accident in April 26, 1986. The men in the two groups had no children.

Subjects from the Kiev group underwent a detailed medical checkup before the course of IHT. All blood and semen investigations were carried out three times in the Kiev group: 2 weeks before IHT, 1 day before IHT, and in the early morning after an overnight fast, 24 h after completing the 14-day IHT program.

18.2.2 Sperm Morphology and Motility

Sperm analysis included sample volume, pH, sperm count, motility, and morphological characteristics. The volume, pH, sperm count, and motility were completed immediately after obtaining the samples. The pH was measured by a RADELKIS meter. For the sperm count, samples were diluted in an isotonic fixative medium (sodium bicarbonate (5 g), formalin (5 mL), and distilled water (95 mL)) in a ratio of 1:200 and analyzed with a light microscope at 400×. Sperm motility was determined with an ATS motility analyzer (J.C. Diffusion International, La Ferte Fresnel) at 37°C.

A minimum of 100 cells was examined for each sample. The number of *motile spermatozoa* (as a percent of total) and the number of *spermatozoa of high motility*, i.e., forward velocity greater than 50 μm/s (as a percent of total), were assessed for each sample.

Morphological characteristics were evaluated using the WHO criteria [35]. A minimum of 100 spermatozoa were evaluated on each stained slide. Spermatozoa were measured with an eye micrometer if there were any uncertainty in the normal morphological parameters. The number of spermatozoa with normal morphology (as a percent of total) was determined.

18.2.3 Chemiluminescence

Blood samples for analyses of ChL and antioxidant enzyme activity in serum were obtained from each subject at three separate times as outlined in the "Design of Study" paragraph. Venous blood was drawn from the median antecubital vein in the early morning after an overnight fast.

Levels of ROS were studied by the chemiluminescence measured on an Analyzer HLMZ-1 (Ukraine) with photoelectric multiplier −130 at −11°C. The lower boundary of sensitivity for the apparatus was 1 mV. For spontaneous ChL (sChL), 2 mL of the fluid to be examined was put in the cuvette and the amount of luminescence generated over a period of 60 s at 37°C was recorded. For initiated ChL (iChL), 0.02 mL of 3% H_2O_2 solution was added to each cell, immediately post-sChL measurement, and this second burst of luminescence generated over the next 60 s was measured. The amount of luminescence generated in the first 4 s after initiation, peak ChL (pChL), was also measured and analyzed.

For sperm analysis, three separate fractions were prepared: whole sperm, seminal plasma (dissolved in physiological saline at a ratio of 1:3), and spermatozoal suspension (12×10^9 cells/mL). Blood serum was diluted in physiological saline at a ratio of 1:3.

The intensity of sChL depends on the amount of recombined hydroxyl radicals. After initiation of iChL by hydrogen peroxide, a recombination growth occurs because of the Fenton reaction, which is catalyzed by free Fe^{3+}. Thus, the iChL reflects the concentration of superoxide and hydroxyl radicals as well as free iron in the sample.

Catalase activity was measured following the method Koroliuk et al. [36]. The activity of SOD was measured following the method Kostiuk et al. [37], while we measured the MDA concentration by the method of Gavrilov et al. [38].

18.2.4 Intermittent Hypoxia Protocols

Intermittent hypoxia sessions were conducted on 14 consecutive mornings between 10:00 and 12:00, 2 h after a light breakfast. For each of the 14 sessions, the subject was seated and normobaric isocapnic hypoxia was created with a Hypoxotron, a modified closed spirometer which allows measured reduction of Po_2 as the subject respires with concomitant CO_2 absorption [18, 39], for four 5–7-min repetitions of induced hypoxia interspersed with 5-min periods of ambient inspiration. Initial inspired gas contained atmospheric (20.9%) O_2. During the procedure, inspired O_2 fell to a value of 5–7% as the subject breathed into the closed system. The final arterial O_2 saturation was typically 84–85%. End-tidal Pco_2 was maintained by soda/lime absorption at the initial pretest value for each subject, typically 38–40 mmHg, throughout the intermittent hypoxia session. Subjects easily tolerated the hypoxia periods without any untoward effects.

18.3 Results and Discussion

18.3.1 Retrospective Comparative Study

A large difference was found between the two geographically separate groups in both sperm count and motility (Table 18.1) for this comparative study carried out in 1995.

Prior to the hypoxic training, the L'viv group's sperm motility was significantly higher than the Kiev group ($p<0.01$). Values for total motile and vital spermatozoal count had identical distribution with the same significance. The L'viv military men's total motile value was 1.7 times higher than Kiev students. How are these differences to be explained? We found no big differences in their mode of life, professional activities, or the use of substances that have a negative influence on spermatozoa (caffeine, alcohol consumption, and smoking). Males from L'viv were a little younger and their frequency of sexual activity was lower than males from Kiev. The spermatozoal concentration in the Kiev group was 40% lower than in the L'viv group. The same relative differences were registered for other sperm parameters: percent motility, percent live/dead, and number of morphologically normal spermatozoa. The data suggest that not only in 1 year but in 10 years after the Chernobyl catastrophe (when studies were done), the influence of radiation contamination factors on spermatogenesis was visible. The group from Kiev with the lower sperm count and motility underwent the 14-day hypoxic training protocol.

Table 18.1 Sperm count and motility in the L'viv and Kiev groups prior to hypoxic training

Parameters	L'viv group	Kiev group
Sperm count	206.3±19.1*	148.0±26.8
Total count of spermatozoa	405.9±53.9*	324.0±53.8
Sperm motility (%)	63.0±4.2*	47.2±3.7
Total motile × 10^6	255.7±26.4*	152.9±23.2

*$p<0.01$

Table 18.2 Sperm characteristics before and after IHT

Collections	Cnt (10^9/mL)	Tot cnt (10^9)	M (%)	Tot M (10^9)	High M (%)	N (%)	Tot N (10^9)
I	148.0±16.8	324.0±53.8	63.6±3.8	207.0±7.5	47.2±3.7	27.8±2.6	91.0±8.3
II	132.0±14.2	296.0±42.5	65.5±5.7	214.0±9.1	50.1±3.3	30.6±3.1	88.0±9.4
III	140.0±20.2	316.0±58.9	72.5±8.4	230.0±11.5	61.3±4.1	29.5±4.8	92.0±11.4
Significance							
I–II	NS	NS	NS	NS	NS	NS	NS
II–III	NS	NS	NS	NS	$p<0.05$	NS	NS

Cnt count, *Tot* total, *M* motile, *N* normal

Table 18.3 ChL of sperm before and after hypoxic training

	Whole sperm			Seminal plasma			Suspension of spermatozoon		
Col	sChL, imp/m	iChL, imp/m	pChL, imp/4 s	sChL, imp/m	iChL, imp/m	pChL, imp/4 s	sChL, imp/m	iChL, imp/m	pChL, imp/4 s
I	147.2±3.0	336.9±37.7	4.6±0.4	168.2±2.4	225.0±22.3	4.6±0.4	150.2±3.4	175.9±25.7	4.3±0.4
II	140.2±3.2	352.8±43.4	4.8±0.5	159.1±9.7	234.5±19.4	4.4±0.5	146.2±2.6	180.3±29.8	3.7±0.4
III	137.2±1.4	310.6±28.7	4.0±0.4	141.2±1.1	190.7±18.8	3.1±0.3	143.1±7.5	170.5±30.2	4.0±0.5
Significance									
I–II	NS	NS	NS	NS	NS	NS	NS	NS	NS
II–III	NS	NS	NS	NS	$p<0.05$	$p<0.05$	NS	NS	NS

Col collections, *imp* impulses, *m* minute, *s* second

18.3.2 Prospective Study

The results from three separate sample collections from the Kiev males are summarized in the following tables: (1) 2 weeks before IHT, (2) the day before IHT, and (3) the day after the 14-day IHT regimen. Data from the first two collections (pre-IHT training) shows no significant differences between any parameters in either sperm or blood samples (Table 18.2).

18.3.3 IHT, Sperm Motility, and Morphology

After the course of IHT, a significant increase (22%) in high-motility spermatozoa was observed (Table 18.2). The percent of motile spermatozoa also increased (11%) but without statistical significance. The pH (7.46–7.54), ejaculate volume (2.5±0.2 mL), sperm count, and morphological characteristics showed no statistically significant change, thus no decrease in any parameters occurred due to IHT.

Therefore, 2 weeks of our IHT training protocol produced no changes in spermatogenesis, and we are confident that IHT does not inhibit the final 2 weeks of spermatogenesis or the normal physiology and anatomy of mature spermatozoa. The observed increase in motility could reflect a metabolic increase due to substrate accumulation or enzymes activation, and/or an improvement in membrane condition. Thus, IHT might be useful as a treatment for men with asthenospermia.

18.3.4 Free Radical Processes in Sperm

The plasma membrane condition is directly related to free radical processes. IHT led to significant decreases in iChL (23%) and pChL (38%) within seminal plasma (Table 18.3).

These changes in ChL parameters are evidence that IHT caused a decrease of hydroxyl radicals in seminal plasma due to either a decreased OH^* production or plasma antioxidant activation. Most antioxidant activity in the ejaculate is concentrated in the seminal plasma, which is rich in antioxidants, including uric acid, α-tocopherol (vitamin E), and ascorbic acid (vitamin C), and it contains high activity levels of superoxide dismutase (SOD) and catalase [40]. In comparison with the seminal plasma, spermatozoa manifest very low antioxidant activity. They contain α-tocopherol, SOD, and glutathione peroxidase [41]. The main source of ROS production in sperm is the respiratory chain and membrane NADPH oxidase. Changes in the ChL of seminal plasma suggest that antioxidant activity was probably stimulated by IHT. This will be verified in future investigations.

18.3.5 Free Radical Processes and Antioxidants in Blood

Changes in ChL of seminal plasma were accompanied by changes of blood free radical processes. After 14 days of IHT, a significant decrease occurred in blood serum iChL (14%),

Table 18.4 ChL of blood serum and MDA concentration before and after IHT

Collections	iChL, imp/m	pChL, imp/4 s	MDA, nmol/L
I	714.4±41.5	74.4±5.6	2.74±0.35
II	720.5±35.7	69.5±4.8	2.67±0.24
III	630.7±28.7	57.2±4.3	2.24±0.21
Significance			
I–II	NS	NS	NS
II–III	$p<0.05$	$p<0.05$	$p<0.05$

imp impulses, *m* minute, *s* second, *L* liter

Table 18.5 Activity of erythrocyte SOD and catalase before and after hypoxic training

Collections	SOD (act/mL m)	Catalase (mc mol/L bld)
I	250.0±45	217.0±13
II	224.0±38	202.0±12
III	318.0±40	178.0±23
Significance		
I–II	NS	NS
II–III	$p<0.05$	NS

act activity, *m* minute, *mc mol* micromole, *L* liter, *bld* blood

pChL (21%), and MDA concentration (19%) (Table 18.4). The activity of erythrocyte SOD (42%) was significantly increased after the IHT course, while the activity of catalase did not change significantly (Table 18.5).

Conclusion

Progressive motility with high velocity that exhibits normal lateral head displacement is one of most important characteristics of spermatozoa, which directly influences their fertilizing capacity. Frequently, a subfertile condition depends more on sperm motility rather than count. Application of noninvasive method of motility stimulation could become an important treatment modality for male infertility. Many reliable studies have been done, beginning over 30 years ago [42, 43], using motility enhancement chemicals with conflicting results on fertility as decades have gone by. The areas of investigation have included naturopathic or homeopathic substances with questionable experimental protocol. Further investigations are necessary to substantiate the often anecdotal reports. Researchers need to study the mechanisms of motility changes relative to treatment and search for better regimens of individual training which would allow for optimal use of hypoxic stimulation.

In our study, sperm count and morphology did not change. Nevertheless, significant increases in the number of spermatozoa with high motility together with a decrease of seminal plasma ChL were observed. These parameters are some of the most labile when compared to other characteristics of male reproductive function, and their response to external influences is very rapid. Sperm count is more inert. The time for one complete cycle of spermatozoon formation is about 2½ months, so the results of spermatogenic stimulation, if it occurs, could only be measured in more longitudinal studies. Our future investigations will include prolonged IHT duration. Of course, sperm count also depends on spermatozoal survival. Lack of MEA or HE phosphates, oxidative stress, or other stress factors can lead to decreased motility and eventually to apoptosis or necrosis. The increase we have found in motility after 2 weeks of IHT implies that in certain cases and regimens, an increase in sperm count could easily be achieved.

We propose that the mechanism of sperm motility augmentation that occurred in our study is due to inhibition of free radical processes. Positive changes in free radical processes should lead to membrane stabilization and improvement of spermatozoal function. Decrease of free radical levels in blood and increase of erythrocyte SOD activity could be two likely causes of decreased free radical oxidation in sperm leading to our improved motility results.

References

1. Okumura A, Fuse H, Kawauchi Y, et al. Changes in male reproductive function after high altitude mountaineering. High Alt Med Biol. 2003;4:349–53.
2. Donayre J, Guerra-García R, Moncloa F, et al. Endocrine studies at high altitude. IV. Changes in the semen of men. J Reprod Fertil. 1968;16:55–8.
3. García-Hjarles MA. Sperm count and seminal biochemistry of high altitude inhabitants and patients with chronic altitude sickness. Arch Biol Med Exp (Santiago). 1989;22:61–7. In Spanish.
4. Yu LK, Gui JH, Feng J, et al. Comparison of sperm parameters between male adults at different altitudes. Zhonghua Nan Ke Xue. 2007;13:122–4. In Chinese.
5. Verratti V, Berardinelli F, Di Giulio C, et al. Evidence that chronic hypoxia causes reversible impairment on male fertility. Asian J Androl. 2008;10:602–6.
6. Tunc O, Tremellen K. Oxidative DNA damage impairs global sperm DNA methylation in infertile men. J Assist Reprod Genet. 2009;26:537–44.
7. Ramya T, Misro MM, Sinha D, et al. Sperm function and seminal oxidative stress as tools to identify sperm pathologies in infertile men. Fertil Steril. 2010;93:297–300.
8. Kumar R, Venkatesh S, Kumar M, et al. Oxidative stress and sperm mitochondrial DNA mutation in idiopathic oligoasthenozoospermic men. Indian J Biochem Biophys. 2009;46:172–7.
9. Saxena DK. Effect of hypoxia by intermittent altitude exposure on semen characteristics and testicular morphology of male rhesus monkeys. Int J Biometeorol. 1995;38:137–40.
10. Cikutovic M, Fuentes N, Bustos-Obregón E. Effect of intermittent hypoxia on the reproduction of rats exposed to high altitude in the Chilean Altiplano. High Alt Med Biol. 2009;10:357–63.
11. Gasco M, Rubio J, Chung A, et al. Effect of high altitude exposure on spermatogenesis and epididymal sperm count in male rats. Andrologia. 2003;35:368–74.
12. Farias JG, Bustos-Obregón E, Orellana R, et al. Effects of chronic hypobaric hypoxia on testis histology and round spermatid oxidative metabolism. Andrologia. 2005;37:47–52.

13. Shevantaeva ON, Kosyuga YI. Effect of acute hypobaric hypoxia on spermatogenesis and lactate concentration in testicular tissue of male albino rats. Bull Exp Biol Med. 2006;141:20–2.
14. Liao WG, Gao YQ, Cai MC, et al. Hypoxia promotes apoptosis of germ cells in rat testes. Zhonghua Nan Ke Xue. 2007;13:487–91. In Chinese.
15. Serebrovskaya TV. Intermittent hypoxia research in the former Soviet Union and the Commonwealth of Independent States: history and review of the concept and selected applications. High Alt Med Biol. 2002;3:205–21.
16. Xie A, Skatrud JB, Puleo DS, et al. Exposure to hypoxia produces long-lasting sympathetic activation in humans. J Appl Physiol. 2001;91:1555–62.
17. Ainslie PN, Poulin MJ. Ventilatory, cerebrovascular, and cardiovascular interactions in acute hypoxia: regulation by carbon dioxide. J Appl Physiol. 2004;97:149–59.
18. Serebrovskaya TV, Manukhina EB, Smith ML, et al. Intermittent hypoxia: cause of or therapy for systemic hypertension? Exp Biol Med. 2008;233:627–50.
19. Hui-guo L, Kui L, Yan-ning Z, et al. Apocynin attenuate spatial learning deficits and oxidative responses to intermittent hypoxia. Sleep Med. 2010;11:205–12.
20. Bertuglia S. Intermittent hypoxia modulates nitric oxide-dependent vasodilation and capillary perfusion during ischemia-reperfusion-induced damage. Am J Physiol Heart Circ Physiol. 2008;294: H1914–22.
21. Honchar OO, Man'kovs'ka IM. Glutathione system adaptation to acute stress in the heart of rats during different regimes of hypoxia training. Ukr Biokhim Zh. 2007;79:79–85. In Ukrainian.
22. O'Flaherty C, de Lamirande E, Gagnon C. Positive role of reactive oxygen species in mammalian sperm capacitation: triggering and modulation of phosphorylation events. Free Radic Biol Med. 2006;41:528–40.
23. de Lamirande E, O'Flaherty C. Sperm activation: role of reactive oxygen species and kinases. Biochim Biophys Acta. 2008;1784:106–15.
24. Baumber J, Ball BA, Gravance CG, et al. The effect of reactive oxygen species on equine sperm motility, viability, acrosomal integrity, mitochondrial membrane potential, and membrane lipid peroxidation. J Androl. 2000;21:895–902.
25. Aitken RJ, De Iuliis GN, Finnie JM, et al. Analysis of the relationships between oxidative stress, DNA damage and sperm vitality in a patient population: development of diagnostic criteria. Hum Reprod. 2010;25:2415–26.
26. Kruger TF, Acosta AA, Simmons KF, et al. Predictive value of abnormal sperm morphology in in vitro fertilization. Fertil Steril. 1988;49:112–7.
27. Sharma RK, Pasqualotto FF, Nelson DR, et al. The reactive oxygen species total antioxidant capacity score is a new measure of oxidative stress to predict male infertility. Hum Reprod. 1999;14:2801–7.
28. Bailey DM, Taudorf S, Berg RM, et al. Increased cerebral output of free radicals during hypoxia: implications for acute mountain sickness? Am J Physiol Regul Integr Comp Physiol. 2009;297: R1283–92.
29. Altan M, Atukeren P, Mengi M, et al. Influence of intermittent hypobaric exposure on SOD and TBARS levels in trained rats. Chin J Physiol. 2009;52:106–12.
30. Zarubina IV, Nurmanbetova FN, Shabanov PD. Bemithyl potentiates the antioxidant effect of intermittent hypoxic training. Bull Exp Biol Med. 2005;140:190–3.
31. Manukhina EB, Downey HF, Mallet RT. Role of nitric oxide in cardiovascular adaptation to intermittent hypoxia. Exp Biol Med. 2006;231:343–65.
32. Caires KC, de Avila J, McLean DJ. Vascular endothelial growth factor regulates germ cell survival during establishment of spermatogenesis in the bovine testis. Reproduction. 2009;138: 667–77.
33. Hägele S, Behnam B, Borter E, et al. TSGA10 prevents nuclear localization of the hypoxia-inducible factor (HIF)-1alpha. FEBS Lett. 2006;580:3731–8.
34. Hwang GS, Wang SW, Tseng WM, et al. Effect of hypoxia on the release of vascular endothelial growth factor and testosterone in mouse TM3 Leydig cells. Am J Physiol Endocrinol Metab. 2007;292: E1763–9.
35. WHO. WHO laboratory manual for the examination of human semen and sperm-cervical mucus interaction. 3rd ed. Cambridge: Cambridge University Press; 1992.
36. Koroliuk MA, Ivanova LI, Maĭorova IG, et al. A method of determining catalase activity. Lab Delo. 1988;1:16–9. In Russian.
37. Kostiuk VA, Potapovich AI, Kovaleva ZhV. A simple and sensitive method of determination of superoxide dismutase activity based on the reaction of quercetin oxidation. Vopr Med Khim. 1990;36:88–91. In Russian.
38. Gavrilov VB, Gavrilova AR, Mazhul' LM. Methods of determining lipid peroxidation products in the serum using a thiobarbituric acid test. Vopr Med Khim. 1987;33:118–22. In Russian.
39. Serebrovska TV, Lopata VA, Roy VV et al. Device for breathing with hypoxic mixtures "Hypoxytron". Patent No. 44179, IPC A61M 16/00. Ukraine, 25 Sept 2009: Bulletin 18; 2009.
40. Baker MA, Aitken RJ. Reactive oxygen species in spermatozoa: methods for monitoring and significance for the origins of genetic disease and infertility. Reprod Biol Endocrinol. 2005;29:67.
41. Williams AC, Ford WC. Functional significance of the pentose phosphate pathway and glutathione reductase in the antioxidant defenses of human sperm. Biol Reprod. 2004;71:1309–16.
42. Mrsny RJ, Waxman L, Meizel S. Taurine maintains and stimulates motility of hamster sperm during capacitation in vitro. J Exp Zool. 1979;210:123–8.
43. Meizel S, Lui CW, Working PK, et al. Taurine and hypotaurine: their effects on motility, capacitation and the acrosome reaction of hamster sperm in vitro and their presence in sperm and reproductive tract fluids of several mammals. Develop Growth Differ. 1980;22: 483–94.

Anticancer Effects of Intermittent Hypoxia in Acute Myeloid Leukemia

19

Guo-Qiang Chen and Wei Liu

Abstract

Acute myeloid leukemia (AML), a commonly developed heterogenous group of hematopoietic malignancies, is characterized by maturation/differentiation block at specific stages during the hematopoietic development. Recently, we reported that moderate hypoxia and hypoxia-mimetic agents could induce the differentiation of human AML cells in culture. Also, hypoxia-mimetic agents enhance differentiation in acute promyelocytic leukemic cells induced by arsenic trioxide (As_2O_3). In vivo studies show that intermittent hypoxia significantly prolongs the survival of transplanted leukemic mice with inhibition of infiltration and differentiation induction of leukemic cells. Further investigations explore the role of hypoxia-inducible factor-1alpha (HIF-1α) in differentiation of myeloid leukemic cell, in which HIF-1α physically interact with so as to increase the activities of two critical hematopoietic transcription factors, CCAAT/enhancer binding protein alpha (C/EBPα) and Runt-related transcription protein 1(Runx1), whereas C/EBPα competes with HIF-1β and significantly inhibits the DNA-binding ability of HIF-1. Besides, HIF-1α has been shown to play a part in all-trans retinoic acid (ATRA)-induced differentiation of leukemic cells. Therefore, these observations disclose the two-edged sword effect of hypoxia/HIF-1α. Additional investigations may uncover ways to mimic the differentiative effects of hypoxia in a manner that will benefit human patients with AML.

Abbreviations

AML	Acute myeloid leukemia
AML1	Acute myeloid leukemia-1
ARNT	Aryl-hydrocarbon receptor nuclear transporter
As_2O_3	Arsenic trioxide
ATRA	All-trans retinoic acid
BM	Bone marrow
C/EBPα	CCAAT/enhancer binding protein alpha
$CoCl_2$	Cobalt chloride
Co-IP	Coimmunoprecipitation
DFO	Desferrioxamine
EMSA	Electrophoretic mobility shift assay
FACS	Flow cytometry analysis
HIF-1α	Hypoxia-inducible factor-1alpha
HRE	Hypoxia-responsive element
HSCs	Hematopoietic stem cells
IL1RA	Interleukin-1 receptor antagonist
LacO array	Lac operator heterochromatic array, Operator (LacO) heterochromatic array
NCF1	Neutrophil cytosolic factor-1
ODD	Oxygen-dependent degradation domain
PHDs	Prolyl hydroxylases
PML-RARα	Promyelocytic leukemia-retinoic acid receptor alpha
PODs	PML oncogenic domains
Runx1	Runt-related transcription protein 1

G.-Q. Chen (✉) • W. Liu
Department of Pathophysiology, Key Laboratory of Cell Differentiation and Apoptosis of Ministry of Education of China, Shanghai Jiao Tong University School of Medicine, Shanghai 200025, China
e-mail: chengq@shsmu.edu.cn

L. Xi, T.V. Serebrovskaya (eds.), *Intermittent Hypoxia and Human Diseases*,
DOI 10.1007/978-1-4471-2906-6_19, © Springer-Verlag London 2012

shRNAs Short-hairpin RNAs
SPP1 Secreted phosphoprotein 1
VEGF Vascular endothelial growth factor
VHL von Hippel-Lindau

19.1 Introduction

19.1.1 Acute Myeloid Leukemia

Hematopoiesis is a finely regulated and controlled process wherein the pluripotential hematopoietic stem cells undergo several successive stages of differentiation, from immature and committed progenitor cells to lymphoid, erythroid, megakaryocytic, or myeloid precursors, which in turn become functional mature progeny that make up the specific cell types in blood [1]. Over the past decade, a number of studies have pointed to the dominant role of lineage-specific transcription factors in normal hematopoietic differentiation [2]. It is recognized that, besides the alterations in oncogenes and tumor suppressors associated with abnormal cellular proliferation and cell death, loss of differentiation is an important component in the pathogenesis of hematopoietic malignancies. Acute myeloid leukemia (AML), a heterogenous group of leukemia commonly developed in adult, is characterized by an increase in the number of myeloid cells in the bone marrow and an arrest in their maturation/differentiation at certain stages, mainly due to specific gene rearrangements and mutations targeting a variety of lineage-specific transcription factors and signaling molecules [3]. A typical example is that most patients who suffer from acute promyelocytic leukemia (APL), the M3 subtype AML, carry the specific reciprocal chromosome translocation t(15;17) which causes the expression of leukemia-promoting promyelocytic leukemia-retinoic acid receptor alpha (PML-RARα) chimeric protein that can interact with transcriptional corepressors such as the nuclear corepressor (N-CoR)-histone deacetylase complex and exerts dominant negative effects on functions of wild type PML and RARα [4].

19.1.2 Development of Cell Differentiation Therapy for AML

Since the 1970s, when research demonstrated that cultured AML cells could be induced to undergo terminal differentiation [5], several groups started to screen for differentiation inducers and this led to the application of *all-trans* retinoic acid (ATRA) in the treatment of APL, which was firstly achieved in the middle of 1980s in Shanghai and became the first-line drug for APL worldwide [6–8]. From then on, the revolutionary concept of differentiation therapy has been viewed as a promising approach for the treatment of AML.

Although ATRA can induce complete remission as a single agent in newly diagnosed APL patients, almost all cases eventually relapsed [9]. In 1992, arsenic trioxide (As_2O_3), a traditional Chinese medicine, was introduced into the treatment arsenal for APL patients who were refractory to ATRA and conventional chemotherapeutic drugs [10–12]. To date, many leukemic cell differentiation-inducing agents (including histone deacetylase inhibitors and novel retinoids) and new therapeutic approaches [such as combinations of biologic agents with defined molecular targets (e.g., monoclonal antibodies, hypomethylating agents, tyrosine kinase inhibitors)] have been explored [13]. However, the successful clinical model of differentiation therapy has still been limited to the application of ATRA/As_2O_3 in the treatment of APL. Therefore, it has become an urgent need to develop novel practicable differentiation-induction therapy in other leukemia subtypes and even solid tumors.

Previous studies showed that clinical concentration of As_2O_3 (1–2 μmol/L) triggers apoptosis not only in APL with the downregulation of bcl-2 gene expression and the modulation of PML-RARα protein [11] but also in a large array of other cancer cells, in which a variety of mechanisms have been documented [14]. However, the clinical effectiveness of As_2O_3 appears to be restricted to APL, which suggests that some other effects besides the apoptosis induction contribute to the efficacy of As_2O_3 in clinic. Further investigation indicates that, after 2–3 weeks of continuous intravenous infusion of As_2O_3, the number of myelocyte-like cells and degenerative cells increases while leukemic promyelocytes decrease in the bone marrow and peripheral blood of APL patients, which probably imply a partial differentiation-induction effect of As_2O_3 [12, 15]. This in vivo action of As_2O_3 is confirmed by other clinical trials and in transplanted APL mice [16, 17]. On the other hand, As_2O_3 has dose-dependent dual effects on cultured APL cell lines: inducing apoptosis preferentially at relatively high concentrations (0.5–2 μmol/L) and inducing partial differentiation at low concentrations (0.1–0.5 μmol/L) [12, 18], the latter, however, appeared to be less significant than its in vivo activity. Together with these observations, it shows that the differentiation-induction activity of As_2O_3 plays a role in its clinical efficacy, and it is also reasonable to speculate that some factors or events in bone marrow (BM) microenvironments may modulate and potentiate the in vivo differentiation-inducing activity of As_2O_3.

19.1.3 Investigative Evolution on the Role of Hypoxia in AML Pathogenesis and Therapy

As we try to figure out the different effects of As_2O_3 existing in vivo and in vitro, some important clues lead us to consider an essential factor: oxygen concentration. As it is well known, in vitro leukemic cells are cultured in ambient O_2 concentration around 21%, while in vivo, tissues are exposed physiologically to lower O_2 tension, ranging from 16% in pulmonary alveoli and artery blood to less than 5% in distal tissues [19]. The O_2 tension of bone marrow in leukemic patients might be much lower due to the rapid proliferation of the leukemic cells [20]. Furthermore, increasing vascular endothelial growth factor (VEGF) levels, which are associated with angiogenesis, growth, dissemination, metastasis, and poor outcome in solid tumors, are reported to be related to shorter survival as the independent predictor of the outcome in diagnosed AML [21–23]. Mammalian bone marrow has been suggested to be relatively hypoxic compared to other tissues, and primitive hematopoietic cells including hematopoietic stem cells (HSCs) are thought to be localized in the most hypoxic microenvironment of the BM [24, 25]. Recently, Takubo et al. [26] reported that normal hematopoietic stem cells (HSCs) maintain intracellular hypoxia and stabilize hypoxia-inducible factor-1alpha (HIF-1α) protein, and HSCs maintain cell cycle quiescence through the precise regulation of HIF-1α level. Accordingly, we began to broaden our view about the regulation of oxygen metabolism in the organism and to investigate whether oxygen concentration influences As_2O_3-induced leukemic cell differentiation.

Cellular and systemic O_2 homeostasis is a tightly regulated process which is essential for energy metabolism as well as the survival of mammalian cells. It is well established that HIF-1, a heterodimeric transcriptional factor composed of the constitutively expressed HIF-1β (also named arylhydrocarbon receptor nuclear transporter, ARNT) subunit and the highly regulated HIF-1α subunit, plays a critical role in cellular adaptation to changes in oxygen availability [27, 28]. Under normoxic conditions, HIF-1α is subjected to hydroxylation by oxygen-activated HIF prolyl hydroxylases (PHDs) in an oxygen-dependent degradation domain (ODD) and rapidly degraded by the von Hippel-Lindau (VHL) tumor suppressor protein-mediated ubiquitin–proteasome pathway. Under hypoxic or hypoxic-mimic conditions, due to the significantly reduced enzymatic activities of PHDs, HIF-1α could be stabilized and then translocate to the nucleus, heterodimerize with HIF-1β, and activate a broad range of genes through binding to the hypoxia-responsive element (HRE) in the cis-acting sequences so as to adapt hypoxic stress [19].

Since HIF-1 was first identified as a key regulator induced under hypoxia, the transcription factor has been attracting a tremendous amount of insight because of its involvement in fundamental biological processes, including but not limited to tumor metabolism, angiogenesis, metastasis, and inflammation [29]. Although the effects of hypoxia and its potential role as a therapeutic target in solid tumors have been widely investigated, few studies have been reported regarding the possible effects of hypoxia on leukemic cells. Therefore, the in vitro and in vivo observations mentioned above drive us to extend research of hypoxia toward leukemia, which, surprisingly, uncover the two-edged sword effect of hypoxia/HIF-1α.

19.2 Hypoxia Induces Differentiation of AML Cells: The In Vitro Evidences

19.2.1 Hypoxia-Mimetic Agents and Environmental Hypoxia Induce Differentiation of AML Cells

The behaviors of murine and human hematopoietic progenitor, regarding self-renewal, proliferation, and differentiation, have been reported to be modulated by severe hypoxia (1% O_2) [30, 31]. On the way to unravel the possible effect of As_2O_3 on APL cells under hypoxic condition, to our surprise, we found that nontoxic concentrations of cobalt chloride ($CoCl_2$, 12.5–50 μM) and desferrioxamine (DFO, 5–20 μM), two commonly used hypoxia-mimetic agents, trigger differentiation in NB4 cells (a PML-RARα-positive human APL cell line), as assessed by morphological criteria (including condensed chromatin, a decreased nuclei/cytoplasm ratio with smaller nuclei although nucleoli remained visible) and myeloid differentiation-associated antigens CD11b and CD11c [32, 33]. Recently, it was also shown that iron chelating therapy induces the differentiation of leukemia blasts and normal bone marrow precursors into monocytes/macrophages in a manner involving modulation of reactive oxygen species expression and the activation of mitogen-activated protein kinases [34]. However, unlike ATRA/As_2O_3, which have been well documented that could cleave/degrade the specific fusion proteins PML-RARα resulting in differentiation of APL cells, treatment with $CoCl_2$ does not modulate the cellular level of PML-RARα, suggesting that the differentiation-induction effect of hypoxia and hypoxia-mimetic agents might not be limited in APL cells. Indeed, the following experiments show that hypoxia and hypoxia-mimetic agents could also differentiate other subtypes of AML cells such as U937, a human leukemic monocyte lymphoma cell line, in a similar manner. Of importance, $CoCl_2$ induces primary leukemic cells from some AML patients to undergo differentiation, which strongly supports the results observed in the cell lines and offers the hope of clinical application. In addition, higher concentrations of $CoCl_2$ and DFO trigger leukemic cells to undergo apoptosis through mitochondrial-dependent and HIF-1α-independent mechanisms [35]. Furthermore, the direct effects of environmental low oxygen tension on differentiation of leukemic cells have also been determined. The results show that 2–3% O_2 hypoxic cultured condition but not equal to or above 5% O_2 concentration can trigger both AML cell lines, U937 and NB4, to undergo differentiation. In parallel, the cell differentiation induced by hypoxia/hypoxia-mimetic agents is accompanied by the increase of HIF-1α protein and its DNA-binding activity, which suggests that HIF-1 may play an active role in the differentiation of AML cells [32, 33].

19.2.2 Hypoxia-Mimetic Agents Selectively Stimulate As_2O_3-Induced Growth Arrest and Cell Differentiation in APL Cells

Since hypoxic condition and hypoxia-mimetic agents have promising effects on AML cells, we began to figure out the original idea: whether hypoxic-mimic condition has something to do with As_2O_3-induced leukemic cell differentiation. The results show that $CoCl_2$ and DFO do potentiate the growth-inhibiting and differentiation-induction effects of low-dose As_2O_3 (0.5 μmol/L), the latter enhances $CoCl_2$ and DFO-induced accumulation of HIF-1α protein in NB4 cells but not in U937 cells. Besides, these two hypoxia-mimetic agents also accelerated As_2O_3-induced modulation and degradation of PML-RARα protein in NB4 cells. Furthermore, inducible expression of PML-RARα fusion gene restored the cooperative effects of As_2O_3 and $CoCl_2$/DFO on U937/PR9 cells (a cell line could express PML-RARα protein in the presence of Zn^{2+}) in terms of growth arrest, differentiation induction, and HIF-1α protein accumulation. Taken together, these results suggest that low oxygen concentration might potentiate the clinical action of As_2O_3 in the treatment of APL, in which HIF-1α and PML-RARα proteins should play an important role [36].

19.3 Anticancer Effects of Intermittent Hypoxia in an Animal Model of AML

Inspired by those in vitro discoveries, we set out to investigate in vivo effects of hypoxia on AML mice [37]. In this series of studies, a transplantable AML mouse model originated from leukemic hMRP8-PML-RARα transgenic mice [38], which has been used to evaluate the efficacy of combined treatment of ATRA and As_2O_3 in APL [16], was employed.

19.3.1 Intermittent Hypoxia Prolongs Survival and Induces Tumor Regression in the Mouse Model of AML

For intermittent hypoxia treatment, mice intravenously implanted with leukemic blasts are caged in a hypoxic chamber equivalent to an altitude of 6,000 m for 18 h every day. Our results show that either normal or leukemic mice present poor activity and anorexia with the reduction of body weight under intermittent hypoxia environment. However, normal mice kept alive under hypoxia for 60 days are tested and do not show evidence for hypoxic damage by pathological examination, indicating that mice could endure such an intermittent hypoxia. Hypoxia-treated early phase (caged in hypoxia from day 1 after transplantation, 39.7 ± 3.02 days) and middle phase leukemic mice (caged in hypoxia from day 7 after transplantation, 36.5 ± 1.96 days) have markedly longer survival than leukemic mice in normal oxygen (29.4 ± 0.84 days). Of note, early phase leukemic mice also show longer survival than middle phase leukemic mice in hypoxia.

Meanwhile, the effects of $CoCl_2$ and DFO on the survival of these leukemic mice have also been evaluated in our study. The results show that $CoCl_2$ (15 μg/g body weight, intraperitoneal injection every other day) slightly prolongs survival of leukemic mice, although this treatment regime fails to cure the disease. However, DFO (50 μg/g body weight, intraperitoneal injection every other day) has no effect on the survival of the mouse model, which is consistent with the previous report that showed the failure of subcutaneous DFO to alter the course of AML in the rat [39]. It was proposed that the short plasma half-life of DFO so as not to achieve effective drug concentration in vivo was a potential reason for this lack of protection. Therefore, potential effects of $CoCl_2$ and novel iron chelators in the treatment of AML deserve to be further evaluated with their proper pharmacokinetics and pharmacodynamics analysis.

Then we examined and compared leukemic infiltration within different tissues between leukemic mice under intermittent hypoxia and those in normoxia. Moribund leukemic mice in normoxia present a marked elevation in WBC count and severe thrombocytopenia in peripheral blood; both early and middle phase leukemic mice have normal WBC and platelet counts in hypoxia. Of note, all mice show the similar RBC counts possibly due to the long half-life of RBC. Furthermore, the WBC in leukemic mice in normoxia is strictly monomorphic, immature promyelocyte-like cells, which could hardly be seen in hypoxia-treated early and middle phase leukemic mice under microscopic observations in peripheral blood smears. Similarly, massive immature leukemic cells could be found in spleen and BM of leukemic mice in normoxia but much fewer in those of hypoxia-treated leukemic mice. In parallel, leukemic mice in normal oxygen present huge spleen while both early and middle phase leukemic mice in hypoxia almost completely normalized the macroscopic appearance of the organ without increased spleen weight (Fig. 19.1a). Also, reduced infiltration of leukemic cells could be seen in livers of hypoxia-treated leukemic mice (Fig. 19.1b, bottom). There are only small remaining tumor masses existing mainly around vessels of the portal tracts or centrilobular veins of livers under microscopic examination in hypoxia-treated early and middle phase leukemic mice. In total, these results from our study indicate that intermittent hypoxia significantly reduce the infiltration of leukemic cells in peripheral tissues.

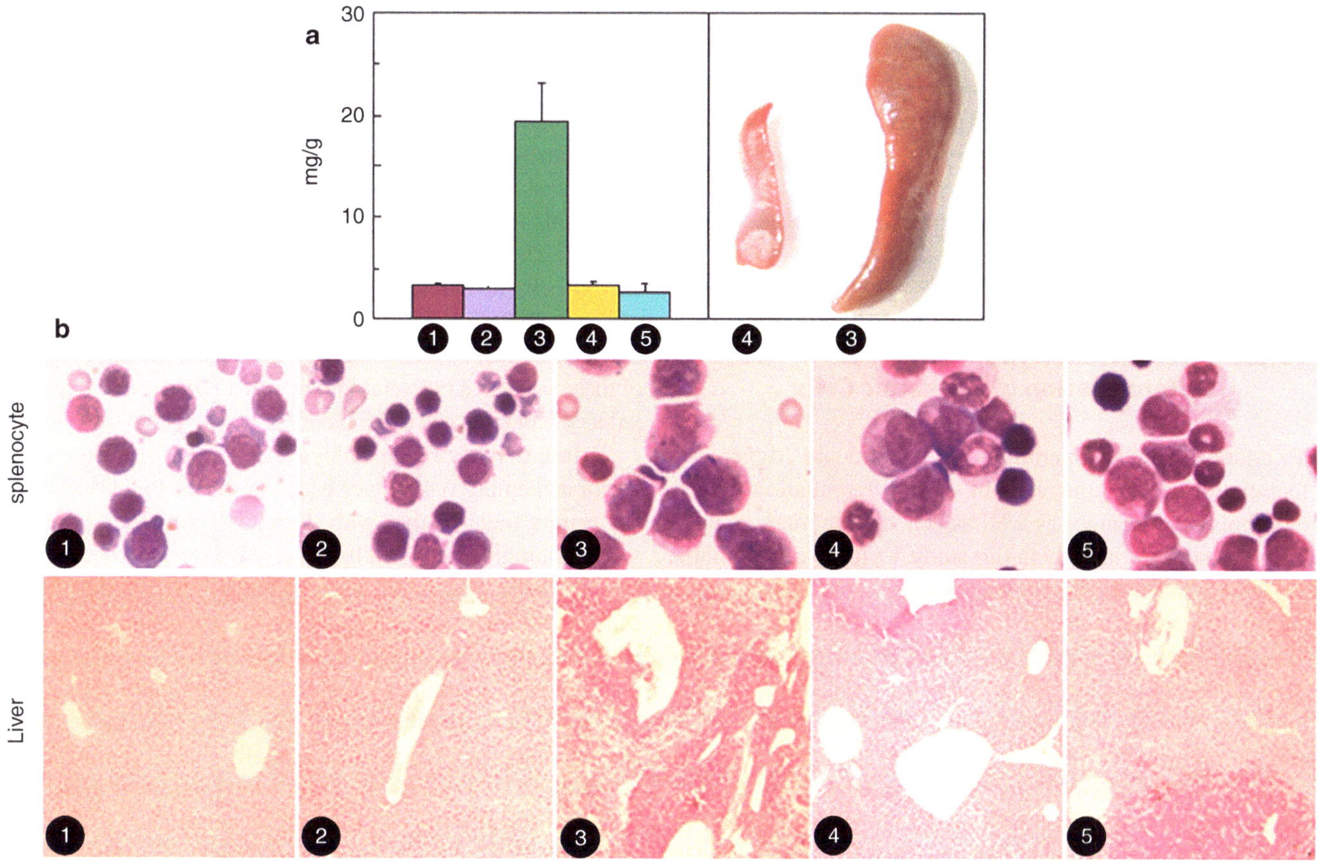

Fig. 19.1 Inhibition of leukemic cell infiltration in bone marrow, spleen, and liver by intermittent hypoxia. (**a**) Leukemic cells (2×10^5) from BM and spleen of hMRP8-PML-RARα transgenic mice were transplanted intravenously into FVB/N mice. Then, these mice were randomly placed into intermittent hypoxia at day 1 (early phase/hypoxia) or at day 7 (middle phase/hypoxia) after transplantation or kept in normal oxygen (leukemia/normoxia). Nontransplanted normal mice in normal oxygen (normal// normoxia) and in intermittent hypoxia (normal/hypoxia) were used as controls. (**a**) The spleen of each mouse was weighed, and data are shown as the ratio of spleen (mg)/body wt (g). (**b**) Splenocytes and liver were collected onto slides by cytospin, stained by Wright's Giemsa, and observed under microscope. ❶ normal mice in normoxia; ❷ normal mice in hypoxia; ❸ leukemic mice in normoxia; ❹ early phase leukemic mice in hypoxia; ❺ middle phase leukemic mice in hypoxia (This figure is partially adapted from Liu et al. [37])

19.3.2 Intermittent Hypoxia Inhibits Proliferation Without Apoptosis Induction of Leukemic Cells

Although the cellular effects of hypoxia in solid tumors have been well documented, the relationship between hypoxia and cell proliferation/apoptosis in hematologic malignancies remains unclear. So we investigated the *in situ* expression of proliferating cell nuclear antigen (PCNA) and terminal deoxynucleotidyl transferase-mediated dUTP nick end labeling (TUNEL), two important indications respectively for proliferating and apoptotic cells, by immunohistochemical assay. The results show that the number of PCNA-positive cells in tissues of leukemic mice in normoxia (70.33±5.51% for liver and 51.33±3.21% for spleen) is far higher than those of hypoxia-treated early phase leukemic mice (3.33±1.53% for liver and 5.50±1.80% for spleen), the latter having no significant difference from those seen in normal mice in normoxia (0.47±0.15% for liver and 2.83±0.76% for spleen) and in hypoxia (0.33±0.58% for liver and 0.93±0.51% for spleen). The percentages of PCNA-positive cells in liver and spleen of hypoxia-treated middle phase leukemic mice are respectively 23.33±6.11% and 16.33±5.13% that are higher than those of normal mice and hypoxia-treated early phase leukemic mice, but are far lower than those of leukemic mice in normoxia.

On the other hand, we found that few TUNEL-positive cells could be seen in all mice with different treatments. In agreement with this, annexin V^+ cells and sub-G_1 cells are rarely found on flow cytometry in spleen and liver suspensions of all mice; PARP cleavage and activated caspase-3, two important hallmarks of apoptosis, were also undetectable. Besides, short-term hypoxia (24 days after transplantation, leukemic mice were caged into intermittent hypoxia chamber for 1–3 days) increases G_1-phase cells with reduction of S-phase cells and without the appearance of sub-G_1 cells.

Taken together, these results strongly indicate that hypoxia can inhibit proliferation but does not induce apoptosis of leukemic cells, and such an inhibitory effect of hypoxia on leukemic mice was not because of hypoxia toxicity because all mice could endure hypoxic condition used in this work without the evidence of tissue damage.

19.3.3 Intermittent Hypoxia Induces Differentiation of Leukemic Cells

To address whether intermittent hypoxia could trigger differentiation of leukemic cells in vivo, differentiation-related morphological changes as well as cell surface markers have been investigated intently in our study. Cytological examination shows that there is low percentage of leukemic blast-like cells in the BM of leukemic mice under hypoxia, which tend to morphologically mature. Most infiltrated leukemic cells in the spleen and liver of hypoxia-treated leukemic mice predominantly consist of maturating myeloid cells that present differentiation-related morphological features such as condensed chromatin with indented, distorted, horseshoed, or circular nuclei, which are significantly different from those seen in normal mice and leukemic mice in normal oxygen. In accord with this, the BM and spleen have much higher percentages of differentiation-related antigens Gr-1^+ and Mac-1^+ cells than those of leukemic mice in normal oxygen by FACS analysis or direct immunofluorescence microscopy. Furthermore, cells in spleen of hypoxia-treated leukemic mice presented Gr-1^+ staining and have normal and even disappeared PML speckles (known as PML oncogenic domains [PODs] or nuclear bodies), whereas infiltrated leukemic cells in the spleen of leukemic mice in normoxia exhibit Gr-1^- staining and hundreds of PML-RARα-related micropunctates in the nuclei. These results propose that intermittent hypoxia could induce in vivo differentiation of leukemic cells, although further investigation is needed.

19.4 The Role of HIF-1α in Leukemic Cell Differentiation

Following investigations provide several convincing evidences that support the role of HIF-1α in leukemic cell differentiation. As showed in above-mentioned in vitro experiments, the differentiation of AML cells induced by hypoxia/hypoxia-mimetic agents is always consistent with the accumulation of cellular HIF-1α protein as well as its DNA-binding activity. By contrast, while $CoCl_2$/DFO-triggered HIF-1α accumulation and HRE-binding activity have been antagonized by small molecular chemical, nitric oxide (NO) donor 3-morpholinosydnonimine (SIN-1) or metavanadate respectively, the growth arrest and differentiation of AML cells are also abrogated [32, 40]. Furthermore, Short-hairpin RNAs (shRNAs) specifically targeting and silencing HIF-1α also remarkably inhibit $CoCl_2$ and 2% O_2-induced differentiation of AML cells [41]. In consistence, Kim et al. also found that tiron, a widely used antioxidant and nontoxic chelator to alleviate an acute metal overload, causes HL-60 cells to induce differentiation-related alterations such as the increase in CD11b and CD14 expression or chromatin condensation through increasing HIF-1α expression [42]. All of these suggest a potential link between HIF-1α and hypoxia-induced leukemic cell differentiation.

To further verify the capability of HIF-1α, HIF-1α-expressing vector and empty vector have been transfected into U937 cells; the results indicate that with decreased proliferative ability, some maturating cells can be observed under microscope and CD11b$^+$ cells are significantly higher in HIF-1α-transfected cells than those in empty vector-transfected cells [33]. Meanwhile, we generated myeloid leukemic U937T transformants, in which HIF-1α is tightly induced by tetracycline withdrawal [41, 43]. The results show that, 3–4 days after the induction of HIF-1α, the proliferation is substantially slowed down and the G1–S-phase transition is blocked. More importantly, HIF-1α induction directly triggers myeloid leukemic cells to undergo differentiation, as determined by differentiation-related morphological changes, increased CD11/NBT reduction, and expressions of differentiation signatures such as neutrophil cytosolic factor-1 (NCF1), interleukin-1 receptor antagonist, (IL1RA) and secreted phosphoprotein 1 (SPP1) [41]. In total, these data indicate the direct contribution of HIF-1α to hypoxia/hypoxia-mimetic agents-induced differentiation of myeloid leukemic cells. Besides, the in vivo work also shows that intermittent hypoxia remarkably and progressively increases HIF-1α protein in peripheral tissues of leukemic mice. It is noteworthy that $CoCl_2$ and DFO at doses used in vivo studies fail to remarkably increase HIF-1α protein as well as the survival of AML mice [37].

As HIF-1α protein has been reported to accumulate in differentiating U937 macrophages under normoxia [44], we also investigated the relationship between HIF-1α and the differentiation effect triggered by ATRA, classical differentiation-induction agent, [45]. To our surprise, the results show that ATRA rapidly accumulates endogenous and inducible expressed or $CoCl_2$-stabilized HIF-1α protein of leukemic cells under normoxic condition. More importantly, suppression of HIF-1α expression by specific shRNAs partially but significantly represses, while conditional HIF-1α induction and HIF-1α-stabilizing greatly enhances, ATRA-induced leukemic differentiation. These observations indicate that, as a protein rapidly responsive to ATRA, HIF-1α does exert a role in the differentiation induction of ATRA on AML cells, which provide a new sight in clinical potential of ATRA.

19.5 Interactions of HIF-1α with Hematopoietic Lineage-Specific Transcription Factors

It is well known that HIF-1α protein exerts its role in a series of biological processes through the transcriptional activation of its target genes, which requires its heterodimerization with HIF-1β [46–49]. Hence, to determine whether HIF-1α-mediated differentiation involves its transcriptional activity, two effective pairs of shRNAs specially against HIF-1β mRNA were transfected into the U937 cells. While the suppression of HIF-1β protein by shRNAs impairs the transcriptional activity of HIF-1, which is evidenced by the inhibition of HIF-1 target genes, 50 μM $CoCl_2$ or 2% O_2 treatment still induces U937 cells to undergo differentiation. Similarly, the silencing of HIF-1β protein does not impinge on HIF-1α-triggered differentiation in U937T cells after tetracycline withdrawal [41]. So it can be concluded that HIF-1β is not necessary for hypoxia/HIF-1α-mediated myeloid cell differentiation.

Fusion genes involving in hematopoietic malignancies have been reported to exhibit inhibitory effects on differentiation of AML cells promoted by a wide spectrum of differentiation-inducing agents [50]. Our study shows that, compared with other leukemic cells, Kasummi-1 cell line, which expresses a high level of AML1-ETO fusion protein generated by t(8;21) chromosomal translocation that is associated with 12% of de novo AML cases and up to 40% of the M2-subtype AML, is much less sensitive to and could hardly be induced to undergo differentiation by hypoxia/hypoxia-mimetic agent [33]. The result probably indicates that the expression of AML1-ETO fusion protein can interfere with hypoxia-induced differentiation. Indeed, inducible AML1-ETO expression inhibits hypoxia-induced cell differentiation in the ecdysone-inducible system from parental U937 cells. More surprisingly, the inducible expression of AML1-ETO increases HIF-1α transcription in U937 cells via an undefined mechanism. Based on these contradictory data, we hypothesize that HIF-1α induces leukemic differentiation by regulating some other differentiation-related factors which might be inhibited by the AML1-ETO protein. It has been reported that AML1-ETO fusion protein leads to the down-regulation of C/EBPα [51], a member of the leucine zipper family of transcription factors that plays a critical role in granulocytic hematopoiesis [52]. So in following studies, the potential role of C/EBPα in HIF-1α-induced differentiation has been investigated [33, 53]. Although inducible expression of HIF-1α protein cannot alter C/EBPα protein/mRNA level, coimmunoprecipitation assay indicates that not only ectopically but also endogenously expressed HIF-1α protein interacts with C/EBPα. GST pull-down assay proposes that the protein–protein interaction is direct and demonstrated that C/EBPα competes with HIF-1β for direct binding to HIF-1α protein. The functional analysis such as EMSA, chromatin immunoprecipitation, luciferase assay, and the expression of HIF-1-targeted genes shows that HIF-1α protein enhances transcriptional activity of C/EBPα while C/EBPα significantly inhibits the DNA-binding ability and transcriptional activity of HIF-1α. Kim et al. also reported that tiron could increase HIF-1α protein and the activity of C/EBPα [42]. These studies propose that C/EBPα plays a certain role in HIF-1α-mediated leukemic cell differentiation. On the other hand, the functional inhibition of HIF-1 mediated by C/EBPα may lead to the reduced expression of VEGF, inhibiting angiogenesis to form a hypoxic microenvironment which facilitate leukemic cell differentiation.

PU.1 and Runt-related transcription protein 1 (Runx1, also known as acute myeloid leukemia-1, AML1) are two other well-documented transcriptional factors, which have been reported not only to play an important role during hematopoiesis but also to participate in angiogenesis process [54]. Our studies show that ectopically expressing Runx1 protein directly interacts with HIF-1α protein as determined by LacO array, Co-IP, and GST pull-down assay. Such interaction can also be detected between endogenously expressed Runx1 and $CoCl_2$-stabilized HIF-1α protein. Like C/EBPα, Runx1 shows inhibitory effect on HIF-1 because overexpression of Runx1 suppresses DNA-binding and transcriptional activity of HIF-1 as well as decreased expression of HIF-1-targeted genes, while abrogation of Runx1 expression by specific shRNAs significantly increases transcriptional activity of HIF-1 protein; vice versa, HIF-1α enhances DNA-binding ability and transcriptional activity of Runx1 protein [55]. Luciferase assay also shows that HIF-1α enhances the transcriptional activity of PU.1, Runx1, C/EBPα, and their synergistic actions. Moreover, knockdown of PU.1, Runx1, and C/EBP alpha greatly inhibits HIF-1α-triggered differentiation as well as the differentiation cooperation of ATRA and HIF-1α induction [41, 45, 56].

Conclusion and Prospection

The results summarized above put forward the notion that hypoxia/hypoxia-mimetic agents can trigger differentiation in myeloid leukemic cells in which HIF-1α plays a critical role independent of its transcriptional activity while C/EBPα and Runx1 act as the effectors downstream to HIF-1α protein through direct interactions to enhance their transcriptional activities (Fig. 19.2). These discoveries would shed new insights for understanding mechanisms underlying leukemogenesis and designing new strategies for differentiation therapy of AML.

Albeit, some directions still deserve further investigation. Firstly, as hypoxia favors leukemic cell differentiation, it could be considered that the alterations of hypoxia-related signaling might contribute to differentiation block of hematopoietic cells. Although no report has shown that knockdown of HIF-1α induces leukemia,

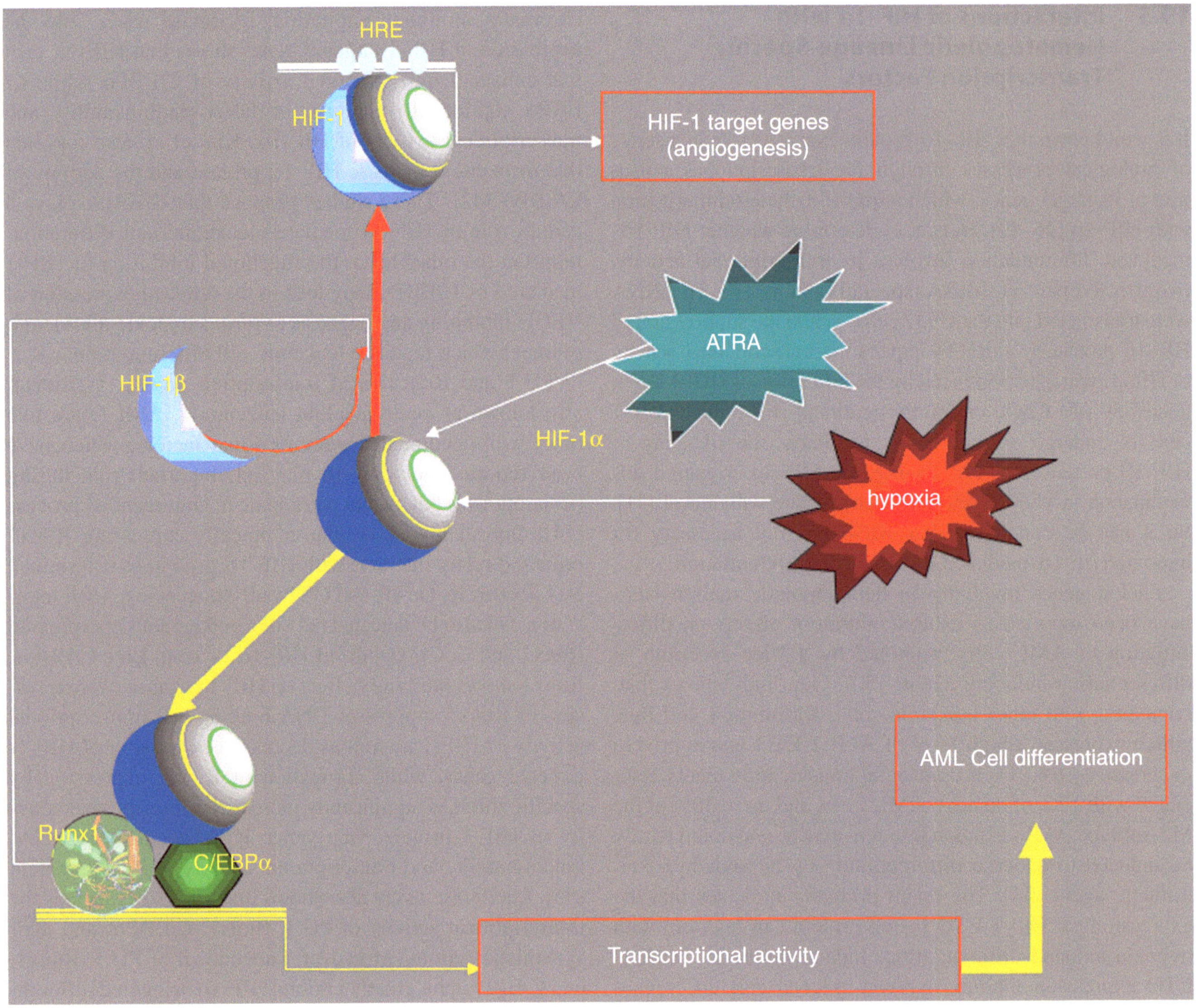

Fig. 19.2 The mechanisms of hypoxia-induced leukemic differentiation. Hypoxia and hypoxia-mimetic agents as well as classical leukemic cell differentiation-inducing agent ATRA stabilize and thus accumulate HIF-1α protein, which physically interacts with and enhances the transcriptional activities of hematopoiesis-associated transcriptional factors C/EBPα and Runx1, which finally induce leukemic differentiation. On the other hand, C/EBPα and Runx1 also antagonize formation of HIF-1α/HIF-1β heterodimer and block transcriptional activity of HIF-1. In the absence of C/EBPα and Runx1 in nonhematopoietic tissues, HIF-1α/HIF-1β heterodimer functions as transcriptional factor and induces expressions of genes related to cellular adaption to hypoxia such as VEGF

a t(1;12)(q21; p13) translocation in an AML-M2 results in the expression of a fusion gene between TEL/ETV6 and essentially all of ARNT, a constitutive subunit for HIF-1α activities. The breakpoint of ARNT loci is also found in 11 out of 36 patients with various hematopoietic disorders. Our studies also show that $CoCl_2$ is capable of inducing apparent differentiation in leukemic cells from some but not all AML patients. So it is worthwhile elucidating the role of abnormal alterations of HIF-1α gene in leukemogenesis. Secondly, besides the three transcriptional factors mentioned above, some other factors might also link HIF-1α protein to leukemic differentiation due to the network of the hematopoietic regulation. Actually, by employing the comparative proteomic analysis, we have identified some proteins which relate to hypoxia and $CoCl_2$ treatment and possess differentiation-induction activity [47]. Finally, the global efficacy of intermittent hypoxia remains to be investigated on additional in vivo models with non-APL leukemia. Also, it would be of interest to investigate whether there is lower incidence of leukemia and better prognosis in populations who live at very high altitudes than those who live near sea level. Following these investigations, it should be considered to use hypoxia as a physical treatment for AML. In addition, other small molecular compounds need to be explored to target the HIF-1α signaling pathway.

References

1. Xie H, Ye M, Feng R, et al. Stepwise reprogramming of B cells into macrophages. Cell. 2004;117:663–76.
2. Speck NA, Gilliland DG. Core-binding factors in haematopoiesis and leukaemia. Nat Rev Cancer. 2002;2:502–13.
3. Scandura JM, Boccuni P, Cammenga J, et al. Transcription factor fusions in acute leukemia: variations on a theme. Oncogene. 2002;21:3422–44.
4. Melnick A, Licht JD. Deconstructing a disease: RARalpha, its fusion partners, and their roles in the pathogenesis of acute promyelocytic leukemia. Blood. 1999;93:3167–215.
5. Fibach E, Hayashi M, Sachs L. Control of normal differentiation of myeloid leukemic cells to macrophages and granulocytes. Proc Natl Acad Sci USA. 1973;70:343–6.
6. Chen GQ, Shen ZX, Wu F, et al. Pharmacokinetics and efficacy of low-dose all-trans retinoic acid in the treatment of acute promyelocytic leukemia. Leukemia. 1996;10:825–8.
7. Huang ME, Ye YC, Chen SR, et al. Use of all-trans retinoic acid in the treatment of acute promyelocytic leukemia. Blood. 1988;72:567–72.
8. Lo Coco F, Nervi C, Avvisati G, et al. Acute promyelocytic leukemia: a curable disease. Leukemia. 1998;12:1866–80.
9. Delva L, Cornic M, Balitrand N, et al. Resistance to all-trans retinoic acid (ATRA) therapy in relapsing acute promyelocytic leukemia: study of in vitro ATRA sensitivity and cellular retinoic acid binding protein levels in leukemic cells. Blood. 1993;82:2175–81.
10. Shen ZX, Chen GQ, Ni JH, et al. Use of arsenic trioxide (As_2O_3) in the treatment of acute promyelocytic leukemia (APL): II. Clinical efficacy and pharmacokinetics in relapsed patients. Blood. 1997;89:3354–60.
11. Chen GQ, Zhu J, Shi XG, et al. In vitro studies on cellular and molecular mechanisms of arsenic trioxide (As_2O_3) in the treatment of acute promyelocytic leukemia: As_2O_3 induces NB4 cell apoptosis with downregulation of Bcl-2 expression and modulation of PML-RAR alpha/PML proteins. Blood. 1996;88:1052–61.
12. Chen GQ, Shi XG, Tang W, et al. Use of arsenic trioxide (As_2O_3) in the treatment of acute promyelocytic leukemia (APL): I. As_2O_3 exerts dose-dependent dual effects on APL cells. Blood. 1997;89:3345–53.
13. Shipley JL, Butera JN. Acute myelogenous leukemia. Exp Hematol. 2009;37:649–58.
14. Zhang TD, Chen GQ, Wang ZG, et al. Arsenic trioxide, a therapeutic agent for APL. Oncogene. 2001;20:7146–53.
15. Jing Y, Wang L, Xia L, et al. Combined effect of all-trans retinoic acid and arsenic trioxide in acute promyelocytic leukemia cells in vitro and in vivo. Blood. 2001;97:264–9.
16. Lallemand-Breitenbach V, Guillemin MC, Janin A, et al. Retinoic acid and arsenic synergize to eradicate leukemic cells in a mouse model of acute promyelocytic leukemia. J Exp Med. 1999;189:1043–52.
17. Kinjo K, Kizaki M, Muto A, et al. Arsenic trioxide (As_2O_3)-induced apoptosis and differentiation in retinoic acid-resistant acute promyelocytic leukemia model in hGM-CSF-producing transgenic SCID mice. Leukemia. 2000;14:431–8.
18. Cai X, Shen YL, Zhu Q, et al. Arsenic trioxide-induced apoptosis and differentiation are associated respectively with mitochondrial transmembrane potential collapse and retinoic acid signaling pathways in acute promyelocytic leukemia. Leukemia. 2000;14:262–70.
19. Semenza GL. Oxygen homeostasis. Wiley Interdiscip Rev Syst Biol Med. 2010;2:336–61.
20. Jensen PO, Mortensen BT, Hodgkiss RJ, et al. Increased cellular hypoxia and reduced proliferation of both normal and leukaemic cells during progression of acute myeloid leukaemia in rats. Cell Prolif. 2000;33:381–95.
21. Hussong JW, Rodgers GM, Shami PJ. Evidence of increased angiogenesis in patients with acute myeloid leukemia. Blood. 2000;95:309–13.
22. Padro T, Ruiz S, Bieker R, et al. Increased angiogenesis in the bone marrow of patients with acute myeloid leukemia. Blood. 2000;95: 2637–44.
23. Di Raimondo F, Palumbo GA, Molica S, et al. Angiogenesis in chronic myeloproliferative diseases. Acta Haematol. 2001;106:177–83.
24. Levesque JP, Winkler IG, Hendy J, et al. Hematopoietic progenitor cell mobilization results in hypoxia with increased hypoxia-inducible transcription factor-1 alpha and vascular endothelial growth factor A in bone marrow. Stem Cells. 2007;25:1954–65.
25. Yoshihara H, Arai F, Hosokawa K, et al. Thrombopoietin/MPL signaling regulates hematopoietic stem cell quiescence and interaction with the osteoblastic niche. Cell Stem Cell. 2007;1:685–97.
26. Takubo K, Goda N, Yamada W, et al. Regulation of the HIF-1alpha level is essential for hematopoietic stem cells. Cell Stem Cell. 2010;7:391–402.
27. Wang GL, Jiang BH, Rue EA, et al. Hypoxia-inducible factor 1 is a basic-helix-loop-helix-PAS heterodimer regulated by cellular O_2 tension. Proc Natl Acad Sci USA. 1995;92:5510–4.
28. Semenza GL. Hypoxia-inducible factor 1: master regulator of O_2 homeostasis. Curr Opin Genet Dev. 1998;8:588–94.
29. Semenza GL. Targeting HIF-1 for cancer therapy. Nat Rev Cancer. 2003;3:721–32.
30. Ivanovic Z, Bartolozzi B, Bernabei PA, et al. Incubation of murine bone marrow cells in hypoxia ensures the maintenance of marrow-repopulating ability together with the expansion of committed progenitors. Br J Haematol. 2000;108:424–9.
31. Ivanovic Z, Dello Sbarba P, Trimoreau F, et al. Primitive human HPCs are better maintained and expanded in vitro at 1 percent oxygen than at 20 percent. Transfusion. 2000;40:1482–8.
32. Huang Y, Du KM, Xue ZH, et al. Cobalt chloride and low oxygen tension trigger differentiation of acute myeloid leukemic cells: possible mediation of hypoxia-inducible factor-1alpha. Leukemia. 2003;17:2065–73.
33. Jiang Y, Xue ZH, Shen WZ, et al. Desferrioxamine induces leukemic cell differentiation potentially by hypoxia-inducible factor-1 alpha that augments transcriptional activity of CCAAT/enhancer-binding protein-alpha. Leukemia. 2005;19:1239–47.
34. Callens C, Coulon S, Naudin J, et al. Targeting iron homeostasis induces cellular differentiation and synergizes with differentiating agents in acute myeloid leukemia. J Exp Med. 2010;207:731–50.
35. Guo M, Song LP, Jiang Y, et al. Hypoxia-mimetic agents desferrioxamine and cobalt chloride induce leukemic cell apoptosis through different hypoxia-inducible factor-1alpha independent mechanisms. Apoptosis. 2006;11:67–77.
36. Yan H, Peng ZG, Wu YL, et al. Hypoxia-simulating agents and selective stimulation of arsenic trioxide-induced growth arrest and cell differentiation in acute promyelocytic leukemic cells. Haematologica. 2005;90:1607–16.
37. Liu W, Guo M, Xu YB, et al. Induction of tumor arrest and differentiation with prolonged survival by intermittent hypoxia in a mouse model of acute myeloid leukemia. Blood. 2006;107:698–707.
38. Brown D, Kogan S, Lagasse E, et al. A PMLRARalpha transgene initiates murine acute promyelocytic leukemia. Proc Natl Acad Sci USA. 1997;94:2551–6.
39. Blatt J, Boegel F, Hedlund BE, et al. Failure to alter the course of acute myelogenous leukemia in the rat with subcutaneous deferoxamine. Leuk Res. 1991;15:391–4.
40. Xue ZH, Jiang Y, Yu Y, et al. Metavanadate suppresses desferrioxamine-induced leukemic cell differentiation with reduced hypoxia-inducible factor-1alpha protein. Biochem Biophys Res Commun. 2005;332:1140–5.
41. Song LP, Zhang J, Wu SF, et al. Hypoxia-inducible factor-1alpha-induced differentiation of myeloid leukemic cells is its transcriptional activity independent. Oncogene. 2008;27:519–27.
42. Kim JS, Cho EW, Chung HW, et al. Effects of tiron, 4,5-dihydroxy-1,3-benzene disulfonic acid, on human promyelotic HL-60 leukemia cell differentiation and death. Toxicology. 2006;223:36–45.
43. Janardhan HP. The HIF-1 alpha-C/EBP alpha axis. Sci Signal. 2008;1:jc2.

44. Knowles HJ, Mole DR, Ratcliffe PJ, et al. Normoxic stabilization of hypoxia-inducible factor-1alpha by modulation of the labile iron pool in differentiating U937 macrophages: effect of natural resistance-associated macrophage protein 1. Cancer Res. 2006;66:2600–7.
45. Zhang J, Song LP, Huang Y, et al. Accumulation of hypoxia-inducible factor-1 alpha protein and its role in the differentiation of myeloid leukemic cells induced by all-trans retinoic acid. Haematologica. 2008;93:1480–7.
46. Chen GQ, Wang LS, Wu YL, et al. Leukemia, an effective model for chemical biology and target therapy. Acta Pharmacol Sin. 2007;28:1316–24.
47. Han YH, Xia L, Song LP, et al. Comparative proteomic analysis of hypoxia-treated and untreated human leukemic U937 cells. Proteomics. 2006;6:3262–74.
48. Liao SH, Zhao XY, Han YH, et al. Proteomics-based identification of two novel direct targets of hypoxia-inducible factor-1 and their potential roles in migration/invasion of cancer cells. Proteomics. 2009;9:3901–12.
49. Zhao XY, Chen TT, Xia L, et al. Hypoxia inducible factor-1 mediates expression of galectin-1: the potential role in migration/invasion of colorectal cancer cells. Carcinogenesis. 2010;31:1367–75.
50. Peterson LF, Zhang DE. The 8;21 translocation in leukemogenesis. Oncogene. 2004;23:4255–62.
51. Pabst T, Mueller BU, Harakawa N, et al. AML1-ETO downregulates the granulocytic differentiation factor C/EBPalpha in t(8;21) myeloid leukemia. Nat Med. 2001;7:444–51.
52. Gao FH, Wang Q, Wu YL, et al. c-Jun N-terminal kinase mediates AML1-ETO protein-induced connexin-43 expression. Biochem Biophys Res Commun. 2007;356:505–11.
53. Yang L, Jiang Y, Wu SF, et al. CCAAT/enhancer-binding protein alpha antagonizes transcriptional activity of hypoxia-inducible factor 1 alpha with direct protein-protein interaction. Carcinogenesis. 2008;29:291–8.
54. Rosmarin AG, Yang Z, Resendes KK. Transcriptional regulation in myelopoiesis: hematopoietic fate choice, myeloid differentiation, and leukemogenesis. Exp Hematol. 2005;33:131–43.
55. Peng ZG, Zhou MY, Huang Y, et al. Physical and functional interaction of runt-related protein 1 with hypoxia-inducible factor-1alpha. Oncogene. 2008;27:839–47.
56. Zhang J, Chen GQ. Hypoxia-HIF-1alpha-C/EBPalpha/Runx1 signaling in leukemic cell differentiation. Pathophysiology. 2009;16: 297–303.

Energotropic Effects of Intermittent Hypoxia: Role of Succinate-Dependent Signaling

20

Ludmila D. Lukyanova, Yu I. Kirova, and Elina L. Germanova

Abstract

This chapter focuses on a bioenergetic mechanism for development of urgent and long-term adaptation to hypoxia. Hypoxia induces reprogramming of respiratory chain function and switching from oxidation of NAD-related substrates (complex I) to succinate oxidation (complex II). Transient, reversible, compensatory activation of respiratory chain complex II is a major mechanism of urgent adaptation to hypoxia, which is necessary for (1) succinate-related energy synthesis in the conditions of oxygen shortage and formation of urgent resistance in the body, (2) succinate-related stabilization of HIF-1α and initiation of its transcriptional activity related with formation of long-term adaptation, and (3) succinate-dependent activation of the succinate-specific receptor GPR91. Therefore, succinate is a signaling molecule, and succinate effects in hypoxia occur at three levels, intramitochondrial, intracellular, and intercellular. In these settings, succinate displays antihypoxic and antiradical activities. Suppression of free-radical processes in early phase of hypoxia potentiates effects of succinate and facilitates development of urgent adaptation to hypoxia. The chapter considers tactics and strategy for development of the antihypoxic defense and of antihypoxants with energotropic properties.

Abbreviations

AHBH	Acute hypobaric hypoxia
ATP	Adenosine triphosphate
CD	Conjugated dienes
FAD	Flavin adenine nucleotides
GPR91	Succinate-related guanine nucleotide binding protein-coupled receptor
GSH	Reduced glutathione
GSSG	Oxidized glutathione
HIF	Hypoxia-inducible factor
HR	High-resistance rats
HSP	Heat shock proteins
INH	Interval normobaric hypoxia
LOOH	Lipid hydroperoxides
LP	Lipid peroxidation
LR	Low-resistance rats
NAD	Nicotine adenine nucleotides
NBH	Normobaric hypoxia
PC	Phosphocreatine
ROS	Reactive oxygen species
SDH	Succinate dehydrogenase
TBARS	Thiobarbituric acid reactive substances.

L.D. Lukyanova (✉) • Y.I. Kirova • E.L. Germanova
Institute of General Pathology and Pathophysiology,
Russian Academia of Medical Sciences,
Moscow, Russia
e-mail: ldlukyanova@gmail.com

20.1 Regulatory Role of Mitochondria in Vital Functions of the Body

Mitochondria play a key role in oxygen homeostasis. This role is determined primarily by the key function of mitochondria in the cell, the function of a self-regulating biological machine that uses oxygen for generation of energy in the form of ATP and mitochondrial membrane potential. Inhaled

L. Xi, T.V. Serebrovskaya (eds.), *Intermittent Hypoxia and Human Diseases*,
DOI 10.1007/978-1-4471-2906-6_20, © Springer-Verlag London 2012

oxygen eventually reflects the state and the oxygen demand of mitochondria because it is mitochondria that are the main oxygen consumers: up to 98% of oxygen delivered to the body is related with mitochondrial respiration. This process provides up to 80–90% of ATP to cells of different mammalian tissues. Due to this function, which is responsible for vital capacity and function of aerobic organisms, evolution has produced most sophisticated physiological systems for oxygen delivery to mitochondria and maintenance of optimal cell oxygenation (breathing, lung system of oxygen transport, cardiovascular circulation, blood mass and transportation system, red cells, hemoglobin). The arrangement of the digestive system including consumption and subsequent stepwise enzymic processing of food is also determined primarily by the necessity to supply substrates to reactions of mitochondrial oxidation and oxidative phosphorylation [6, 11, 45].

In addition to energy production, mitochondria play a leading role in cell metabolism. They contain many key and limiting enzymes for steroid biosynthesis and gastric juice secretion (carbonic anhydrase). Mitochondria perform a coordinating function in complex signal pathways of calcium and potassium metabolism, especially in specialized cells. A constant, intensive flow of inorganic ions and metabolites continuously circulates between cytosol and mitochondria. As the inner mitochondrial membrane is permeable only for H_2O, O_2, CO_2, and NH_3, other hydrophilic metabolites and all biologically significant organic ions are transported through the membrane due to the availability of specific channels and protein carriers. Among the latter, carriers of phosphates, adenine nucleotides (ATP and ADP), and respiratory mono-, di-, and tricarbonates are most important.

Mitochondria participate in regulation of various physiological functions by providing energy for most of intracellular processes necessary for vital functions of the body including, first of all, contractility of the heart and smooth muscles in the gastrointestinal tract, blood vessels, and lungs, maintenance of ion gradients in excitable tissues, accumulation of secretables in vesicles, and maintenance of hormonal and neurotransmitter functions. Nevertheless, the major function of mitochondria is their *regulatory role in oxygen homeostasis*, which is evident at both systemic and cellular levels.

At the systemic level, mitochondria determine the concentration gradient of oxygen arriving from the environment because just mitochondria represent the final step of molecular oxygen interactions [6, 11, 40]. *At the cell level*, the mitochondrial respiratory chain functions as a signal-transforming metabolic system which activates the physiological response to hypoxia. Apparently, we can say therefore that mitochondria are involved in intra- and extracellular signaling mechanisms, which actively participate in information transmission via various intracellular signaling pathways.

20.2 Peculiarities of Respiratory Chain Performance in the Conditions of Hypoxia: Role of Respiratory Chain in Adaptation to Hypoxia

It is known that hypoxia is associated with disturbances of ATP synthesis resulting from depressed functions of electron transport and phosphorylation in the respiratory chain. The determinative factor of hypoxic states is disorders of oxygen delivery from the environment to the cell. In the cell, oxygen participates in reactions of aerobic energy synthesis as the substrate for cytochrome oxidase, the terminal enzyme of mitochondrial respiratory chain. Therefore, oxygen deficiency in the extracellular environment may lead to either reduction or total inhibition of aerobic energy synthesis involving a decrease in the content of high-energy molecules (ATP and PC), the main marker of hypoxic conditions. This results in inhibition of multiple energy-dependent reactions such as membrane potential formation, ion transport, electrogenic cell function, muscle contraction, receptor function, etc. Mitochondrial dysfunction inevitably leads to different pathologies and even death.

Responses to hypoxia include various adaptive reactions aimed at eliminating functional and metabolic disturbances typical for this condition. Two types of mechanisms exist, emergency *short-term compensatory mechanisms* aimed at preventing consequences of acute hypoxia and at fast recovery after the hypoxia exposure. The other type is *long-term mechanisms of adaptation* to hypoxia; these mechanisms occur within relatively long periods of hypoxia to enhance the body resistance to oxygen shortage. These mechanisms are based on regulatory modulation of the mitochondrial respiratory chain function.

In normoxic conditions, performance of the respiratory chain is usually related with oxidation of NAD-related substrates, the major suppliers of reduction equivalents to the respiratory chain through mitochondrial complex I. The complex I contribution as estimated by oxygen consumption may reach 55–65% in intact cells. At the same time, 25–30% of mitochondrial respiration under these conditions is attributed to succinate (complex II) oxidation [34–37] although the succinate level in mitochondrial matrix is very low (0.2–0.4 mM) [24, 29]. The ratio between two oxidation pathways depends primarily on properties of the principal enzyme complexes I and II. Kinetic characteristics of two major enzymes of these complexes, NAD-ubiquinone oxidoreductase and succinate dehydrogenase (SDH), are tissue-specific and differ in intact animals with different sensitivity to hypoxia [12, 13, 33–37, 39–41].

Hypoxic environments induce reversible depression of complex I function and compensatory activation of complex II and succinate oxidation, with increased contribution of the

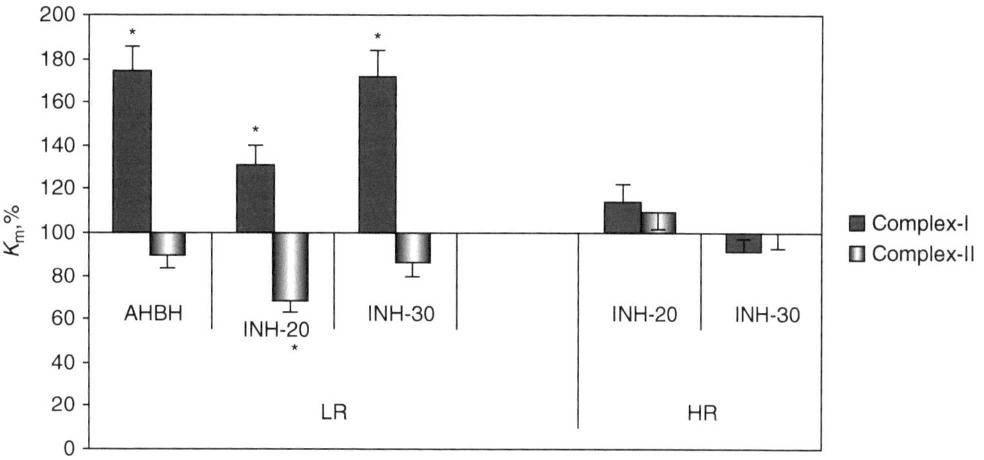

Fig. 20.1 Effects of different hypoxia regimens on K_m values (% of control) for enzymes of complex I (NADH-ubiquinone oxidoreductase, upregulated) and complex II (succinate-cytochrome c reductase, downregulated) in rat cortex 2 h after a hypoxic exposure (1 h). Any regimen of hypoxic exposure with any level of oxygenation results in increased K_m values for complex I and decreased K_m values for complex II. *AHBH* acute hypobaric hypoxia (time of survival to the second agonal breath at critical altitude (11,500, 2–4% O_2)), *INH* intermittent normobaric hypoxia training consisting of passive breathing a hypoxic gas mixture (10% O_2) at constant pressure for 5 min and interspersed with breathing atmospheric air (21% O_2) for 3 min. These sessions were repeated 6–7 times (a training cycle) and lasted for about 1 h in total, *INH-30* intermittent normobaric hypoxia training consisting of passive breathing a hypoxic gas mixture (10% O_2) at constant pressure for 5 min and interspersed with breathing 30% O_2 for 3 min, *LR* low-resistance rats, *HR* high-resistance rats. *$p<0.05$

latter to respiration and energy production. When substrate is abundant, the contribution of succinate-dependent oxidation to total respiration may reach 70–80%.

Hypoxia-induced reprogramming of the respiratory chain substrate region is the first of three phases in the hypoxia-induced mitochondrial disturbances. Twenty-five years ago, we have described these disturbances as those correlating with phase changes occurring at the systemic level [33, 37]. At present time, a great wealth of experimental evidence confirms the reversible inactivation of complex I electron transport function in hypoxic conditions, which persists and even increases in the posthypoxic period (first 30 min–2 h of reoxygenation) [1, 10, 16, 33–36], (Lukyanova 2009a, b); [44, 49, 51, 54, 68]. Many studies have documented a special role of succinate in tissue oxidative metabolism at the early phase of hypoxia. For example, in 1966, Goldberg et al. found that after 30 s of global brain ischemia, succinate level increased 1.5 times in the setting of reduced concentrations of certain NAD-dependent substrates [19]. Similar data were also obtained by other researchers. In the first 30 min of anoxic incubation, formation of succinate increases by an order of magnitude, reaches 4–7 mM, and continues to grow for the first 30 min of reoxygenation [24, 26, 27, 29, 64]. Hypoxia is also associated with activation of SDH and succinate oxidation and with increased contribution of succinate to respiration and energy production [3, 10, 20, 27, 30, 31, 33, 34, 37, 39–41, 64, 68]. Therefore, hypoxic changes are associated with succinate accumulation in tissues and blood, where succinate level increases by two orders of magnitude, and with suppressed oxidation of NAD-related substrates. Kinetic properties of both enzymes change simultaneously (Fig. 20.1). Any regimen of hypoxic exposure with any level of oxygenation (acute hypobaric hypoxia 11,500 m; intermittent normobaric hypoxia at about 10% or 30% concentration in inhaled air) results in pronounced changes in K_m values for both enzymes: increased K_m values for complex I and decreased K_m values for complex II. This process reflects impaired and enhanced efficiency of enzyme performance, respectively.

It should be noted that pheno- and genotypic peculiarities of the response to hypoxia are essential; these changes are relatively more pronounced in the brain of low-resistance rats and are not statistically significant for the neocortex of high-resistance rats (Fig. 20.1) [41].

Therefore, different forms of hypoxia are associated with switching of mitochondrial substrate oxidation. Activation of succinate oxidation constitutes a regulatory and compensatory mechanism, which occurs in the conditions of oxygen shortage in most tissues (brain, myocardium, liver, kidneys, lymphocytes) [31, 34]. This mechanism prevents or attenuates disorders in ATP synthesis, exerts a normalizing effect on the adenylate pool and vital functions of the body, stabilizes and normalizes pH to eliminate hypoxia-characteristic acidosis, and increases the resistance to oxygen shortage. If such switching does not occur in hypoxia, the complex I dysfunction leads to severe de-energizing (decreased membrane potential; ATP loss and changes in the adenine nucleotide pool) and disturbed

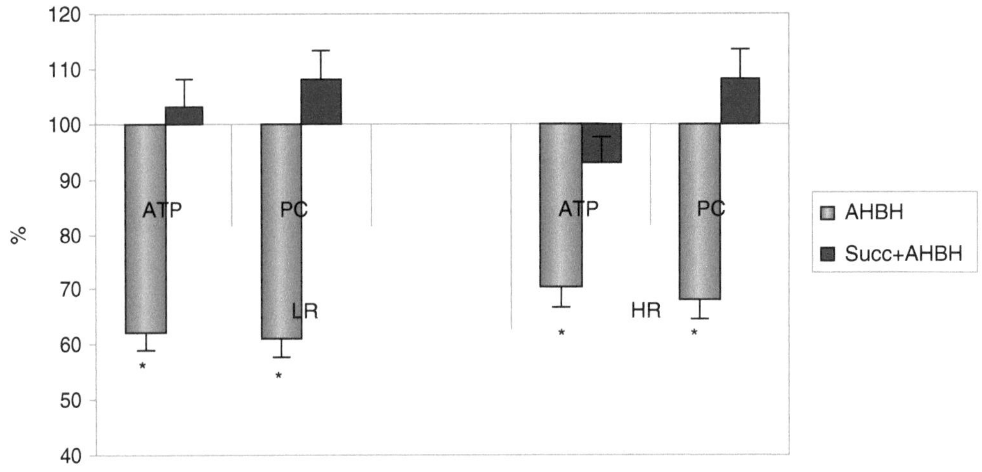

Fig. 20.2 Normalizing effect of the succinate-containing drug proxipin (3-oxypyridine, 40 mg/kg, i.p., 15 min prior to hypoxic exposure) on *ATP* and phosphocreatine (*PC*) levels (% to control) in the neocortex of rats exposed to altitude chamber hypoxia (acute hypobaric hypoxia, *AHBH*) at a simulated extreme altitude (11,500 m, 18 m/s). *AHBH* without proxipin, *Succ+AHBH* with proxipin, *LR* low-resistance rats, *HR* high- resistance rats. $^*p<0.05$

respiration due to oxidation of NAD-related substrates (electron donors for complex I) [12, 13, 18, 26, 27, 37, 40, 41, 64, 68]; (Lukyanova 1999). All these events precede changes in other functional and metabolic parameters that control cell vital activity including condensation of mitochondrial matrix, disturbance of calcium and potassium homeostasis, loss of oxygen sensitivity, disordered expression of mitochondrial genome, appearance of mitochondria-derived reactive oxygen species, CoQ loss, initiation of cytochrome *c* exit to the intermembrane space, apoptosis, and impaired capability of cells for adaptation to low pO_2. In this process, the lactate/pyruvate ratio increases, cell redox potential changes, and metabolic acidosis develops. Also different energy-dependent processes become affected (e.g., electrogenic function of excitable cells, and anabolic processes such as urea synthesis and stage 2 biotransformation reactions.) [13, 17, 37, 40, 41].

Depending on tissue-specific peculiarities of energy metabolism, pathways of endogenous succinate formation are different in hypoxia. However, all these pathways are based on aspartate- and glutamate-dependent aminotransferase reactions, substrate-level α-ketoglutarate phosphorylation during the conversion of α-ketoglutarate to succinate by α-ketoglutarate dehydrogenase, reversal of tricarbonic cycle, and oxidative phosphorylation reactions (substrate-level phosphorylation in citric acid cycle via 2-oxoglutarate dehydrogenase and fumarate reductase reactions) [7, 19, 24, 26, 30, 55, 64, 68].

However, the rate of endogenous succinate formation in hypoxia apparently may not be sufficient for complete compensation for the energy deficiency. This may explain the fact that exogenous succinate or succinate-containing medicines exert a pronounced antihypoxic effect in the setting of oxygen shortage. Such medicines expand the intracellular ATP pool and prevent disorders of energy metabolism (energotropic effect of succinate). For instance, a single injection of the succinate-containing compound proxipin, a 3-hydroxypyridine derivative, 15 min prior to the exposure of rats to extreme, life-incompatible simulated altitude (11,500 m, 2–4% O_2) prevented the loss of high-energy compounds (ATP and phosphocreatine) in rat neocortex (Fig. 20.2). Furthermore, in this process, animal tolerance of acute hypoxia also increases [34–37, 41].

The accumulation of succinate in tissues during hypoxia and the reprogramming of respiratory enzyme performance develop fast and in different levels of oxygenation. However, indirect evidence shows that this process begins much earlier, virtually within the first minutes of a one-hour hypoxic exposure, and reaches the maximum intensity in about 2 h after completion of the exposure. Thereby, the reversible reprogramming of respiratory chain during hypoxia (switching oxidation of NAD-related substrates to succinate oxidation) *is an obligatory, evolutionarily developed, urgent signaling compensatory mechanism.* Due to this mechanism, the energy synthesizing function of respiratory chain is preserved in disturbed oxygen homeostasis.

Mitochondrial disorders induced by hypoxia correlate with phase changes in the content of the adenine nucleotide pool components, ATP, ADP, and AMP [12, 13]. The first step is characterized by a relatively minor, mild (within 6–10%) increase in ATP level followed by transition to a somewhat reduced (by 10–15%), steady-state ATP level (second step), which reflects ATP hydrolysis. This reduction is accompanied by a rise of intracellular ADP content and a decrease in ATP/ADP ratio, accordingly. However, in parallel with the ongoing slight reduction of intracellular ATP level, the intracellular AMP content gradually raises. The regulatory role of ATP/ADP ratio gradually decreases and gets replaced by control of ATP synthesis through the ATP/AMP ratio. At the last stage of hypoxia, when a linear decrease in

ATP content is observed, the controlling role of ATP/ADP and ATP/AMP ratios becomes minimal, and a decrease in total adenine nucleotides plus energetic charges are observed [37, 40]. The changes in adenine nucleotides pool under hypoxia exposure resulting from disturbances in electron flow, and oxidative phosphorylation reactions precede changes in other functional and metabolic parameters controlling the cell vital activity. Thus, increased membrane permeability and lipid peroxidation can be observed only during the terminal stage. Contrastingly, the compensatory role of glycolysis as an ATP supplier is effective only in early hypoxia. During the terminal period, despite a sharp glycolysis activation, glycolysis fails to prevent the decrease in ATP content [37, 40].

The phase rearrangement of mitochondrial enzyme function is associated with and contribute to virtually any kind of hypoxia or ischemia as a basic molecular (bioenergetic) mechanism [36, 37]. Inadequate oxygen delivery to tissues and organs occurs in both exogenous hypoxia and different pathologies associated with injuries of the respiratory and cardiovascular systems and oxygen-transport function of blood. The oxygen shortage inevitably leads to phase changes in activities of mitochondrial enzyme complexes, depression of aerobic energy production, and dysregulation of energy-dependent functions and cell metabolism. Therefore, the body response to oxygen shortage reflects a very sophisticated, multifunctional cell response coordinated by neurohumoral mechanisms, with *energy metabolism playing a trigger role* in the general hierarchy of intracellular processes. The knowledge about the intracellular functional and metabolic mechanisms of adaptation to hypoxia is essential not only for development of science-based principles of pharmacotherapy for disorders caused by acute hypoxia. It is also important for optimizing the conditions of nonspecific resistance where hypoxia is used as a nondrug preventive and therapeutic factor.

20.3 Succinate and Intracellular Signaling for Initiation of Urgent and Long-Term Adaptive Responses to Hypoxia

Significance of succinate for formation of protective responses in hypoxia is not limited to the role of succinate as a mitochondrial energy substrate for the tricarbonic acid cycle, which possesses an advantage of oxidation under the conditions of hypoxia. Multiple facts show that succinate contributes to the formation of urgent adaptive mechanisms. For instance, a succinate injection prior to any hypoxic exposure provides a greater increase in the resistance than hypoxia or succinate alone. Moreover, succinate accelerates formation of resistance to hypoxia. For example, a single hypobaric hypoxia exposure in the regimen of preconditioning results in a significant increase in the resistance of rats within 30 min. However, a prior addition of succinate compounds induces the development of resistance within 5 min (Fig. 20.3). Taken together, these facts suggest that succinate participates in the development of urgent resistance of the body to hypoxia.

In addition, evidence suggests a special role of succinate in transcriptional activity and development of mechanisms underlying long-term adaptation to hypoxia. It is known that the process of adaptation to low oxygen level is controlled mostly by a specific transcription protein factor induced in all tissues under hypoxia, hypoxia-inducible factor 1 (HIF-1) [60, 61]. This factor is a heterodimeric transcription protein composed of HIF-1α and HIF-1β subunits that functions as a master regulator of oxygen homeostasis. The regulation of HIF-1 activity is attributed mostly to α subunit. There are two pathways of HIF −1α accumulation.

In normoxia, the regulatory oxygen-dependent process of prolyl hydroxylation and proteasomal HIF-1α degradation occurring in cell cytosol is associated with utilization of α-ketoglutarate, a NAD-related substrate for the tricarbonic

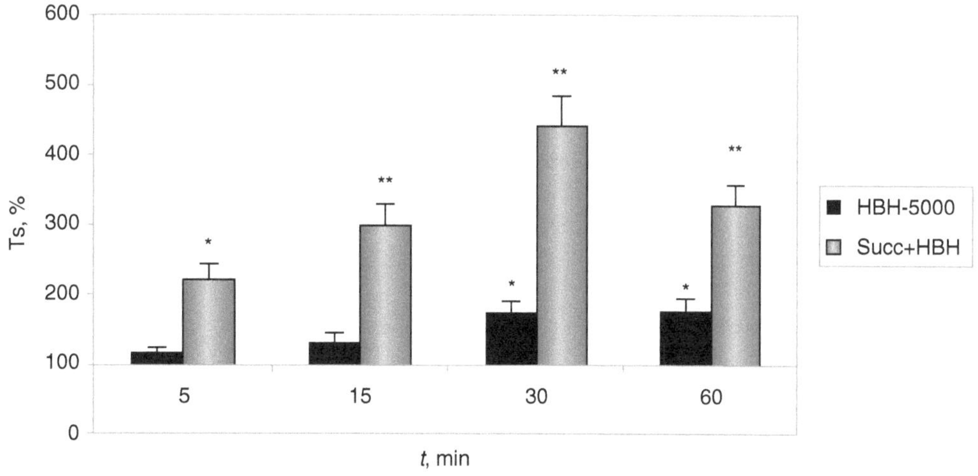

Fig. 20.3 Effects of the succinate-containing drug proxipin on rat resistance (Ts, % to control) after hypobaric hypoxia preconditioning (*HBH*, 5,000 m, 10% O_2). Time of preconditioning: 5, 15, 30 and 60 min. *HBH* without proxipin, *Succ + HBH* with proxipin (40 mg/kg, i.p., 15 min prior to hypoxic exposure). $*p<0.05$; $**p<0.01$

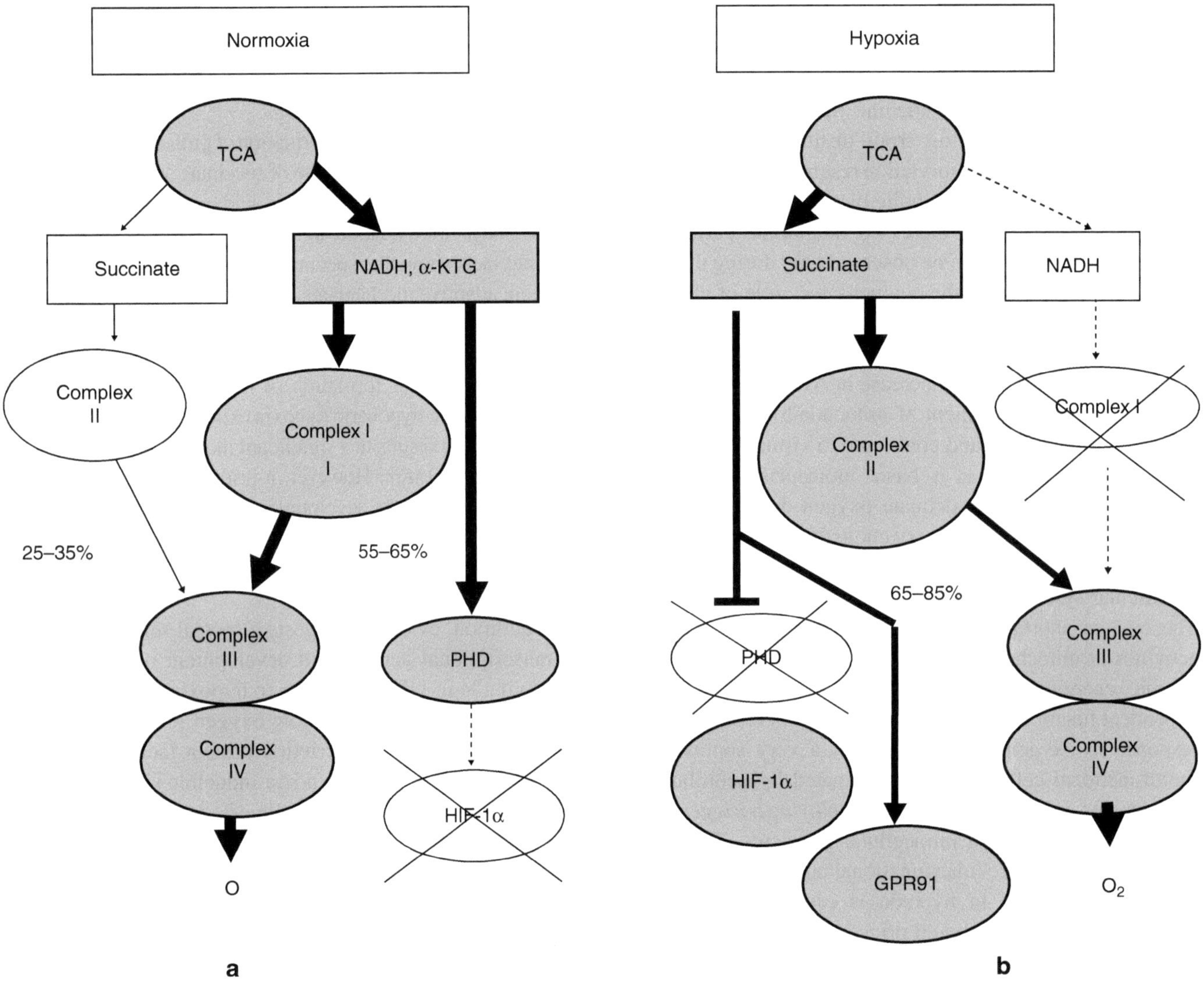

Fig. 20.4 Reprogramming of the respiratory chain function and switching from oxidation of NAD-related substrates (complex I) in normoxia to succinate oxidation (complex II) in hypoxia. (Regulatory role of the respiratory chain complex II in formation of urgent and long-term mechanisms of adaptation to hypoxia). (**a**) normoxia, high activity of complex I, low activity of complex II, and degradation of HIF-1α; (**b**) hypoxia, depression of complex I, activation of complex II and GPR91, accumulation of HIF-1α. *TAC* tricarbonic acid cycle

acid cycle (Fig. 20.4a). Hypoxia increases the HIF-1α level by reducing the proteasomal degradation of HIF-1α. Succinate is an inhibitor of prolyl hydroxylases. The increased succinate synthesis in hypoxia should provide depression of prolyl hydroxylase activity, accumulation of HIF −1α in cytosol, and enhancement of HIF-1α activity responsible for the transcriptional activity of many genes contributing to the formation of adaptive features (Fig. 20.4b) [25, 28, 59, 66].

According to literature, stabilization of HIF-1α is directly related to the activation of succinate oxidase oxidation. For instance, it was shown that even a partial (20%) suppression of complex I activity almost completely inhibited the hypoxic induction of HIF-1α. However, it recovered in the presence of succinate [1, 2, 9]. Hence, there must be a direct relationship between activation of the succinate oxidase pathway and synthesis of HIF-1α.

However, another oxygen-independent way to increase HIF-1α exists, HIF-1α synthesis. HIF-1α protein synthesis is regulated by activation of the phosphatidylinositol 3-kinase (PI3K) and ERK mitogen-activated protein kinase (MAPK) pathways. These pathways can be activated by signaling via receptor tyrosine kinases, nonreceptor tyrosine kinase, or G-protein-coupled receptors [61]. After the discovery of GPR-91 receptor [23] with succinate being its specific ligand, it was demonstrated that succinate signaling through GPR91 was a physiological mechanism regulating the ROS activity [22, 23, 65].

By the present time, conclusive evidence has demonstrated a direct correlation between inactivation of complex I and activation of complex II and formation of HIF-1α [1, 2, 9, 66]. We also showed that activation of HIF-1α synthesis after a single hypoxic exposure in the regimen of preconditioning correlated with increased efficiency of complex II performance and was associated with a multiple increase in the resistance of animals to acute hypoxia. This process was accompanied by a sharp increase in HSP70 level of activated reparation [40, 41]. In the absence of activated succinate oxidation, for example, in the neocortex of high-resistance rats, HIF-1α was undetectable, and neither the resistance to hypoxia nor the tissue level of HSP-70 increased [40].

Therefore, succinate plays a trigger role in initiating urgent adaptive processes related with HIF-1α. However, succinate oxidase oxidation gradually loses its significance during long-term adaptation to hypoxia [36, 39, 41]. For instance, during a course of intermittent normobaric hypoxia (INH), the maximum change in kinetic properties of complex II (reduced K_m values) occurs only on the first day with normalization on subsequent days (Fig. 20.5). In contrast, K_m values for complex I increase reaching the maximum in several days, remain at this level for 10–15 days, and then go down although not returning to baseline values (Fig. 20.5). As we have demonstrated earlier [36, 39], this process is associated with appearance of new isoforms of the major complex I enzyme with new kinetic properties. The appearance of new isoforms enables the recovery of electron transport function in the NAD-related oxidation pathway under the conditions of high reduction of the pyridine nucleotide pool typical for hypoxia. Therefore, the process of long-term adaptation is associated with transcriptional remodeling of properties of the main complex I enzyme [34, 36, 39, 41]. Since the succinate-related oxidation pathway is an alternative to the NAD-related oxidation pathway, preserving a high activity of complex II would hamper the NAD-related oxidation. This is why the activity of succinate-related oxidation pathway gradually decreases in the course of adaptation to hypoxia, and kinetic parameters of the complex I enzymes return to baseline values.

The reduced role of succinate oxidase oxidation pathway may have an additional and important regulatory implication in the course of long-term adaptation to hypoxia. This implication is related with the need to restrict the transcriptional function of HIF-1α and, thus, to prevent possible uncontrolled enhancement of cell proliferation activity and tumor growth [60, 61, 67]. Therefore, it is obvious that the response of the respiratory chain substrate region to a single hypoxic exposure and long-term adaptation to hypoxia have essential differences.

Urgent adaptation to hypoxia develops in the first few minutes and hours of a single hypoxic exposure. The major mechanism of adaptation is a transient, reversible, and compensatory activation of respiratory chain complex II necessary for (1) succinate-related energy production in the conditions of oxygen deficiency and formation of urgent resistance in the body and (2) succinate-related stabilization of HIF-1α and initiation of its transcriptional activity.

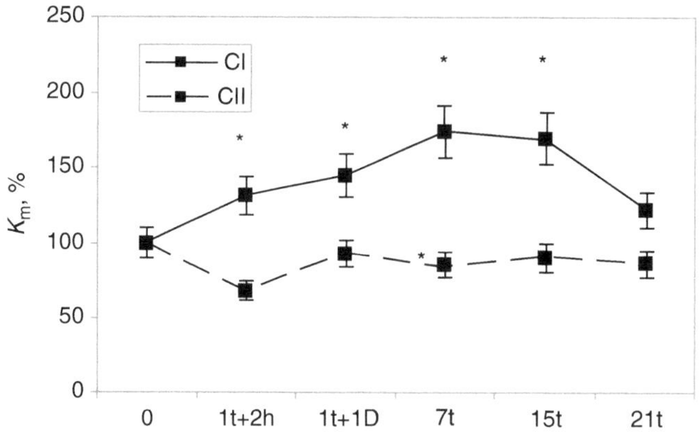

Fig. 20.5 Effect of intermittent hypoxia (INH) course on K_m values for complex I and complex II in LR neocortex. A daily training cycle consisted of passive breathing a hypoxic gas mixture containing 10% O_2 at constant pressure (5 min) interspersed with breathing atmospheric air (21% O_2) (3 min) repeated 6–7 times per hour. Enzyme K_m values were measured 2 h after the first training cycle (1t+2 h); 24 h after the first training cycle (1t+1D); 24 h after 7, 15, and 21 training cycles. *$p<0.01$

Long-term adaptation to hypoxia develops after hours and days as a result of multiple, lengthy application of hypoxic exposures. Such adaptation is based on HIF-1α-related formation of adaptive genes and generation of a new set of enzymes (including mitochondrial enzymes) capable to ensure vital activity and energy supply in the conditions of high reduction and low oxygen concentration in cells. This process is associated with formation of a set of stable adaptive features responsible for the long-standing increase in body resistance to hypoxia.

Mandatory components of this process include (1) transcriptional remodeling of mitochondrial complex I kinetic properties, which allows restoration of mitochondrial electron transport and coupling function in the setting of hypoxia, (2) alternative limitation of the complex II role in the processes of mitochondrial oxidation, and (3) changes in kinetic properties of the respiratory chain cytochrome region, which allows transition to a more efficient level of energy production [12, 13, 34, 36, 37, 39–42]. Earlier, we have shown that this process is associated with simultaneous development of a new population of small mitochondria [34, 37].

Therefore, a hypoxic exposure initiates a sophisticated, multistep rearrangement of respiratory chain function triggered by succinate-related processes. Furthermore, mitochondria and cytosol establish a very close cross talk where succinate plays a role of a signaling molecule.

20.4 Free-Radical Activity in Early Phase of Hypoxia

At present time, the concept on a signaling role of free radicals in the mechanisms of urgent and long-term adaptive reactions is very important [5, 8, 10, 21, 54, 57, 58, 63]. According to this concept, free radicals generated in hypoxia or during the posthypoxic reoxygenation period are a primary cause for inactivation of prolyl hydroxylase reactions responsible for proteasomal degradation and hampered accumulation of HIF-1α. Therefore, free-radical processes presumably may act as a trigger mechanism that initiates transcriptional and adaptogenic HIF-1α functions.

At the same time, available controversial data show that a single hypoxic exposure in the preconditioning mode suppresses free radical activity and decreases redox oxidative changes [14, 15, 45, 62, 67]. In other words, hypoxia may protect the cell from oxidative injuries under certain conditions. Such opposite points of view may be due to methodological issues. Indeed, according to our early data, decreased oxygen levels result in a gradual decline of lipid peroxidation in tissues. However, at very low oxygen tension (2–4% of normoxic level), secondary intensification of free-radical activity can be observed [38]. A similar dynamics was observed for superoxide anion (data not shown). The increased free-radical activity in the range of low oxygen concentrations results from proteolytic conversion of the cytosolic enzyme xanthine dehydrogenase into xanthine oxidase. The latter becomes activated in this range due to its kinetic properties (K_m $(O_2)=10$ μM) [37, 40]. Therefore, activation or suppression of reactive oxygen species depends on the extent of hypoxic exposure. This may explain contradictory data of literature. Evidence for the free-radical inactivation of HIF-1α transcriptional function is generally based on either results of experiments performed on cell models using either very lengthy, many-hour exposures to nonphysiological, low levels of oxygen (1% O_2) or long-term, many-day exposures to acute hypoxia. In any case, the posthypoxic period is associated with oxidative stress with concomitant ROS generation along with increased free-radical production, nitric oxide level, and lipid peroxidation (LP).

Different results can be obtained using milder hypoxic conditions. Our experiments showed that a single exposure to hypobaric hypoxia (HBH, 5,000 m, 1 h) or INH in the preconditioning regimen was associated with an instant increase in resistance of animals to acute hypoxia, activation of complex II, and accumulation of HIF-1α [38], but either did not significantly influence LP or even suppressed this process within the first day of exposure (Fig. 20.6). The level of hydroperoxides (LOOH), especially conjugated diens (CD), the primary LP products, decreased to the greatest extent. Maximum changes were observed as soon as after 15 min of hypoxic exposure. Significant changes in malonic dialdehyde (measured as thiobarbituric acid-reactive substances, TBARS), a secondary LP product, were absent.

The content of oxidized glutathione (GSSG), a marker for cell redox state, remained virtually unchanged or sharply fell in the same period (Fig. 20.7). Therefore, formation of urgent mechanisms for adaptation to hypoxia occurs during this period in the absence of pronounced oxidative stress and increased LP, but with activation of complex II. Hence, it is just succinate, the inhibitor of prolyl hydroxylase reactions, rather than free-radical processes that can claim the role of an initiator of transcriptional processes.

Experiments with the classic antihypoxant ionol have also demonstrated that formation of mechanisms for urgent adaptation does not depend on free-radical processes. Ionol

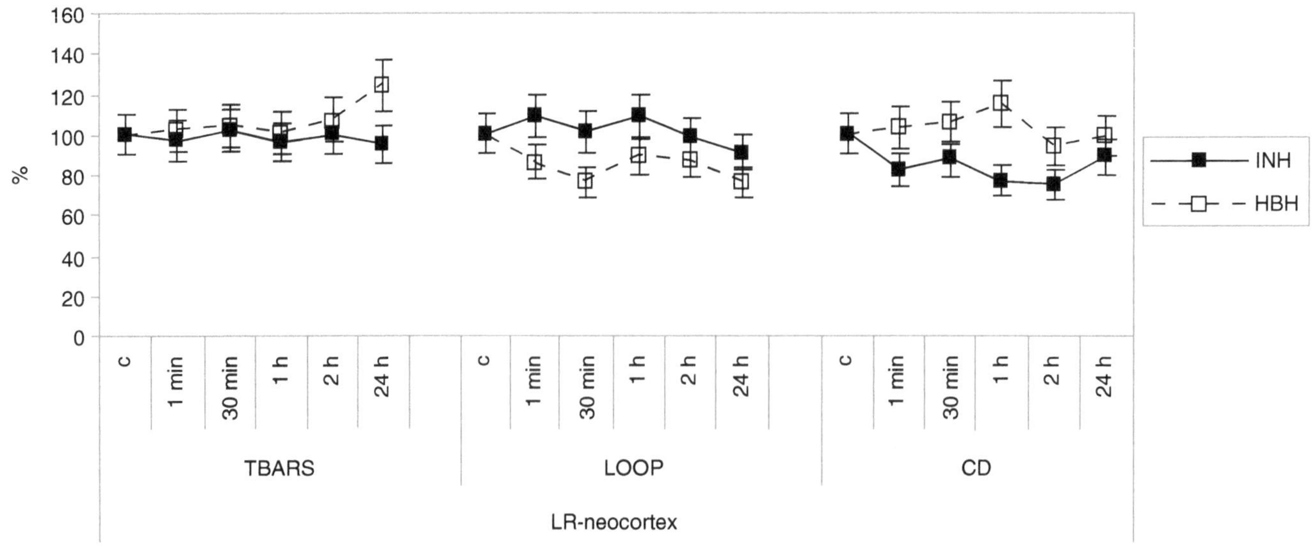

Fig. 20.6 Effect of a single exposure to intermittent normobaric hypoxia (*INH*) or hypobaric hypoxia (*HBH*) in the preconditioning regimen on parameters of lipid hydroperoxidation in the early posthypoxic period. *TBARS* thiobarbituric acid-reactive substances, *LOOH* lipid hydroperoxides, *DC* conjugated dienes (neocortex of low resistant rats)

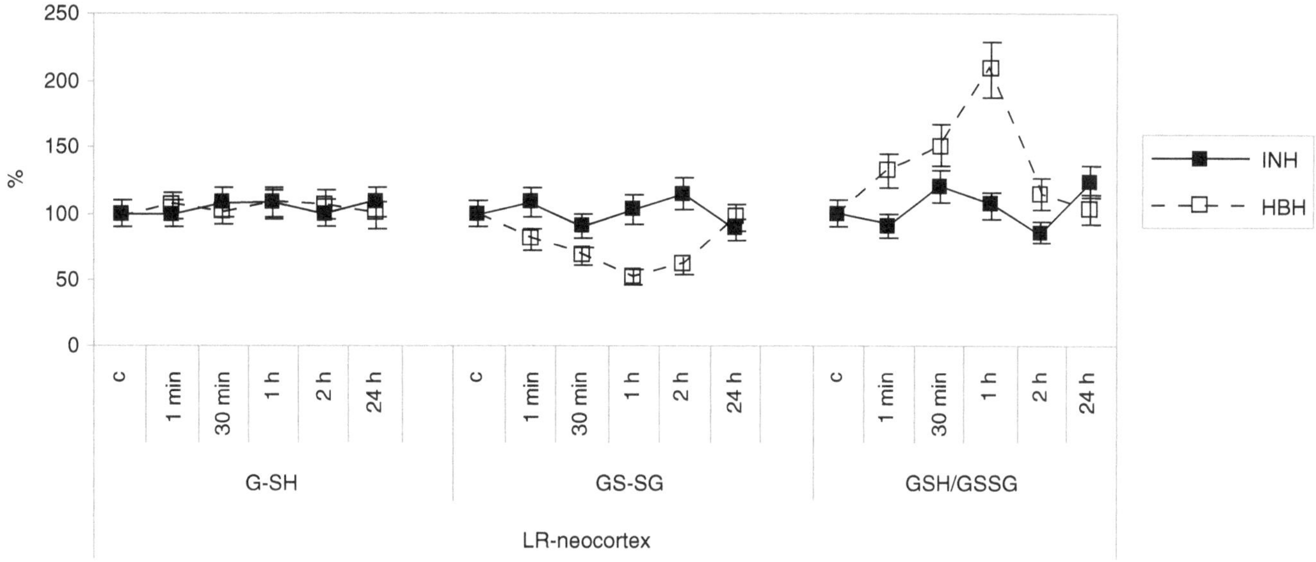

Fig. 20.7 Effects of a single exposure to hypobaric hypoxia HBH and INH in the preconditioning regimen on parameters of glutathione pool in the early posthypoxic period (neocortex of low-resistance rats). *GSH* reduced glutathione, *GSSG* oxidized glutathione

Fig. 20.8 Additive effect of ionol and succinate on rat resistance after preconditioning in the regimen of hypobaric hypoxia (HBH, 5,000 m/1 h) (by Ts, %). $*p<0.05$; $**p<0.01$

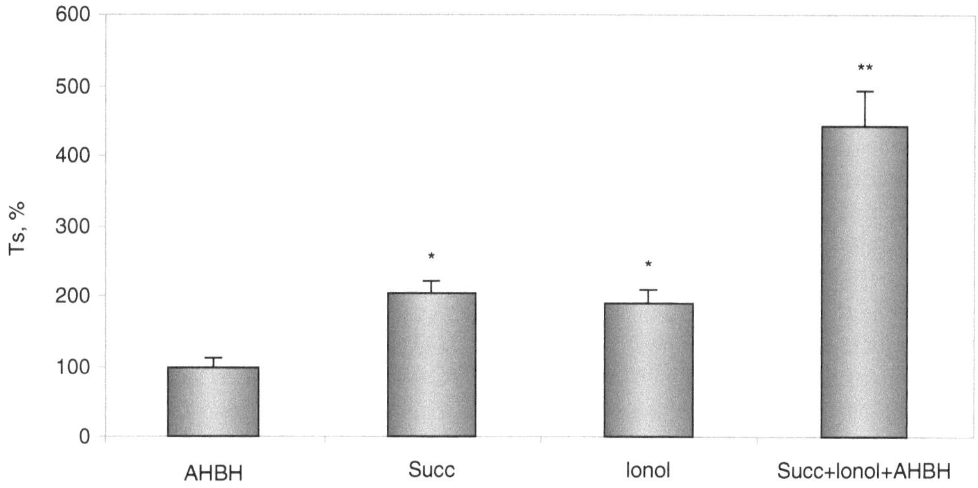

administered to animals prior to hypobaric hypoxic preconditioning not only exerted pronounced antioxidant activity, depressed ROS, and decreased GSSG (not shown) but also increased resistance of animals to hypoxia (Fig. 20.8). The effect of ionol was similar to the effect of succinate in the same conditions. However, their combination (ionol + succinate) increased the animal resistance even more, i.e., ionol and succinate exerted additive effects, suggesting that these drugs have different targets for their antihypoxic action (Fig. 20.8).

Therefore, (1) formation of urgent adaptation to hypoxia can occur in the absence of oxidative stress and (2) protective effect of succinate during hypoxia is not related with amplification of free-radical processes, and this effect increases when free-radical processes are suppressed.

20.5 Role of Succinate in Cell-to-Cell Interactions

The increased level of succinate in blood and cytoplasm allows considering succinate a marker for hypoxic states [29]. It means that succinate may participate in cell-to-cell interactions and regulatory, functional, and metabolic processes at the systemic level. For instance, it has long been known that succinate contributes to regulation of blood pressure. Succinate stimulates renin formation in renal tubules and thereby produces a vasodilatory effect in hypoxia [4].

Studies show that a succinate-controlled electron bypass exists between peripheral cells and lungs. In hypoxia, blood transports succinate from peripheral hypoxic tissues to lungs, where succinate synthesis is depressed by high level of oxygenation. Delivered succinate is used in lungs as an energy substrate needed for pulmonary vasoconstriction. In this process, succinate is oxidized to fumarate which is again transported with blood to peripheral cells and again forms succinate through the fumarate oxidase reaction [7, 47].

In the recent two decades, data on receptor function of succinate have appeared. Maria Kondrashova of Russia has demonstrated a regulatory connection of the sympathetic system with succinate and the parasympathetic system with α-ketoglutarate. She has shown that stimulation of physiological functions with epinephrine involves selective activation of succinate dehydrogenase. Succinate, in its turn, acts in micromolar concentrations as a signaling molecule that stimulates adrenalin and noradrenalin release [32].

Studies have shown that complex II contributes to gene expression of glutamate and dopaminergic signaling systems [46].

A sensational discovery was made by a research group in San Francisco in 2004. The study demonstrated that succinate was a specific ligand of GPR91 [23]. This receptor belongs to a group of guanine nucleotide binding protein-coupled receptors which form large and diverse gene families translating extracellular signals into intracellular ones, but the sequence similarity among the most distant GPCRs is minimal [48]. It has been established that GPR91 is localized in plasma membranes. GPR91 was found in more than 20 tissue types, and the array of its localizations is continuously expanding. Kidneys, liver, spleen, small intestine, and bladder possess the best capability for expression of this receptor. Only succinate activates GPR91 in a receptor-specific way and also induces GPR91 internalization [22].

Succinate-dependent receptor activation induces (1) accumulation of inositol phosphate and increases $[Ca^{2+}]_i$; (2) extracellular signal-regulated kinase (Erk); (3) mitogen-activated protein kinase, p38, and cyclooxygenase; and (4) synthesis and release of prostaglandin E2 and NO.

Taken together, these results suggest that GPR91 activation by succinate couples to at least several signaling pathways [22, 65]. However, the succinate signal is apparently tissue-specific, and these pathways may not work in all tissues.

In kidneys, the succinate-induced expression of GPR91 associated with GPR91 internalization involves the renin-angiotensin system and precipitates renovascular hypertension, a disease closely related to atherosclerosis, diabetes mellitus, and renal insufficiency [22, 53]. This process is absent in GPR91-deficient rats [22]. It has been demonstrated recently that this activation is a part of kidney-specific paracrine signal pathway initiated by high glucose levels. The signaling cascade includes local accumulation of succinate as well as expression and internalization of GPR91 receptors in endothelial cells of renal tubules. This GPR91 signal cascade can modulate renal function and provide elimination of different metabolic products through renal hyperfiltration. The GPR91 cascade is apparently a connecting link to pathologies such as diabetes mellitus, syndrome of renin-angiotensin system hyperactivity, systemic hypertension, and organ injury. This succinate receptor signaling cascade can modulate renal function and provide elimination of different metabolic products through renal hyperfiltration [65].

In hepatic ischemia associated with intensive succinate release, the GPR91 receptor is expressed only in hepatic stellate cells. However, the fact that succinate does not increase hepatic perfusion pressure suggests that activities of succinate in the liver do not contribute to its hypertensive effects. The GPR91 receptor transforms the signal related with increased extracellular levels of succinate into an intracellular signal providing activation of stellate cells in response to organ injury. Therefore, the effect of succinate should be regarded as a paracrine signal in this instance as well.

Succinate-dependent expression of GPR91 in ischemia was observed in dendritic cells; it results in production of various angiogenic factors including VEGF. In these cells, succinate triggers mobilization of intracellular calcium, induces migratory responses, and acts in synergy with Toll-like receptor ligands to produce proinflammatory cytokines [52].

Succinate also enhanced antigen-specific activation of human and mouse helper T cells. GPR91-deficient mice had less migration of Langerhans cells to draining lymph nodes and impaired tetanus toxoid-specific recall T cell responses [62].

Studies show that succinate accumulates in hypoxic retina of rodents and, via GPR91, acts as a potent mediator of vessel growth in the settings of both normal retina development and proliferative ischemic retinopathy. The effects of GPR91 are mediated by retinal ganglion neurons. These neurons respond to increased succinate levels to regulate production of numerous angiogenic factors including VEGF. Accordingly, succinate did not display any angiogenic effects in RGC-deficient rats [56].

As a GPR91 ligand, succinate can regulate lipolysis in white adipose tissue, suggesting that the succinate signaling may regulate energy homeostasis [50].

The receptor function along with the participation of succinate in cell-to-cell signaling and systemic regulation can explain many fast effects of this metabolite including the role of succinate in development of urgent adaptation. Data on the interaction of GPR91 with other receptors help to understand also the regulatory participation of catecholamines and acetylcholine in the activation of succinate dehydrogenase.

Therefore, the response to hypoxia initially develops at the subcellular, mitochondrial level through compensatory potentiation of enzyme complex II and involves activation of a specific succinate-dependent receptor. This receptor initiates cytoplasmic signaling pathways which coordinate and facilitate formation of adaptive processes, as well as cell-to-cell interactions at the systemic level.

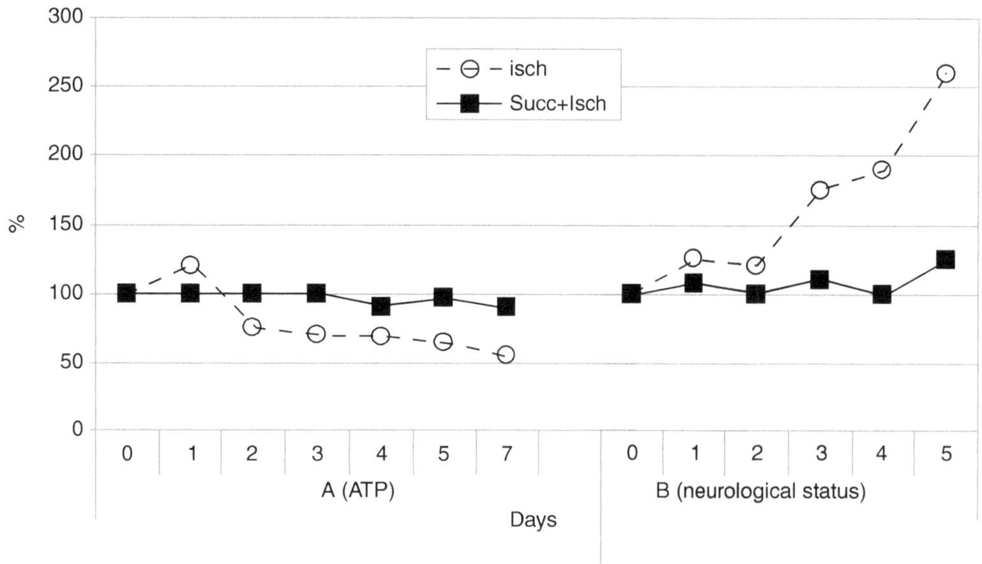

Fig. 20.9 Normalizing effects of three daily injections of the succinate-containing drug proxipin on the ATP content in neocortex (**a**) and disturbances of neurological status (**b**) in rats during chronic brain global ischemia (*isch*). Proxipin (*Succ*) was injected once daily (40 mg/kg, i.p) for the first 3 days of global cerebral ischemia

20.6 Use of Succinate-Containing Drugs as Energotropic Medicines in Clinical Practice

Prevalence of pathologies bearing a hypoxic component defines the exceptional importance and social significance of protecting the body from oxygen shortage and related energy deficiency. The above data also show that understanding the role of succinate signaling in the electron transport function of respiratory chain in hypoxia is an essential practical challenge that has defined the tactics and strategy for antihypoxic defense and the development of antihypoxants with energotropic action.

The *energotropic therapy* implies using as medicines the substances that are able to interact with the mitochondrial respiratory chain and to prevent disorders of energy metabolism up to its complete recovery in the conditions of pathology. The principles of energotropic therapy are based on the concept of phase nature of mitochondrial dysfunction in hypoxia related with changes in activities of mitochondrial enzymes.

The central role among such medicines belongs to succinate-containing drugs which have been successfully used in Russia as effective antihypoxic and energotropic therapy [31, 35, 37, 41, 43]. Several different kinds of succinate-containing drugs are used in Russian clinical practice. The most effective of these drugs are structural derivatives of vitamin B_6, which belongs to 1-hydroxypyridine derivatives (mexidole, proxipin). These drugs are used in the early period of acute disorders induced by oxygen shortage [43].

Mechanistic studies showed that the succinate moiety of these drugs is used by the respiratory chain as an energy substrate according to the schedule classic for succinate. In this process, respiration becomes stimulated, and the electron flow switches from complex I to complex II (succinate monopolization of the respiratory chain as demonstrated by the increased sensitivity of respiration to malonate and the decreased rotenone-sensitive respiration due to oxidation of NAD-dependent substrates) [40, 41, 43].

The obtained results suggest that succinate-containing drugs, proxipin and mexidole, are succinate donors for the respiratory chain. In hypoxic conditions, they function as antihypoxants potentiating activation of the succinate oxidase oxidation pathway to facilitate recovery and normalization of aerobic energy production. Furthermore, it has been demonstrated than the energotropic effect of succinate-containing drugs is due to oxidation of succinate included into the structure of 3-oxypyridine by a pathway classic for succinate in the respiratory chain [43]. All succinate-containing drugs are very rapidly absorbed in different types of hypoxia/ischemia. They exert a stabilizing or restoring effect on intracellular ATP as soon as 15 min after administration.

Energotropic and antihypoxic effects of succinate-containing compounds are associated with (1) modification and resynthesis of phospholipids; (2) normalizing effect on calcium metabolism; (3) catecholamine-mimetic, antiteratogenic, anti toxic, hepatoprotective, antiketogenic, and anticholesterolemic effects; (4) removal of excessive acetyl-Co-A associated with decreases in excessive lipids and their metabolites; and (5) reduction and normalization of pH and elimination of metabolic acidosis [41].

Proxipin and mexidole are characterized by a broad range of physiological actions. Succinate-containing drug therapies used during the phase of formation of urgent compensatory adaptive mechanisms, i.e., in the first 1–3 days of global cerebral ischemia, stroke, myocardial infarction, acute heart failure, traumatic shock, resuscitation after heart arrest, early postoperative period, after anesthesia, etc., exert pronounced protective, antihypoxic effects and increase ATP in tissues (Fig. 20.9a).

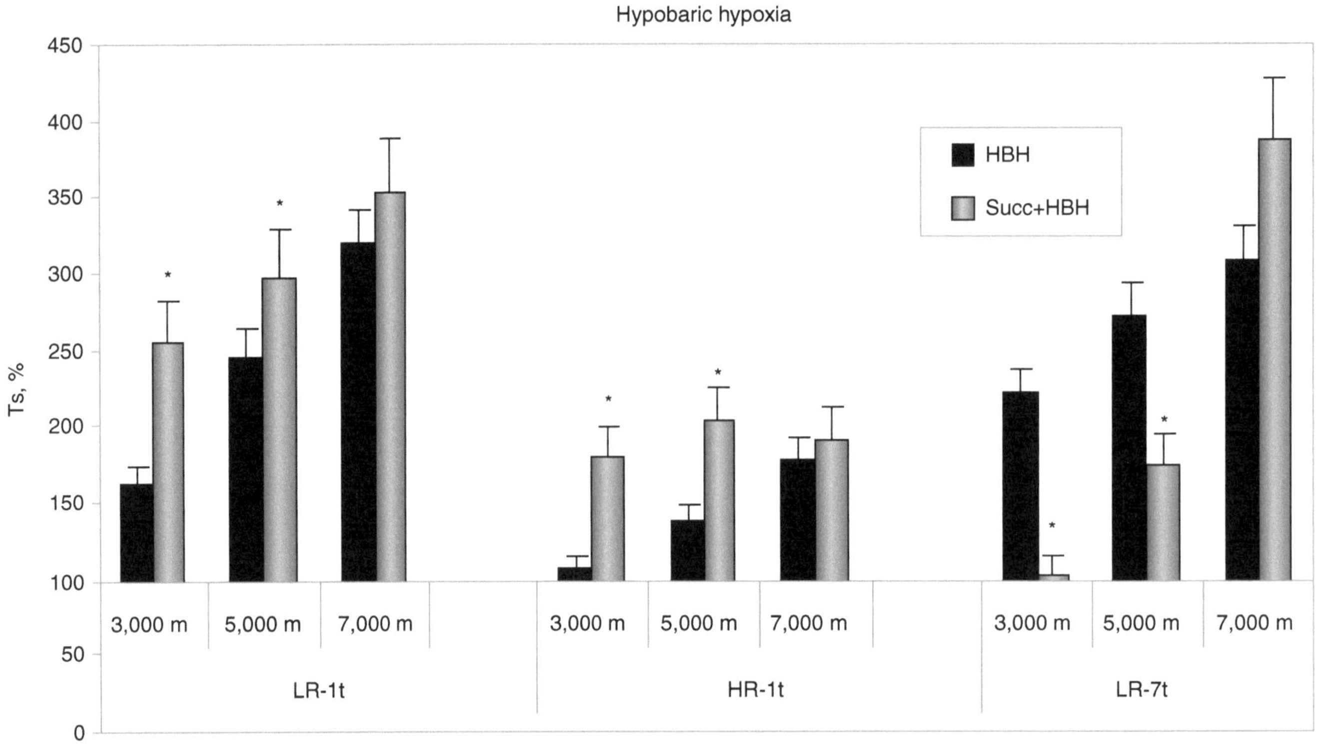

Fig. 20.10 Antihypoxic effects of the succinate-containing drug proxipin (Succ) on resistance of rats (Ts, % to control), exposed to preconditioning in the regimen of hypobaric hypoxia (*HBH*) (3,000, 5,000 and 7,000 m/1 h). LR-1t and HR-1t, a single injection of proxipin (40 mg/kg, i.p.) 15 min prior to the first hypoxic exposure (HBH 3,000, 5,000 and 7,000 m); LR, low-resistance rats; HR, high-resistance rats; LR-7t, a course of administration of proxipin (40 mg/kg, i.p.) 15 min prior to subsequent HBH exposure (7 HBH training sessions during 7 days). *$p<0.05$

Along with the energotropic and antihypoxic effects, proxipin and mexidole beneficially influence multiple vital functional parameters in hypoxia and ischemia. These drugs reduce the death rate, recover the ability of the body for gaining weight, decrease severity of neurological disorders (Fig. 20.9b) and aggression typical of hypoxia, and exert antistress and normalizing effects on locomotor, exploratory, and emotional activities of animals [35, 36, 40, 41].

Timely use of this drug decreases mortality and provides a faster and more complete regression of general and focal cerebral symptoms in the majority of patients. Therefore, a single preventive or therapeutic administration of succinate-containing drugs in the setting of hypoxic therapy will improve the development of urgent resistance in the body, and therefore, it may be used in practice for activation of urgent adaptive mechanisms [41–43]. However, a longer use of succinate-containing drugs loses its protective effects. Figure 20.10 shows that succinate administered prior to the first hypoxic exposure (HBH 3,000 m, 5,000 m) exerts a pronounced antihypoxic effect and increases the resistance of animals to hypoxia. However, a course administration (7 days daily prior to each hypoxic session) was unfavorable for the resistance of rats (Fig. 20.10) because it began to hamper the formation of long-term mechanisms of adaptation. Therefore, the optimal therapeutic effect of succinate can be achieved with its no more than three injections at early stages of hypoxic exposure.

Conclusion

The role of mitochondria as a cell "power station" is well known. However, the chapter shows that mitochondria also play an important regulatory role in the conditions of hypoxia. In hypoxia, the mitochondrial respiratory chain not only directly participates in formation of both early and late adaptive signs, but it is also involved in the sophisticated system of intra- and inter-cellular signaling. This system provides systemic responses to oxygen shortage. At least three regulatory functions of this system can be distinguished: (1) *compensatory* function, which is responsible for development of urgent adaptive responses and resistance to hypoxia; this function is associated with changes in kinetic properties of mitochondrial enzymes and pathways of energy substrate oxidation; (2) *transcriptional* function, which provides HIF-1 dependent expression of genes responsible for development of mechanisms of long-term adaption to low pO_2; and (3) *receptor* function, which is related with the participation of mitochondria in the system of intercellular signaling.

The tricarbonic acid cycle intermediate, succinate, plays a special role in these processes. Succinate is a signal molecule that is involved in this process during various kinds and regimens of hypoxic exposure. In early hypoxia, for example, the ability of respiratory chain for reprogramming (transition from NAD-dependent substrate oxidation to succinate oxidation, which is energetically more efficient in these conditions) maintains both aerobic energy production and development of urgent resistance in the body. If such transition fails, urgent mechanisms of adaptation cannot develop. Increases in intracellular succinate provide succinate-dependent stabilization of HIF-1α and initiation of its transcriptional activity. Therefore, long-term adaptation to hypoxia is a succinate-dependent process, during which the HIF-1α-dependent formation of adaptive genes and the generation of a new enzyme spectrum (including mitochondrial enzymes) can ensure vital activity of and energy supply to cells in conditions of high reduction and low oxygen concentration.

Another no less important signaling mechanism in hypoxia is the succinate activation of a succinate-specific and very common tissue GPR91 receptor. The receptor signaling function provides initiation and coordination of a broad spectrum of other signaling pathways which may not only facilitate formation of adaptive processes but also provide cell-to-cell interactions at the systemic level. The succinate signaling function is unrelated with the signaling function of free-radical processes in early hypoxia. Suppression of free-radical processes in early hypoxia potentiates effects of succinate and facilitates development of urgent adaptation to hypoxia.

Understanding of biological mechanisms for adaptation to hypoxia has substantiated the development of a new strategy for antihypoxic defense. A single preventive or therapeutic administration of succinate-containing drugs in the setting of hypoxic therapy enhances development of urgent resistance in the body, and therefore, it may be used in practice for activation of urgent adaptive mechanisms.

References

1. Agani FH, Pichiule P, Chavez JC, et al. The role of mitochondria in the regulation of hypoxia-inducible factor 1 expression during hypoxia. J Biol Chem. 2000;275:35863–7.
2. Agani FH, Pichule P, Chavez JC, et al. Inhibitors of mitochondrial complex I attenuate the accumulation of hypoxia-inducible factor-1 during hypoxia in Hep3B cells. Comp Biochem Physiol. 2002;132: 107–9.
3. Aithal HN, Ramasarma T. Activation of liver succinate dehydrogenase in rats exposed to hypobaric conditions. Biochem J. 1969;115: 77–83.
4. Baumbach L, Leyssac PP, Skinner SL. Studies on rennin release from isolated superfused glomeruli: effects of temperature, urea, ouabain and ethacrynic acid. J Physiol. 1976;258:243–56.
5. Bell EL, Klimova TA, Eisenbart J, et al. Mitochondrial reactive oxygen species trigger hypoxia-inducible factor-dependent extension of the replicative life span during hypoxia. Mol Cell Biol. 2007;27:5737–45.
6. Brunk UT, Terman A. The mitochondrial-lysosomal axis theory of aging. Eur J Biochem. 2002;269:1996–2002.
7. Cascarano J, Ades IZ, O'Conner JD. Hypoxia: a succinate-fumarate electron shuttle between peripheral cells and lung. J Exp Zool. 1976;2:149–53.
8. Chandel NS, Schumacker PT. Cellular oxygen sensing by mitochondria: old questions, new insight. J Appl Physiol. 2000;88: 1880–9.
9. Chavez JC, Agani FH, Pichule P, et al. Expression of hypoxia-inducible factor – 1α in the brain of rats during chronic hypoxia. J Appl Physiol. 2000;89:1937–42.
10. Da Silva MM, Sartori A, Belisle E, et al. Ischemic preconditioning inhibits mitochondrial respiration, increase H_2O_2 release, and enhances K+transport. Am J Physiol Heart Circ Physiol. 2003;285: H154–62.
11. Das J. The role of mitochondrial respiration in physiological and evolutionary adaptation. Bioessays. 2006;28:890–901.
12. Dudchenko AM, Chernobaeva GN, Belousova VV, et al. Bioenergetic parameters of rat brain with different resistance to hypoxia. Bull Exp Biol Med. 1993;115:251–4.
13. Dudchenko AM, Lukyanova LD. The parameters of adenylate pool as predictors of energetic metabolism disturbances in hepatocytes during hypoxia. Bull Exp Biol Med. 2003;136:41–4.
14. Fan J, Cai H, Yang I, et al. Comparison between the effects of normoxia and hypoxia on antioxidant enzymes and glutathione redox state in ex vivo culture of $CD34^+$ cells. Comp Biochem Physiol B Biochem Mol Biol. 2008;151:153–8.
15. Fandrey J, Frede S, Jelkman W. Role of hydrogen peroxide in hypoxia-induced erythropoetin production. Biochem J. 1994;303: 507–10.
16. Feldkamp T, Kribben A, Roeser NF, et al. Preservation of complex I function during hypoxia-reoxygenation-induced mitochondrial injury in proximal tubules. Am J Physiol Renal Physiol. 2004;286: F749–59.
17. Gamboa JI, Boero JA, Monge-C C. Energetic metabolism in mouse cerebral cortex during chronic hypoxia. Neurosci Lett. 2001;301:171–4.
18. Genova MI, Casteluccio C, Fato R, et al. Major changes in complex I activity in mitochondria from aged rats may not be detected by direct assay of NADH-coenzymeQ reductase. Biochem J. 1995;311: 105–9.
19. Goldberg ND, Passonneau JV, Lowry OH. Effects of changes in brain acid cycle intermediates. J Biol Chem. 1966;241:3997–4003.
20. Gutman M. Modulation of mitochondrial succinate dehydrogenase activity, mechanism and function. Mol Cell Biochem. 1978;20:41–60.
21. Guzy RD, Hoyos B, Robin E, et al. Mitochondrial complex III is required for hypoxia-induced ROS production and cellular oxygen sensing. Cell Metab. 2005;1:401–8.
22. Hakak Y, Lehmann-Bruinsma K, Phillips S, et al. The role of GPR91 ligand succinate in hematopoiesis. J Leukoc Biol. 2009;85:837–43.
23. He W, Miao FJ, Lin DC. Citric acid cycle intermediates as ligands for orphan-G-protein-coupled receptors. Nature. 2004;429:188–93.
24. Hems DA, Brosnan JT. Effects of ischaemia on content of metabolites in rat liver and kidney in vivo. Biochem J. 1970;120:105–11.
25. Hewitson KS, Lienard BM, McDonough MA, et al. Structural and mechanistic studies on the inhibition of the hypoxia-inducible transcription factor hydroxylases by tricarbonic acid cycle intermediates. J Biol Chem. 2007;282:3293–301.
26. Hochachka PW, Dressendorfer RH. Succinate accumulation in man during exercise. Eur J Appl Physiol Occup Physiol. 1976;35: 235–42.
27. Hohl C, Oestreich R, Rösen P, et al. Evidence for succinate production by reduction of fumarate during hypoxia in isolated adult rat heart cells. Arch Biochem Biophys. 1987;259:527–35.
28. Kolvunen P, Hirsila M, Remes AM, et al. Inhibition of hypoxia-inducible factor (HIF) hydrolases by citric acid cycle intermediates: possible links between cell metabolism and stabilization of HIF. J Biol Chem. 2007;282:4524–32.
29. Komaromy-Hiller G, Sundquist PD, Jacobsen LJ, et al. Serum succinate by capillary zone electrophoresis: marker candidate for hypoxia. Ann Clin Lab Sci. 1997;27:163–8.
30. Kondrashova MN. Interaction of carbonic acid reamination and oxidation processes at various functional states of tissue. Biokhimiia. 1991;56:388–405 [In Russian].

31. Kondrashova MN. The formation and utilization of succinate in mitochondria as a control mechanism of energization and energy state of tissue. In: Chance B, editor. Biological and biochemical oscillators. New York: Academic; 1993.
32. Kondrashova MN, Doliba NM. Polarographic observation of substrate-level phosphorylation and its stimulation by acetylcholine. FEBS Lett. 1989;243:153–5.
33. Lukyanova LD. Limiting steps of energy metabolism in brain in hypoxia. Neurochem Int. 1988;13:146–7.
34. Lukyanova LD. Molecular, metabolic and functional mechanisms of individual resistance to hypoxia. In: Sharma BK, Takeda N, Ganguly NK, Singal PK, editors. Adaptation biology and medicine. New Delhi: Narosa Publishing House; 1997. p. 261–79.
35. Lukyanova LD. Cellular mechanism responsible for beneficial effects of hypoxic therapy. In: Moraveč J, Takeda N, Singal PK, editors. Adaptation biology and medicine. New Delhi: Narosa Publishing House; 2002. p. 290–303.
36. Lukyanova LD. Novel approaches to the understanding of molecular mechanisms of adaptation. In: Hargens A, Takeda N, Singal PK, editors. Adaptation biology and medicine. New Delhi: Narosa Publishing House; 2004. p. 11–22.
37. Lukyanova LD, Dudchenko AM. Regulatory role of the adenylate pool in the formation of hepatocyte resistance to hypoxia. In: Pandolf N, Takeda KB, Singal PK, editors. Adaptation biology and medicine. New Delhi: Narosa Publishing House; 1999. p. 156–64.
38. Lukyanova LD, Kirova YuI. Effect of hypoxic preconditioning on free radical processes in tissues of rats with different resistance to hypoxia. Bull Exp Biol Med. 2011;151:292–6.
39. Lukyanova LD, Dudchenko AM, Tsybina TA, et al. Effect of intermittent normobaric hypoxia on kinetic properties of mitochondrial enzymes. Bull Exp Biol Med. 2007;144:795–801.
40. Lukyanova LD, Dudchenko AV, Tsybina TA, et al. Mitochondrial signaling in adaptation to hypoxia. In: Lukyanova L, Takeda N, Singal P, editors. Adaptation biology and medicine. New Delhi: Narosa Publishing House; 2008. p. 245–60.
41. Lukyanova LD, Dudchenko AM, Germanova EL, et al. Mitochondria signaling in formation of body resistance to hypoxia. In: Xi L, Serebrovskaya TV, editors. Intermittent hypoxia: from molecular mechanisms to clinical applications. New York: Nova; 2009. p. 423–50.
42. Lukyanova LD, Germanova EL, Kopaladze RA. Development of resistance of an organism under various conditions of hypoxic preconditioning: role of the hypoxic period and reoxygenation. Bull Exp Biol Med. 2009;147:400–4.
43. Lukyanova LD, Germanova EL, Tsybina TA, et al. Energotropic effect of succinate-containing drugs. Bull Exp Biol Med. 2009;148:587–91.
44. Maklashinas E, Sher Y, Zhou HZ, et al. Effect of anoxia/reperfusion on the reversible active/de-active transition of NADH-ubiquinone oxidoreductase (complex I) in rat heart. Biochim Biophys Acta. 2002;1556:6–12.
45. Michiels K. Physiological and pathological responses to hypoxia. Am J Pathol. 2004;164:1875–82.
46. Napolitano M, Centoze D, Gubellini P, et al. Inhibition of mitochondrial complex II alters striatal expression of genes involved in glutamatergic and dopaminergic signaling: possible implications for Huntington's disease. Neurobiol Dis. 2004;15:407–14.
47. Paddenberg R, Ishak B, Goldenberg A, et al. Essential role of complex II of the respiratory chain in hypoxia-induced ROS generation in pulmonary vasculature. Am J Physiol Lung Cell Mol Physiol. 2003;284:1710–9.
48. Peers Ch, Kemp PJ. Acute oxygen sensing: diverse but convergent mechanisms in airway and arterial chemoreceptors. Respir Res. 2001;2:145–9.
49. Pitkänen S, Merante F, McLeod DR, et al. Familial cardiomyopathy with cataracts and lactic acidosis: a defect in complexes I of the mitochondrial respiratory chain. Pediatr Res. 1996;39:513–21.
50. Regard JB, Sato IT, Coughlin SR. Anatomical profiling of G protein-coupled receptor expression. Cell. 2008;135:561–71.
51. Robinson BH. Human complex I deficiency: clinical spectrum and involvement of oxygen free radicals in the pathogenicity of the defect. Biochim Biophys Acta. 1998;1364:271–86.
52. Rubic T, Lametschwandtner G, Hinteregger S, et al. Triggering the succinate receptor GPR91 on dendritic cells enhances immunity. Nat Immunol. 2008;9:1261–9.
53. Sadagopan N, Roberds SL, Major T, et al. Circulating succinate is elevated in rodent models of hypertension and metabolic disease. Am J Hypertens. 2007;20:1209–15.
54. Sadek HA, Sweda PA, Sweda LI. Modulation of mitochondrial complex I activity by reversible Ca^{2+} and NADH mediated superoxide anion dependent inhibition. Biochemistry. 2004;43:8494–502.
55. Sanborn T, Gavin W, Berkowitz S, et al. Augmented conversion of aspartate and glutamate to succinate during anoxia in rabbit heart. Am J Physiol. 1979;237:H535–41.
56. Sapieha P, Sirinyan M, Hamel D, et al. The succinate receptor GPR91 in neurons has a major role in retinal angiogenesis. Nat Med. 2008;14:1067–76.
57. Schumacker PT. Hypoxia-inducible factor-1 (HIF-1). Crit Care Med. 2005;33:S423–5.
58. Schroedel C, McClintock DS, Budinger S, et al. Hypoxic but not anoxic stabilization of HIF-1α requires mitochondrial reactive oxygen species. Am J Physiol Lung Cell Mol Physiol. 2002;283:L922–31.
59. Selak MA, Armour SM, McKenzie ED. Succinate links TCA cycle dysfunction to oncogenesis by inhibiting HIF-prolyl hydroxylase. Cancer Cell. 2005;7:77–85.
60. Semenza GL. Expression of hypoxia-inducible factor 1: mechanisms and consequences. Biochem Pharmacol. 2000;59:47–53.
61. Semenza GL. Targeting HIF-1 for cancer therapy. Cancer. 2003;3:721–31.
62. Serviddio G, Di Venosa N, Agostino D, et al. Brief hypoxia before normoxic reperfusion (postconditioning) protects the heart against ischemia-reperfusion injury by preventing mitochondria peroxide production and glutathione depletion. FASEB J. 2005;19:354–61.
63. Shu X, Zuo L, Cardounel AJ, et al. Characterization of in vivo tissue redox status, oxygenation, and formation of reactive oxygen species in postischemic myocardium. Antioxid Redox Signal. 2007;9:447–55.
64. Taegtmeyer H. Metabolic responses to cardiac hypoxia: increased production of succinate by rabbit papillary muscles. Circ Res. 1978;43:808–15.
65. Toma I, Kang JJ, Sipos A, et al. Succinate receptor GPR91 provides a direct link between high glucose levels and renin release in murine and rabbit kidney. J Clin Invest. 2008;118:2526–34.
66. Vaux EC, Metzen E, Yeates KM, et al. Regulation of hypoxia-inducible factor is reserved in the absence of a functioning respiratory chain. Blood. 2001;98:296–302.
67. Wartenberg M, Ling FC, Muschen M, et al. Regulation of the multidrug resistance transporter P-glycoprotein in multicellular tumor spheroids by hypoxia-inducible factor HIF-1 and reactive oxygen species. FASEB J. 2003;17:503–5.
68. Weinberg JM, Venkatachalam MA, Roeser NF, et al. Anaerobic and aerobic pathways for salvage of proximal tubules from hypoxia-induced mitochondrial injury. Am J Physiol Renal Physiol. 2000;279:F927–43.

Intermittent Hypoxia and Health: From Evolutionary Aspects to Mitochondria Rejuvenation

21

Arkadi F. Prokopov

Abstract

Mitochondrial aging manifests as gradual depletion of energy reserves at cellular and systemic levels, as well as lowered stress resistance. Vital functional state of mitochondria is essential to reduce burden of age-dependent degenerative diseases and prolong health span. Two mitochondria-rejuvenating interventions: intermittent hypoxic training (IHT) and extended morning fasting (EMF), as engineered derivates of naturally occurred intermittent oxygen restriction (IOR) and intermittent calorie restriction (ICR), have been already in clinical practice. IHT and EMF utilize the familiar developmental and adaptational genetic programs, evolutionarily "preinstalled" in all aerobic organisms. Both ICR and IOR employ a common mitochondria-rejuvenating pathway, the mitoptosis – a selective elimination of the mitochondria that excessively produce reactive oxygen species in the cells. Mitoptosis is a natural process that maintains quality of mitochondria in the female germinal cells during early embryogenesis and can be stimulated and maintained by IOR and ICR also in postmitotic cells of adult organisms. ICR and IOR synergistically diminish the basal level of mitochondria-dependent oxidative stress that is supposed to be the key factor modulating life span and health span in aerobes. Furthermore, ICR and IOR influence longevity and tempo of development of age-related diseases via several mitochondria-independent pathways, such as suppressed protein glycation, enhanced DNA repair, accelerated protein turnover, stimulation of erythropoetin, growth hormone, heat shock protein 70, and other functional proteins. In addition, the IOR specifically intensifies stem cells-dependent tissue repair. The synergistic application of IOR- and ICR-based protocols, accompanied by nutrigenomical adjustment and individualized nutraceutical supplementation, brings multiple health benefits and alleviation or cure in numerous chronic degenerative and age-related diseases. Further development of engineered ICR and IOR protocols should help their advanced clinical implementation and user-friendly, self-help applications.

A.F. Prokopov
La Balance Clinic, Avda. Jaume lll, 18 - 1b,
07008 Palma de Mallorca,
Baleares, Spain
e-mail: ark1860@gmail.com

L. Xi, T.V. Serebrovskaya (eds.), *Intermittent Hypoxia and Human Diseases*,
DOI 10.1007/978-1-4471-2906-6_21,

Abbreviations

ADCR	Alternate day calorie restriction
ADF	Alternate day fasting
ATP	Adenosine triphosphate
BMI	Body mass index
BW	Bowhead whale (*Balaena mysticetus*)
CNS	Central nervous system
CR	Calorie restriction
EMF	Extended morning fasting
EPO	Erythropoetin
GH	Growth hormone
HIF-1	Hypoxia-inducible factor-1
HSP70	Heat shock protein 70
ICR	Intermittent caloric restriction
IHT	Intermittent hypoxic therapy/training
IOR	Intermittent oxygen restriction
MSC	Mesenchymal stem cells
mtDNA	Mitochondrial DNA
NO	Nitric oxide
nuDNA	Nuclear DNA
OSA	Obstructive sleep apnea
OXPHOS	Oxidative phosphorylation
RNS	Reactive nitrogen species
ROS	Reactive oxygen species
SC	Stem cells
SOD	Superoxide dismutase

21.1 Introduction

Complementary to the multilevel definition (The WHO world report 2008 http://www.who.int/whr/2008/en/index.html), the biological meaning of wide-ranging term "health" is related to the individual's healthy life span, as well as to reproductive health span, both of which could be measured and compared among individuals and species. It is generally agreed that the vital cellular and, ultimately, mitochondrial functional fitness constitute the fundament of biological health in aerobes.

This chapter aims to elucidate the role of intermittent hypoxia in health maintenance, focusing on its utility as a multifunctional tool of a natural mitochondria-rejuvenative strategy and to discuss its current derivative clinical use. The interrelated evolutionary strategies and metabolic pathways that underlie exceptionally lengthy and healthy life span of some mammals will be explored. It is neither a systematic review nor a summary of controlled randomized clinical studies; it is rather an eclectic attempt to clarify the whole picture by "connecting the dots," as well as an unfolding reflection of author's thoughts and experiences, accumulated during more than two decades of practicing therapeutic hypoxia.

Commonly, it is agreed that an efficient preventive and therapeutic strategy aiming to prolong healthy life span, slow down aging process, and reduce age-related pathology in humans shall address a better preservation and continuous rejuvenation of mitochondrial populations in the postmitotic cells [14, 26]. Mitochondria carry multiple functions, different from ATP production [136]. These include participation in apoptosis and cellular proliferation, generation, and transmission of the transmembrane potential, oxygen sensing, regulation of the cellular redox state and the level of second messengers, heme and steroid syntheses, calcium storage and release, detoxification, and heat production. In the majority of listed functions, reactive oxygen species (ROS) and reactive nitrogen species (RNS) modulate vitally important physiological cellular activities, hence the importance of integrity of the mitochondrial DNA.

On the other hand, the oxidative mutational damage to nuclear genome (nuDNA) and particularly to the mitochondrial genome (mtDNA) is believed to be the culprit of aging-related genomic instability that underlies degenerative disease and frailty of old age. ROS and RNS are constantly produced in oxidative phosphorylation (OXPHOS) in the mitochondria, inducing mutational deletions in the mtDNA [69]. Suppressing the mitochondrial ROS production prolongs healthy life span in numerous studies on different species [45, 110].

Currently applied mitochondria-supportive interventions confined to attempts in slowing down ROS/RNS-induced damage, either by dietary supplementation with antioxidants [74] or by engineered overexpression of genes encoding endogenous antioxidant enzymes (e.g., SOD, catalase, glutathione-peroxidase). However, the antioxidative supplementation provided, until now, controversial results [43], whereas the engineered enhancement of antioxidant enzyme-encoding genes is still far away from practical use.

In the meantime, the analysis of exceptional longevity phenomenon, found in some animals, is also worthwhile if we want to evaluate the late-life-onset interventions aiming to postpone aging and alleviate age-related pathology in humans [96]. Elucidating constituting pathways may help increase effectiveness of current therapies and outline prospective interventions, either behavioral, or straightforwardly pharmaceutical, or genomic.

21.2 The Challenge of Bowhead Whales

Extraordinary longevity of bowhead whales (BWs, *Balaena mysticetus*), as well as their remarkable resistance to cancer, attracted attention recently. These diving mammals have at least two key denominators: (1) they occupy ecological niche in rather unproductive environment that offers season-dependent nutrition and have relatively few predators (killer whales and humans), and (2) they continuously experience significant oscillations of cellular O_2 and CO_2 tensions (diving hypoxia - hypercapnia), combined with seasonal (in winter months) severe calorie restriction or total fasting.

21.2.1 Enhanced Longevity and Low Cancer Morbidity

George et al. [37] conducted aspartic acid racemization measurements of the eye lenses of 48 BWs harvested between 1978 and 1996 in order to estimate the whale's age at the time of death. It was found that four animals were older than 100 years, and one was estimated to be 211 years old. The method has an accuracy range of about 16%, which means this whale could have been from 177 to 245 years old. Amazingly, one of the 100+ males was killed during mating. The oldest living person with a verified birth certificate was a 122-year-old French woman, Jeanne Calment, who died in 1997. Elephants have lived to 70 years in captivity, so BW appears to hold "the longevity record" for mammals.

Of 130 harvested BWs examined between 1980 and 1989, only one exemplar had a benign tumor, found in the liver. According to Philo et al. [93], "It is unlikely that tumors are major contributors to bowhead whale morbidity or mortality." In general, the necropsy studies of numerous baleen whales and odontocetes, harvested during decades of industrial whale hunting in the north and Antarctic regions, or stranded on the shores, show inexplicably low cancer morbidity compared to humans or terrestrial mammals. Thus, "A single cancer was found in over 1,800 other cetaceans examined, and tumors were not found in approximately 50 beluga examined in the Canadian Arctic" [27]. Similarly, a single benign tumor was observed in 55 slaughtered pilot whales in Newfoundland [20], and only two benign tumors (0.1%) were reported in 2000 baleen whales hunted in South African waters [121]. Only three cases of cancers (0.7%) were found during the postmortem examination of 422 odontocetes from British waters [60]. Among few cancerous tumors ever discovered in baleen whales, there were no metastatic ones and those found were small and encapsulated [39].

21.2.2 Life Span, Cancer, and Mitochondria

All metazoans face the problem of controlling cancer, which is a by-product of one of the major evolutionary events, the advent of multicellularity [77]. Theoretically, the chance of malignant transformation is proportional to the number of cells multiplied to the life span of the organism [92]. So humans have much higher cancer-control capacity than mice (about two thirds of wild mice, kept in a laboratory setting, naturally die from cancer). Prevention and suppression of malignancy in constantly proliferating tissues (e.g., epithelial, liver, bone marrow) become progressively more difficult as body size increases, requiring the accelerated recruitment of additional controls that are supposed to operate efficiently during initiation, promotion, and progression – at all three levels of cancerous genome evolution in the host. Therefore, BWs that can weight 2,000 times more and live twice longer than humans obviously have much better cancer control.

It is recognized that malignous cells and tumors in an organism are products of multistage evolution of instable copies of the "selfish" mutated genome that escape immune surveillance and apoptosis [89]. Characteristically, most of these events are mediated by mitochondria-produced ROS and RNS. On the other hand, it is assumed that each somatic cell initially contains a pool of mtDNA copies, having various degrees of oxidative/mutational deletions (*heteroplasmy*). It was found that under normal, affluent in fuel and oxygen, stable metabolic conditions, the damaged, partially deleted mtDNA copies acquire replicative advantage and increase their number more rapidly than the intact and less damaged ones, thus progressively escalating accumulative ROS burden [83].

What biological mechanisms provide such an extraordinary combination of increased cancer resistance and extended health span in BW? Here, I hypothesize that the intermittent hypoxia in the form of continuous, lifelong oscillations of tensions of O_2 and CO_2 and the general pattern of oxygen metabolism, together with habitual intermittent calorie restriction, are the factors synergizing in this phenomenon.

21.2.3 Peculiarities of Bowhead Whale Physiology

In their natural habitats, BWs continuously undergo the intermittent hypoxia, or *intermittent oxygen restriction* (*IOR*), which is characterized by oscillating systemic hypercapnic hypoxia that all mammals are normally exposed to during embryonic and prenatal period. IOR is dubbed to emphasize its deep interrelation with the established term: *intermittent calorie restriction* (*ICR*). The behavioral IOR in BW may induce and maintain a phenotypic adaptation to intermittent hypoxia or a lifelong phenomenon of hypoxic preconditioning that is well known to reduce oxidative stress and prevent apoptotic and necrotic damage caused by acute hypoxia reoxygenation [78, 102].

21.2.4 Intermittent Calorie Restriction (ICR) and Fat-Based Oxidative Metabolism

Bowhead whales are the only baleen whales that spend their entire lives near polar ice edge; they do not migrate to temperate or tropical waters to calve. BWs are well adapted for living in cold waters – they have very thick (up to 0.5 m) blubber, which provides insulation and energy storage. Nutritional and energy balance in BW is characterized by depletion of stored nutrients, particularly fat, during winter months, followed by summer periods of great abundance. This pattern of ICR makes BW fully dependent on the affluent nutrients buildup in summer, while their survival throughout winter months under extreme fasting relies on autophagy (especially in pregnant and nursing females). The autophagy is a well-recognized natural mechanism of mitochondrial as well as cellular rejuvenation and cancer suppression [28, 72, 90].

As all baleen whales, BW thrives on fat- and protein-rich zooplankton. Fat-based OXPHOS has distinctive advantages compared to glucose-dependent OXPHOS (the later prevails in mitochondrial energy pathways in terrestrial herbivores). Marine mammals do not drink seawater; instead, they produce it metabolically (oxidation of 1 g fat gives 1.07 g water). Remarkably, in summer periods of affluent nutrition, as well as during fasting months, the blood glucose in BW corresponds to the levels found in terrestrial animals [48]. Due to absence of carbohydrates in their food, glucose in BW is synthesized from glycerin, amino acids, and lactate in gluconeogenesis, thus providing mitochondria with optimal amount of this essential energy substrate and important metabolic precursor.

However, under starvation-induced hypoglycemia, mitochondria switch to metabolizing fat-derived ketones for energy production. This is a highly conserved adaptation to fasting and prolonged food restriction that evolved to enhance survival and maintain adequate functions while sparing proteins [12, 84, 91]. Ketone bodies, consisting of acetoacetate and β-hydroxybutyrate, originate from fat metabolism in the liver, and their concentration in blood is inversely related to that of glucose. Ketone bodies are more energetically efficient than either pyruvate or fatty acids because they are more reduced (greater hydrogen/carbon ratio) than pyruvate and do not uncouple the mitochondrial proton gradient as occurs with fatty acid metabolism [124]. In contrast to glucose, ketone bodies bypass cytoplasmic glycolysis and directly enter the mitochondria where they are oxidized to acetyl-CoA. The amount of acetyl-CoA formed from ketone body metabolism is also greater than that formed from glucose metabolism, which increases ATP production. Remarkably, the ketone body-induced boost in the ATP production is accomplished with diminished oxygen consumption [104]. In addition to increasing ATP production while sinking oxygen consumption, ketone metabolism also lessens production of free radicals, which suppresses tissue inflammation provoked by ROS [30]. It is noteworthy that compared to oxidation of fat acids and ketones, glucose oxidation in mitochondria results in significantly higher ROS production [103].

Conversely, physiological hypoglycemia selectively induces mitochondria-triggered apoptosis of malignant cells, while mitochondria of normal cells easily tolerate even deeper hypoglycemia [57]. Thus, fat-derived ketone bodies are not only a more efficient metabolic fuel than glucose, but also provide mitochondria-protective, anti-inflammatory, and antineoplastic effects.

Bowheads grow to about 8 m during their first year then they grow very slowly after weaning. Affluent, protein- and fat-rich nutrition during weaning and growing period, followed by a lifelong, rhythmically predictable, season-dependent ICR results in downregulation of longevity-modulating genes daf-2 and daf-16 [33, 53], a highly conserved genomic response found in yeasts, *C. elegans*, mice, and men. Hsu et al. [53] have found that in adulthood, only daf-2-deficient *C. elegans* are both longer lived and resistant to oxidative stress. It is noteworthy that ICR induce daf-2 product deficiency.

21.2.5 Genomocentristic Viewpoint

In contrast to often prevailing cellulocentristic picture of an organism, the following argumentation employs the evolutionary-based genomocentristic viewpoint. Would it be a mistake to believe that bodies, cells, and cellular organelles can be logically viewed as molecular machines that are designed, assembled, used, and maintained by their genomes with the single purpose of enabling transfer of derivative genome copies into the next generations? [24]. The theory of integration of anaerobic cells and aerobic protomitochondria and their genomes via endocytosis, which happened about two billion years ago and consequently evolved into mutual symbiosis, is widely accepted. The sequence of evolutionary coadaptative steps created the multitude of aerobic species. According to Dawkins' "The Selfish Gene" theory, "adaptations are the phenotypic tools through which genes secure their propagation."

The mutual cooperation and cross-talk between huge nuclear genome (about 3.3 Gb in size) and tiny mitochondrial genomes (16.6 Kb) in human cells, is similar to that one of a shepherd and his cattle. Both benefit from each other, but it is the shepherd who governs his herd and controls the cattle's quantity and quality.

21.3 Evolutionary Preservation of mtDNA

Since uncorrected accumulation of mtDNA mutations would, within a very small number of generations, become incompatible with survival, it is hypothesized that there should exist some common mechanisms for preservation of innate, wild-type mtDNA and selection against harmful, ROS-enhancing mtDNA deletions. According to Allen [2], the mtDNA evolutionary maintenance mechanism relies on the repressed oxidative function of female germ line mitochondria (promitochondria). The obligatory matrilineal mitochondria inheritance is found in the vast majority of species. They delegate to egg cells to contain, transmit, and preserve from oxidative mutational damage the germinal line promitochondria, which do not enter postmitotic oxidative phosphorylation.

mtDNA of oxidatively functional mitochondria is more vulnerable to oxidative damage than nuclear DNA because it is not protected by histones and mitochondria are the primary sites of ROS generation [127]. This leads to accelerated mutations and deletions in mtDNA, involving the genes coding for respiratory chain proteins, and also may disturb the continuous fission and fusion of mitochondria, followed by their enlargement. Larger mitochondria are slowly autophagocytosed and undergo further oxidative damage, as well as produce more ROS [118]. As the oxidative mtDNA damage gradually progresses, the proportion of deleted mtDNA to wild-type mtDNA (heteroplasmy) increases [59]. Critically damaged mitochondria undergo *mitoptosis* (self-destruction of deleted and "worn-out" mitochondria) [111] and *mitophagy*; whereas the less damaged mtDNAs multiply continuously and more rapidly than wild-type mtDNAs, thus achieving selective replicative advantage. This manifests as clonal expansion of deleted mtDNA – a phenomenon consistently found both in inherited and acquired mitochondrial diseases [59, 86, 117].

In addition, it was suggested that *microheteroplasmy* (accumulation of acquired mutations in mitochondria of somatic and germinal cells that begins already in early embryonic period) is the primary cause of the exhaustion of the tissue renewal capacity in advanced age [113]. Another mechanism underlying cellular senescence is telomere erosion [47]. It is found that higher level of ROS accelerates telomere shortening and triggers senescence [126].

Energy demand and increased functional activity stimulate mitochondrial biogenesis in the postmitotic cells. The primary messenger NO and thyroid and steroid hormones, as well as mitochondria-specific nutrients and cofactors (L-carnitine, alpha-lipoic acid, taurine, coenzyme Q10, etc.), may stimulate and support mitochondrial proliferation nonspecifically, irrespective of the degree of mutational burden presented in a particular clone of mtDNA.

This is a common clinical situation seen in many patients suffering from inborn or acquired mitochondrial disorders. Patients are stabilized when supplemented with large amounts of mitochondrial nutrients, but usually experience an immediate exacerbation of the disease, as soon as supplementation balance is changed. Additionally, the excessive antioxidative supplementation may suppress signaling functions of mitochondrial ROS and hinder adaptive response to exercise [43], consequently diminishing quality of life. Thus, mitochondrial supplementation alone does not prevent and probably may even support the clonal expansion of mutated, deleted mtDNA.

21.4 Natural Selection of Better Quality Mitochondria

Natural mtDNA selection and purification mechanism is presented by the follicular atresia [25] that is common in all vertebrates. This phenomenon is suggested to be responsible for maintenance of germ line mtDNA quality in vertebrates. Follicular atresia, executed via apoptotic and/or necrotic elimination of about 90% of germinal cells in the ovaries of early female embryos, presents an efficient "quality control" tool [65]. It eliminates the majority of ROS-producing mitochondria in the female germinal cell lines, thus preventing them from entering future generations, which would definitely reduce offspring evolutionary fitness. For the same reason, the mitochondria of a sperm cell undergo annihilation in the egg cell immediately after fertilization, since to start a new life with foreign, oxidatively damaged mitochondria (to succeed in competition, winner sperm cells have to sacrifice them) would be a great disadvantage that was sorted off at the earlier evolutionary stages.

The clonal expansion of mutated and partially deleted mtDNA copies that is found in more intensively ROS-producing mitochondria correlates with advance of senescence and aging. It is discovered that with *ad libitum* available nutrition and uninterrupted supply of sea level O_2 (21%, 160 torr), the damaged, deleted mtDNA enjoys replicative advantage over wild-type, nondeleted mtDNA, which ultimately accelerates senescence [83]. This phenomenon employs the chemokinetic advantages of replication of shorter mtDNA molecules in the postmitotic mitochondria reproduction cycle: smaller molecules need shorter time to make their own copies (Fig. 21.1).

Clonal expansion of mutated mtDNA ultimately increases oxidative stress, thus accelerating senescence. Uninterrupted oxygen supply and affluent nutrition help mutated mitochondria outcompete the wild-type mitochondria for room and resources, thus further increasing oxidative stress. This vicious circle underlies advent of age-related pathology (Fig. 21.2).

However, there is evidence that nuclear genome is capable to indirectly maintain better quality of subordinated mitogenome not only in gametes but also in somatic cells of adult animals, such as bowhead whales, which may, at least partially, explain their significantly increased healthy life span. This would be typically achieved as a beneficial "side effect" of behavioral adaptation, described as the "extended phenotype" [23]. Such evolutionary-conserved strategies as adaptation to intermittent hypoxia and ICR provide survival in hostile environments characterized by predictable, rhythmic fluctuations in the availability of oxygen and nutrients.

Notably, similar strategy makes possible the extraordinary life span extension in plants that grow in hostile, oscillating in temperature and altitude environments. Thus, Bristlecone pines (*Pinus longaeva and Pinus aristata*) are among the oldest living organisms on earth. Bristlecone pines grow in Californian mountain isolated groves at and just below the tree line. Because of cold temperatures, dry soils, high winds, and short growing seasons, the trees grow very slowly. The wood is very dense and resinous, and thus resistant to invasion by insects, fungi, and other potential pests. The oldest living tree is 4,765 years old (http://www.nps.gov/brca/naturescience/

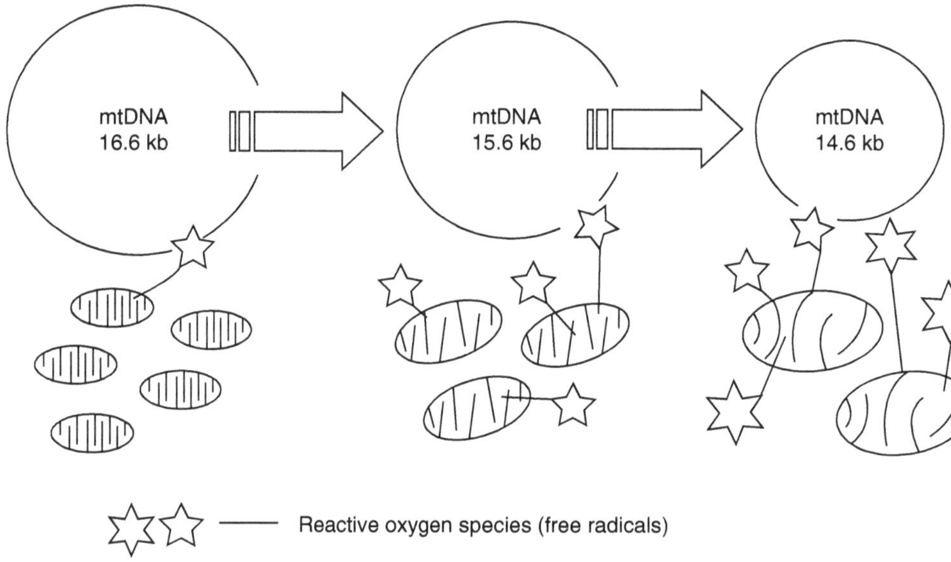

Fig. 21.1 mtDNA mutations/deletions produce inefficient, more ROS-producing mitochondria. mtDNA (*ring-shaped* molecule, approximate size in kb.) suffers about a magnitude higher oxidative mutational damage compared to nuDNA. During insufficient self-repair, the mutated segment of mtDNA ring would be excised/deleted and free ends merged together. The mtDNA loses information, its ring molecule becomes smaller, and the mutated mitochondrion turns to be less efficient and more polluting. Wild-type mitochondria are small and dense; they move and fuse easily into the mitochondrial network. The mutated mitochondria are large and sluggish; they do not fuse and abundantly produce of ROS

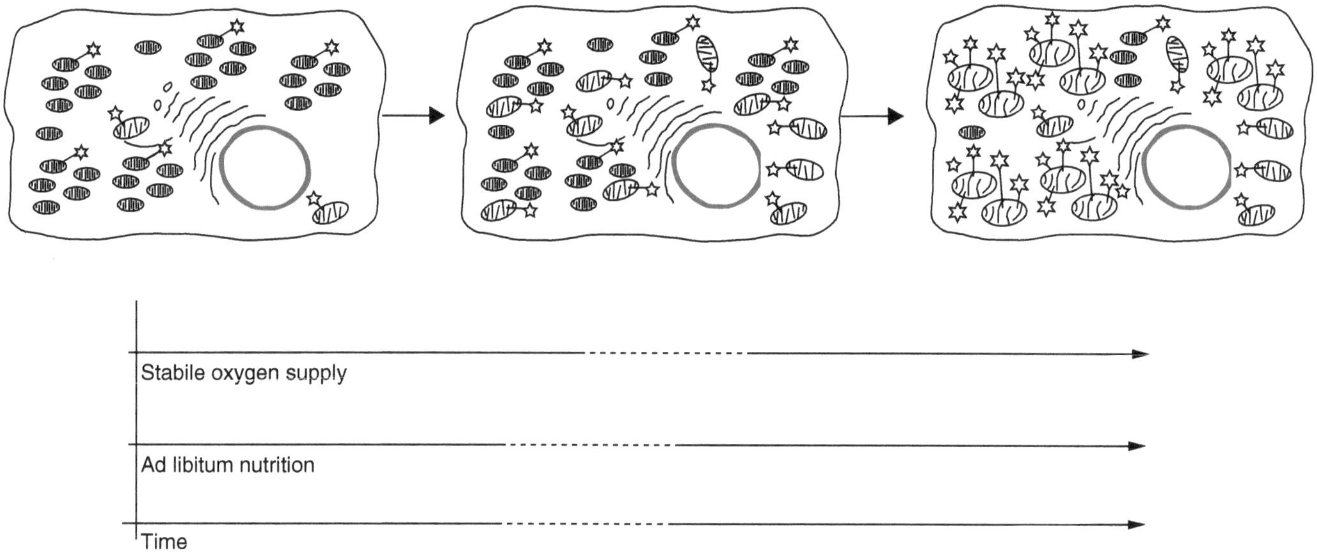

Fig. 21.2 Affluent and uninterrupted supply of oxygen and calories accelerates mtDNA deletions and clonal expansion of mutated mtDNA. Stabile oxygen supply and *ad libitum* nutrition help mutated mitochondria outcompete the wild-type mitochondria for room and resources. Mutated mitochondria multiply faster because their deleted mtDNA molecules are shorter. This vicious circle brings up the basal ROS output, which accelerates cellular senescence and development of age-related pathology

bristleconepine.htm). An even older tree was discovered in Sweden. Scientists from Umeaa University discovered it on Fulu Mountain in Dalarna province while carrying out a census of tree species there in 2004. A tree believed to be the oldest on the planet – nearly 10,000 years old (http://www.onlineweblibrary.com/blog/?p=511).

21.5 Intermittent Hypoxia in Ontogenesis

Combined hypoxia-hypercapnia is a primary physiological state in a developing mammalian embryo and is essential to support its growth [31, 108]. The corresponding redox potential of embryonic tissues differs significantly from that of

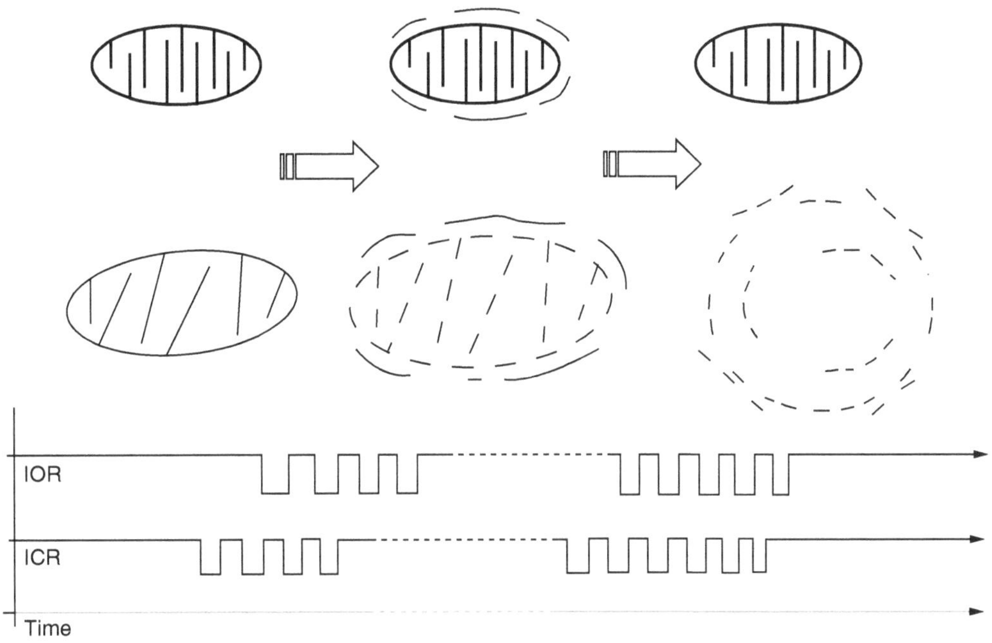

Fig. 21.3 Mitoptosis as a physiological response to hypoxia-reoxygenation and intermittent calorie restriction. Oscillations of oxygen and nutrients (intermittent oxygen restriction, *IOR* and intermittent calorie restriction, *ICR*) stimulate impulse ROS production in mitochondria, consequently overloading mitochondrial antioxidative defense. Wild-type mitochondria (*above*) respond with increased production of antioxidative enzymes and survive. Mutated mitochondria (*below*) are more vulnerable to oxidative stress; they would be selectively eliminated in mitoptosis

newborn and adult and is a necessary condition for growth and development. On the other hand, the gradual increase of cellular oxygen tension during the later phases of fetal development correlates with differentiation and maturation of tissues and organs [54, 55]. Yet, the first observations of life under increased oxygen partial pressure by J. Priestley in 1775 revealed that: "Oxygen might burn the candle of life too quickly, and soon exhaust the animal power within."

One possible strategy to slow down the ongoing oxidative mtDNA damage in postmitotic cells could employ maintaining and/or constantly returning back to more economical, embryonic-type pattern of oxidative metabolism, with its hypoxia-resistant and more youthful, chronologically earlier gene-expression profile. This type of metabolism is known to protect both germinal and somatic cells from excessive mutational damage and to support their proliferative potential [22, 35].

A complementary strategy, useful in selection of mtDNA clones for fitness, would be a periodical exposure of populations of heteroplasmic mitochondria in somatic cells to a critical functional load, such as increased energy demand combined with limited availability of fuel and/or oxygen, for instance, by exposing an adult organism to a controlled multiple ischemia-hypoxia-reoxygenation episodes, which yet remain under threshold of a massive apoptotic damage.

Oxygen oscillations boost mitochondrial ROS production that consequently stimulates enhanced enzymatic antioxidative defense in healthy mitochondria [1], whereas mutated mitochondria that are not able to endure ROS oscillation would be self-eliminated via *mitoptosis* [111]. Mitoptosis is not only a key mechanism behind germinal follicles atresia [67], but also plays an important role in the erythrocyte maturation cycle [36] and underlies apoptotic remodeling in normal growth, development, and tissue healing (Fig. 21.3).

One can assume that mitoptosis, being repeatedly induced by IOR and ICR in an adult organism, could continuously purify mitochondrial populations in postmitotic somatic cells from the constantly appearing, oxidatively damaged, ROS-producing mtDNA copies (Fig. 21.4). This would shift replicative advantage in favor of wild-type, nonmutated mtDNAs that are more efficient, significantly less ROS-producing, but replicate slower than mutated mtDNA copies [83, 132].

21.6 The IOR Stimulates Multiple Genome-Stabilizing and Cellular Stress-Reducing Mechanisms

It is recognized that within the physiological range, hypoxia is a universal challenge rapidly triggering multiple compensatory strategies that support genome integrity [7, 94]. Most eukaryotic cells maintain biological functions under hypoxia by switching energy source from fat acids to glucose and shutting down mitochondria. The shift is virtually instant and occurs simultaneously at the level of enzyme activity and gene expression. The first-line antioxidative defense is triggered by hypoxia-induced mitochondrial ROS production and employs the glucose metabolism alteration. The underlying mechanism is based on a redirection of the metabolic flux from glycolysis to the pentose phosphate pathway, altering the redox equilibrium of the cytoplasmic NADP(H) pool [8]. The reversion to hypoaerobic metabolism is not limited to bioenergetic pathways, it stimulates expression of

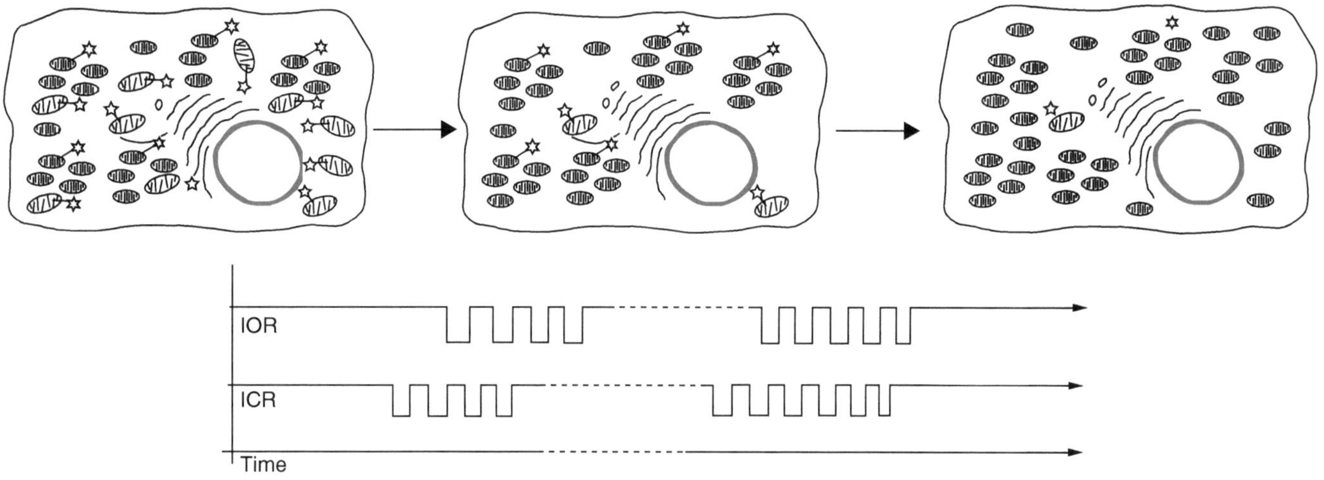

Fig. 21.4 Oscillations of oxygen partial pressure and nutrients availability selectively eliminate the most ROS-producing mitochondria. Multiple oscillations of availability of O_2 and nutrients purify postmitotic cells from mutated mitochondria via mitoptosis. In the absence of clonal competition of mutated mitochondria, wild-type mitochondria rapidly repopulate cells

multiple genes and their products; numerous systems integrate to provide improved oxygen absorption, transportation, and utilization. Generally, it is found that under lower oxygen tension, the mitochondrial ROS production is suppressed significantly, OXPHOS is more efficient, and the mitochondrial maintenance energy expenses are reduced because of notably lesser proton leak [41].

The IOR in the various forms of physiological intermittent hypoxia evokes especially beneficial adaptations, not seen in continuous hypoxia. On the other hand, the obstructive sleep apnea (OSA) that obliterates physiological sleep presents a pathological IOR pattern, which consists of multiple uncontrolled anoxic episodes that induce systemic oxidative stress and chronic sympathetic overactivity [32].

There are multiple pathways, which constitute health beneficial effects, specific for the adaptation to intermittent physiological hypoxia, distinct from mitochondrial rejuvenation. Nevertheless, they all mediated by mitochondria-based ROS signaling.

For instance:

1. Adaptation to IOR elicits upregulation of cytoglobins (myoglobin and neuroglobin), which function as intracellular O_2 buffer and provide protection against RNS [116].
2. IOR stimulates insulin-independent glucose transport and accumulation of glycogen in the oxygen-sensitive cells, including cardiomyocytes and neurons, thus increasing instantly available intracellular energy reserves [10].
3. IOR is more efficient than chronic hypoxia in stimulating activator protein-1 and HIF-1, the master proteins responsible for numerous adaptational pathways [94].
4. IOR efficiently stimulates erythropoietin (EPO) production [50]. EPO is not only the main regulator of erythropoiesis, but also provides multiple adaptogenic and protective effects, particularly in the CNS [29].
5. HSP70, one of the key members in the chaperons family, is also stimulated by IOR [133, 134]. It was demonstrated that lifelong overexpression of HSP70 in skeletal muscle provided protection against injury and facilitated successful recovery after damage in muscles of old mice [9].
6. IOR is shown to stimulate growth hormone and IGF-1 release, while chronic hypoxia suppresses both [128].
7. IOR stimulates increased production of endogenous antioxidative enzymes [135].
8. IOR modulates humoral and cellular immunity [38, 64].
9. IOR stimulates brain-derived growth factor (BDGF) and glial cell-derived growth factor (GDNF) that provide neuronal protection and regeneration [40].

21.7 Hypoxia Facilitates Stem Cell-Based Tissue Repair

Remarkably, IOR modulates production and release of not only hematopoietic, but also stromal stem cells. Stromal or mesenchymal stem cells (MSC) can convert into specialized postmitotic cells (neurons, myocytes, cardiomyocytes, chondrocytes, and osteocytes) in damaged tissues [66]. Normal autoreparative processes in the body seem to be highly dependent on MSC. Thus, progeria particularly affects stem cells, reducing their resistance to oxidative stress and preventing stem cell-dependent repair of tissues damaged with age [46].

Physiological hypoxia universally protects stem cells and stimulates release and homing of MSC [101]. It is found that MSC reside not only in the bone marrow but also in perivascular tissues [21]; thus, their activation by IOR seems to be a part of natural tissue-repair mechanism. At least in some occasions, MSC may donate wild-type mtDNA by fusion with alternated cells without actually transforming into them [114].

Therefore, intermittent hypoxia opens opportunity for enhanced MSC-dependent mitochondrial rejuvenation of the damaged postmitotic, nonreplaceable cells [87].

21.8 Protective Hypercapnic Hypoxia and Deleterious Hypocapnic Altitude Hypoxia

In diving animals, IOR is combined with intermittent hypercapnia. Compared to humans, diving mammals have increased basal CO_2 values but similar hypercapnia tolerance limit (37–60 vs. 45–60 torr, respectively) [11]. Physiological hypercapnia in vivo prevents damaging effects of ischemia or extreme hypoxia, which is investigated in models and used in clinic [70, 73]. Several mechanisms may explain the protective role of CO_2 in vivo. One of the most significant appears to be the stabilization of the iron-transferrin complex, which prevents the involvement of iron ions in the initiation of free-radical reactions [125]. It is found that even moderately elevated pCO_2 directly suppresses mitochondrial ROS production [61]. This was shown in human blood phagocytes and alveolar macrophages, in the cells of liver, brain, myocardium, lungs, kidneys, stomach, and skeletal muscle, as well as in mice tissue phagocytes and liver mitochondria. Generation of ROS was measured in the cell cultures and biopsies using different methods after exposure of cells and whole body to hypercapnia. CO_2 at a tension close to that observed in the blood (37.0 torr) and higher (60 or 146 torr) is a potent inhibitor of mitochondrial ROS generation. The mechanism of CO_2 effect appears to depend, partially, on the inhibition of NADPH-oxidase activity. In addition, increased CO_2 efficiently scavenges peroxynitrite, which diminishes or prevents relevant nitration and oxidative damage, particularly in neurons [123].

In contrast to hypercapnic IOR in diving mammals, the continuous altitude hypoxia (such as in high mountains) is coupled with persistent hypocapnia caused by altitude hyperventilation. Furthermore, compared to consistently intermittent diving hypoxia, the constant altitude hypoxia pose significantly higher "price of adaptation" due to the combined hypocapnia, hypohydration, UV rays, low temperatures, and insufficient rest, additionally aggravated by nutritional deficiencies, typical in mountains. It was shown that many mountain climbers that completed the Everest trail without supplementary oxygen suffer long-term CNS damage. The extent of this damage was proportional to the degree of altitude hypocapnia [34, 129]. It was found that continuous hypoxia caused accelerated mitochondrial damage, seen as accumulating lysosomal mitochondrial "junk" – lipofuscin [52].

Compared to beneficial effects of IOR, the continuous exposure to high altitude hypoxia, combined with hypocapnia, accelerates development of age-related pathology in humans, as it was demonstrated in a study focused on the relationship linking human aging and altitude [17]. The author examined cardiovascular, respiratory, neurological, immune, and endocrine systems of the subjects at different altitudes. The study showed that memory (in particular, short-term memory) declined with altitude. The age of memory loss at high altitude began several years earlier than that of the subjects in lowland areas. The altitude also negatively influenced cardiac functions. The lung function of middle- and old-aged subjects living at high altitude and then moving to lowland areas for 4–7 years was still lower than those of lowlanders. Their immune and endocrine functions were suppressed as well. These changes indicated that environmental stresses at high altitude and particularly chronic hypoxia result in accelerated aging.

The underlying molecular mechanisms have been elucidated [56]. The authors verified that oxidative stress is increased in both acute exposures to high altitude without exercise and with chronic residence at high altitude. The limit of human altitude hypoxia adaptability is believed to be around 3,500–4,000 m. These data indicate that chronic hypocapnic hypoxia at high altitude might cause oxidative distress, disadaptation, functional overload of mitochondria, and their accelerated structural degradation.

21.9 Adaptation to IOR Extends Health Span in Nondiving Animals

Whereas longevity-inducing and health-benefiting effects of ICR have been extensively demonstrated in numerous studies and in diverse species, there is also mounting data on similar effects of IOR. Experiments show that beneficial adaptations and extension of healthy life span may be induced by IOR in species that habitually live in normoxic and normocapnic atmosphere.

It was shown [51] that changes in the generation and destruction of free radicals could modulate *C. elegans* life span. The life spans under high and low oxygen partial pressures were shorter and longer, respectively, than those under normoxic conditions. Short-term exposure to high and low oxygen concentration also lengthens the life span. This is considered to be the result of an increase in enzymatic antioxidant defense induced by short-term oxidative stress, caused by oscillations of oxygen partial pressure.

Since the pioneer publication of Meerson [80], multiple aspects of adaptation to IOR were elucidated in detail. A number of animal studies show that beneficial effects of IOR would be achieved during short and/or multiple hypoxic exposures, varying from half an hour to several hours a day [85, 105]. IOR was also shown to directly prevent mtDNA deletions and mitochondrial structure damage in ischemia-reperfusion in vivo [88]. Milano et al. [82] focused on the difference in adaptation to continuous, compared with intermittent, hypoxia. Authors tested the hypothesis that repeated brief reoxygenation episodes interspersed with chronic hypoxia improve myocardial tolerance to hypoxia-induced dysfunction. Three groups of male rats were exposed for 2 weeks to chronic hypoxia (10% O_2 and 90% N_2), intermittent hypoxia (same as chronic hypoxia, but 1 h/day exposure to room air), or remained in normoxia (room air, 21% O_2). To evaluate myocardial tolerance to reperfusion, hearts of sacrificed animals were isolated and perfused for 30 min, initially with hypoxic and then with hyperoxic medium. Exposure to either chronic hypoxia or intermittent hypoxia increased hematocrit, hemoglobin concentration, and erythrocytes count. Hypoxia decreased food and water intake with respect to normoxia. As a result, normoxic rats experienced net weight gain in 2 weeks. In contrast, chronically hypoxic rats underwent weight loss, whereas intermittent hypoxia rats neither gained nor lost weight. As the energy expenditure in caged rats can be assumed to be the same in all animals, the efficiency in food assimilation should have been greater in intermittent hypoxia group. In normoxia and especially in intermittent hypoxia group, the deleterious effect of reperfusion stress was apparently less than in continuous hypoxia group. Thus, despite differing only for 1 h daily exposure to room air, chronic and intermittent hypoxia induced different responses in animal homeostasis, markers of oxidative stress, and myocardial tolerance to reoxygenation. These authors conclude that the protection in rats exposed to intermittent hypoxia appears conferred by the hypoxic preconditioning due to the repetitive reoxygenation rather than by hypoxia per se.

There are contrasting differences in physiological outcomes of various intermittent hypoxic regiments and protocols. Persistent hypertension is a common disorder found in patients and animals exposed to the severe, uncontrolled, brief episodes of IOR, as occurs in obstructive sleep apnea (OSA). Alternatively, the adaptation to the mild, physiological, normo- or hypobaric IOR has been repeatedly demonstrated to prevent development of experimental hypertension and reduce blood pressure of hypertensive animals and human patients [107].

21.10 The Ontogenetic Basis of Therapeutic Intermittent Hypoxia

The physiological justification of the most efficient intermittent hypoxia protocols stems from the study of naturally occurring IOR (hypoxic cycles) in nonpregnant and pregnant mammalian uterus [15, 16]. The authors discovered series of rhythmical plummeting of oxygen tension in the uterus (−4±2 torr from 6 to 8 torr baseline of pO_2, duration for 3–5 min) with subsequent return to baseline that appeared several times a day and continued for about an hour in each series. It is suggested that these oscillations serve as an evolutionary-conserved cellular "hypoxic training" mechanism that assists embryogenesis, development, and maturation of embryo's enzymatic antioxidative defense. Logically, one can presume that these O_2 oscillations, caused by rhythmical spasms of uterine arteries, may serve as an instrument of mitoptosis execution in the follicular atresia phenomenon. Similar spontaneous pO_2 oscillations were also found in the various tissues of adult mammals [44, 68].

The IOR protocols based on this discovery are currently known under the name of "intermittent hypoxic training/therapy" (IHT) [106]. The IHT efficiently induces hypoxic preconditioning or long-term adaptation to hypoxia in oxygen-sensitive organs [131, 135]. Hypoxic preconditioning or hypoxia adaptation presents a common physiological pathway that involves adaptive gene expression and synthesis of corresponding proteins; it modulates multitude of cellular functions both in health and disease. The mitochondria-produced ROS and RNS trigger adaptation in hypoxic preconditioning [75, 122]. The role of messenger nitric oxide (NO) that participates in hypoxia adaptation was suggested [76]. The NO-dependent protective mechanisms activated by IOR include stimulation of NO synthesis, dynamic NO storage, and restriction of NO overproduction. The availability of NO precursors and donors (arginine and ornithine) and negative feedback may optimize NO production. The adaptive enhancement of NO synthesis activates other protective factors, such as heat shock proteins, enzymatic antioxidants, and prostaglandins, making the adaptation to hypoxia multilevel and sustained.

The unified positive effect of physiological IOR on the body is called cross adaptation (induction of nonspecific resistance to multiple stressors) and is a highly conserved characteristic that employs fundamental regulatory pathways that were established at the beginning of evolution of aerobes [79].

21.11 Therapeutic Hypoxia in Clinic

Therapeutic hypoxia, physiologically optimized as designed intermittent hypoxia protocols (historically known as various forms of altitude training) that vary in periodicity, duration, and intensity of hypoxic challenge, is used for a long time in humans to accomplish particular aims, such as preacclimatize to high altitude and improve athletic performance [62].

Clinical experience shows that the IHT, as "engineered natural intervention" presents a feasible, compliant protocol that is effective in prevention, treatment, and rehabilitation of chronic degenerative diseases [119]. The IHT technology has been gradually developed during the last decades [5]. Ultimately, this intervention belongs to the tools of evolutionary medicine [120], which harnesses the process of adaptation to challenging environmental conditions or response to physical stimuli. A completed and sustained hypoxia adaptation, induced by IHT, provides multiple health benefits.

Technically, an IHT session consists of 6–10 repeated 2–6-min-duration intervals of hypoxic (9–12% O_2) air inhalation, interspersed with 3–6-min-duration inhalations of normoxic or hyperoxic air. Optimally, such daily sessions shall be consequently repeated 3–6 days a week. Throughout each session, a patient experiences controlled multiple hypoxia-reoxygenation episodes, and in the course of 2–6 weeks of treatment, a systemic, long-lasting hypoxia adaptation can be gradually induced.

During the last decades, the IHT was gradually progressing as a nonmedication treatment and revealing its notable preventative, curative, and rehabilitative potential. While theoretical basis of IHT has been consolidating through several decades of academic research in the former USSR, the practical knowledge of curative power of moderately hypoxic "mountain air," as well as familiarity with breathing techniques that induce a temperate hypoxia+hypercapnia, accounts for millennia and runs through various cultures and civilizations. Current technology advancement catalyzed the evolution and development of hypoxic treatment from esoteric concepts and costly mountain sanatoriums to molecular biological insights and high-tech, user-friendly equipment that supports individualized treatment protocols.

The IHT centers in Russia and CIS, Europe and the USA, China, Japan, Australia, and New Zealand accumulated nearly three decades of physiological, sport medicine, and clinical research in this modality. Up to date, only in Russia, clinical scientific research in IHT resulted in hundreds of dissertations, as well as numerous publications and presentations at international conferences. In the light of accumulated evidence, the effectiveness and safety of IHT is unquestionable. The statistics of treatment of 46,723 patients (including 4,716 children) revealed good and satisfactory results in 75–95% of cases treated during a standard 2- to 3-week cure [42].

Contraindications to IHT include acute infections, intoxications, exacerbations of chronic inflammatory diseases, fever, acute somatic conditions and trauma (crash syndrome, myocardial infarction, stroke, asthma attack, etc.), and decompensated chronic conditions.

21.12 A Multiple-Modality Rejuvenative Intervention

The IHT influences several underlying mechanisms of aging, such as expression of p53 and p66 proteins that modulate apoptosis and inflammation, as well as DNA maintenance and tissue repair [6, 75]. These pathways underlie the pathogenesis of aging and also function as the key players in a host of common degenerative or "civilization" diseases. Those include atherosclerosis and its main manifestations (cardiovascular disease, myocardial infarction, stroke), as well as Type 2 diabetes, arterial hypertension, inflammatory diseases of joints and respiratory ways, allergy, gastrointestinal problems and autoimmune conditions, cancer, and neurodegenerative diseases. Figure 21.5 illustrates the influence of intermittent hypoxia on the evolution of mitochondria in human body.

The potential of IHT in future rejuvenative therapies has been discussed [63, 97]. In one study, using the biochemical parameters (levels of ROS and antioxidative enzymes) and psychometric tests, researchers demonstrated that in average, a single completed course of IHT results in reversal of selected markers of aging on 3–5 years [42].

21.13 Using Synergism of IOR and ICR in the Clinic

While a lifelong caloric restriction remains a golden standard in life-extending interventions, it is recently demonstrated that various forms of ICR can have even higher efficiency in inducing favorable gene-expression changes and corresponding health benefits. Anson et al. [3] compared intermittent fasting and continuous calorie restriction in mice. A control group was fed *ad libitum*; another group was fed 60% of the calories that the control group consumed. A third group was fasted for 24 h and then permitted to free-feed. The intermittently fasting mice did not cut total calories at the beginning and the end of the observation period and only slightly cut calories in between. A fourth group was fed the average daily intake of the fasting mice every day. Both the fasting mice and those on a restricted diet had significantly lower blood sugar and insulin levels than the free-fed controls. Kainic acid, a toxin that damages neurons, was injected into the dorsal hippocampus of all mice. Hippocampal damage is associated with Alzheimer's disease. Interestingly, less damage was found in the brains of the intermittently fasting mice than in those that were on a restricted diet, and most damage occurred in the mice with an unrestricted diet. In addition, ICR decreases incidence and increases latency of mammary tumors in mice to a greater extent than does chronic caloric restriction does [19].

Human studies confirm the efficiency of ICR. A 6-month caloric restriction protocol resulted in improvement of biomarkers of longevity and oxidative stress in overweight subjects [49]. Similar results were obtained in obese diabetic patients [109]. Johnson and colleagues investigated the efficiency of alternate day calorie restriction (ADCR) protocol in asthma patients [58]. The study aimed to determine if overweight asthma patients would adhere to this dietary regimen and to establish the effects of the protocol on their symptoms, pulmonary function, markers of oxidative stress, and inflammation. Ten subjects with BMI>30 were maintained for 8 weeks on a dietary regimen in which they ate

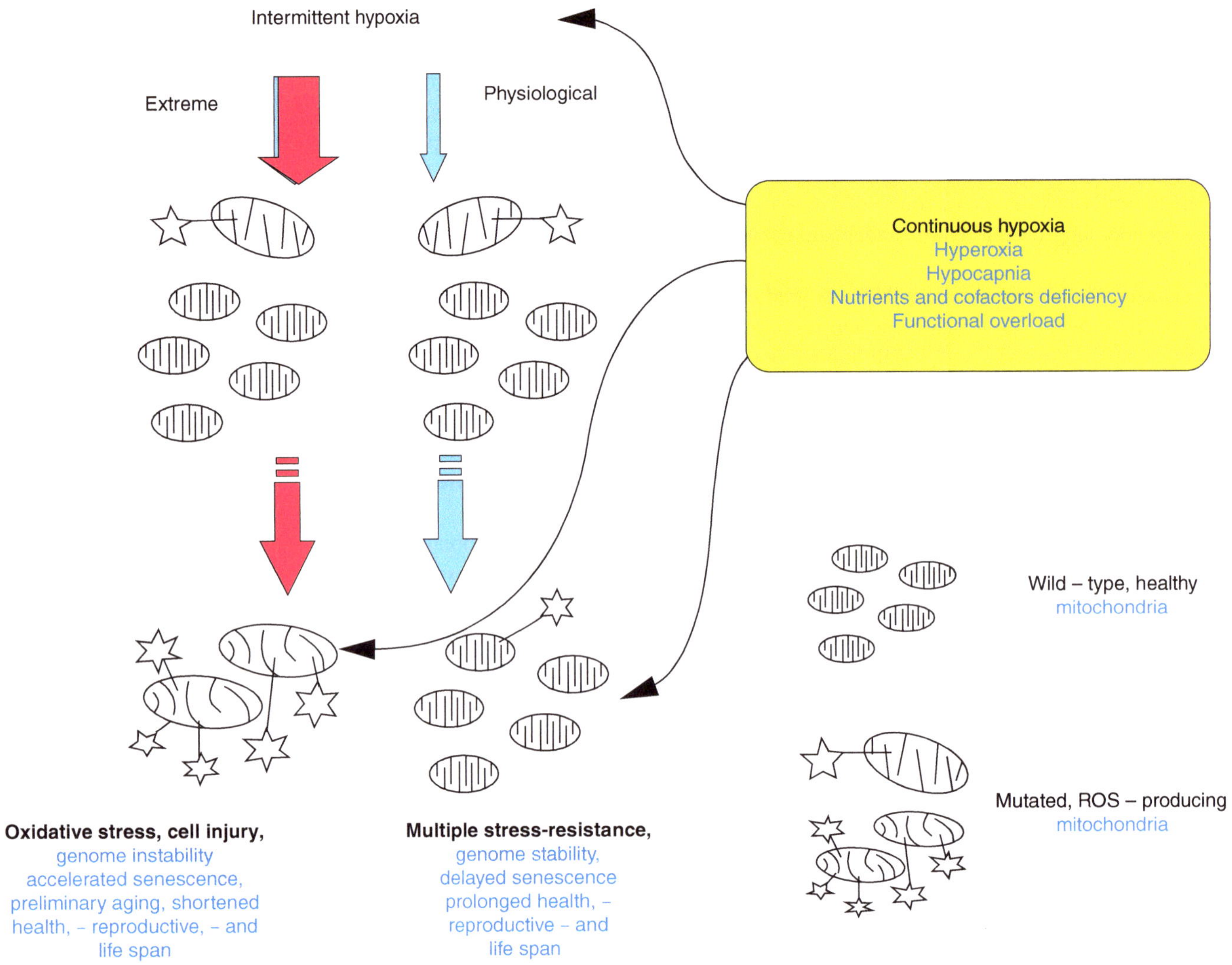

Fig. 21.5 Intermittent hypoxia governs evolution of mitochondria in postmitotic cells. *Left*: extreme intermittent hypoxia accelerates mtDNA mutation rate, ensuing clonal expansion of mutated, ROS-producing mitochondria; *Right*: physiological intermittent hypoxia facilitates multiplication of wild-type, healthy mitochondria, eliminating mutated, ROS-producing mitochondria. Note other important players

ad libitum every other day, while consuming less than 20% of their normal calorie intake on the intervening days. Nine of the subjects adhered to the diet and lost an average of 8% of their initial weight during the study. Their asthma-related symptoms, asthma control, and quality of life improved significantly within 2 weeks of diet initiation. These changes persisted for the duration of the study. Levels of serum beta-hydroxybutyrate were increased, and leptin were decreased on the calorie restriction (CR) days, indicating a shift in energy metabolism toward utilization of fatty acids and confirming compliance with the diet. The improved clinical findings were associated with decreased levels of serum cholesterol and triglycerides, notable reductions in markers of oxidative stress (8-isoprostane, nitrotyrosine, protein carbonyls, and 4-hydroxynonenal adducts), and increased levels of the endogenous antioxidant uric acid. Indicators of inflammation, including serum tumor necrosis factor-alpha, were also significantly decreased by ADCR. Compliance with the ADCR diet was high, symptoms and pulmonary function improved, and oxidative stress and inflammation declined.

In the human calorie restriction study by Civitarese et al. [18], mitochondrial DNA content increased by 35 ± 5% in the CR group and 21 ± 4% in the CR + exercise group, with no change in the control group. The authors demonstrated that in the overweight nonobese humans, short-term calorie restriction lowers whole-body energy expenditure and oxygen consumption in parallel with an induction of mitochondrial biogenesis, PPARGC1A and SIRT1 mRNA, and a decrease in DNA damage with a tendency toward lower SOD activity. Authors conclude that caloric restriction directly stimulates biogenesis of more efficient mitochondria in human skeletal muscle, which diminishes basal oxidative stress. It was also found that acute CR partially or completely reverses age-related alterations of liver, brain, and heart proteins [115].

CR also rapidly and reversibly mitigates biomarkers of aging in adult rhesus macaques and humans.

The IOR and ICR may synergistically modulate OXPHOS in the mitochondria and stimulate mitochondrial turnover and biogenesis. Similarly to ICR, the short-term IOR (as intermittent exposure to mountain altitude) induced clinical improvements in patients with metabolic syndrome and related conditions [71]. Current research together with earlier observations clearly indicates a spectacular similarity in mechanisms and outcomes of adaptation to ICR and IOR and justifies concomitant use of both. In our own practice, we have found that a combination of modified IHT and fasting shows synergism in the accelerated recovery of Type 2 diabetes patients and other degenerative diseases [95]. Earlier clinical research [4] has demonstrated that ICR in 5–7 days clinical setting induces a significant improvement in Type 2 diabetes patients. We also found that outpatients could be more conveniently treated with a partial (early daytime) fasting regime, which we dubbed extended morning fasting (EMF) [99]. To achieve the optimum results from combining of IHT and EMF, it is necessary to individualize the intensity, dose, frequency, and timing between the applications of hypoxic stimuli and carefully monitor the patient's response. Fluctuations of blood oxygen saturation (SpO_2) and heart rhythm variability during an IHT session serve as a valuable indicator of responsiveness to treatment. An interesting case of functional and morphological brain recovery of an Alzheimer's-type dementia patient, achieved with the combined IHT–EMF protocol, was presented by the author recently [98].

Recently, Dr. B. Loeffler reported on the enhanced mitochondrial energy potential and increased up to 60% endogenous coenzyme Q10 production as a result of IHT course (Berlin, IPAM, personal communication and unpublished presentation). Coenzyme Q10 (ubiquinone) is a naturally occurring mitochondrial compound, an electron carrier in the mitochondrial respiratory chain. Q10 is one of the most important lipophilic antioxidants, preventing the generation of free radicals as well as oxidative modifications of proteins, lipids, and DNA. It can also regenerate the other powerful lipophilic antioxidant, alpha-tocopherol. Decreased levels of Q10 in humans are found in many diseases (e.g., cardiac disorders, neurodegenerative diseases, AIDS, cancer) associated with intensive generation of free radicals and their action on cells and tissues. Supplementation with cofactors (i.e., folic acid and B-group vitamins) only insignificantly increased mitochondria-dependent ubiquinone biosynthesis in the organism. Improved mitochondrial energy production, resulting from IHT course, may explain the observed effect on Q10.

Currently, the ultimate test of mitochondrial-oxidative stress theory of aging is under way [112]. Mitochondria-specific antioxidant SkQ, which selectively accumulates in mitochondria, applied in nanomole concentrations inhibited development of such age-related conditions such as osteoporosis, involution of thymus, cataract, retinopathy, some tumors, etc. SkQ1 has a strong therapeutic action on some retinopathies, in particular, congenital retinal dysplasia. With drops containing SkQ1, vision is recovered in 50 of 66 animals that became blind because of retinopathy. SkQ1-containing drops instilled in the early stage of the disease prevent the loss of sight in rabbits with experimental uveitis and restore vision to animals that had already become blind. Alleviation is also achieved in experimental glaucoma in rabbits. Further, the pretreatment of rats with SkQ1 significantly decreases the H_2O_2-induced arrhythmia of the isolated heart. SkQ1 strongly reduces the damaged area in myocardial infarction or stroke and prevents the death of animals from kidney infarction. In p53-deficient mice, SkQ1 decreases the ROS level in the spleen cells and inhibits appearance of lymphomas, which are the main cause of death of such animals.

According to the theory of stress-induced premature senescence [13], sublethal doses of various noxious agents (such as environmental and behavioral stress, H_2O_2, hypoxia and hyperoxia, ionizing irradiation, UV light, etc.) lead to the exhaustion of the replicative potential of the proliferative normal cell types and the accumulation of senescent cells, which might be responsible for the creation of a microinflammatory state, thereby participating in tissue aging. On the other hand, the same agents and interventions being applied in smaller doses and proper timing may induce increased nonspecific resistance to multiple stressors and increase healthy life span in various species via hormetic effect [100]. This is fully relevant to both IOR and ICR and their synergistic combination.

The oscillating character of the IOR and ICR, as well as their synergism, seems to be crucial for the observed effects. Oscillating stress/relaxation, damage/recovery interval patterns, in contrast to constant, uninterrupted functional load, diminishes risk of pathological outcome. Thus, interval physical training in general is significantly safer and more efficient than continuous aerobic training [81, 130]. Species adapted to a rhythmic, oscillating pattern of accumulation and depletion of structural and energy reserves constantly exercise their storage and mobilization mechanisms, according to the universal principle of "Use it or lose it." Exercising energy-accumulating and energy-mobilizing systems, as well as continuous training of endogenous cellular antioxidative defense network functions as is the evolutionarily developed maintenance and repair tool that slows down aging process and prolongs healthy life span.

21.14 Concluding Remarks

At the molecular level, any physiological activity causes a certain degree of functional damage and depletion of reserves, which would be repaired and, under favorable conditions, should be consequently supercompensated, thus increasing the amount of available cellular reserves. The same pathways and same cellular energy and structural reserves are depleted in the normal aging; they may decline if not challenged and do not undergo continuous functional damage, repair, and supercompensation. On the other hand, they would degrade if overused and chronically underrepaired. In both cases, the mitochondria-modulated oxidative stress seems to be the culprit. It would not be a big exaggeration saying that we prematurely kill experimental animals, as well as ourselves, by *ad libitum* feeding. But it is also true for any aerobic organism, which is constantly and unlimitedly supplied with oxygen or, in contrary, being exposed to chronic hypoxia. The common "U" – or bell – curve scientifically validates the old wisdom: "Sola dosis facit venenum" (only the dose makes the poison; Paracelsus, 1538).

Nature offers a universal mitochondria-rejuvenating and tissue-regenerative approach that modulates life span in the evolutionary-distanced species, such as *C. elegans* and bowhead whale via cycling availability of O_2 and nutrients. This natural strategy incorporates affluent nutrition during postnatal development, followed by continuous ICR and IOR in adulthood. The underlying mechanisms and pathways synergistically influence oxygen absorption, transportation, and utilization, resulting in improved mitochondrial efficiency and reduction of basal oxidative stress level. This, in turn, results in improved genome stability, postponed senescence, and retarded development of age-related pathology, which ultimately increases healthy life span. While the underlying conserved evolutionary pathways have been found at all levels of aerobes organization, there is little doubt that the same strategy is equally efficient in humans. Historically, different forms of ICR and IOR have an impressive account of empiric and evidence-based use in health and spiritual practices of various human cultures.

Mitochondria-rejuvenating interventions, IHT and EMF, as engineered derivates of naturally occurred IOR and ICR, have been already in use in clinic. The synergistic application of such protocols, accompanied by individualized nutraceutical supplementation, brings multiple health benefits and alleviation or cure in numerous chronic degenerative and age-related diseases. Maintaining vital physiological functions and building up and regularly emptying the bodily reserves is a common advice, which becomes more difficult to follow with each passed year of an individual's life, particularly when a person does not exercise regularly. Certainly, there is a demand for the cost-efficient, naturally based rejuvenative interventions that could be used in clinical settings, as well as incorporated into modern demanding and challenging lifestyle. The engineered derivatives of IOR and ICR seem to fulfill this requirement.

References

1. Ahmad S, Ahmad A, Gerasimovskaya E, et al. Hypoxia protects human lung microvascular endothelial and epithelial-like cells against oxygen toxicity. Role of phosphatidylinositol 3-kinase. Am J Respir Cell Mol Biol. 2003;28:179–87.
2. Allen JF, et al. Separate sexes and the mitochondrial theory of ageing. J Theor Biol. 1996;180:135–40.
3. Anson RM, Guo Z, de Cabo R, et al. Intermittent fasting dissociates beneficial effects of dietary restriction on glucose metabolism and neuronal resistance to injury from calorie intake. Proc Natl Acad Sci USA. 2003;100:6216–20.
4. Balobolkin MI, Nedosugova LV, Gavriluk LI, et al. The influence of fasting on the interaction between insulin and insulin receptors in diabetic patients. Ther Arch. 1983;9:136–40 [In Russian].
5. Bassovitch O, Serebrovskaya TV. Equipment and regimes for intermittent hypoxia therapy. In: Xi L, Serebrovskaya TV, editors. Intermittent hypoxia: from molecular mechanisms to clinical applications. New York: Nova Science Publ Inc; 2009. p. 589–601.
6. Bianchi G, Di Giulio C, Rapino C, et al. p53 and p66 proteins compete for hypoxia-inducible factor 1 alpha stabilization in young and old rat hearts exposed to intermittent hypoxia. Gerontology. 2006;52:17–23.
7. Bickler PE, Donohoe PH. Adaptive responses of vertebrate neurons to hypoxia. J Exp Biol. 2002;205:3579–86.
8. Breitenbach M, Lehrach H, Krobitsch S. Dynamic rerouting of the carbohydrate flux is key to counteracting oxidative stress. J Biol. 2007;6:10. doi:10.1186/jbiol6.
9. Broome CS, Kayani AC, Palomero J, et al. Effect of lifelong overexpression of HSP70 in skeletal muscle on age-related oxidative stress and adaptation after non-damaging contractile activity. FASEB J. 2006;20:1549–51.
10. Brucklachera RM, Vannuccia RC, Vannucci SJ. Hypoxic preconditioning increases brain glycogen and delays energy depletion from hypoxia-ischemia in the immature rat. Dev Neurosci. 2002;24:411–7.
11. Butler PJ, Jones DR. Physiology of diving of birds and mammals. Physiol Rev. 1997;77:837–99.
12. Cahill Jr GF. Starvation in man. N Engl J Med. 1970;282:668–75.
13. Chen J, Patschan S, Goligorsky MS. Stress-induced premature senescence of endothelial cells. J Nephrol. 2008;21:337–44.
14. Chinnery PF, Pagon RA, Bird TD, Dolan CR, et al. Mitochondrial disorders overview. In: Gene reviews. Seattle: University of Washington; 2000–2010.
15. Chizhov AI. Physiologic bases of the method to increase nonspecific resistance of the organism by adaptation to intermittent normobaric hypoxia. Fiziol Zh. 1992;38:13–7 [In Russian].
16. Chizov AI, Filimonov VG, Karash YM, et al. Biorhythm of oxygen tension in uterine and fetal tissues. Biull Eksp Biol Med. 1981;10:392–4 [In Russian].
17. Chu Y-D. High altitude and aging. High Alt Med Biol. 2004;5:350.
18. Civitarese AE, Carling S, Heilbronn LK, et al. Calorie restriction increases muscle mitochondrial biogenesis in healthy humans. PLoS Med. 2007;4:e76. doi:10.1371/journal.pmed.0040076.
19. Cleary MP, Jacobson MK, Phillips FC, et al. Weight-cycling decreases incidence and increases latency of mammary tumors to a greater extent than does chronic caloric restriction in mouse mammary tumor virus-transforming growth factor-alpha female mice. Cancer Epidemiol Biomarkers Prev. 2002;11:836–43.
20. Cowan DF. Pathology of the pilot whale. *Globicephala melaena* a comparative survey. Arch Pathol. 1966;82:178–89.
21. da Silva-Meirelles L, Chagastelles PC, Nardi NB. Mesenchymal stem cells reside in virtually all post-natal organs and tissues. J Cell Sci. 2006;119:2204–13.
22. Danet GH, Pan Y, Luongo JL. Expansion of human SCID-repopulating cells under hypoxic conditions. J Clin Invest. 2003;112:126–35.
23. Dawkins R. The extended phenotype. Oxford: Oxford University Press; 1982.
24. Dawkins R. The selfish gene. Oxford: Oxford University Press; 1976.
25. de Bruin JP, Dorlandb M, Spekc ER, et al. Ultrastructure of the resting ovarian follicle pool in healthy young women. Biol Reprod. 2002;66:1151–60.

26. de Grey AD. Inter-species therapeutic cloning: the looming problem of mitochondrial DNA and two possible solutions. Rejuvenation Res. 2004;7:95–8.
27. de Guise S, Lagacé A, Béland P. Tumors in St. Lawrence beluga whales (*Delphinapterus leucas*). Vet Pathol. 1994;31:444–9.
28. Dhahbi J, Kim HJ, Mote PL, et al. Temporal linkage between the phenotypic and genomic responses to caloric restriction. Proc Natl Acad Sci USA. 2004;101:5524–9.
29. Erbayraktar S, Yilmaz O, Gökmen N, et al. Erythropoetin is a multifunctional-tissue-protective cytokine. Curr Hematol Rep. 2003;2: 465–70.
30. Evans JL, Goldfine ID, Maddux BA, et al. Ketones metabolism increases the reduced form of glutathione thus facilitating destruction of hydrogen peroxide. Endocr Rev. 2002;23:599–622.
31. Fischer B, Bavister BD. Oxygen tension in the oviduct and uterus of rhesus monkeys, hamsters and rabbits. J Reprod Fertil. 1993;99:673–9.
32. Foster GE, Poulin MJ, Hanly PJ. Intermittent hypoxia and vascular function: implications for obstructive sleep apnoea. Exp Physiol. 2007;92:51–65.
33. Gami MS, Wolkow CA. Studies of *Caenorhabditis elegans* DAF-2/ insulin signaling reveal targets for pharmacological manipulation of lifespan. Aging Cell. 2006;5:31–7.
34. Garrido E, Castello A, Ventura JL, et al. Cortical atrophy and other brain magnetic resonance imaging (MRI) changes after extremely high-altitude climbs without oxygen. Int J Sports Med. 1993;14:232–4.
35. Gassmann M, Fandrey J, Bichet S, et al. Oxygen supply and oxygen-dependent gene expression in differentiating embryonic stem cells. Proc Natl Acad Sci USA. 1996;93:2867–72.
36. Géminard C, de Gassart A, Vidal M. Reticulocyte maturation: mitoptosis and exosome release. Biocell. 2002;26:205–15.
37. George JC, Bada JL, Zeh J, et al. Age and growth estimates of bowhead whales (*Balaena mysticetus*) via aspartic acid racemization. Can J Zool. 1999;77:571–80.
38. Geppe NA, Kurchatova TV, Dairova RA, et al. Interval hypoxic training in bronchial asthma in children. Hypoxia Med J. 1995;3:11–4.
39. Geraci JR, Palmer NC, St Aubin DJ. Tumors in cetaceans: analysis and new findings. Can J Fish Aquat Sci. 1987;44:1289–300.
40. Gidday JM. Cerebral preconditioning and ischaemic tolerance. Nat Rev Neurosci. 2006;7:437–48.
41. Gnaiger E, Méndez G, Hand SC. High phosphorylation efficiency and depression of uncoupled respiration in mitochondria under hypoxia. Proc Natl Acad Sci USA. 2000;97:11080–5.
42. Golikov MA. Health, endurance, longevity: the role of hypoxic stimulation. In: Strelkov RB, editor. Intermittent normobaric hypoxytherapy. Annals of international academy of problems of hypoxia. Vol 5. 2005. p. 164–200. [In Russian].
43. Gomez-Cabrera MC, Domenech E, Romagnoli M, et al. Oral administration of vitamin C decreases muscle mitochondrial biogenesis and hampers training-induced adaptations in endurance performance. Am J Clin Nutr. 2008;87:142–9.
44. Grechin VB, Krauz EI. Spontaneous fluctuations of oxygen tension in human brain structures. Biull Eksp Biol Med. 1973;75:20–2 [In Russian].
45. Gredilla R, Barja G. Minireview: the role of oxidative stress in relation to caloric restriction and longevity. Endocrinology. 2005;146:3713–7.
46. Halaschek-Wiener J, Brooks-Wilson A. Progeria of stem cells: stem cell exhaustion in Hutchinson-Gilford progeria syndrome. J Gerontol A Biol Sci Med Sci. 2007;62:3–8.
47. Harley CB, Futcher AB, Greider CW. Telomeres shorten during ageing of human fibroblasts. Nature. 1990;345:458–60.
48. Heidel JR, Philo LM, Albert TF, et al. Serum chemistry of bowhead whales (*Balaena mysticetus*). J Wildl Dis. 1996;32:75–9.
49. Heilbronn LK, de Jonge L, Frisard MI, et al. Effect of 6-month calorie restriction on biomarkers of longevity, metabolic adaptation, and oxidative stress in overweight individuals: a randomized controlled trial. JAMA. 2006;295:1539–48.
50. Heinicke K, Cajigal J, Viola T, et al. Long-term exposure to intermittent hypoxia results in increased hemoglobin mass, reduced plasma volume, and elevated erythropoietin plasma levels in man. Eur J Appl Physiol. 2003;88:535–43.
51. Honda Y, Honda S. Oxidative stress and life span determination in the nematode *Caenorhabditis elegans*. Ann N Y Acad Sci. 2002;959: 466–74.
52. Hoppeler H, Kleinert E, Schlegel C, et al. Morphological adaptations of human skeletal muscle to chronic hypoxia. Int J Sports Med. 1990;11:S3–9.
53. Hsu AL, Murphy CT, Kenyon C. Regulation of aging and age-related disease by DAF-16 and heat-shock factor. Science. 2003;300:1142–5.
54. Huckabee W, Metcalfe J, Prystowsky H, et al. Blood flow and oxygen consumption of the pregnant uterus. Am J Physiol. 1961;200:274–8.
55. Jauniaux E, Watson A, Ozturk O. In-vivo measurement of intrauterine gases and acid-base values early in human pregnancy. Hum Reprod. 1999;14:2901–4.
56. Jefferson J, Ashley J, Simoni J, et al. Increased oxidative stress following acute and chronic high altitude exposure. High Alt Med Biol. 2004;5:61–9.
57. Jelluma N, Yang X, Stokoe D, et al. Glucose withdrawal induces oxidative stress followed by apoptosis in glioblastoma cells but not in normal human astrocytes. Mol Cancer Res. 2006;4:319–30.
58. Johnson JB, Summer W, Cutler RG, et al. Alternate day calorie restriction improves clinical findings and reduces markers of oxidative stress and inflammation in overweight adults with moderate asthma. Free Radic Biol Med. 2007;42:665–74.
59. Khrapko K, Nekhaeva E, Kraytsberg Y, et al. Clonal expansions of mitochondrial genomes: implications for in vivo mutational spectra. Mutat Res. 2003;522:9–13.
60. Kirkwood JK, Bennett PM, Jepson PD, et al. Entanglement in fishing gear and other causes of death in cetaceans stranded on the coasts of England and *Wales*. Vet Rec. 1997;141:94–8.
61. Kogan AKh, Grachev SV, Eliseeva SV, et al. Carbon dioxide – a universal inhibitor of the generation of active oxygen forms by cells. Izv Akad Nauk Ser Biol. 1997;2:204–17 [In Russian].
62. Kolchinskaya AZ, Tsyganova TN, Ostapenko LA. Normobaric interval hypoxic training in medicine and sports. Moscow: Meditsina; 2003 [In Russian].
63. Kolesnikova EE, Serebrovskaya TV. Parkinson's disease and intermittent hypoxia training. In: Xi L, Serebrovskaya TV, editors. Intermittent hypoxia: from molecular mechanisms to clinical applications. New York: Nova Science Pub Inc; 2009. p. 577–88.
64. Kotlyarova LA, Stepanova EN, Tkatchouk EN, et al. The immune state of the patients with rheumatoid arthritis in the interval hypoxic training. Hypoxia Med J. 1994;2:11–2.
65. Krakauer DC, Mira A. Mitochondria and germ cell death. Nature. 1999;400:125–6.
66. Krause DS, Theise ND, Collector MI, et al. Multi-organ, multilineage engraftment by a single bone marrow-derived stem cell. Cell. 2001;105:369–77.
67. Krysko D, Mussche S, Leybaert LD, et al. Gap junctional communication and connexin 43 expression in relation to apoptotic cell death and survival of granulosa cells. J Histochem Cytochem. 2004;52:1199–207.
68. Kunze K. Spontaneous oscillations of pO_2 in muscle tissue. Adv Exp Med Biol. 1976;75:631–7.
69. Lacza Z, Kozlov AV, Pankotai E, et al. Mitochondria produce reactive nitrogen species via an arginine-independent pathway. Free Radic Res. 2006;40:369–78.
70. Laffey J, Motoschi T, Engelberts D. Therapeutic hypercapnia reduces pulmonary and systemic injury following in vivo lung reperfusion. Am J Respir Crit Care Med. 2000;162:2287–94.
71. Lee W-C, Chen J-J, Ho H-Y, et al. Short-term altitude mountain living improves glycemic control. High Alt Med Biol. 2003;4: 81–91.

72. Lemaster JJ. Selective mitochondrial autophagy, or mitophagy, as a targeted defense against oxidative stress, mitochondrial dysfunction and aging. Rejuvenation Res. 2005;8:3–5.
73. Li A-M, Quan Y, Guo Y-P, et al. Effects of therapeutic hypercapnia on inflammation and apoptosis after hepatic ischemia-reperfusion injury in rats. Chin Med J. 2010;123:2254–8.
74. Liu J, Ames B. Reducing mitochondrial decay with mitochondrial nutrients to delay and treat cognitive dysfunction, Alzheimer's disease, and Parkinson's disease. Nutr Neurosci. 2005;8:67–89.
75. Lukyanova LD, Dudchenko AV, Germanova EL, et al. Mitochondrial signaling in formation of body resistance to hypoxia. In: Xi L, Serebrovskaya TV, editors. Intermittent hypoxia: from molecular mechanisms to clinical applications. New York: Nova Science Pub Inc; 2009. p. 423–50.
76. Manukhina EB, Downey FH, Mallet RT. Role of nitric oxide in cardiovascular adaptation to intermittent hypoxia. Exp Biol Med. 2006;231:343–65.
77. Maynard-Smith J, Szathmary E. The major transitions in evolution. Oxford: Freeman; 1995.
78. Meerson FZ, Gomzakov OA, Shimkovich MV. Adaptation to high altitude hypoxia as a factor preventing development of myocardial ischemic necrosis. Am J Cardiol. 1973;31:30–4.
79. Meerson FZ. Adaptation to intermittent hypoxia: mechanisms of protective effects. Hypoxia Med J. 1993;3:2–8.
80. Meerson FZ. Mechanism of phenotypic adaptation and the principles of its use for prevention of cardiovascular disorders. Kardiologiia. 1978;18:18–29 [In Russian].
81. Meyer K, Foster C, Georgakopoulos N, et al. Comparison of left ventricular function during interval versus steady-state exercise training in patients with chronic congestive heart failure. Am J Cardiol. 1998;82:1382–7.
82. Milano G, Corno A, Lippa S, et al. Chronic and intermittent hypoxia induce different degrees of myocardial tolerance to hypoxia-induced dysfunction. Exp Biol Med. 2002;227:389–97.
83. Moraes CT, Kenyon L, Hao H. Mechanisms of human mitochondrial DNA maintenance: the determining role of primary sequence and length over function. Mol Biol Cell. 1999;10:3345–56.
84. Morris AA. Cerebral ketone body metabolism. J Inherit Metab Dis. 2005;28:109–21.
85. Neubauer JA. Physiological and pathophysiological responses to intermittent hypoxia. J Appl Physiol. 2001;90:1593–9.
86. Nicholasa A, Kraytsberga GX, et al. On the timing and the extent of clonal expansion of mtDNA deletions: evidence from single-molecule PCR. Exp Neurol. 2009;218:316–9.
87. Nikolsky I, Serebrovskaya TV. Hypoxia and stem cells. In: Xi L, Serebrovskaya TV, editors. Intermittent hypoxia: from molecular mechanisms to clinical applications. New York: Nova Science Pub Inc; 2009. p. 469–87.
88. Ning Z, Yi Z, Hai-Feng Z, Zhao-Nian Z. Intermittent hypoxia exposure prevents mtDNA deletion and mitochondrial structure damage produced by ischemia/reperfusion injury. Acta Physiologica Sinica Oct. 2000; 52 (5): 375-380.
89. Nunney L. Lineage selection and the evolution of multistage carcinogenesis. Proc Biol Sci. 1999;266:493–8.
90. Ogier-Denis E, Codogno P. Autophagy: a barrier or an adaptive response to cancer. Biochim Biophys Acta. 2003;1603:113–28.
91. Owen OE, Morgan AP, Kemp HG, et al. Brain metabolism during fasting. J Clin Invest. 1967;46:1589–95.
92. Peto R. Epidemiology, multistage models, and short-term mutagenicity tests. In: Hiatt HH, Watson JD, Winsten JA, editors. The origins of human cancer. Cold spring harbor conferences on cell proliferation. New York: Cold Spring Harbor Laboratory Press; 1977. p. 1403–28.
93. Philo LM, Shotts EB, George JC. Morbidity and mortality. In: Burns JJ, Montague JJ, Cowles CJ editors. The bowhead whale. Vol 2. Soc Mar Mamm Spec Publ; 1993. p. 275–312.
94. Prabhakar NR. Oxygen sensing during intermittent hypoxia: cellular and molecular mechanisms. J Appl Physiol. 2001;90:1986–1994. [PubMed]http://www.ncbi.nlm.nih.gov/pubmed/11299293.
95. Prokopov A, Voronina T. Intermittent hypoxic therapy/training (IHT): the aetiologic and pathogenetic anti-aging treatment. Rejuvenation Res. 2007;10(S1):45.
96. Prokopov A. Exploring overlooked natural mitochondria – rejuvenative intervention. The puzzle of bowhead whales and naked mole rats. Rejuvenation Res. 2007;10:543–59.
97. Prokopov A, Kotliar I. The perspectives of hypoxic treatment in the anti-aging medicine. Hypoxia Med J. 2001;3:37.
98. Prokopov A. A case of recovery from dementia following rejuvenative treatment. Rejuvenation Res. 2010;13:217–9.
99. Prokopov A, Voronina T. Engineered natural longevity – enhancing interventions. In: Bentely JV, Keller MA, editors. Handbook on longevity: genetics, diet, and disease. New York: Nova Science Publ Inc; 2009.
100. Rattan S. Hormetic interventions in aging. Am J Pharmacol Toxicol. 2008;3:27–40.
101. Rochefort GY, Delorme B, Lopez A, et al. Multipotential mesenchymal stem cells are mobilized into peripheral blood by hypoxia. Stem Cells. 2006;24:2202–8.
102. Ruscher K, Isaev N, Trendelenburg G, et al. Induction of hypoxia inducible factor-1 by oxygen glucose deprivation is attenuated by hypoxic preconditioning in rat cultured neurons. Neurosci Lett. 1998;254:117–20.
103. Russell JW, Golovoy D, Vincent AM, et al. High glucose-induced oxidative stress and mitochondrial dysfunction in neurons. FASEB J. 2002;16:1738–48.
104. Sato K, Kashiwaya Y, Keon CA, et al. Insulin, ketone bodies, and mitochondrial energy transduction. FASEB J. 1995;9:651–8.
105. Sazontova TG, Arkhipenko YuV, Lukyanova LD. Comparative study of the effect of adaptation to intermittent hypoxia on active oxygen related systems in brain and liver of rats with different resistance to oxygen deficiency. In: Sharma BK, Takeda N, Ganguly NK, et al., editors. Adaptation biology and medicine. New Delhi: Narosa Publishing House; 1997. p. 260–6.
106. Serebrovskaya TV. Intermittent hypoxia research in the former Soviet Union and the Commonwealth of Independent States: history and review of the concept and selected applications. High Alt Med Biol. 2002;3:205–21.
107. Serebrovskaya T, Manukhina EB, Smith ML, et al. Intermittent hypoxia: cause of, or therapy for systemic hypertension? Exp Biol Med. 2008;233:627–50.
108. Singer D. Neonatal tolerance to hypoxia: a comparative-physiological approach. Comp Biochem Physiol A Mol Integr Physiol. 1999;123:221–34.
109. Skrha J, Kunesova M, Hilgertova J. Short-term very low calorie diet reduces oxidative stress in obese type-2 diabetic patients. Physiol Res. 2005;54:33–9.
110. Skulachev V, Longo V. Aging as a mitochondria-mediated atavistic program: can aging be switched off? Ann N Y Acad Sci. 2005;1057:145–64.
111. Skulachev V. Mitochondrial physiology and pathology: concepts of programmed death of organelles, cells and organisms. Mol Aspects Med. 1999;20:139–84.
112. Skulachev VP. A biochemical approach to the problem of aging: "mega project" on membrane-penetrating ions. Biochemistry (Moscow). 2007;72:1385–96.
113. Smigrodzki RM, Khan SM. Mitochondrial microheteroplasmy and a theory of aging and age-related disease. Rejuvenation Res. 2005;8:172–98.
114. Spees JL, Olson SD, Whitney MJ, et al. Mitochondrial transfer among cells can rescue aerobic respiration. Proc Natl Acad Sci USA. 2006;103:1283–8.

115. Spindler S. Rapid and reversible induction of the longevity, anticancer and genomic effects of caloric restriction. Mech Ageing Dev. 2005;126:960–6.
116. Sun Y, Jin K, Mao XO. Neuroglobin is up-regulated by and protects neurons from hypoxic-ischaemic injury. Proc Natl Acad Sci USA. 2001;98:15306–11.
117. Taylor D, Zeyl C, Cooke E. Conflicting levels of selection in the accumulation of mitochondrial defects in *Saccharomyces cerevisiae*. Proc Natl Acad Sci USA. 2002;99:3690–4.
118. Terman A, Dalen H, Eaton JW, et al. Mitochondrial recycling and aging of cardiac myocytes: the role of autophagocytosis. Exp Gerontol. 2003;38:863–76.
119. Tkatchouk EN, Gorbatchenkov AA, Kolchinskaya AZ, et al. Adaptation to interval hypoxia for the purpose of prophylaxis and treatment. In: Meerson FZ, editor. Essentials of adaptive medicine: protective effects of adaptation. Moscow: Hypoxia Medical Ltd; 1994. p. 200–21.
120. Trevathan WR. Evolutionary medicine. Ann Rev Anthropol. 2007;36:139–54.
121. Uys CJ, Best PB. Pathology of lesions observed in whales flensed at Saldanha Bay, South Africa. J Comp Pathol. 1966;76:407–12.
122. Vanden Hoek T, Becker L, Shao Z, et al. Reactive oxygen species released from mitochondria during brief hypoxia induce preconditioning in cardiomyocytes. J Biol Chem. 1998;273: 18092–8.
123. Vanucci RC, Towfigi J, Heitjan DF, et al. Carbon dioxide protects the perinatal brain from hypoxic-ischemic damage: an experimental study in the immature rat. Pediatrics. 1995;95:868–74.
124. Veech RL. The therapeutic implications of ketone bodies: the effects of ketone bodies in pathological conditions, ketosis, ketogenic diet, redox states, insulin resistance, and mitochondrial metabolism. Prostagl Leukot Essent Fatty Acids. 2004;70:309–19.
125. Vesela A, Wilhelm J. The role of carbon dioxide in free radical reactions of the organism. Physiol Res. 2002;51:335–9.
126. von Zglinicki T. Oxidative stress shortens telomeres. Trends Biochem Sci. 2002;27:339–44.
127. Wallace DC. Mitochondrial DNA in aging and disease. Scientific Am. 1997;8:40–7.
128. Wang X, Deng J, Boyle D, et al. Potential role of IGF-I in hypoxia tolerance using a rat hypoxic-ischemic model: activation of hypoxia-inducible factor 1α. Pediatr Res. 2004;55:385–94.
129. West JB. Do climbs to extreme altitudes cause brain damage? Lancet. 1986;2:387.
130. Wisløff U, Støylen A, Loennechen JP, et al. Superior cardiovascular effect of aerobic interval training versus moderate continuous training in heart failure patients: a randomized study. Circulation. 2007;115:3086–94.
131. Yellon DM, Downey JM. Preconditioning the myocardium: from cellular physiology to clinical cardiology. Physiol Rev. 2003;83: 1113–51.
132. Yoneda M, Chomyn A, Martinuzzi A. Marked replicative advantage of human mtDNA carrying a point mutation that causes the MELAS encephalomyopathy. Proc Natl Acad Sci USA. 1992;89: 11164–8.
133. Zhong N, Yi Z, Fang Q, et al. Intermittent hypoxia exposure-induced heat-shock protein 70 expression increases resistance of rat heart to ischemic injury. Acta Pharmacol Sin. 2000;21: 467–72.
134. Zhong N, Zhang Y, Zhu HF, et al. Intermittent hypoxia exposure prevents mtDNA deletion and mitochondrial structure damage produced by ischemia/reperfusion injury. Sheng Li Xue Bao. 2000;52:375–80.
135. Zhuang J, Zhou Z. Protective effects of intermittent hypoxic adaptation on myocardium and its mechanisms. Biol Signals Recept. 1999;8:316–22.
136. Zorov DB, Krasnikov BF, Kuzminova AE, et al. Mitochondria revisited. Alternative functions of mitochondria. Biosci Rep. 1997;17: 507–20.

Part V

Methods and Equipment for Therapeutic Use of Intermittent Hypoxia in Humans

22 Benefits and Risks of Different Regimen of Intermittent Hypoxic Training

Katerina Rozova, Olga Gonchar, and Iryna N. Mankovska

Abstract

Intermittent hypoxia could effectively stimulate various metabolic processes, and this phenomenon is increasingly used in sport and medicine practice. However, the mode of intermittent hypoxia training (IHT) is important for achieving adequate protective effects. It is known that the short and chronic intermittent hypoxia may have serious pathophysiological consequences in organism's tissues, depending on severity and duration of the hypoxia insult. This chapter investigates the effects of various modes of IHT differing by the intensity and duration of hypoxic exposure on morphology and antioxidant status of the heart and lung tissues. The results showed that the IHT mode with more severe but shorter hypoxic component led to the prooxidant/antioxidant imbalance in the myocardial and lung tissues, which was accompanied with significant disorders in their morphology and function. Moderate hypoxic exposure of different durations promoted the maintenance of optimal antioxidant homeostasis and development of compensatory adaptive changes in tissue structure.

Abbreviations

IHT	Intermittent hypoxic training
LPO	Lipid peroxidation
RTLF	Respiratory tract lining fluid
TBARS	Thiobarbituric acid-reactive substances

22.1 Introduction

The effects of periodic hypoxia/reoxygenation have attracted considerable interest for many years. The repetitive cycles of hypoxia/reoxygenation are the basis of intermittent hypoxia training (IHT) that is one of the adaptive training types. Numerous studies have reported that intermittent hypoxia might activate various metabolic processes and cause a complex of adaptive changes in the organism [1–3]. IHT increased resistance to damaging factors such as ischemia, severe and sustained hypoxia, and exhaustive endurance exercise and is now widely used in sports as well as in treatment and prophylaxis of various human diseases [4–6]. Adaptation to intermittent hypoxia has been employed to treat patients with coronary heart disease, arrhythmias, post-myocardial infarction heart failure, as well as chronic obstructive pulmonary disease, bronchitis, bronchial asthma, etc. [7, 8]. At the same time, a recent study showed that the duration, frequency, and severity of hypoxic episodes in the IHT program are important for achieving adequate protective effects [9, 10]. It is known that both short and chronic intermittent hypoxia may also have serious pathophysiological consequences, including pulmonary and systemic hypertension, stroke, and cognitive dysfunction, depending on the severity and duration of the hypoxia insult [11]. Experimental data concerning the degree and duration of hypoxic exposure during IHT as critical factors determining whether hypoxia is a beneficial or a noxious agent are contradictory [12, 13].

K. Rozova (✉) • O. Gonchar • I.N. Mankovska
Department of Hypoxia, Bogomoletz Institute of Physiology,
National Academy of Sciences of Ukraine,
Kiev, Ukraine
e-mail: erozova@ukr.net

L. Xi, T.V. Serebrovskaya (eds.), *Intermittent Hypoxia and Human Diseases*,
DOI 10.1007/978-1-4471-2906-6_22, © Springer-Verlag London 2012

It is known that short periods of H/R are associated with induction of antioxidant response [14], in which first-line antioxidant defense enzymes (superoxide dismutase and catalase) and the glutathione system play an important role [15]. Changes in the reduced (GSH) to oxidized glutathione (GSSG) ratio reflect the level of nonspecific resistance to any stress exposure, including hypoxia [16, 17]. Numerous studies have demonstrated that antioxidant capacity is changed as a result of hypoxia as well as reoxygenation and the ultimate balance between production of free radicals and antioxidative processes at intermittent hypoxia directly depends on the experimental hypoxic regimen and tissue-specific resistance to hypoxia/reoxygenation [18]. Changes in prooxidant-antioxidant balance under IH are paralleled by changes in energy metabolism, tissue morphology and functions, specifically, in the state of biological barriers, mitochondrial system, and capillary endothelium.

Here, we have conducted the comparative analysis of morphological characteristics as well as the antioxidant status parameters of the heart and lung tissues at different regimen of IHT that might have interest for clinicians in choice of the intensity and duration of hypoxic exposure during treatment by hypoxic training.

22.2 Materials and Methods

The study was carried out on adult male Wistar rats that were divided into four groups (ten rats each): (1) control (normoxia), (2) animals breathing gas mixture with 7% O_2 in N_2 during 5 min with 15-min normoxic intervals (protocol I), (3) animals breathing gas mixture with 12% O_2 in N_2 during 5 min with 15-min normoxic intervals (protocol II), and (4) animals breathing gas mixture with 12% O_2 in N_2 during 15 min with 15-min normoxic intervals (protocol III). The total duration of exposure in all trained groups was 65 min, and duration of IHT course was 14 days. The animals were decapitated 24 h after the end of IHT course. Lung and heart tissue preparations for electron microscopy were prepared routinely with double fixation in glutaraldehyde and OsO_4, dehydrated in ascending alcohols, and embedded in epon [19]. Ultrathin section (40–60 nm) were fixed in uranyl acetate and lead citrate and examined in a JEM 100-CX electron microscope. Morphometric studies were carried out after Weibel [19]. For biochemical analysis, the heart and lungs were rapidly removed, washed in saline, and frozen in liquid nitrogen. Lipid peroxidation (LPO) was measured from the formation of thiobarbituric acid-reactive substances (TBARS) using the method of Buege and Aust [20]. Activities of Cu/Zn-SOD and catalase were estimated by the methods of Misra and Fridovich [21] and Korolyuk et al. [22]. Reduced and oxidized glutathione were measured by the method of Anderson [23]. Protein concentration was estimated by the Lowry method, using bovine serum albumin as a standard. The results were processed using Student's *t* test, and the differences were considered significant at $p < 0.05$.

22.3 Results and Discussion

Hypoxic training performed after protocol I caused of LPO processes intensification: an increase in TBARS level by 22% ($p < 0.05$) in the myocardium and by 33% ($p < 0.05$) in lungs in comparison with control (Fig. 22.1a). This increase accompanied by a rise in GSSG content and a reduction in GSH content in the heart and lung tissues (Fig. 22.2). The shift of the GSH/GSSG balance toward disulfide accumulation indicated the retained activity of oxidative processes and decreased reduction potential of glutathione under conditions of this training mode. Accumulation of GSSG during oxidative stress can lead to imbalance of the antioxidant system, because GSSG, as a toxic compound, easily forms mixed disulfides with the thiol-containing enzymes impairing their activity [16, 17]. IHT according to protocol I led to a reduction of Cu/Zn-SOD activity and an increase in catalase activity in the heart and lung tissues (Fig. 22.1b, c), which is important, because catalase plays the key role in cell protection from active oxygen metabolites during oxidative stress [15].

Changes in antioxidant system in response to more severe hypoxic exposure were paralleled by significant changes in tissue ultrastructure. Changes in the lung tissue involved mainly the surfactant system and the cell mitochondrial system. They manifested in inhibited synthesis (devastation of lamellar bodies in type II pneumocytes) and secretion (no free surfactant on alveolar surface) of surfactant, mosaic vacuolation and swelling of mitochondria, and dyscomplectation and destruction of cristae in 25–30% organelles (Fig. 22.3a). Hypoxic edema of the lungs was mild, and the thickness of the blood-air barrier exhibited a trend to an increase (Table 22.1), while intra-alveolar edema and destruction of individual layers of the blood-air barrier were observed in just solitary alveoles. Electron microscopy investigation of myocardium showed vast areas impregnated with fluid and proteins, which indicated increased permeability of cytoplasmic membranes. This was associated with swelling, disorganization, and destruction of the myofibrils, pronounced edema of the blood-tissue barrier (Table 22.1) with marginal localization, and cardiomyocyte destruction without significant disorders in the capillary endothelial ultrastructure. Partial vacuolation was rarely seen in myocardial mitochondria, but in the majority of cases, the matrix was condensed, which can be regarded as an indirect evidence of inhibited glycolysis under this mode of hypoxic exposure (Fig. 22.3b). These data are in line with the opinion that more intense and longer hypoxia stimulates

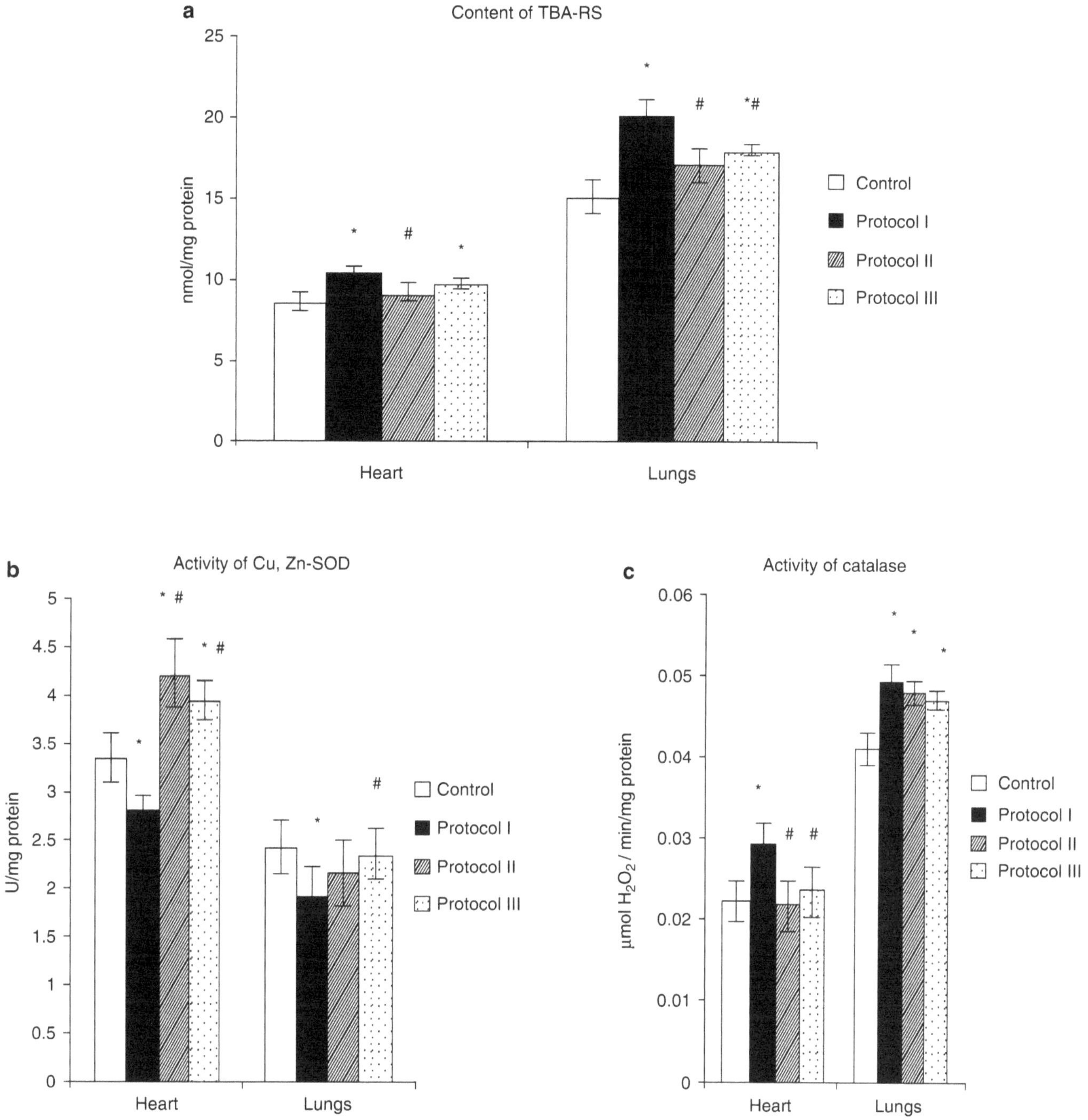

Fig. 22.1 Effect of different regimen of intermittent hypoxic training on lipid peroxidation (**a**) and activities of antioxidant enzymes (**b** and **c**) in the heart and lung tissues. Values are mean ± SEM, $n = 10$ in each group. *$p < 0.05$ vs. control; #$p < 0.05$ vs. protocol I

free radical processes and causes morphofunctional changes in various tissues [18].

IHT performed after protocol II caused just a trend to an increase in the level of LPO products in the heart and lung tissues, in contrast to protocol III, when these parameters surpassed the control level by 13% and 19%, respectively ($p < 0.05$). Activity of Cu/Zn-SOD in the myocardium increased by 26% under using of IHT by protocol II and by 18% in response to IHT by protocol III ($p < 0.05$), while catalase activity remained unchanged. Catalase activity in the lungs increased by 15–17%, while Cu/Zn-SOD activity maintained at the control level (Fig. 22.1a, b, c). Analysis of the glutathione pool in the studied tissues showed that hypoxic training according to protocols II and III led to an increase in GSH content in the lungs, while in the myocardium, the increased level of GSSG was retained in comparison with control (Fig. 22.2). The lungs, unlike other tissues, have a wide range of antioxidant

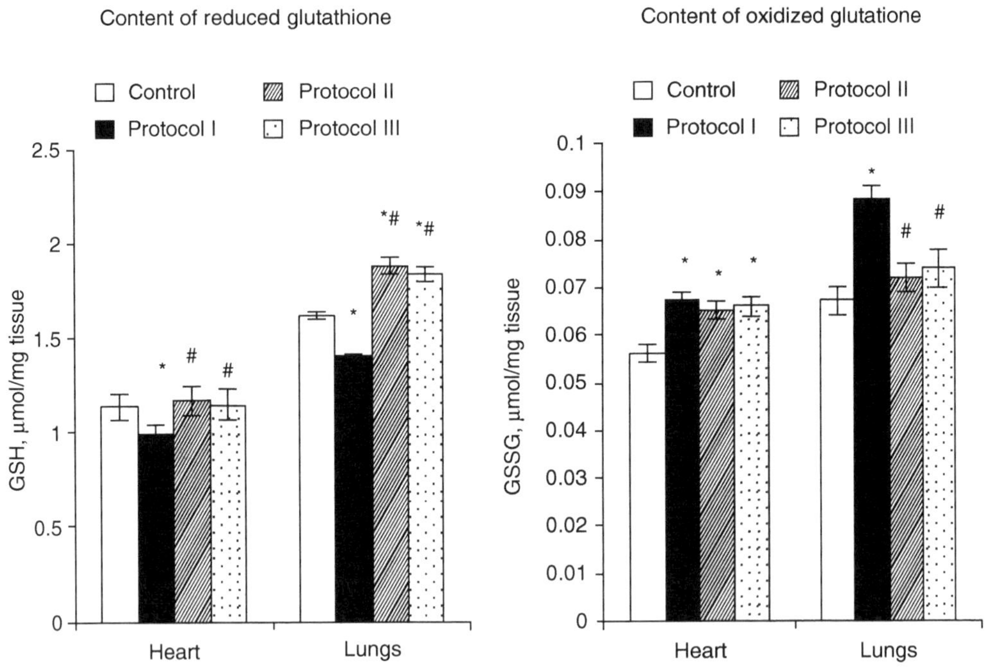

Fig. 22.2 Effect of different regimen of intermittent hypoxic training on glutathione pool in the heart and lung tissues. (**a**) Content of reduced glutathione, (**b**) content of oxidized glutathione. Values are mean ± SEM, $n = 10$ in each group. *$p < 0.05$ vs. control; #$p < 0.05$ vs. protocol I

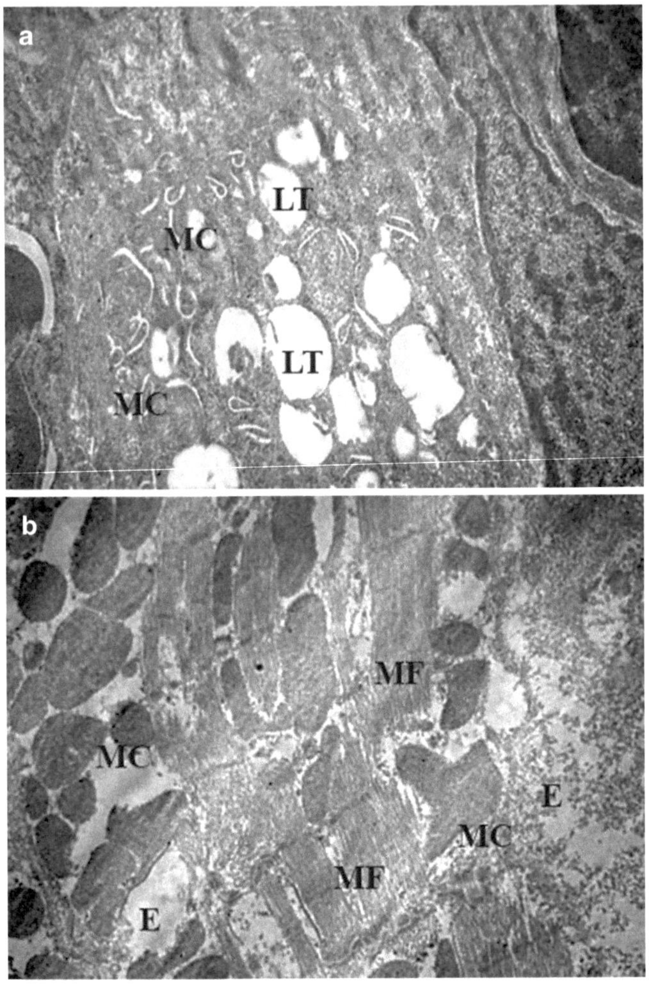

Fig. 22.3 Effects of IHT (protocol I) on lung (**a**) and heart (**b**) tissue ultrastructure. *MC* mitochondria, *LT* lamellar bodies, *E* edema, *MF* myofibrils. ×9,600

defense tools which help to maintain a balanced redox status under various extreme conditions. Enzymatic and nonenzymatic antioxidants are present in the intracellular, the vascular, and extracellular respiratory tract lining fluid (RTLF) of lung, but the reduced glutathione content of RTLF is particularly high (100-fold higher than in the blood plasma) [24].

Changes in the morphofunctional state of the studied tissues in response to IHT with a hypoxic component of moderate intensity (protocol II) were largely compensatory and adaptive. Mild hypoxic edema of the blood-tissue barrier (23–29% increase in the thickness; $p < 0.05$; Table 22.1) in cardiac tissue was paralleled by an increase in the total number of mitochondria in comparison with the control (by 8–10/μ—2, $p < 0.05$) and by twofold decreased number of structurally changed organelles in comparison with their level under IHT according protocol I. Mosaic disorders of myocardial ultrastructure with cardiomyocyte edema, myofibrillar swelling, and sometimes disorganization were also seen (Fig. 22.4a). These changes were characteristic for tissue reaction to hypoxic exposure [25]. Activation of the surfactant synthesis

Table 22.1 Mean thickness of blood-air and blood-tissue barriers under different IHT modes (nm, $M \pm m$)

Experiment conditions	Blood-air barrier	Blood-tissue barrier
Control	163 ± 8	221 ± 14
IHT		
Protocol I	198 ± 21	396 ± 29*
Protocol II	186 ± 19	285 ± 21*+
Protocol III	194 ± 28	272 ± 17*+

*P < 0.05 vs Control; *+ P < 0.05 vs Protocol I

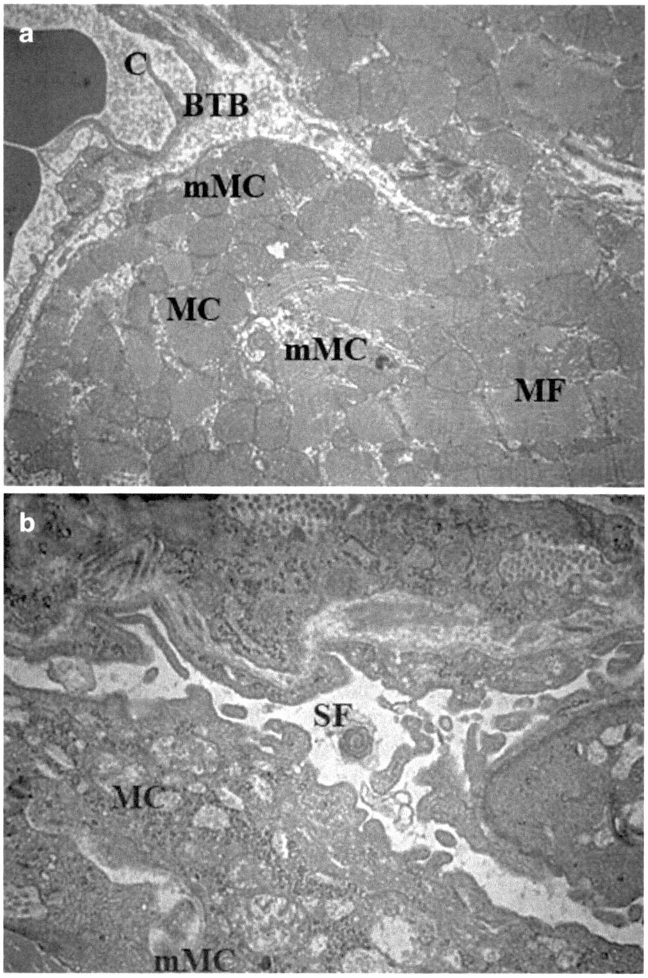

Fig. 22.4 Effects of IHT (protocol II) on heart (**a**) and lung (**b**) tissue ultrastructure. *A* alveolar lumen, *BTB* blood-tissue barrier, *C* capillary lumen, *MF* myofibrils, *SF* free surfactant, *MC* mitochondria, *mMC* "mitochondria in mitochondria." ×9,600

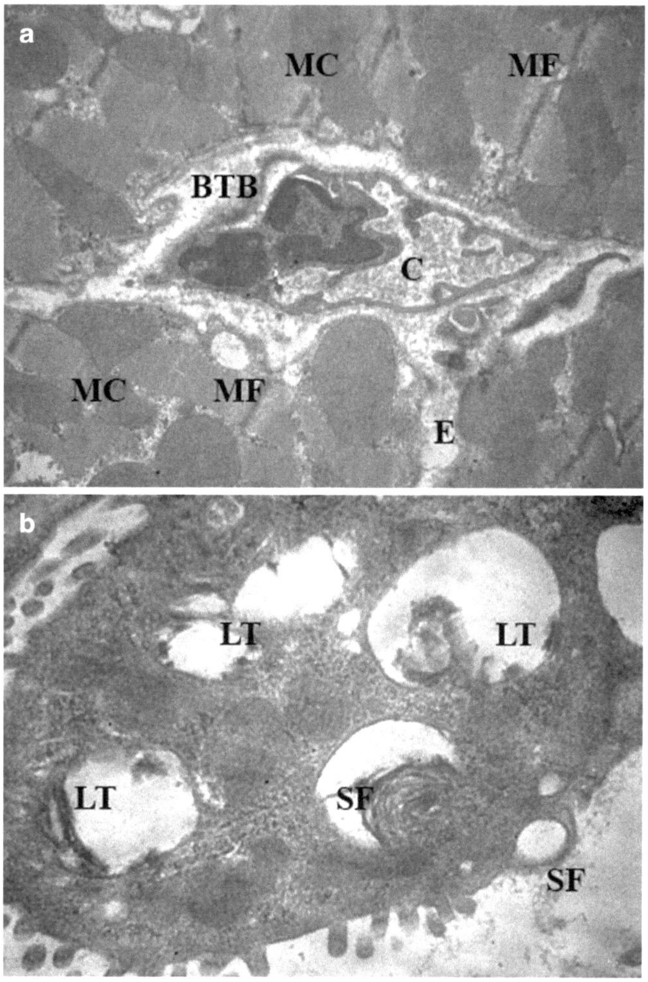

Fig. 22.5 Effects of IHT (protocol III) on heart (**a**) and lung (**b**) tissue ultrastructure. *A* alveolar lumen, *C* capillary lumen, *BTB* blood-tissue barrier, *E* edema, *LT* lamellar bodies, *MF* myofibrils, *SF* free surfactant. ×11,000

and secretion with restoration of the surfactant lining in the greater part of the alveoles was observed in the lung tissue. The ultrastructure of the blood-air barrier and lung stroma corresponded to intact tissue in the majority of regions (Fig. 22.4b). For certain, the displays of edema of blood-air barrier also diminished that was expressed in the decline of the barrier thickness in relation to this parameter measured at a protocol I. Partial vacuolation and swelling of the mitochondria and low (up to 10%) level of organelles with manifestations of crist dyscomplectation and destruction were observed. These results indicate that the effects of IHT on the ultrastructure of the studied tissues are, at first, organ specific. Secondly, their positive influence on morphofunctional state of the heart and lungs tissues shows up at a moderate force of hypoxic stimuli.

The mode III of IHT was also accompanied by the less expressed changes in ultrastructure of the studied tissues in comparison with the training in the hard mode, but at the same time, they were more expressed than at training according to protocol II: in particular, separate areas were saved from destructive changes, both in the whole tissues and in their mitochondria apparatus (Fig. 22.5a, b). Thus, in this case, the hyperhydratation of blood-air barrier, estimated on this thickness, for certain did not differ from the known changes after protocol I of IHT. So, in respect of blood-tissue barrier, a diminished thickness in response to severe hypoxia sustained, confirming an organ-specific manner of IHT influences.

We would further speculate the possible mechanism of the increased resistance to unfavorable influences of IHT. We have shown under IH, as well as under acute hypoxic hypoxia, an increase of the stake of apoptotic changes, especially in mitochondria of cardiomyocytes. It is known that this process is physiological and was stated by many researchers as a positive sign under the different influences on organism [26–28]. The conducted research allows us to educe a new type of apoptosis in lung and heart tissues under acute moderate hypoxia – formation of micromitochondria within the mitochondria structurally broken due to hypoxia (Fig. 22.6a, b). According to the work of Russian researches,

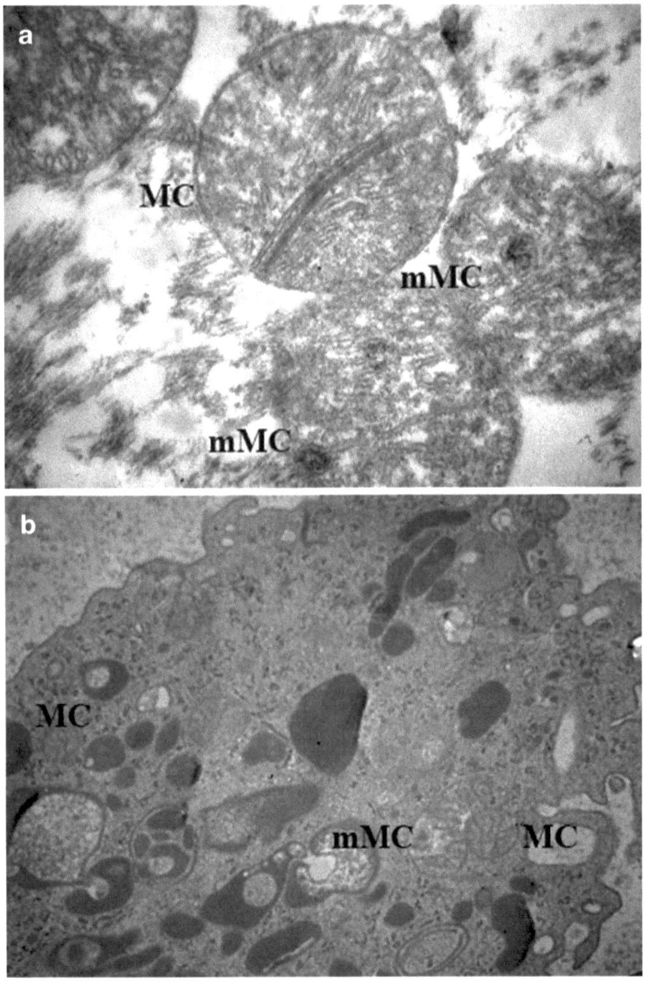

Fig. 22.6 Ultrastructure of mitochondria in heart (**a**) and lung (**b**) tissue under hypoxic hypoxia. *MC* mitochondria, *mMC* "mitochondria in mitochondria"; ×32,000 (**a**), ×18,000 (**b**)

in micromitochondria not only a structure, peculiar for these organelles, but also their function, were saved [29, 30]. We incline to examine formation of intramitochondrial mitochondria as one of ways of apoptosis, directed to maintain of the mitochondrial apparatus energy power under hypoxic condition, and, consequently, to form the additional adaptive mechanism at the hypoxic training.

Conclusion

Different regimen of IHT, in terms of duration and intensity, lead to the different morphological and functional responses to ROS and to the different changes in the balance between the pro- and antioxidant systems. Highly intensive repetitive free radical signal under the mode I of IHT acts as a destructive factor for antioxidant homeostasis and for tissue structure, while more or less compensated induction of ROS under the modes II and III of IHT stimulates the defense systems including endogenous antioxidative systems and development of the adaptive organ-specific changes in ultrastructure of the lung and heart. According to our results, we consider that the mode II of IHT is more effective and less dangerous for the studied organs and tissues (i.e., heart and lung) and may be recommended for prophylaxis and treatment of cardiac and lung pathology.

References

1. Cai Z, Manalo D, Wei G, et al. Hearts from rodents exposed to intermittent hypoxia or erythropoietin are protected against ischemia-reperfusion injury. Circulation. 2003;108:79–85.
2. Clanton T, Klawitter P. Adaptive responses of skeletal muscle to intermittent hypoxia: the known and the unknown. J Appl Physiol. 2001;90:2476–87.
3. Gonchar O, Mankovska I. Glutathione system adaptation to acute stress in the heart of the rats during different regimes of hypoxia training. Ukr Biokhim Zh. 2007;79:79–85 [In Ukrainian].
4. Tkachouk E, Gorbachenkov A, Kolchinskaya A, et al. Adaptation to interval hypoxia for prophylaxis and therapy. Moscow: Hypoxia Med. Ltd; 1994.
5. Belaidi E, Ramond A, Joyeux-Faure M, et al. Contrasting effects of intermittent hypoxia on myocardial ischemic tolerance. In: Xi L, Serebrovskaya TV, editors. Intermittent hypoxia: from molecular mechanisms to clinical application. New York: Nova Science Publishers; 2009. p. 3–18.
6. Serebrovskaya T, Manukhina E, Smith M, et al. Intermittent hypoxia: cause of or therapy for systemic hypertension. Exp Biol Med. 2008;233:627–50.
7. Burtscher M, Pachinger O, Ehrenbourg I, et al. Intermittent hypoxia increases exercise tolerance in elderly men with and without coronary artery disease. Int J Cardiol. 2004;96:247–54.
8. Serebrovskaya T, Swanson R, Kolchinskaya A. Intermittent hypoxia: mechanisms of action and some applications to bronchial asthma treatment. J Physiol Pharmacol. 2003;54(suppl):35–41.
9. Chen L, Einbinder E, Zhang Q, et al. Oxidative stress and left ventricular function with chronic intermittent hypoxia in rats. Am J Respir Crit Care Med. 2005;172:915–20.
10. Suzuki Y, Jain V, Park A, et al. Oxidative stress and oxidant signaling in obstructive sleep apnea and associated cardiovascular diseases. Free Radic Biol Med. 2006;40:1683–92.
11. Neubauer J. Physiological and pathophysiological responses to intermittent hypoxia. J Appl Physiol. 2001;90:1593–9.
12. Zong P, Setty S, Sun W, et al. Intermittent hypoxic training protects canine myocardium from infarction. Exp Biol Med. 2004;229:806–12.
13. Joyeux-Faure M, Stanke-Labesque F, Lefebvre B, et al. Chronic intermittent hypoxia increases infarction in the isolated rat heart. J Appl Physiol. 2005;98:1691–6.
14. Gulyaeva NV, Tkatchouk EN. Antioxidative effects of interval hypoxic training. Hypoxia Med J. 1997;5:18–21.
15. Yu B. Cellular defenses against damage from reactive oxygen species. Physiol Rev. 1994;74:139–62.
16. Saez GT, Bannister WH, Bannister JV. Oxidative stress and glutathione. In: Vina J, editor. Glutathione: metabolism and physiological functions. Boca Raton: CRC Press; 1990. p. 237–54.
17. Hayes J, McLellan L. Glutathione and glutathione-dependent enzymes represent a coordinately regulated defense against oxidative stress. Free Radic Res. 1999;31:273–300.
18. Gonchar O, Mankovska I. Antioxidant system in adaptation to intermittent hypoxia. J Biol Sci. 2010;10:545–54.
19. Karupu VYa. Electron microscopy. Kiev: Naukova Dumka; 1984 [In Russian].
20. Buege A, Aust S. Microsomal lipid peroxidation. Methods Enzymol. 1978;52:302–8.

21. Misra H, Fridovich I. The role of superoxide anion in the autoxidation of epinephrine and a simple assay superoxide dismutase. J Biol Chem. 1972;247:3170–5.
22. Korolyuk M, Ivanova L, Maiorova I, et al. A method for measuring catalase activity. Lab Manuals. 1988;1:16–9 [In Russian].
23. Anderson M. Determination of glutathione and glutathione disulfide in biological samples. Methods Enzymol. 1985;113:548–51.
24. Kelly F. Glutathione: in defense of the lung. Food Chem Toxicol. 1994;37:963–6.
25. Kolchinskaya AZ, Khatsukov BKh, Zakusilo MP. Oxygen insufficiency, destructive and constructive effects. Nalchik: RASc; 1999 [In Russian].
26. Rozova EV. Changes of morphofunctional state of mitochondria of the rat lung and heart tissues in hypoxia of various genesis. J Acad Med Sci Ukr. 2008;14:752–65 [In Russian].
27. Sudakova JV, Bakeeva LE, Tsyplenkov VG. Energy-dependent changes of ultrastructure of cardiomyocytes mitochondria of man at the alcoholic defeat of heart. Arch Pathol. 1999;2:15–20 [In Russian].
28. Sudakova JV, Bakeeva LE, Tsyplenkov VG. Destructive changes of cardiomyocytes mitochondria of man at the alcoholic defeat of heart. Arch Pathol. 1999;9:19–23 [In Russian].
29. Saprunova VB, Solodovnikova IM, Bakeeva LE. Exposure of cytochrome c-oxidase activity in mitochondria of cardiomyocytes of the isolated tissues of myocardium at the prolonged effect of hypoxia. Cytology. 2008;50:268–74 [In Russian].
30. Solodovnikova IM, Saprunova VB, Bakeeva LE, et al. Dynamics of changes of ultrastructure of cardiomyocytes mitochondria in the isolated myocardium of rat during the protracted incubation in the conditions anoxia. Cytology. 2006;48:848–55 [In Russian].

Individualized Intermittent Hypoxia Training: Principles and Practices

23

Tatiana V. Serebrovskaya and Lei Xi

Abstract

Individual variation of homeostatic response to hypoxia has been recognized by investigators from the former Soviet Union as well as Western countries. The proven influence of both hereditary and environmental parameters on physiological responses must drive the selection of individual regimes for athletic training, disease treatment, and outcome prognostication. Our longitudinal examinations of identical twins both at sea level and altitudes have shown that the ventilatory response to hypoxic stimulus is a rigid, genetically determined, physiological characteristic reflecting an organism's overall nonspecific reactivity. On the basis of our twin investigations, we have designed a nomogram to estimate individual nonspecific reactivity and functional reserves for prognosis of subject adaptation to hypoxia. Various strategies of adaptation were identified for persons with differing hypoxic ventilatory sensitivity. Intermittent hypoxic training (IHT) regimes can be customized to match this known individual reactivity. Mechanisms that mediate interindividual variation of adaptation to hypoxia were primarily determined by making measurements in animals with high (HR) and low (LR) resistance to acute hypoxia. Although there are several possible causes for such variation, much of the interest in Russian/Ukraine has focused on mitochondria. The researchers found that, when compared to LR rats, HR rats had: (1) greater mitochondrial enzyme complex I activity, (2) increased nitric oxide inhibition of Ca^{2+}-ATPase activity with concomitant decreased intracellular Ca^{2+}, (3) enhanced antioxidant activity, and (4) increased gene expression. Differential selective oxidation of two Krebs cycle substrates, alpha-ketoglutarate versus succinate, acts more intensively in HR animals, thereby enhancing cholinergic status. Our investigations have shown that L-arginine injections as well as IHT increase mitochondrial calcium capacity in LR rats to the same level as HR rats. Mitochondrial ATP-dependent potassium channel openers affected mitochondrial respiration differently in HR and LR rats. These differences were similar to the IHT effects. Nevertheless, there is a continued search for potential universal marker(s) for individual prognosis of adaptation to hypoxia. Future investigations will shed light on this very important question. Collectively, we can envisage a bright future for individualized IHT, which may play a significant role in the fast-developing field of personalized preventive medicine against various human diseases.

T.V. Serebrovskaya (✉)
Department of Hypoxia, Bogomoletz Institute of Physiology, National Academy of Sciences of Ukraine, Kiev 01024, Ukraine
e-mail: sereb@biph.kiev.ua

L. Xi
Division of Cardiology, Department of Internal Medicine, Virginia Commonwealth University, Richmond, VA, 23298-0204, USA
e-mail: lxi@vcu.edu

Abbreviations

CIS	Commonwealth of Independent States
EPO	Erythropoietin
HCVR	Hypercapnic ventilatory sensitivity
HIF-1	Hypoxia-inducible factor 1

L. Xi, T.V. Serebrovskaya (eds.), *Intermittent Hypoxia and Human Diseases*,
DOI 10.1007/978-1-4471-2906-6_23, © Springer-Verlag London 2012

HR	High resistant
HVR	Hypoxic ventilatory response
IHT	Intermittent hypoxic training
LHTL	Live high-train low
LR	Low resistant
mK_{ATP}	Mitochondrial ATP-dependent potassium channels
MR	Medium resistant
NO	Nitric oxide
VO_2max	Maximal oxygen uptake

23.1 Introduction

No matter is common to all nature but nature exists in a multitude of matters and a multitude of forms.
Sir Francis Bacon (1561–1626)

Human functions have rates of reaction with exceedingly broad ranges. This inherent variability underlies the plasticity and high adaptability of all organisms. The genetic information in DNA does not provide a fixed program of adaptation but rather presents a smorgasbord of possible responses that are only realized in the changeable environmental conditions that produce the highly individual response, which can eventually determine the individual development in both physiological and pathological states. As the tremendous advances in human genome information and our understanding on molecular mechanisms of diseases progresses, personalized medicine has become a broad and rapidly advancing field of healthcare that is informed by each person's unique clinical, genetic, genomic, and environmental information [23]. Personalized medicine now allows healthcare professionals to create optimized care plans at every stage of a disease, shifting the focus from reactive to preventive medical strategies. Physicians may now use a patient's genetic variation or expression profile as well as protein and metabolic markers to guide the selection of individual treatment plans with greater precision [1, 23].

The fact of individual variations in an organism's resistance to hypoxia has been confirmed by numerous investigations, in both humans and animals, conducted in the former Soviet Union and the Commonwealth of Independent States (CIS) as well as the Western countries. In particular, the economic development of high-altitude areas has increased and thus reinforced the importance of understanding the ecological factors influencing human health with added emphasis on analyzing and comprehending individual human adaptive responses. The answers to this fundamental question could also reveal risk factors for diseases and help in the selection of individualized intermittent hypoxia training (IHT) regimes during sport training or disease treatment. It will also be instrumental in selection of professionals whose job functions correspond to their innate hypoxic resistance. In general, individualized IHT can be classified as a promising approach within the fast-growing field of personalized preventive medicine.

23.2 History and Evolution of Individualized IHT

Hypoxic training of individual pilots in a barochamber was suggested by Holdein in 1919. Variations of individual subject response to hypoxia had captivated the attention of former Soviet Union and CIS scientists for many decades. Crafting an individual dose prescription for IHT was first applied in the training of pilots, mountaineers, and athletes. Basic research in this field was initiated by Egorov [31], Streltsov [73], Sirotinin [72], Rozenblyum [62], and others. Since 1970s, a large volume of work had been published by Berezovskiy et al. [10–16], Lukiyanova (Lukyanova – in different spelling) et al. [45–47], Agadzhanyan et al. [2, 3], Aidaraliev and Maksimov [4, 5], Kolchinskaya et al. [38, 39], Serebrovskaya (Serebrovska, Serebrovskaia, Serebrovs'ka – in different spellings) et al. [64–69], and many others. Important contributions in developing the underlying principles and in understanding the physiological processes of individual peculiarities of adaptation to hypoxia involved a number of research centers, including (1) Institute of Medico-Biological Problems in Moscow, (2) Army Medical College in St. Petersburg, (3) Institute of High Altitude Physiology in Kirgizia, and (4) Bogomoletz Institute of Physiology in Kiev. Unfortunately, many Russian and Ukrainian discoveries did not become a "common property" of the international scientific community. During the Soviet period, the "iron curtain" cut off most of the paths of communication with Western scientists. In spite of the negative impact, isolation may have actually promoted the development of some original ideas in this particular field of IHT.

The individualized character of ventilatory reaction to hypoxia – from hypersensitivity up to a complete absence of response – has been well described [12, 64, 66]. Obviously, genetically based individual differences exist in an organism's resistance to hypoxia. These differences are based on a unique and complex combination of the functional and metabolic features of the major regulatory systems of the body. To confirm the existence of genetically determined characteristics that would lead to the discovery of markers for individual reactivity and adaptability, a series of investigations were conducted along several lines of research including studies of (1) twins, (2) human family relationships including longitudinal data, and (3) animal experiments on such variability using both intra- and interspecies protocols.

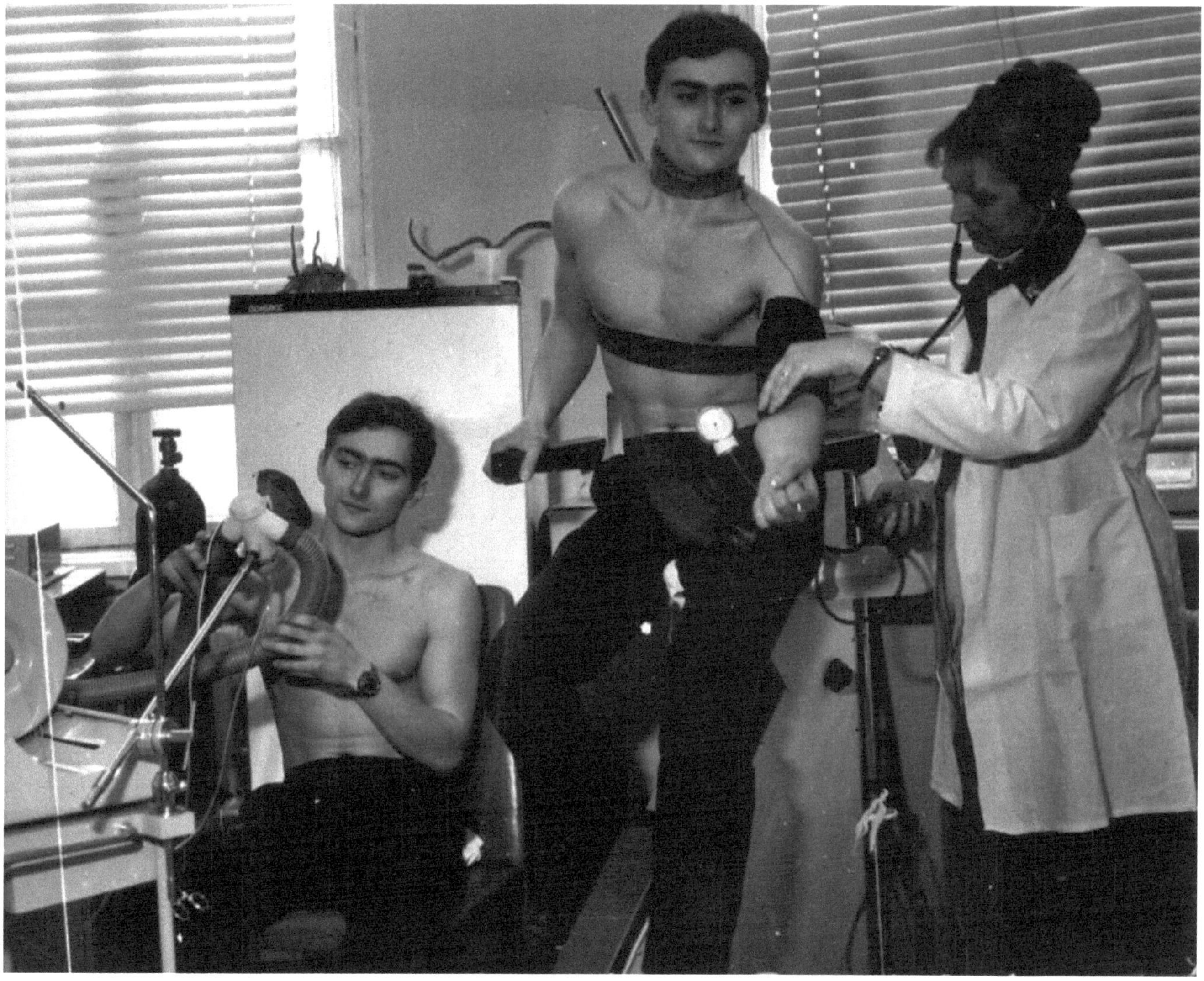

Fig. 23.1 Twins investigation at the Bogomoletz Institute of Physiology, Kiev, Ukraine, 1979 (Researcher: Tatiana Serebrovskaya)

Phenotypic and genotypic differences in the development of individual adaptations were determined in the twins study [15, 64, 66] (Fig. 23.1). Concurrent investigations in both the Western and Eastern countries [26, 36] were independently conducted by researchers without knowing anything of what happen on another side of the "iron curtain." Results obtained by Ukrainian researchers were later confirmed by investigators from outside of the former Soviet Union. Information about the extent of the genetic determination of different functional and biochemical factors accumulated during these years. Use of the twin method did not reveal the mechanisms of interindividual difference, but these studies did disclose parameters useful for individual prognosis and career guidance. In particular, results confirm that ventilatory responses to hypoxic and hypercapnic stimuli are rigid, genetically determined physiological parameters, which reflect an organism's overall nonspecific reactivity (Fig. 23.2). Longitudinal investigation of monozygotic twins during 8 years (i.e., from age of 10–11 until 18–19 years old) showed that the indices of Holzinger hereditary scale for these parameters did not change significantly over this time period. The studies also pointed out that the ability of humans to maintain relatively constant oxygen consumption levels under short-term moderate hypoxia (11% oxygen in nitrogen for 15 min) is largely determined genetically (70–80%) and depends on both hypoxic (HVR) and hypercapnic (HCVR) ventilatory sensitivity. Factor analysis has shown HVR (to a lesser extent) and HCVR (to a greater extent) closely correlate with reactions of physiological systems after adequate stimuli and can serve as a criterion for individual reactivity estimation. For example, young healthy men were studied in the paper by Berezovskii et al. [14]. These young natives of sea-level land lived and worked for 1 year under chronic hypoxia (at altitude of 3,650 m with $PO_2=90$ mmHg). Those subjects with a higher rate of anaerobic metabolism in a low PO_2 environment displayed diminished sensitivity to hypoxic stimulation

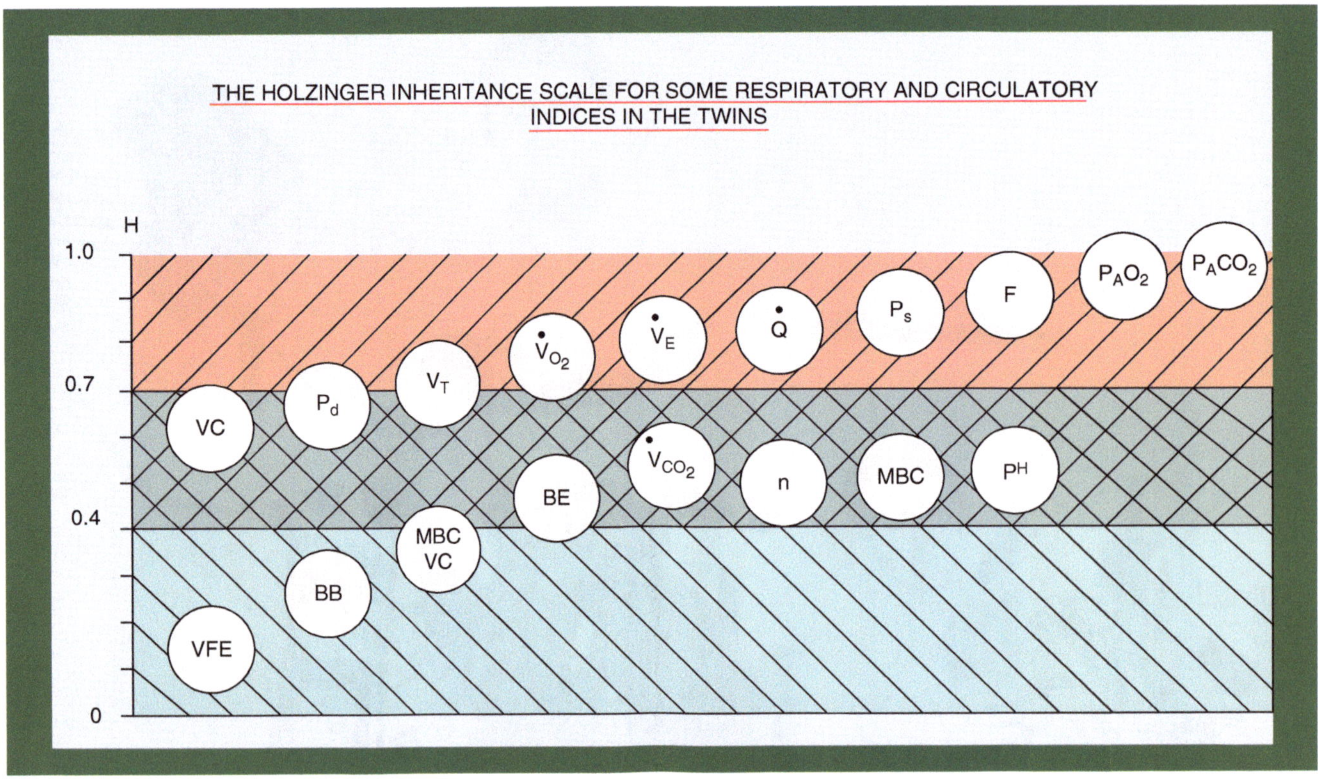

Fig. 23.2 Holzinger inheritance scale for some respiratory and circulatory indices. *VC* lung vital capacity, P_d diastolic blood pressure, V_t tidal volume, VO_2 minute oxygen consumption, V_E minute ventilation, *Q* minute cardiac output, P_s systolic blood pressure, *F* respiratory rate, P_AO_2 oxygen partial pressure in alveolar gas, P_ACO_2 carbon dioxide partial pressure in alveolar gas, *VFE* FEV1, *BB* buffer base, *MBC/VC* chirographic index, *BE* base excess, VCO_2 minute CO_2 excretion, *n* HR (heart rate), *MBC* maximal lung ventilation, *pH* arterial blood pH. The *Y*-axis indicates: *H* Holzinger inheritance scale, in which, 0–0.4 prevalence of environmental factors; 0.4–0.7 combined influence of hereditary and environmental factors; 0.7–1 prevalence of hereditary factors

of respiration, increased tolerance to very low PaO_2, and reduced work capacity in chronic hypoxia.

Comparative research-based relationships between (1) respiratory reactions to weak and strong hypercapnic stimuli and (2) reactions to acute and chronic hypoxia combined with physical load allowed us to characterize three main types of responses [11]. Persons expressing higher ventilatory responses both to weak (slope one, S_1) and severe (slope two, S_2) hypercapnia (hyperreactive type) are characterized by (1) higher minute ventilatory parameters, (2) increased heart rate and minute cardiac output, (3) increased resting gas exchange, (4) greater reactions to quick ascent to altitudes and physical load, (5) strongly pronounced skin reactions to irritants, (6) more labile neurological function, (7) good working capacity at middle altitudes with low economy of cardiorespiratory functions, and (8) low resistance to extreme hypoxia and physical load. In persons with reduction in both S_1 and S_2, ventilatory and circulatory reactions to stimuli are weakly expressed. During moderate hypoxia, acidosis can occur and work capacity can fall (hyporeactive type). Optimal reactions were observed in persons with low S_1 and high S_2 (normoreactive type), producing a reduced response to stimuli of small value and an increased response to intense stimuli. Longitudinal investigations of twins have demonstrated relatively permanent group reactivity assignment, i.e., hyper-, normo-, or hyporeactivity during the 8-year period.

On the basis of these studies, a method for determining individual reactivity of the respiratory system was designed with development of a prognostic monogram to define reactivity types (i.e., hypo-, normo-, and hyperreactivity). This research also allowed differentiating persons within one reactivity type with having either high, average, or low functional reserves [13] (Fig. 23.3, two extreme classes are presented).

Respiratory reactivity types had strong positive correlation with indices of the higher nervous activities, such as (1) functional ability of nervous processes, (2) rate of visual information processing, and (3) volume of short-term memory at both sea level and high altitude [50]. Application of this method for estimating human individual reactivity had produced positive results in athletic performance, professional career selection, and clinical practice. The researcher, trainer, or clinician could correctly choose an individual IHT regime approach for physical development or disease treatment. For an effective IHT treatment in the persons with

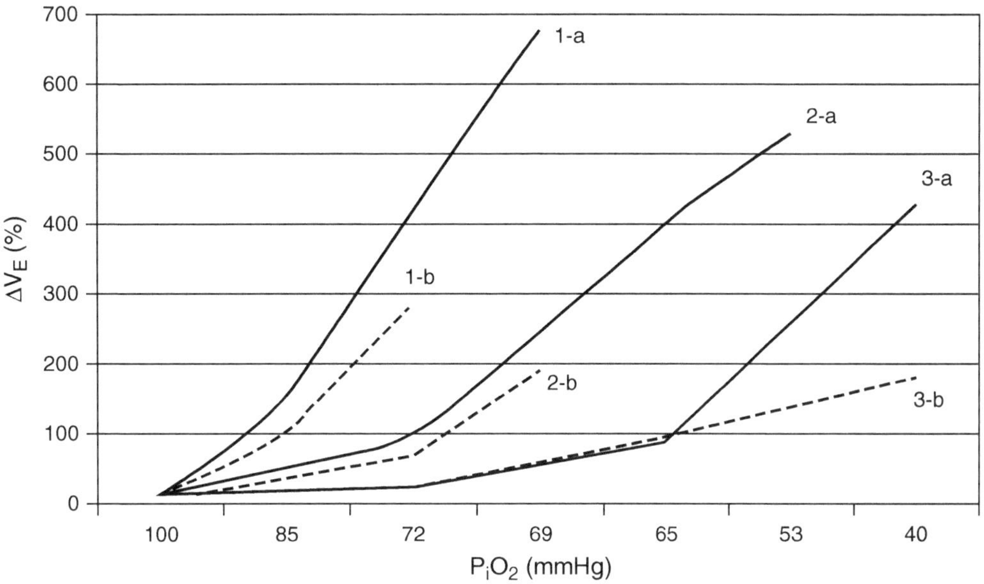

Fig. 23.3 Different types of respiratory system reactivity to growing hypoxic stimulus with due account for its reserve capabilities: (1) hyperreactive type with high (*1-a*) and weak (*1-b*) reserve capabilities; (2) normoreactive type with high (*2-a*) and weak (*2-b*) reserve capabilities; 3- hyporeactive type with high (*3-a*) and weak (*3-b*) reserve capabilities. *Ordinate*: ΔV_E, % is calculated in accordance with diagram of pulmonary ventilation (V_E) dependence on P_iO_2 level at point where P_iO_2 = 75 mmHg and when maximum ventilation (ΔV_{Emax}) is reached at the end of the test

abnormally high sensitivity, a moderate regime is needed. And for individuals with low sensitivity, a more severe regime must be applied. Tables for selection of individual IHT regimes have been published [49].

The prognostic significance of physiological, biochemical, or hormonal parameters in evaluating human tolerance to hypoxia has been described by Vasin [75], Berezovskii and Levashov [12], and Aidaraliev and Maksimov [4]. Aydaraliev et al. [7] reported that prior to their ascent to the high mountain area, volunteers were divided into two groups with a high or low level of hypoxic tolerance based on the work capacity index calculated by standard bicycle ergometry tests. By the day 30 of adaptation, the subjects with low hypoxic tolerance and nonspecific resistance experienced biorhythm changes in both amplitude and phase with a 12-h ultradian component. By contrast, the subjects with high hypoxic tolerance retained normal circadian patterns.

As early as 1976, Eckes declared: "No parameters exist which could allow a prognosis as to what kind of individuals will or will not tolerate altitude" [29]. However, most Russian and Ukrainian scientists considered that exposure to hypoxia and/or hypercapnia elicits a number of compensatory changes that can serve as the markers for such prognosis [4, 5, 12, 13, 32, 52, 66]. More recent studies in Western countries have also confirmed this conclusion [18, 36, 57, 78]. Furthermore, Waters and Gozal [77] found significant correlations for those hypoxia markers and glycolytic enzyme mRNAs that previously have been linked to hypoxia-specific muscle adaptations.

Also other markers are used for prognosis of individual adaptation to hypoxia and for the selection of optimal treatment regimes. In Moscow's "Hypoxia Medical" scientific-clinical laboratory, a special program was developed to couple hypoxic training with concurrent data collection of hemodynamic parameters during a steady decrease in blood oxygen saturation [74]. The independent variables for the training program were SaO_2 and heart rate. Estimation of individual patient sensitivity to hypoxia for selecting an individual IHT regime has also been elaborated by Berezovskii and Levashov [12]. A number of different markers have been proposed to predict individual reactivity, including (1) the use of sympathetic and parasympathetic nervous system parameters [17, 59, 70]; (2) individual personality indices (psychomotor performance, mental efficiency with personality traits, etc.) [4, 6, 19, 20, 22, 51, 54, 60, 61]; and (3) cardiovascular indexes (e.g., heart rate, ECG) [4, 8, 9, 21, 28, 37, 55, 56, 58, 72, 74, 79].

More recently, investigators from the United States have also well recognized the individual variability in response to certain forms of interval high-altitude training (such as the living high-training low strategies), and they indicated that the exact mechanisms behind this variability remain obscure [24, 44]. Future research efforts clearly need to focus on defining the optimal dosing strategy for these devices, and determining the underlying mechanisms of the individual variability, in order to enable the individualized "prescription" and appropriate "dose" of altitude exposure to optimize the performance of each athlete.

23.3 Cellular and Molecular Basis of Individualized IHT

As the above-described historical survey, major physiological parameters within the respiratory, cardiovascular, endocrine, and others systems have been extensively studied in the field of intermittent hypoxia research for over a half of century [68]. Many of these investigations presented data that linked molecular biology to the physiological control of the body's response to hypoxia. During the past decades, this field has been rapidly transformed into the cellular and molecular levels, which would lead to a more accurate understanding of the organelles and their biochemical reactions at the subcellular level.

Studies of the mechanisms of individual variation to hypoxia have largely involved animal experiments following the demonstration that even within a single strain of rats, there was substantial variability in hypoxic tolerance. Using the endpoint of asphyxiation, animals could be separated at a specific barochamber-produced altitude (11,000 m) into high-resistant (HR), medium-resistant (MR), and low-resistant (LR) responders to acute hypoxia. The period of time up to the onset of the second agonal breath was recorded as the time needed for high-altitude asphyxia for each animal, after which animals were allowed to recover by adjusting the pressure in the chamber back to sea level. The average values of rat asphyxiation time were approximately 3 min in LR, 6 min in MR, and 10 min in HR [16, 47].

Although there are several possible causes for the variation of individual response to hypoxia (e.g., ventilatory sensitivity, circulatory adjustments, acid–base balance), much of the interest in the CIS has focused on mitochondria. In 1977, Lukyanova showed that rats with greater hypoxic resistance had a more active complex I mitochondrial enzyme than rats with low tolerance. In the more tolerant rat's brains, maximum activity and K_m of NADH-cytochrome c oxidoreductase were significantly higher than in rats with low hypoxia tolerance. Similar results were obtained in Kiev [16]. More recent data have been presented by Lukyanova and colleagues [48] and also in Chap. 20 (Lukyanova et al.).

Several concepts for how this theory could work were reviewed in details [68]. Briefly, the idea of mitochondrial involvement could be coupled to the NADH-cytochrome c oxidoreductase enzyme and its inactivation due to substrate saturation. This pathway can be influenced by mitochondrial parameters such as complex I mitochondrial enzyme activity or electron transport chain function in the NAD-cytochrome-b area. The enzyme α-ketoglutarate may also be involved by acting within the Krebs cycle to enhance the cholinergic status.

More recent research has shown that physiological mechanisms maintaining resistance to hypoxia and other extreme environmental stressors possess a common mitochondrial respiratory chain limit for free radical oxidation by means of nitric oxide. During hypoxic adaptation, nitric oxide (NO) production increases, leading to the generation of an active "reserve" for later needs [43]. NO reduces intracellular Ca^{2+} concentration, thereby inhibiting Ca^{2+} ATP-ase and raises the activity of antioxidant enzymes with concomitant expression of genes encoding them. Endogenous NO is capable of raising the K(m) of endothelial cytochrom-C-oxidase, and this suggests [30, 67] that endothelial cells can "feel" hypoxia and mediate hypoxic vasoconstriction through changing NO levels. NO can raise mitochondrial Ca^{2+} capacity of LR rats during IHT to control levels of HR animals. The mitochondrial Ca^{2+} capacity is one of the maintenance factors for calcium homeostasis during hypoxia [40].

Blood flow to tissues is controlled on a global scale by sympathetic tone and locally by factor that influence precapillary sphincters. However, at the cellular level, absorption and use of oxygen, which influences cell metabolism, is regulated by the reciprocal sympathetic and parasympathetic systems. A sharp PO_2 decrease causes changes in adreno- and cholinoreceptor sensitivity. In this autonomic system, NO modulates the sympathetic-parasympathetic ratio, thereby regulating oxygen consumption [33]. The adreno- and cholinoreceptor influence on plasma membranes is associated with selective oxidation of two Kreb's cycle substrates, succinate and alpha-ketoglutarate. Sympathetic regulation is predominant in LR rats while parasympathetic tone predominates in HR animals [41]. These results were confirmed by another comparative study in rats and guinea pigs [42]. Guinea pigs have a greater expression of cholinergic status in comparison to rats. Guinea pigs are more resistant to severe hypoxia during acute exposures to 7% O_2 for 30 min. This O_2 level provokes sharp augmentation of epinephrine, norepinephrine, and DOPA concentration in the rat blood but produces a decrease in catecholamines in guinea pigs. Examination of mitochondrial respiration revealed that the better adaptability of guinea pigs to acute hypoxia may be attributed to a decrease in oxygen consumption coupled with an increase in oxygen's effectiveness for ATP synthesis.

Mitochondrial ATP-dependent potassium channels (mK_{ATP}) play a significant role in interindividual differences in hypoxia resistance. To investigate the effects of mK_{ATP}, we used the fluorine-containing channel-opener flocalin while measuring miocardial tissue respiration in HR and LR rats [69]. In LR rats, intraperitoneal injection of flocalin provoked a sharp augmentation of ADP-stimulating mitochondrial respiration with an increased phosphorylation rate in the presence of succinate, i.e., the transition to an oxygen-preserved regimen. No changes in V_3/V_4 and ADP/O ratios were observed. In the HR rats, an identical manipulation did not produce changes in V_3, thus decreasing V_3/V_4 and ADP/O ratios. In the presence of α-ketoglutarate, an NAD-dependent substrate, the effects of flocalin became apparent in LR rats.

Both V_3 and V_4, in addition to the rate of phosphorylation increased with a concomitant decrease in the V_3/V_4 ratio and no change in the ADP/O ratio. Conversely, in HR rats, a significant inhibition of mitochondrial respiration was observed in the presence of α-ketoglutarate: (1) a decrease in V_3/V_4 by 50%, (2) a twofold augmentation of V_4, (3) a diminution of ADP/O by 25%, and (4) inhibition of the phosphorylation rate by 38%. The results indicate variable controls for mK_{ATP} channel opening in myocardial respiration for the animals with high and low resistance to acute hypoxia. These effects mirror the outcome of IHT on mitochondrial respiration in LR and HR animals.

Hypoxia-inducible factor 1 (HIF-1) has been identified as a master regulator for the expression of genes involved in the hypoxic response [63, 76]. HIF-1 has been suggested as a marker for the successful adaptation to different types of hypoxia [27, 34, 35, 71]. Some data showed that HIF-1 reflects individual variability of cardiorespiratory reactions of subjects overwintering in the Ukrainian Antarctic station "Academician Vernadsky." Therefore, HIF-1 could be used as a marker for selecting qualified individuals who would be able to work in critical hypoxic conditions [53]. This question demands further attention.

As one of well-known gene targets of HIF-1, erythropoietin (EPO) has been studied in relation to the individual response to the so-called Live High-Train Low (LHTL) mode of IHT, which resulted in a significantly greater improvement in maximal oxygen uptake (VO_2max) and performance than its equivalent sea-level training mode [24, 44]. A wide variability of the individual response to the IHT was reported in the examined athletes. In a retrospective analysis, the responders displayed a significantly larger increase in circulating EPO concentration after 30 h at altitude as compared with the nonresponders. After 14 days at altitude, EPO was still elevated in the responders but not in the nonresponders. The EPO response led to a significant increase in total red cell volume and VO_2max in responders, and such beneficial changes were not seen in the nonresponders. Furthermore, the acute increases in EPO and VO_2max following LHTL were also significantly higher in a prospective cohort of responders, compared with nonresponders [24]. Interestingly, a recent study in 26 US national class distance runners (17 males and 9 females) by the same group of investigators [25] demonstrated that the magnitude of EPO release at moderate altitude was not correlated with HVR (r=–0.17), regardless of genders. These authors concluded that the variability in the acute EPO response to moderate altitude cannot be explained by the differences in peripheral chemoresponsiveness in the elite distance runners [25]. Apparently, the factors acting downstream from the lung (most likely in the kidney) would influence the magnitude of the acute EPO response to altitude and in turn control the variable effects of IHT in different individuals.

Conclusion

Compelling results from various research groups suggested individual variability in response to hypoxia in humans and laboratory animals. The high hypoxic-resistant animals are characterized by (1) lower oxygen consumption at rest and during hypoxia, (2) prevalence of parasympathetic links to vegetative regulation, (3) increased kinetic properties of mitochondrial enzyme complex I, (4) predominance of NAD-dependent substrates for oxidation, (5) a higher level of NO production, (6) a more powerful antioxidant defense system, and (7) an increased mitochondrial capacity for calcium accumulation. However, there is a continued search for the potential universal marker(s) for individual prognosis of adaptation to hypoxia. Future investigations will shed light on this very important question. Collectively, we can envisage a bright future for individualized IHT, which may play a significant role in the fast-developing field of personalized preventive medicine against various human diseases.

References

1. Abrahams E, Silver M. The case for personalized medicine. J Diabetes Sci Technol. 2009;3:680–4.
2. Agadzhanyan NA, Mirrakhimov MM. Mountains and resistance. Moscow: Nauka Publishers; 1970 [In Russian].
3. Agadzhanyan NA. Adaptation and an organism's reserves. Moscow: Fizkultura i Sport; 1983 [In Russian].
4. Aidaraliev AA, Maksimov AL. Human adaptation to extreme conditions. The experience of prognosis. Leningrad: Nauka; 1988 [In Russian].
5. Aidaraliev AA, Maksimov AL, Chernook TB. Adaptation capabilities of polar explorers in Antarctic mountains. Kosm Biol Aviakosm Med. 1987;21(6):62–6 [In Russian].
6. Aydaraliev AA, Maksimov AL. Physical capacity estimation in the mountains. Methodical recommendations. Moscow: Nauka; 1980 [In Russian].
7. Aydaraliev A, Baevsky R, Berseneva T, et al. A framework for evaluating an organism's functional reserves. Frunze: Ilim; 1988. 195 pp [In Russian].
8. Baevsky RM. Prognosis of the body's position between normal and pathological condition. Moscow: Meditsina; 1979 [In Russian].
9. Baevsky RM. Principals of astronauts' health predictions and results of prognostic examinations during prolonged space expeditions. In: Physiological investigations of imponderability. Moscow: Nauka; 1983. p. 200–28 [In Russian].
10. Berezovski VA, Boyko A, Klimenko C, et al. Hypoxia and individual peculiarities of reactivity. Kiev: Nfukova Dumka; 1978 [In Russian].
11. Berezovski VA, Serebrovskaia TV. Ventilatory response to a hypercapnic stimulus as an index of the reactivity of the human respiratory system. Fiziol Zh. 1987;33(3):12–8 [In Ukrainian].
12. Berezovskii VA, Levashov MI. The build-up of human reserve potential by exposure to intermittent normobaric hypoxia. Aviakosm Ekolog Med. 2000;34(2):39–43 [In Russian].
13. Berezovskii VA, Serebrovskaia TV. Individual reactivity of the human respiratory system and its evaluation. Fiziol Zh. 1988; 34(6):3–7 [In Russian].

14. Berezovskii VA, Serebrovskaia TV, Ivashkevich AA. Various individual features of human adaptation to altitude. Kosm Biol Aviakosm Med. 1987;21(1):34–7 [In Russian].
15. Berezovskii VA, Serebrovskaia TV, Lipskii PI. Respiratory function in twins under different gas mixtures. Fiziol Zh. 1981;27(1):20–5 [In Russian].
16. Berezovsky VA, editor. Hypoxia: individual sensitivity and reactivity. Kiev: Naukova Dumka; 1978 [In Russian].
17. Bernardi L, Passino C, Serebrovskaya Z, Serebrovskaya T, Appenzeller O. Respiratory and cardiovascular adaptations to progressive hypoxia. Effect of interval hypoxic training. Eur Heart J. 2001;22:879–86.
18. Bhaumik G, Sharma RP, Dass D, et al. Changing hypoxic ventilatory responses of men and women 6 to 7 days after climbing from 2100 m to 4350 m altitude and after descent. High Alt Med Biol. 2003;4:341–8.
19. Bolmont B, Bouquet C, Thullier F. Relationships of personality traits with performance in reaction time, psychomotor ability, and mental efficiency during a 31-day simulated climb of Mount Everest in a hypobaric chamber. Percept Mot Skills. 2001;92:1022–30.
20. Burov A. System for valuation of the operators professional aging rates. Human factors in organizational design and management-VI. In: Proceedings of the sixth international symposium on human factors in organizational design and management. Hague, Netherlands; 19–22 Aug 1998.
21. Burtscher M, Bachmann O, Hatzl T, et al. Cardiopulmonary and metabolic responses in healthy elderly humans during a 1-week hiking programme at high altitude. Eur J Appl Physiol. 2001;84:379–86.
22. Bushov IuV, Makhnach AV, Protasov KT. Analysis of individual differences of psychological reactions to combined hypoxic exposure. Fiziol Cheloveka. 1993;19:97–103 [In Russian].
23. Chan IS, Ginsburg GS. Personalized medicine: progress and promise. Annu Rev Genomics Hum Genet. 2011;12:217–44.
24. Chapman RF, Stray-Gundersen J, Levine BD. Individual variation in response to altitude training. J Appl Physiol. 1998;85:1448–56.
25. Chapman RF, Stray-Gundersen J, Levine BD. Epo production at altitude in elite endurance athletes is not associated with the sea level hypoxic ventilatory response. J Sci Med Sport. 2010;13:624–9.
26. Collins DD, Scoggin CH, Zwillich CW, et al. Hereditary aspects of decreased hypoxic response. J Clin Invest. 1978;62:105–10.
27. Deindl E, Kolar F, Neubauer E, et al. Effect of intermittent high altitude hypoxia on gene expression in rat heart and lung. Physiol Res. 2003;52:147–57.
28. Dembo AR, Zemtsovski EV, Frolov BA. Echocardiogram and correlative rhythmography in sport. Leningrad: Nauka; 1979 [In Russian].
29. Eckes L. Altitude adaptation. Part III. Altitude acclimatization as a problem of human biology. Gegenbaurs Morphol Jahrb. 1976; 122:535–69 [In German].
30. Edmunds NJ, Moncada S, Marshall JM. Does nitric oxide allow endothelial cells to sense hypoxia and mediate hypoxic vasodilatation? in vivo and in vitro studies. J Physiol. 2003;546:521–7.
31. Egorov PI. Effect of high altitude flight on a pilot's body systems. Moscow: Medgiz; 1937 [In Russian].
32. Gurvich HE. Influence of high-altitudes on an organism. In: Krotkov FG, editor. Physiology and hygiene of high-altitude flights. Moscow-Leningrad: State Publishing House of the Biological and Medical Literature; 1938. p. 17–24 [In Russian].
33. Henry Y, Guissani A. Interactions of nitric oxide with hemoproteins: roles of nitric oxide in mitochondria. Cell Mol Life Sci. 1999;55:1003–14.
34. Hochachka PW, Rupert JL. Fine tuning the HIF-1 'global' O_2 sensor for hypobaric hypoxia in Andean high-altitude natives. Bioessays. 2003;25:515–9.
35. Hopfl G, Ogunshola O, Gassmann M. Hypoxia and high altitude. The molecular response. Adv Exp Med Biol. 2003;543:89–115.
36. Kawakami Y, Yamamoto H, Yoshikawa T, et al. Chemical and behavioral control of breathing in adult twins. Am Rev Respir Dis. 1984;129:703–7.
37. Kaznacheev VP, Baevsky RM, Berseneva AP. Prenosological diagnostics during screening tests of a specific human population. Leningrad: Nauka; 1980 [In Russian].
38. Kolchinskaya AZ. Mechanisms of interval hypoxic training effects. Hypoxia Med J. 1993;1:5–7.
39. Kolchinskaya AZ, Hatsukov BH, Zakusilo MP. Oxygen insufficiency: destructive and constructive actions. Nalchik: Kabardino-Balkaria Scientific Center; 1999 [In Russian].
40. Kurhaliuk NM. State of mitochondrial respiration and calcium capacity in livers of rats with different resistance to hypoxia after injections of L-arginine. Fiziol Zh. 2001;47:64–72 [In Ukrainian].
41. Kurhalyuk NM, Serebrovskaya TV, Kolesnikova EE. Role of cholino- and adrenoreceptors in regulation of rat antioxidant defense system and lipid peroxidation during adaptation to intermittent hypoxia. Probl Ecol Med Genet Cell Immunol, Kiev-Lugansk-Kharkiv. 2001;7(39):126–37 [In Ukrainian].
42. Kurhalyuk NM. Role of L-arginine on guinea pigs mitochondrial respiration in myocardium under acute hypoxia. Bull L'viv Univ ser Biol. 2002;29:177–86 [In Ukrainian].
43. Lapshin AV, Manukhina EB, Meerson FZ. Adaptation to short stress exposures prevents the enhancement of the endothelium-dependent reactions of the aorta in myocardial infarct. Fiziol Zh SSSR Im I M Sechenova. 1991;77(3):70–8 [In Russian].
44. Levine BD, Stray-Gundersen J. Dose-response of altitude training: how much altitude is enough? Adv Exp Med Biol. 2006;588:233–47.
45. Luk'ianova LD. Molecular mechanisms of tissue hypoxia and organism adaptation. Fiziol Zh. 2003;49(3):17–35 [In Russian].
46. Lukyanova LD. Molecular, metabolic and functional mechanisms of individual resistance to hypoxia. In: Sharma BK, Takeda N, Ganguly NK, et al., editors. Adaptation biology and medicine. New Dehli: Narosa Publishing House; 1997. p. 236–50.
47. Lukyanova LD, Korablev AV. Some physiological and metabolic characteristics of an animal's individual resistance to hypoxia. In: Proceedings of the third Soviet Union conference of adaptation. Moscow; 1982. p. 73–6.
48. Lukyanova LD, Dudchenko AV, Germanova EL, et al. Mitochondrial signaling in formation of body resistance to hypoxia. In: Xi L, Serebrovskaya TV, editors. Intermittent hypoxia: from molecular mechanisms to clinical applications. New York: Nova; 2009. p. 391–417.
49. Lysenko GI, Serebrovskaya TV, Karaban IN, et al. Use of the method of gradually increasing normobaric hypoxia in medical practice. Methodical recommendations. Kiev: Ukrainian Ministry of Healthcare; 1998 [In Ukrainian].
50. Maidikov YL, Makarenko NV, Serebrovskaya TV. Human mental activity during high altitude adaptation. Pavlov's J Higher Nerv Act (USSR). 1986;36(1):12–9.
51. Makarenko NV. Psychophysiological human functions and operator's work. Kiev: Naukova Dumka; 1991 [In Russian].
52. Malkin VB, Gora EP. Participation of respiration in rhythmic interactions in the body. Usp Fiziol Nauk. 1996;27(2):61–77 [In Russian].
53. Mankovska I, Bakunovsky O, Vargatiy C. Oxygen-transport systems in humans at rest and during physical work after a long-term wintering sojourn at Ukrainian Antarctic station "Academician Vernadsky". In: Proceeding of the 2nd Ukrainian Antarctic conference. Kiev; 22–24 June 2004. p. 11 [In Ukrainian].
54. Medvedev VI. Constancy of human physiological and pathological functions under extreme conditions. Leningrad: Nauka; 1982 [In Russian].
55. Mirrakhimov MM, Khamzamulin RO, Ragozin ON. Features of the ECG in acute altitude sickness. Kardiologiia. 1986;26(2):32–4 [In Russian].

56. Mirrakhimov MM, Aidaraliev AA, Maksimov AL. Prognostic aspects of physical activity at high altitudes. Frunze: Ilim; 1983 [In Russian].
57. Moore LG. Comparative human ventilatory adaptation to high altitude. Respir Physiol. 2000;121:257–76.
58. Navakatikyan AO, Kapshuk AP. Mathematical analysis of heart rhythm during work of different intensity. In: Mathematical methods of research planning, data analysis and prognosis in hygiene. Kiev: Zdorov'e; 1977. p. 34–41 [In Russian].
59. Negoescu R, Filcescu V, Boanta F, et al. Hypobaric hypoxia: dual sympathetic control in the light of RR and QT spectra. Rom J Physiol. 1994;31:47–53.
60. Nicolas M, Thullier-Lestienne F, Bouquet C, et al. A study of mood changes and personality during a 31-day period of chronic hypoxia in a hypobaric chamber (Everest-Comex 97). Psychol Rep. 2000;86:119–26.
61. Noel-Jorand MC, Joulia F, Braggard D. Personality factors, stoicism and motivation in subjects under hypoxic stress in extreme environments. Aviat Space Environ Med. 2001;72:391–9.
62. Rozenblyum DE. Adaptation to oxygen deficiency in short-term, repetitive exposure to low barometric pressure. Bull Exp Biol Med. 1943;21(7–8):6–9 [In Russian].
63. Semenza GL. HIF-1: mediator of physiological and pathophysiological responses to hypoxia. J Appl Physiol. 2000;88:1474–80.
64. Serebrovskaia TV. Hereditary defect of sensitivity to hypoxia in normal sensitivity to hypercapnia. Patol Fiziol Eksp Ter. 1982;4:80–3 [In Russian].
65. Serebrovskaia TV, Ivashkevich AA, Maidikov IL. The relation of the reactivity of the human respiratory system, mental and physical work capacity and metabolic characteristics during a 1-year stay in the mountains. Fiziol Zh. 1989;35(4):61–9 [In Russian].
66. Serebrovskaia TV, Lipskii PI. Levels of hereditary determination of human cardiorespiratory system functional indices. Fiziol Zh. 1982;28(3):267–73 [In Russian].
67. Serebrovskaya TV, Kurhalyuk NM, Nosar VI, et al. Combination of intermittent hypoxic training with exogenous nitric oxide treatment improves rat liver mitochondrial oxidation and phosphorilation under acute hypoxia. Fiziol Zh. 2001;47(1):85–92 [In Ukrainian].
68. Serebrovskaya TV. Intermittent hypoxia research in the former Soviet Union and the Commonwealth of Independent States (CIS): history and review of the concept and selected applications. High Alt Med Biol. 2002;3:205–21.
69. Serebrovskaya TV, Kurhalyuk NM, Moibenko AA et al. Effects of mitochondrial K_{ATP} stimulation on myocardial energy supply in rats with different resistance to hypoxia. In: Proceedings of the 5th international conference "Hypoxia in Medicine", Innsbruk; 2003. Hypoxia Medical J. 2003; 3:36.
70. Shakhtarin VV, Kiriachkov IuIu, IaM K, et al. The autonomic reaction of the body to stress and its prognostic value. Vestn Akad Med Nauk SSSR. 1990;3:33–7 [In Russian].
71. Shen C, Powell-Coffman JA. Genetic analysis of hypoxia signaling and response in *C. elegans*. Ann N Y Acad Sci. 2003;995:191–9.
72. Sirotinin NN. Effect of acclimatization to high mountain climate on adaptation to decreased atmospheric pressure using a decompression chamber. Arkh Pat Anat Pat Physiol. 1940;6:35–42 [In Russian].
73. Streltsov VV. Physiological validation of decompression chamber training for high altitude flights. Abstract of report at the All-Union conference on aerospace medicine. Leningrad; 1939. p. 18 [In Russian].
74. Tsvetkova AM, Tkatchouk EN. "Hypoxia user": the opportunity of individual programming of interval hypoxic training. In: Hypoxia: mechanisms, adaptation, correction. Moscow: BEBIM; 1999. p. 83–4.
75. Vasin MV, Petrova TV, Bobrovnitskii IP, et al. Human biochemical status and its relation to body resistance when exposed to acute hypoxic hypoxia. Aviakosm Ekolog Med. 1992;26(5–6):43–9 [In Russian].
76. Vogt M, Billeter R, Hoppeler H. Effect of hypoxia on muscular performance capacity: "living low-training high". Ther Umsch. 2003;60:419–24 [In German].
77. Waters KA, Gozal D. Responses to hypoxia during early development. Respir Physiol Neurobiol. 2003;136:115–29.
78. Weil JV. Variation in human ventilatory control: genetic influence on the hypoxic ventilatory response. Respir Physiol Neurobiol. 2003;135:239–46.
79. Zagryadsky VP. Selected lectures on physiology during military labor. Leningrad: Nauka; 1972 [In Russian].

Hypoxicators: Review of the Operating Principles and Constructions

24

Viktor A. Lopata and Tatiana V. Serebrovskaya

Abstract

Traditional treatment protocols for intermittent hypoxia training/therapy (IHT) comprises repeated exposures to low oxygen atmosphere breathing, altered with breathing ambient air. The rapid advance of IHT has led to the development of different medical equipment – hypoxicators – for its implementation in sport practice, military operations and also for clinical application. A variety of technical implementations for this treatment has been tested and used in recent decades, including hypobaric chambers, normobaric reduced oxygen rooms and mask-system hypoxicators, which produce hypoxic air in various ways. On the basis of hypoxicators classification, the overview of their design, medical and technical requirements is presented, and the perspectives of their development and industry trends are described as well as advantages and disadvantages of their operation.

Abbreviations

HGM Hypoxic gas mixture
IHT Intermittent hypoxic training/treatment

24.1 Introduction

Increasing use of intermittent hypoxic training/treatment (IHT) methods in sports, military and medical practices has stimulated active development of special devices for IHT implementation such as hypoxicators. The term of "hypoxicator" was suggested by Soviet scientists decades ago to describe a new class of devices for simulated altitude training of pilots, alpinists, mountain military personnel and sportsmen, as well as for drug-free treatment of a wide range of human disorders [34, 13, 23]. They are assigned for the forming and supply of a patient with hypoxic gas mixture (HGM) of the controlled composition. Variety of principles and constructive solutions have distinguished hypoxicators as a separate class of respiratory equipment, classified their designs and set medical and technical requirements for main parameters of hypoxicators.

Hypoxicators are classified based on three main criteria [11]: (1) methods for HGM supply; (2) methods for HGM formation; and (3) methods for regulation and maintenance of HGM composition.

24.2 Designs of the Hypoxicators

First division is based on the criterion of methods for HGM supply to a patient, i.e. mask or chamber (Fig. 24.1). The mask method stipulates the presence of flow circuit containing face mask with valves for inspiration/expiration and a buffer container for HGM in the line of inspiration. When using the chamber method, a patient's body or his head is placed directly into a chamber connected to HGM formation unit. Such chambers can be either hermetic (closed), filled with HGM, or nonhermetic (flow) through which HGM is blown into the chamber [3, 4, 5]. The chambers can be in a form of stationary devices, working rooms and portable tents, as well as movable devices.

V.A. Lopata • T.V. Serebrovskaya (✉)
Department of Hypoxia, Bogomoletz Institute of Physiology, National Academy of Sciences of Ukraine, Kiev 01024, Ukraine
e-mail: sereb@biph.kiev.ua

L. Xi, T.V. Serebrovskaya (eds.), *Intermittent Hypoxia and Human Diseases*,
DOI 10.1007/978-1-4471-2906-6_24, © Springer-Verlag London 2012

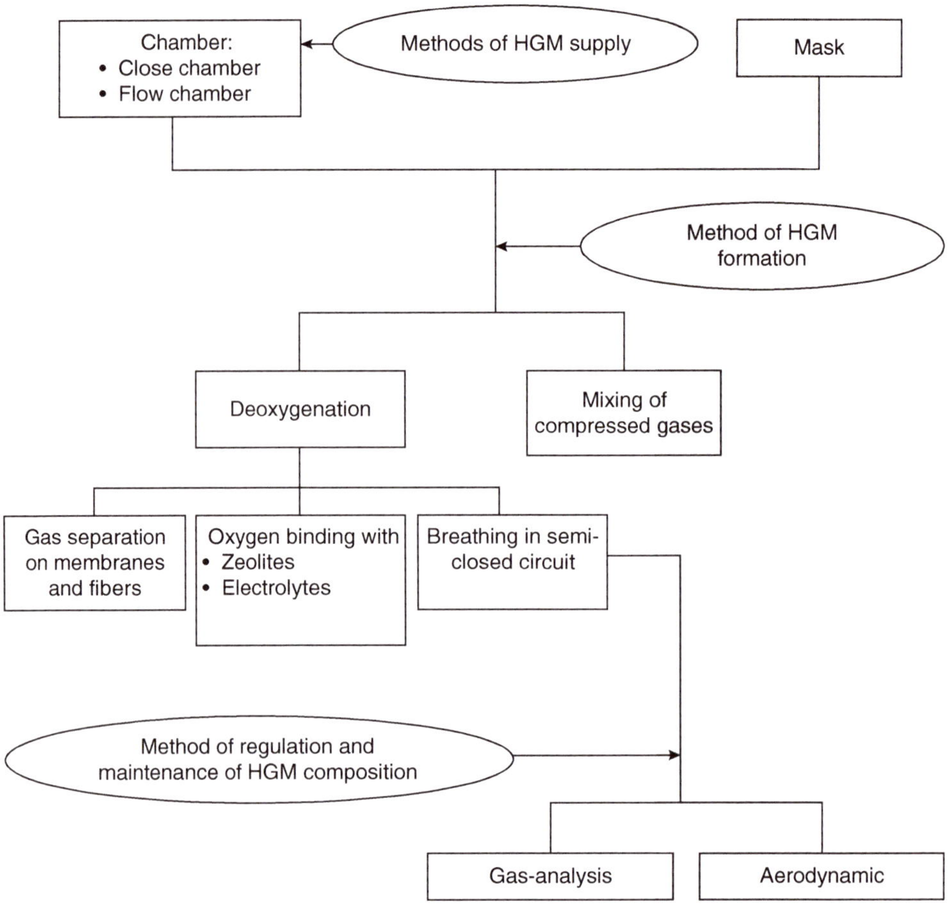

Fig. 24.1 Hypoxicators classification scheme

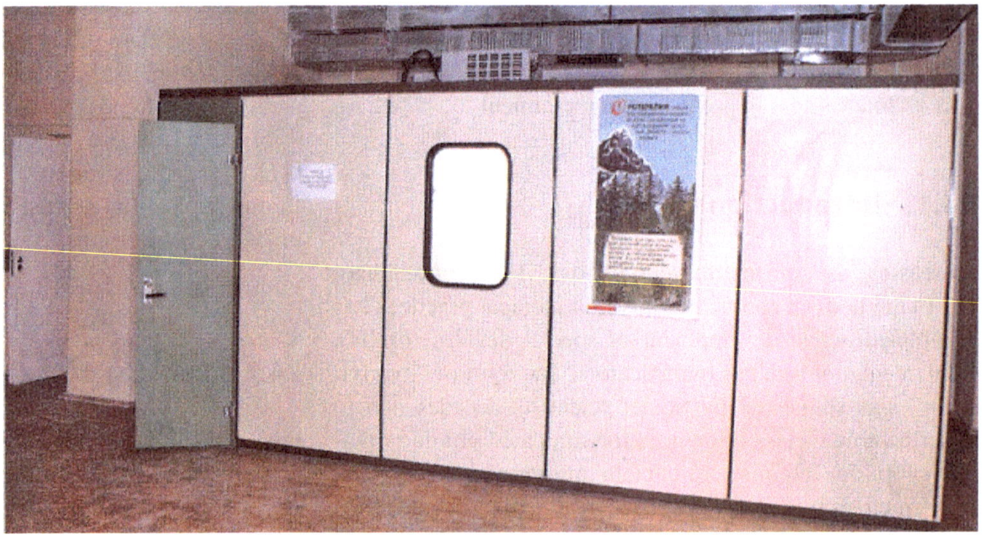

Fig. 24.2 Device "Orothron" (NORT, Kiev, Ukraine)

Device "Orothron" (NORT Company, Ukraine) has an overall dimension of 1,900 × 5,780 × 2,200 mm and volume of 19.9 m^3 and allows holding hypoxic therapy sessions for up to six patients simultaneously (Fig. 24.2).

Hypoxico Inc. (New York, USA) produces altitude sleeping systems like working rooms or portable tents (Fig. 24.3). The Altitude Chamber (home office or bed) offers the utmost in spacious and air-conditioned comfort and it is adjustable to 12,500 ft/3,800 m of simulated altitude. The portable Bed-Tent is Hypoxico's most universal altitude training system. It fits on the box spring of a queen size bed with the mattress inside, or on the floor with a twin/double/queen mattress inside.

Movable device "Borei-5" (NORT Company, Ukraine) consists of four main units: (1) control unit, (2) isolation

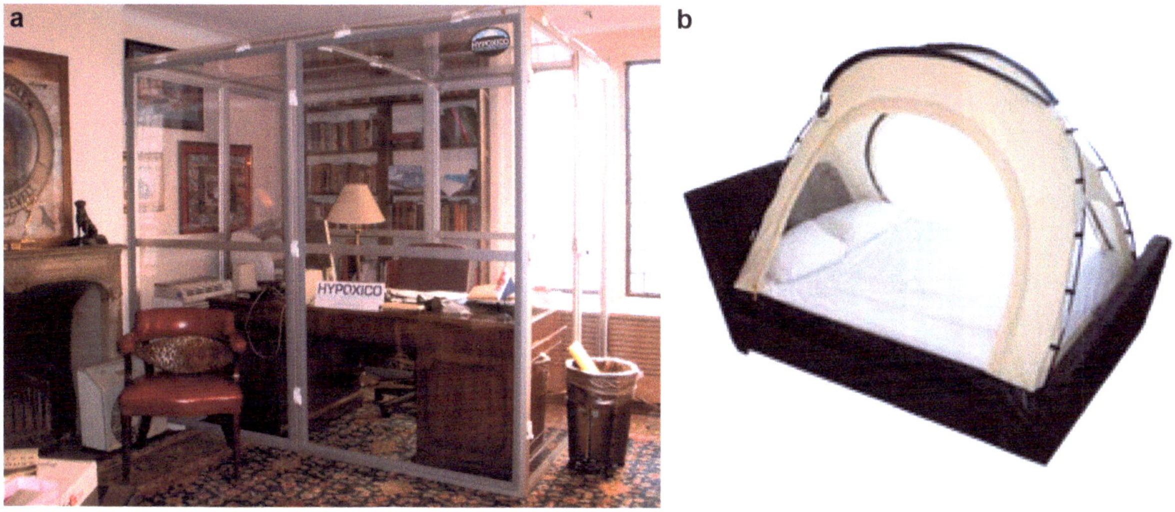

Fig. 24.3 Exterior view of working room (**a**) and portable tent for hypoxic therapy (**b**) (Hypoxico, Inc., USA, New York, USA) (http://www.hypoxico.com/altitude-sleeping-systems.shtml#DelBT)

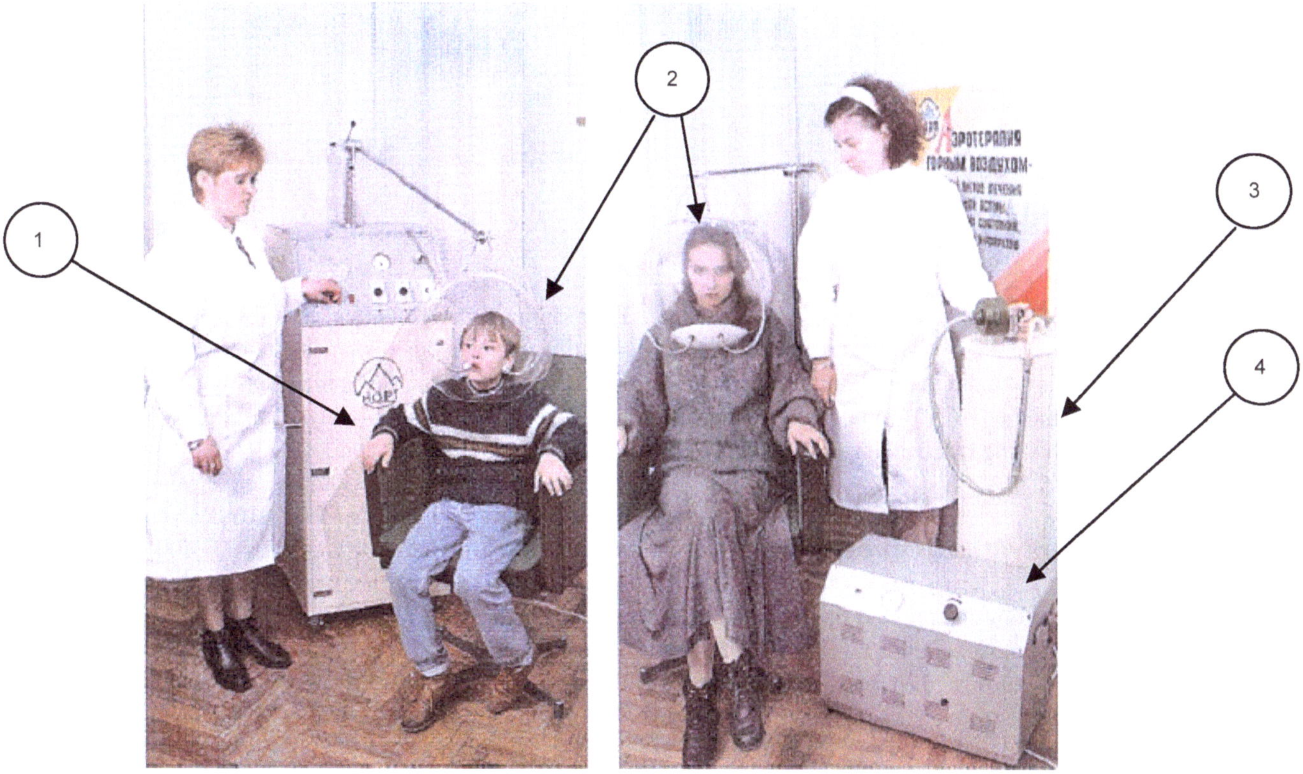

Fig. 24.4 Device "Borei-5" [14]

helmet, (3) gas-separating column and (4) compressor (Fig. 24.4). The device forms HGM no less than 40 L/min with oxygen content in the range of 10–16%. The overall dimensions are control unit, 1,300 × 600 × 600 mm; gas-separating column – ø 225 × 1,180 mm.

Hypoxic treatment complex "Edelweiss" (NVF METAKS Company, Moscow, Russian Federation), which uses membrane technologies, is equipped with monitoring system of internal environment and patient's physiological parameters (ECG, pO_2, arterial pressure, body temperature, respiratory rate, pulse oximetry) (Fig. 24.5). The complexes are produced in portable (for one patient) and stationary (for two, four, six and eight patients) variants. Device for one patient has the following technical characteristics: (1) air pressure in gas-separating unit is 0.5 ± 0.05 MPa; (2) percentage of oxygen in hypoxic mixture is 11 ± 2; (3) output is 15 ± 3 L/min; (4) power

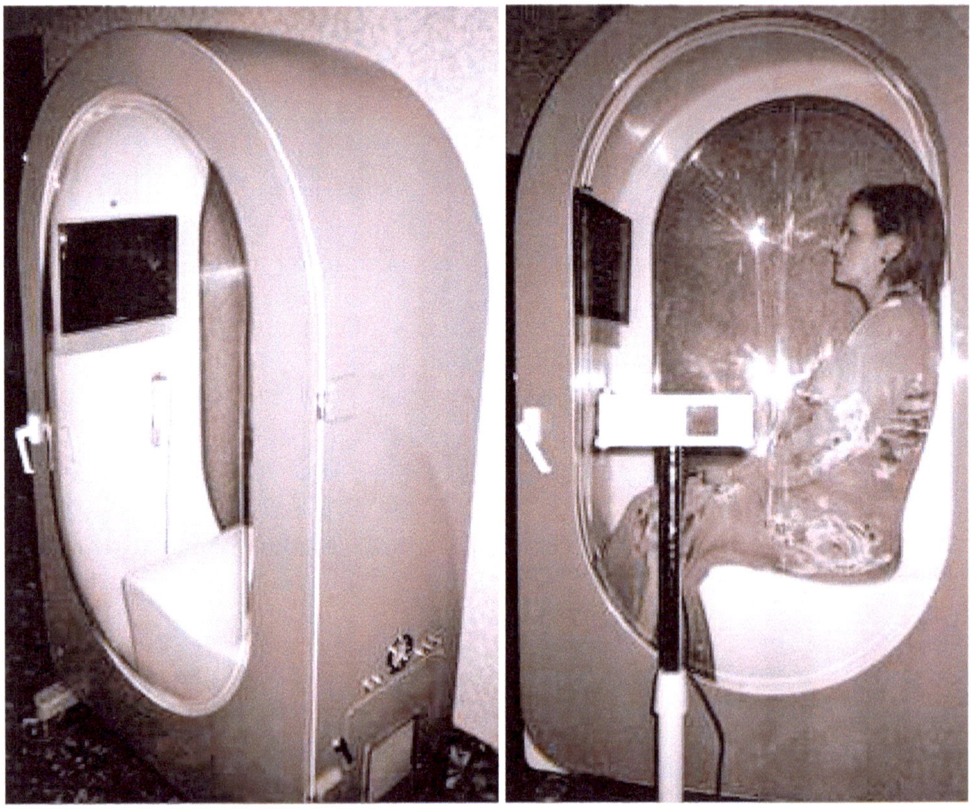

Fig. 24.5 Portable device "Edelweiss" (http://www.metax.ru/index.php?option=com_content&view=category&layout=blog&id=3&Itemid=9)

consumption is no more than 800 W; (5) weight of device without spare parts and accessories is no more than 25 kg; and (6) overall dimensions is no more than 700×250×550 mm.

Based upon the method of HGM formation, hypoxicators are divided into the following two categories (Fig. 24.1).

24.2.1 Hypoxicators with Compressed HGM

Gas mixture is formed from compressed or liquefied gases through the ejection of atmospheric air by the flow of compressed nitrogen in 1:1 ratio or through direct feeding of stable composition mixture from gas cylinder [13, 33]. Such devices are also called generative devices (NTO Bio-Nova Company, Moscow, Russian Federation, http://www.bion-ova.ru/?page=2). Ejection method of HGM formation with oxygen content in the range from 18% to 13.5% is used in AltiTrainer200 device (Fig. 24.6) produced by SMTEC S.A. (Nyon, Switzerland). Overall dimensions of the device are 650×400×580 mm; its weight (without nitrogen cylinder under the pressure of ≥0.3 MPa) is no more than 15 kg. However, while having certain technological advantages [5, 9], direct HGM feeding method is connected with the risk to use containers under 12–15 MPa pressure [11] and requires regular and expensive certification of mixture composition. For ensuring safety, a buffer reservoir is used in current constructions of hypoxicators. Such arrangement is used in 2-in-1 High Performance GO2Altitude Hypoxicator device produced by Biomedtech Australia Pty. Ltd., Melbourne, Australia (http://www.go2altitude.com) (Fig. 24.7). The device with power consumption of 1,500 W delivers IHT modes with HGM in oxygen range from 9% to 16%. Overall dimensions of microprocessor control unit are 400×400×230 mm and weight is 7 kg, whereas the overall dimensions and weight of ERA-II gas mixtures generator are 800×240×500 mm and 37 kg in weight.

24.2.2 Hypoxicators with Deoxygenation Process

Gas mixture is formed from atmospheric air using deoxygenating method. Deoxygenation can be carried out by one of the following approaches: (1) gas separation on membranes [31] or fibres [14], (2) separation of oxygen and nitrogen by solid electrolytes [13], (3) temporary binding of nitrogen by zeolites with further emission of nitrogen into the mixture [13], and (4) breathing in semi-closed flow circuit (rebreathing) [11, 19, 20]. Most of the currently manufactured hypoxicators use the methods of gas separation or rebreathing.

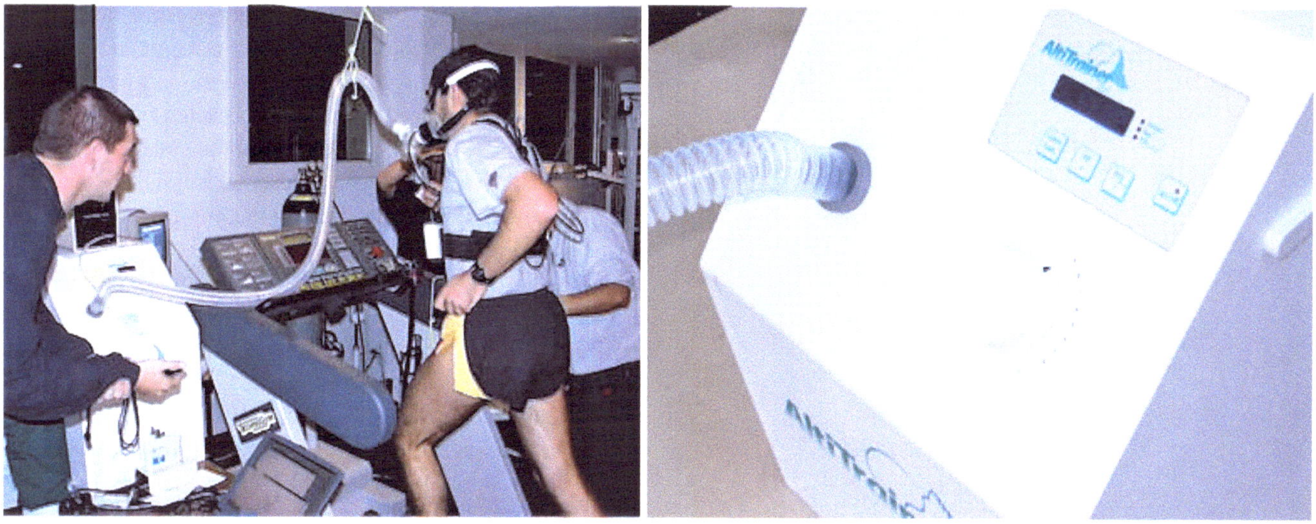

Fig. 24.6 Hypoxicator AltiTrainer200 (http://www.smtec.net/en/documents/altitrainer200_en.pdf)

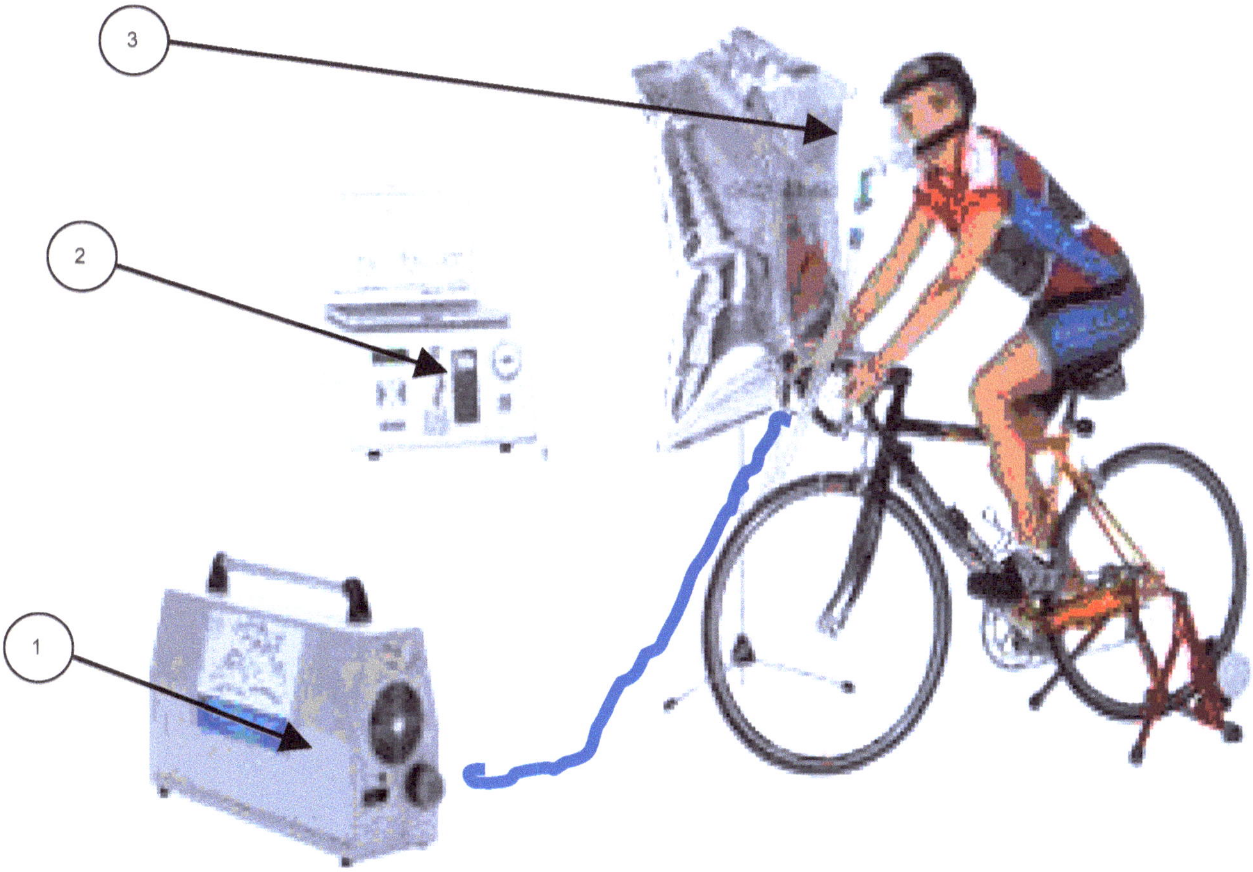

Fig. 24.7 2-in-1 High Performance GO2Altitude Hypoxicator: *1* – ERA-II gas mixtures generator; *2* – microprocessor control unit; *3* – 120 L buffer container

The speed of oxygen molecules transition through flat membrane or package of hollow fibres depends on the contact area with gas and differential pressure, which can reach 0.4 MPa to ensure necessary device output (12–15 L/min) [13]. Desired conditions require the inclusion of compressors to hypoxicators (Fig. 24.8). These compressors must be able to produce sufficiently high pressure and output while having low noise level without using piston-type devices (in order to

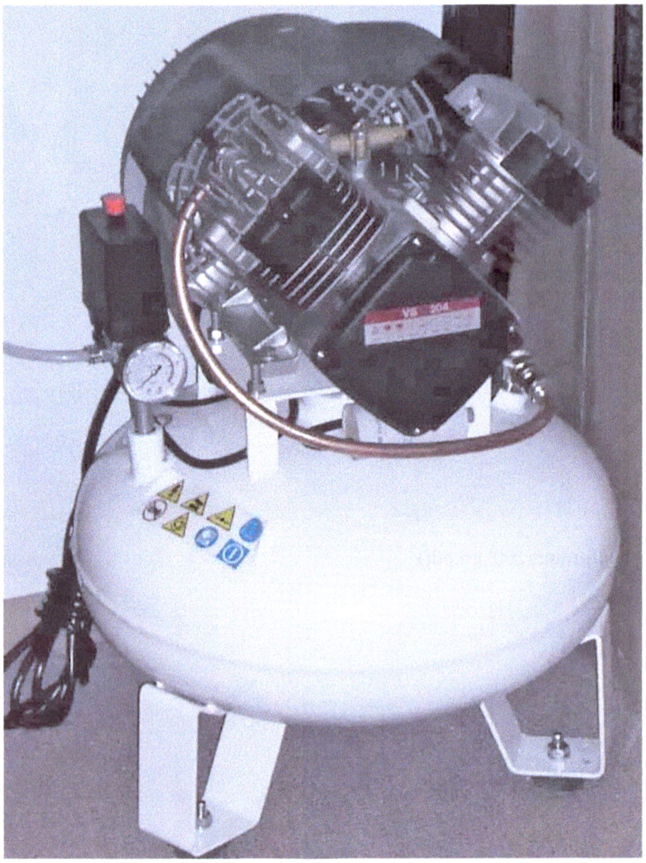

Fig. 24.8 Oil-free compressor as a part of hypoxicator with gas separation

avoid the contamination of gas-separating membranes and formed HGM by oil aerosol). The high price of such devices caused by the necessity to include compressor, gas analyzer and oxygen regulation system is compensated by their ability to work with up to eight patients simultaneously. The "Bio-Nova-204" device (Bio-Nova, Moscow, Russian Federation) has the embodiments depending on the number of simultaneously served patients (from 1 to 8) and the presence of additional standard equipment (Fig. 24.9). Individual IHT regimens are set and controlled by special computer programmes.

In addition, Climbi Company (Moscow, Russian Federation) offers a range of "Everest" hypoxicators in the market (Fig. 24.10). These hypoxicators allow to obtain oxygen concentration in HGM in the range from 10% to 18% and to serve up to four patients. Overall dimensions and weight of "Everest-1" model 08 M are 400 × 460 × 700 mm and 50 kg.

Among the various hypoxicators, a group of devices applying rebreathing principle in semi-closed flow circuit deserve special attention. In these devices named "autohypoxicators" [13], the line of expiration contains carbon dioxide absorber, while the circuit has pneumatic connection to the atmosphere through buffer reservoir, rigid or elastic [1]. In such devices, the process of HGM formation depends on three factors: (1) patient's oxygen consumption, (2) binding of carbon dioxide and (3) atmospheric air inflow into the circuit during inspiration. During rebreathing session the oxygen concentration gradually falls with time, which is very effective for sportsmen training and use at home [28].

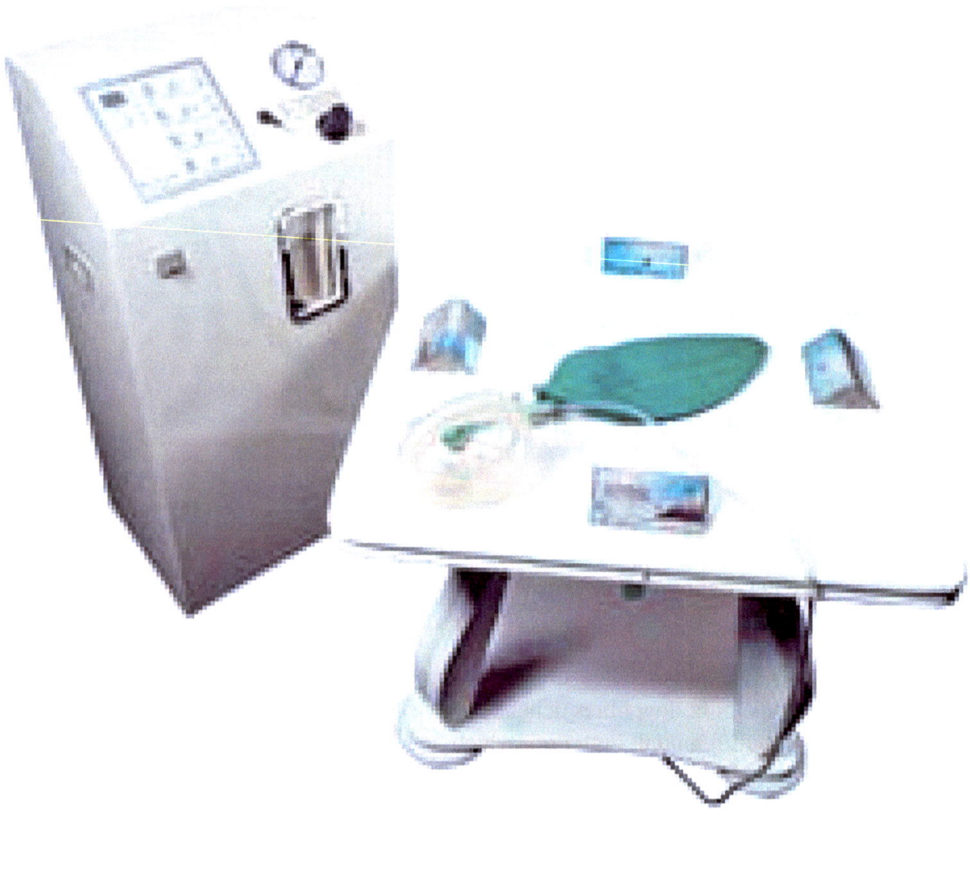

Fig. 24.9 Four-person device for hypoxic therapy "Bio-Nova-204"

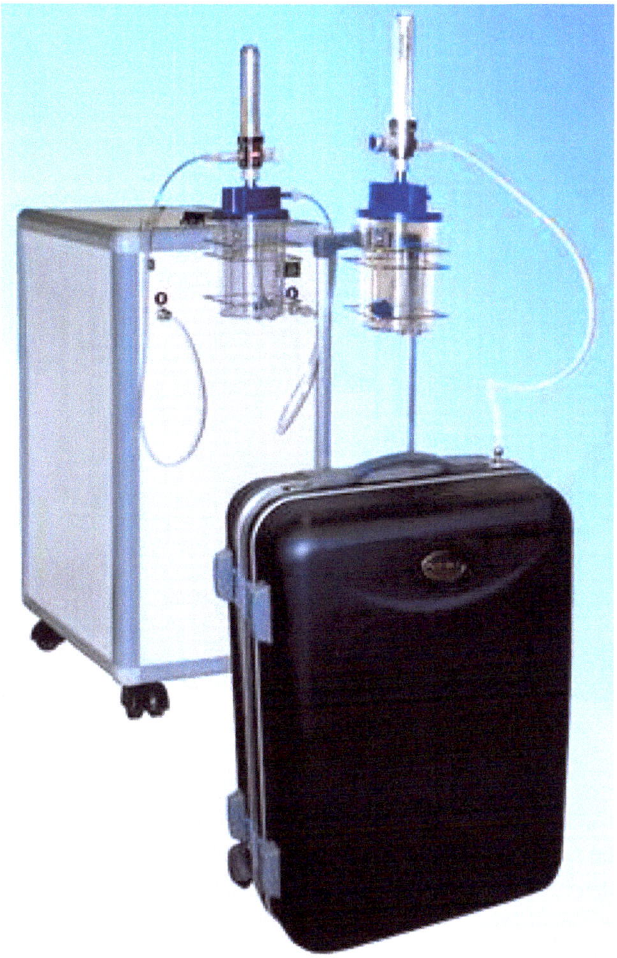

Fig. 24.10 Overview of "Everest-1" Hypoxicators: models 05 M and 08 M

In case of rigid buffer reservoir, which is many times bigger than breathing volume and has an outlet to the atmosphere [13], deoxygenation of gas mixture and its oxygenation by atmospheric air take place simultaneously during the process of breathing. Autohypoxicator with elastic buffer reservoir (Douglas bag or sylphon bellows) differs in certain special features of HGM formation, which depends on the parameters of patient's breathing and technical features of the device [15]. Significant advantage of such scheme is the possibility to use sylphon bellows as a spirometer to control the process of patient's pulmonary ventilation. This possibility is realized by the lines of oxygen feeding and control of oxygen content, which are included in the circuit as well as the transmitter of sylphon volume changes [24, 25].

The evolution of autohypoxicator constructions, which is reflected by the number of relevant patents awarded from 1987 to 2011, was aimed at simplifying the constructions and decreasing their weight and overall dimensions, as well as enhancing the safety for users. According to patents analysis, the safety is achieved due to the regulation and maintenance of HGM composition in the circuit at given level and a decrease of its respiratory resistance. These patented methods of regulation and maintenance of HGM composition can be classified as either gas analytic or aerodynamic. The gas-analysis-based method functions by the use of oxygen gas analyzer with the system of circuit blow-off when critically low level of oxygen content in HGM is reached [15]. For example, Biomedtech Australia PTY Ltd. (Melbourne, Australia) offers AltiPower Pro portable autohypoxicator, which was developed on the basis of a recent patent application [2] (Fig. 24.11). This type of hypoxicator is equipped with oxygen sensor and

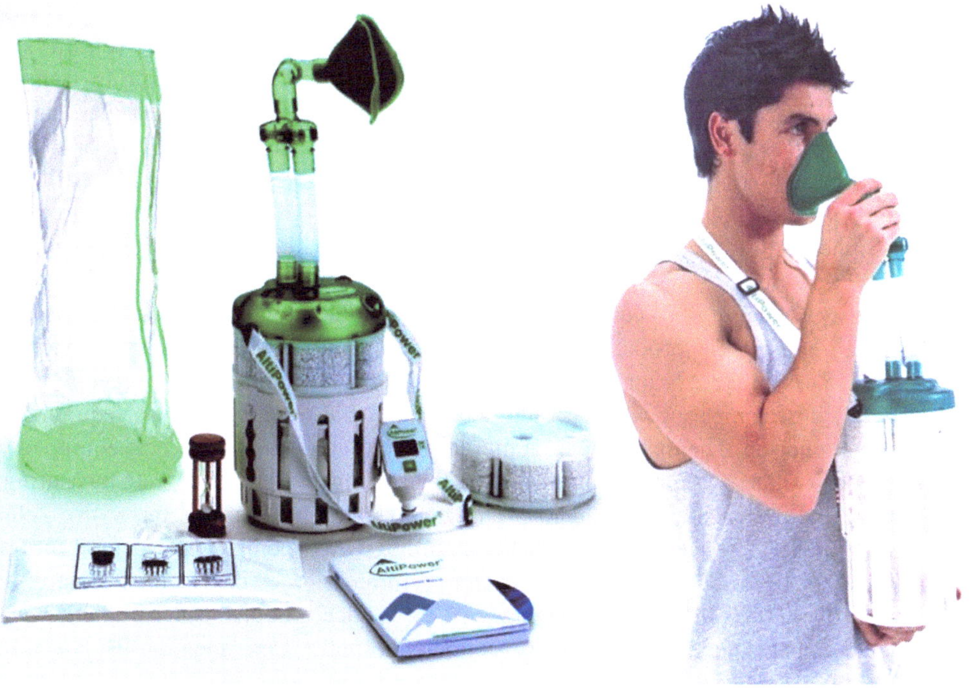

Fig. 24.11 AltiPower Pro autohypoxicator

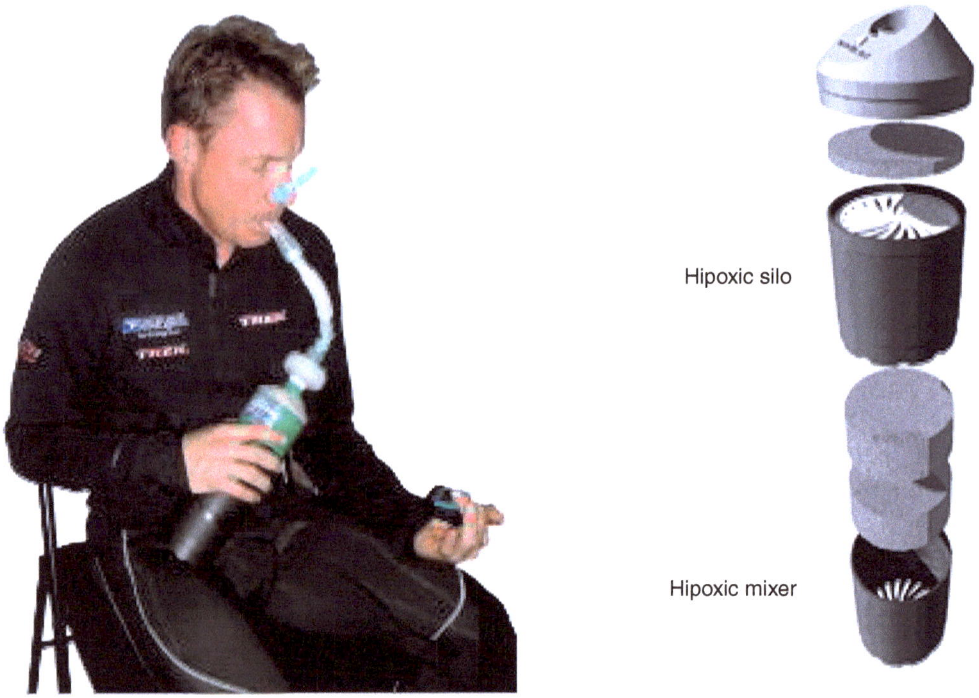

Fig. 24.12 AltoLab autohypoxicator

pulse oximeter to control the training mode. When the device is cyclically connected to gas analyzer, the arrangement of multi-seat IHT room on the basis of one gas analyzer is possible [13]. Similar device was also developed by AltoLab USA LLC (Phoenix, USA) (Fig. 24.12). Breathing circuit of the autohypoxicator includes a hypoxic unit (Hypoxic Silo) and a set of mixers (AltoMixer). The level of hypoxia generated depends on the number of mixers in the set.

There are various constructed components to regulate and maintain the HGM composition by aerodynamic resistance that connect buffer reservoir to the atmosphere. The ratio of resistance values, either constant or regulated, allows maintaining HGM composition within necessary range. Calibrated orifices of diaphragms [18, 26] or removable cap with calibrated holes [27, 30], spool valve air flow [17], movable flaps [35], change of cross-section of vent line which connects flow circuit to the atmosphere [6] are used as resistances.

The most widely used equipment in Russia is the "Vershyna" hypoxicator produced by METOM Company (Moscow, Russian Federation). This device consists of absorber with two nipples to which breathing bag and facial mask are connected. The mask is put on nipple, which has several open orifices with regulating numbers, thus changing the level of hypoxia (Fig. 24.13). The hypoxicator allows holding IHT sessions with oxygen content in HGM from 21% to 10%, CO_2 content <1.5% and respiratory resistance of up to 150 Pa. The advantages of the device include maximal simplicity of its construction, minimal overall dimensions and weight, and convenience of use. At the same time, there are several disadvantages, such as the difficulty to regulate precisely the oxygen concentration in HGM and the burden of changing absorbent after each IHT session.

24.3 Development of the Autohypoxicators

Autohypoxicators [22] advance the regulation of buffer reservoir volume (elastic sylphon bellows or flexible membrane with spring framework) according to the patient's anthropometric parameters by fixing sylphon bellows in certain position or by spiral movement of the spring (Fig. 24.14). The main trend of autohypoxicators perfection is the inclusion of biological feedback [9]. It presupposes the development of new basic schemes which must include (1) Devices for monitoring of respiratory function and cardiovascular system parameters and (2) IHT microprocessor control system. Advanced hypoxicators are adequately equipped with metrological channels and microprocessor equipment [2, 7]. As to autohypoxicators, they are at best equipped with oxygen analyzer and device for air flow rate measuring.

One of innovative solutions which foresees the use of comprehensive number of monitoring channels for microprocessor IHT mode control is patent application [21], which is implemented in the Device for Individual Hypoxic Regime Determination "Hypoxytron-Complex 2011" (Kiev, Ukraine).

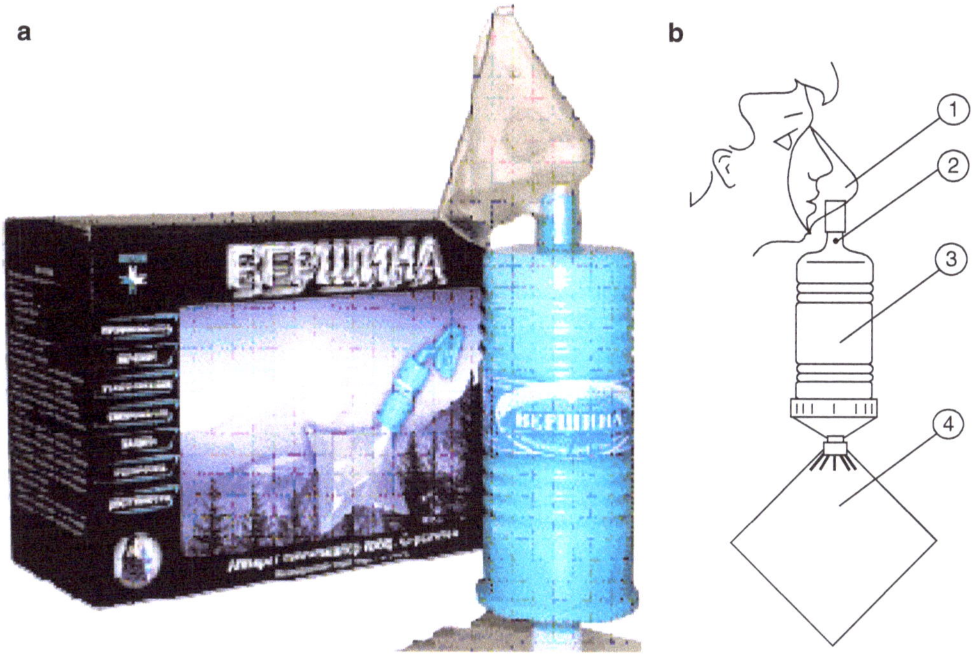

Fig. 24.13 Exterior view (**a**) and scheme (**b**) of "Vershyna" hypoxicator: *1* – mask; *2* – connection branch pipe; *3* – adsorber; *4* – breathing bag

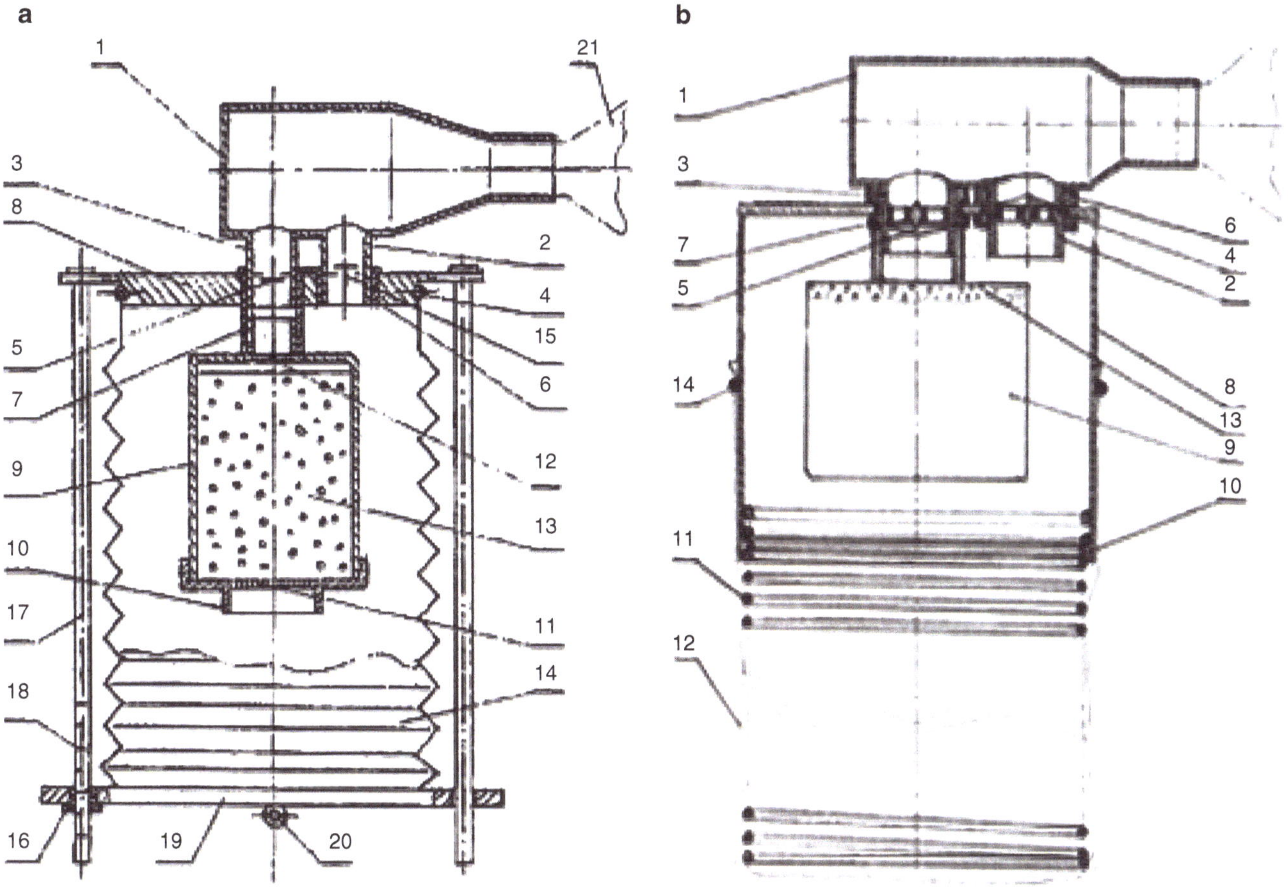

Fig. 24.14 Autohypoxicators with possibility of buffer container volume regulation: (**a**) "Hypoxydoz" with elastic sylphon [22]; (**b**) "Hypoxytron" with flexible membrane [20]

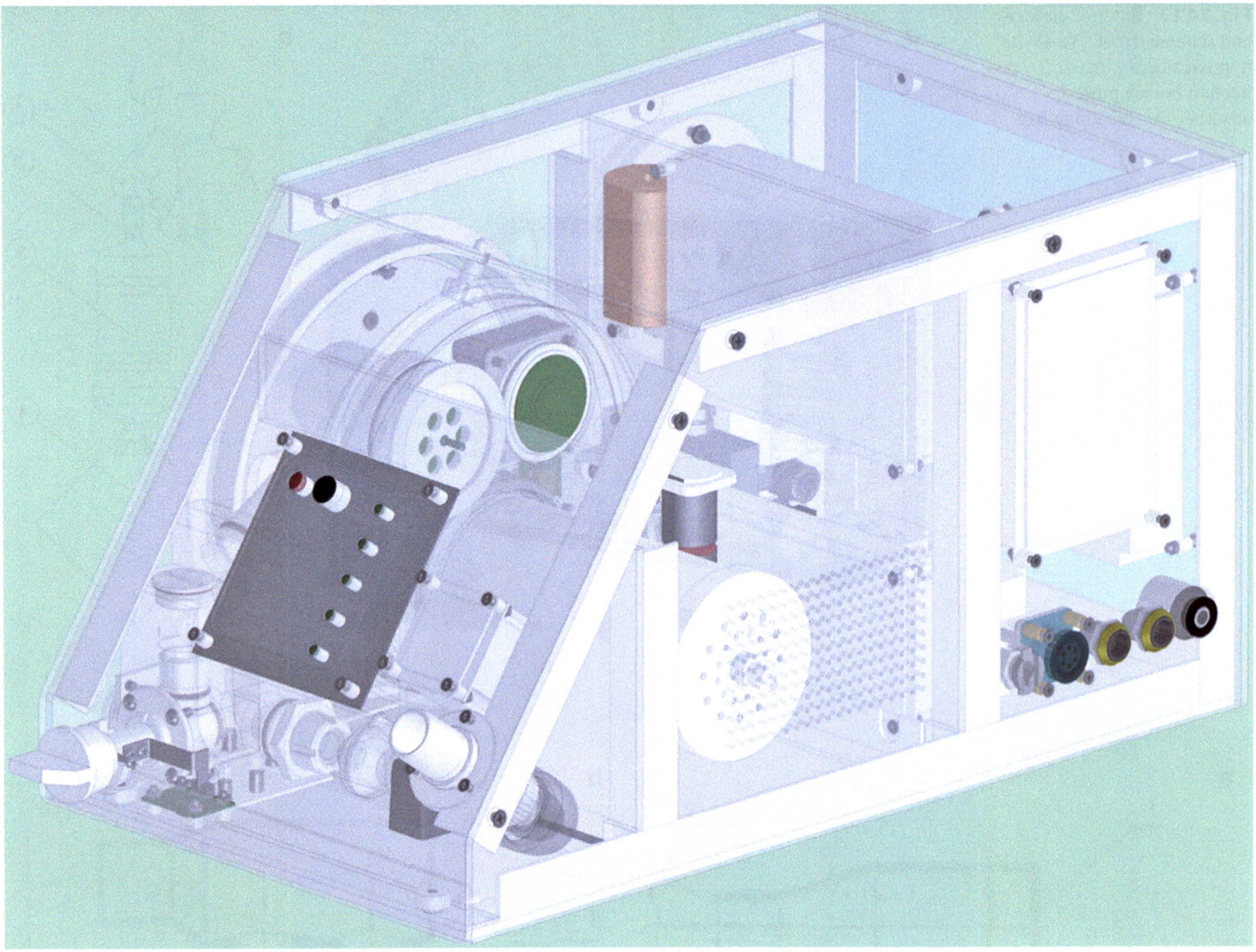

Fig. 24.15 Medical and diagnostic device "Hypoxytron-Complex 2011" (Kiev, Ukraine)

In this device, new methods for individual hypoxic training modes are introduced based upon patient's individual sensitivity to hypoxia (Fig. 24.15). "Hypoxytron-Complex 2011" device has the following scheme of diagnostics, prescription of IHT regimen and providing IHT:

1. *Preparatory stage*: Registration of a patient; questionnaire of health, spirography, hand dynamometry, squatting test; selection of inspired O_2 concentration for standard hypoxic test (14%, 12%, 10%, 9% or 8% O_2)
2. *Standard hypoxic test*: Conducting of the test (with the setting of alarm scopes for monitoring channels); estimation of results
3. *Hypoxic ventilatory response* (HVR, eucapnic rebreathing): Conducting of the test; estimation of results; selection of training regimen
4. *Conducting of Training/treatment sessions* (constant or increasing hypoxia) according to prescribed regimen.

24.4 Development and Use of the Advanced Autohypoxicators

The medical and diagnostic device "Hypoxytron-Complex 2011" can function perfectly together with the portable device "Hypoxytron-Simplex" (Kiev, Ukraine - IHT INTERNATIONAL LTD, New Zealand) for home or field usage (Fig. 24.16). After a subject goes through the testing using the Diagnostic Complex in medical or sports facility and receives the recommendations concerning the most efficient individual training mode, he or she masters the procedure using the Simplex device (which does not take long to do). Then it is possible to continue training at home, sports field, work place or any other environment with periodic testing at the Complex, so the hypoxic dose and training regime can be adjusted.

When defining areas of preferable hypoxicators usage, it should be noted that autohypoxicators are convenient virtually in all operating conditions for individual usage. Ejection

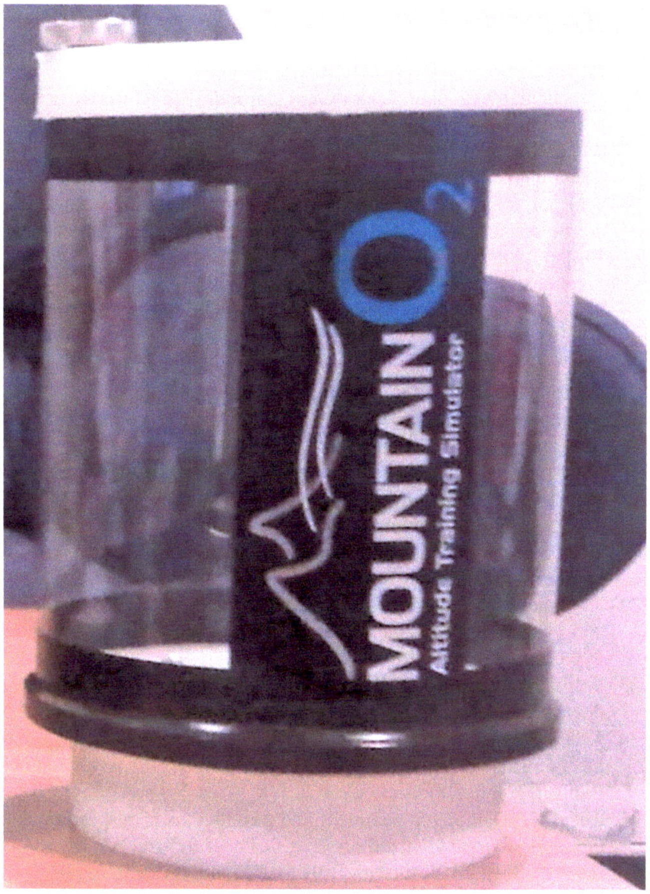

Fig. 24.16 Portable device "Hypoxytron-Simplex" (Kiev, Ukraine - IHT INTERNATIONAL Ltd, New Zealand) for home or field usage

devices are most suitable for use at organizations which can be constantly supplied with compressed nitrogen. Gas separation devices are suitable for the in-patient facilities that are not supplied with compressed nitrogen.

Based upon the methodical recommendations [10, 12, 16, 29, 32] and conditions of ensuring the patient's comfort while breathing with HGM, the main parameters and features of the hypoxicators described above must be set on the basis of the following norms and precautions [11]: (1) inspired oxygen content in HGM, from 8% to 20%; (2) respiratory resistance of flow circuit not more than 150 Pa•sec/l; (3) HGM productivity per one patient, from 9 to 20 L/min; (4) margin of error of oxygen content measurement, ± 0.5%; (5) excessive pressure at the inlet of HGM formation unit, 0.1–0.5 mPa; (6) excessive pressure of HGM at the outlet of mixture formation unit, 0.002–0.005 mPa; (7) excess of relative humidity of HGM over atmospheric air relative humidity, no less than 5%; (8) presence of threshold levels alarm system: content of oxygen in HGM, HGM productivity, oxygen saturation of patient's arterial blood (SpO_2) and heart rate; and (9) patient's minute ventilation must be ensured up to 100 L/min.

24.5 Summary

All the set of formulated medical and technical requirements can be applied to the most complex and multifunctional devices for conducting IHT, but in any case, the above-mentioned requirements 1–3 and 9 must be complied during the development of hypoxicators. Further development of the equipment for hypoxic therapy will be favoured by (1) improvement of gas analysis methods to better maintain HGM composition; (2) combination of IHT process with diagnostics of patient's respiratory and cardiac functions, which require inclusion of spirometrical and electrocardiographic measurement channels; (3) toughening of medical and technical requirements to the devices on criteria of flow circuit respiratory resistance, acceptable error of oxygen content measurement, safety of use; and (4) standardization of medical and technical requirements for hypoxic therapy equipment and software.

References

1. Basovich SN, Sergeev PV, Strelkov RB. Breathing device for hypoxia creation. Inventors certificate 1335294, A61M 16/00. Patent USSR, 07.09.87. Bulletin # 33; 1987 [In Russian].
2. Bassovitch O. Breathing apparatus for hypoxic pre-acclimatization and training. Patent Application Publication US 2006/0130639 A1, A62B 7/10, A62B 23/02. 22 June 2006.
3. Berezovski VA, Deinega VG, Zhuravlenko VJa et al. Device for climatotherapy. Inventors certificate 1526688, A 61 G, 10/00 Patent USSR, 7 Dec 1989. Bulletin #45; 1989 [In Russian].
4. Berezovski VA, Levashov MI. Introduction in orotherapy. Kiev: APG; 2000 [In Russian].
5. Berezovski VA, Rozhanchuk VN, Puh NN et al. Equipment for climatotherapy. Inventors certificate 1801440, A61G 10/00. 15 Mar 1993. Bulletin #10; 1993 [In Russian].
6. Henkin ML. Breathing method and apparatus simulating high altitude conditions. US Patent 4,334,533, A62B 7/10. 15 June 1982.
7. Kalakutski LI, Polyakov VA. Equipment for hypercapnic – hypoxic therapy. See http://eliman.ru/Lit/may96.html (1996) [In Russian].
8. Karash YuM, Strelkov RB, Chizhov AYu. Normobaric hypoxia in treatment, prophylaxis, and rehabilitation. Moscow: Meditsina; 1988 [In Russian].
9. Kolchinskaya A, Hatsukov B, Zakusilo M. Oxygen insufficiency – destructive and constructive action. Nalchik; 1999. p. 208.
10. Korkushko OV, Serebrovskaya TV, Shatilo VB et al. Selection of the optimal modes for intermittent hypoxia training in medical practice and sports medicine. Methodical recommendations. Kiev; 2010 [In Ukrainian].
11. Lopata VO, Berezovs'ky VIa, Levashov MI, et al. Classification and review of technical devices for hypoxia therapy. Fiziol Zh. 2003;49:100–5 [In Ukrainian].
12. Lysenko GI, Serebrovskaya TV, Karaban IN, et al. Use of the method of gradually increasing normobaric hypoxia in medical practice. Methodical recommendations. Kiev: Ukrainian Ministry of Health Care; 1998 [In Ukrainian].
13. Nemerovski LI. Construction principles of apparatus for intermittent normobaric hypoxia. Med Technika. 1992;1:3–8 [In Russian].

14. Orotherapy. Lectures of academy of hypoxia problems. Logos; 1998 [In Russian].
15. Reiderman EN, Trushin AI, Nemerovski LI et al. Device for breathing of hypoxic mixtures. Inventors certificate 1456161, A61M 16/00. Patent USSR, 7 Feb 1989. Bulletin #5; 1989 [In Russian].
16. Sakharchuk II, Denisenko GT, Serebrovskaya TV et al. Use of device "Hypotron" for prophylaxis and treatment of diseases in the conditions of radiation contamination. Methodical recommendations. Kiev; 1993 [In Russian].
17. Samolovov JuI, Strelkov RB. Breathing apparatus for hypoxytherapy. Inventors certificate 1599026, A61M 16/00. Patent USSR, 15 Oct 1990. Bulletin #38; 1990 [in Russian].
18. Scherbakova GN, Shnirev AP, Ksenofontov MI. Hypoxicator Inventors certificate 2167677, A61M 16/00. Patent USSR, Bulletin #15; 2001 [In Russian].
19. Serebrovska TV. Method for nonspecific body resistance increasing by means of intermittent hypoxic influences "Hypotron". Author's certificate PA #32, 6 Dec 1995 [In Ukrainian].
20. Serebrovska TV, Lopata VA, Roy VV et al. Device for breathing with hypoxic mixtures "Hypoxytron". Patent #44179, M A61M 16/00, Ukraine, 25 Sep 2009, Bulletin #18; 2009 [In Ukrainian].
21. Serebrovskaya T, Lopata V. Apparatus for breathing with hypoxic gaseous mixtures. Patent international application to all countries of PCT; PCT/UA 2010/000071, 7 Oct 2010, Completion of written opinion on 9 Mar 2011.
22. Serebrovskaya TV, Roitman EM, Lopata VA et al. Device for breathing with hypoxic mixtures "Hypoxydoz". Patent of the Ukraine #57257A, application #2002054442, 16 June 2003, Bulletin #6; 2003 [In Ukrainian].
23. Serebrovskaya TV. Intermittent hypoxia research in the former soviet union and the commonwealth of independent States (CIS): history and review of the concept and selected applications. High Alt Med Biol. 2002;3:205–21.
24. Slipchenko VG, Serebrovskaya TV, Sakcharchuk II et al. Mode of nonspecific body resistance improvement. Patent USSR #179958, A61M 16.00, 7 Mar 1993 [In Russian].
25. Slipchenko VG, Shulzhenko OF, Denisenko GT et al. Device for breathing with hypoxic mixtures "Hypotron". Author's certificate 45082 A, A61M16/00. 15 Mar 2002, Bulletin #3; 2002 [In Ukrainian].
26. Smirnov VF, Kamenev EA, Feldfebeleva GK. Breather. Inventors certificate 1526699, A61M 16/00. Patent USSR, 7 Dec 1989, Bulletin #45; 1989 [In Russian].
27 Stepanov SL. Breather for hypoxia creation. Inventors certificate 2070064, A61M 16/00. Patent USSR, 10 Dec 1996, Bulletin #34; 1996 [In Russian].
28. Strelkov RB, Chizhov AJa. Normobaric hypoxitherapy and hypoxiradiotherapy. Moscow: Nauka; 1998 [In Russian].
29. Strelkov RB. Normobaric hypoxia. Medical recommendations. Moscow; 1994 [In Russian].
30. Strelkov VB. Strelkov's breather. Patent 2040279, A61M 16/00. Patent USSR, 27 Jul 1995, Bulletin #21; 1995 [In Russian].
31. Tkachouk EN, Tsyganova TN, Staebler R. Apparatus for producing a hypoxic gaseous mixture using hollow fibers of poly-4-methilpenthene-1. US Patent 5,383,448, A62B 7/10, 24 Jan 1995.
32. Tsyganova TN, Egorova EB. Interval hypoxic training in obstetric and gynecologic practice. Methodical recommendations. Moscow; 1993 [In Russian].
33. Wartman R, Stiney M, Bower E et al. Reduced oxygen breathing device. US Patent 6,871,645 B2, A61M 16/00. 29 Mar 2005.
34. Xi L, Serebrovskaya TV. Intermittent hypoxia: from molecular mechanisms to clinical applications. New York: Nova Science Publishers Inc; 2009.
35. Zuev EG. Device for treatment and prophylaxis of respiration and circulation organs. Inventors certificate 1607817, A61M 16/00. Patent USSR, 23 Nov 1990, Bulletin #43; 1990 [In Russian].

25 Method of Combined Intermittent Hypoxia and Surface Muscle Electrostimulation for Enhancing Peripheral Stem Cells in Humans

Ginés Viscor, Casimiro Javierre, Teresa Pagès, Luisa Corral, Joan Ramon Torrella, Antoni Ricart, and Josep Lluis Ventura

Abstract

Short-term intermittent hypoxia exposure, at a level well tolerated by healthy humans and previously shown by our group to increase erythropoietin and erythropoiesis, could mobilize hematopoietic stem cells (HSC) and increase their presence in peripheral circulation. Four healthy male volunteers were subjected to three protocols: one with only hypoxic stimulus (OH), another with hypoxic stimulus plus muscle electrostimulation (HME), and the third with only muscle electrostimulation (OME). Intermittent hypobaric hypoxia exposure consisted of three sessions of 3 h inside a hypobaric chamber at a barometric pressure 535 hPa (equivalent to an altitude of 5,000 m) for 3 consecutive days. Muscular electrostimulation was performed in two separate periods of 25 min within each session. Blood samples were obtained from an antecubital vein on 3 consecutive days immediately before the experiment and 24, 48 h, 4, and 7 days after the last day of hypoxic exposure. There was a clear increase in the number of circulating $CD34^{+}$ cells but only after the experimental program combining hypobaric hypoxia and muscular electrostimulation. This response was not observed after the isolated application of the same stimuli. Our results open a new application field for intermittent hypobaric hypoxia as a way to increase peripheral HSC concentration. Muscle electrostimulation combined with hypoxia can be a useful tool for patients with a wide variety of conditions limiting classical physical exercise.

G. Viscor (✉) • T. Pagès • J.R. Torrella
Departament de Fisiologia i Immunologia, Universitat de Barcelona, Av. Diagonal, 643, E-08028, Barcelona, Spain
e-mail: gviscor@ub.edu

C. Javierre
Departament de Ciències Fisiològiques II, Universitat de Barcelona, IDIBELL, Feixa Llarga s/n, E-08907 L'Hospitalet de Llobregat, Barcelona, Spain

L. Corral
Departament de Ciències Fisiològiques II, Universitat de Barcelona, IDIBELL, Feixa Llarga s/n, E-08907 L'Hospitalet de Llobregat, Barcelona, Spain

Servei de Medicina Intensiva, Hospital Universitari de Bellvitge, IDIBELL, Feixa Llarga s/n, E-08907 L'Hospitalet de Llobregat, Barcelona, Spain

A. Ricart • J.L. Ventura
Servei de Medicina Intensiva, Hospital Universitari de Bellvitge, IDIBELL, Feixa Llarga s/n, E-08907 L'Hospitalet de Llobregat, Barcelona, Spain

Abbreviations

CXCR4	CXC receptor 4
EPO	Erythropoietin
FITC	Fluorescein isothiocyanate
G-CSF	Granulocyte colony-stimulating factor
HME	Hypoxic stimulus plus muscle electrostimulation
HSCs	Hematopoietic stem cells
IH	Intermittent hypoxia
OH	Only hypoxic stimulus
OME	Only muscle electrostimulation
SCs	Stem cells
SDF1	Stromal-derived factor 1

L. Xi, T.V. Serebrovskaya (eds.), *Intermittent Hypoxia and Human Diseases*, DOI 10.1007/978-1-4471-2906-6_25, © Springer-Verlag London 2012

25.1 Introduction

Stem cells (SCs) are primitive cells with the potential to differentiate into mature cells [2]. An increase in SCs is observed after various events such as myocardial infarction [15], dilated myocardiopathy [45], cardiac surgery with cardiopulmonary bypass [36], 12 weeks of physical exercise [19, 44], menstruation [27], cessation of smoking [22], and in animals or human cells subjected to deep hypoxia conditions in vitro [16, 17, 34, 53].

Several studies have found that elevated concentrations of SCs correlate with better clinical outcomes [51], since they have a general regenerative capacity in blood vessel disorders [28]. Various methods of SC delivery have been shown to be beneficial, mostly with autologous bone marrow cell transplantation [10, 33, 43]. No significant differences were found when bone marrow cells or SCs from peripheral blood were compared [3], nor when bone marrow cells were compared with adipose tissue-derived SCs [49].

An erythropoietin (EPO)-induced increase in hematopoietic stem cells (HSCs) has been detected in healthy individuals and in patients with renal anemia at 2 weeks after administration of EPO [4], correlating with physiological and hematological improvements [9, 35, 37, 38]. Moreover, EPO-induced mobilization and homing of HSCs and their mediated neovascularization have also been reported in rats after post-myocardial infarction heart failure after 6 weeks of treatment [52].

Intermittent hypoxia (IH) has been shown to be physiologically beneficial in various groups of healthy and ill people [8, 20, 41].

IH exposure sessions have been used to improve the physical condition and to treat several illnesses, mostly in the countries of the former Soviet Union, although this was done without a clear understanding of their holistic effects [40]. At all events, this practice has now become widespread in the world of competitive sport, and there are even several commercialized forms of IH exposure available. Hypoxia exposure has been combined with normal athletic training according to different patterns [26], the most widely adopted being the living-high training-low model [25]. Different types and intensities of physical exercise have been showed to be capable of mobilizing SCs [6, 29, 46]. However, various forms of standard physical exercise can be difficult to apply with hypoxic procedures, especially in patients with severe obesity, osteoarticular conditions, neurological sequelae, etc. In contrast, muscle electrostimulation is easier to apply and has been shown to be as efficient in reproducing training effects [7, 11, 23]. On the other hand, intermittent hypobaric hypoxia exposure is an efficient stimulus for eliciting different adaptive responses to improve peripheral oxygen supply [12, 13, 30, 31].

The objective of this chapter is to describe a new hypobaric hypoxia application to increase blood SC concentration. The IH application tested here consisted of few short-term sessions at levels well tolerated by healthy humans and previously shown by our group to be capable of increasing EPO and stimulate erythropoiesis [37]. The effect of the hypoxic stimulus is considered both alone and in combination with muscular electrostimulation.

25.2 Short Intermittent Hypobaric Hypoxia Exposure Protocol and Surface Muscle Stimulation

25.2.1 Subjects and Procedures

Subjects were four healthy males, without toxic habits or medication and with different levels of habitual physical activity (one jogger, 4 days/week; one gym user, also 4 days/week; and two without regular physical training). Their mean age was 54.3 (range 46–60), mean height 175 cm (range 170–182), and mean body mass 85.5 kg (range 75–89). They were each subjected to three different protocols: one with only hypoxic stimulus (OH), another with hypoxic stimulus plus muscle electrostimulation (HME), and the third with only muscle electrostimulation (OME). In order to avoid undesired interactions, each experimental protocol was performed at least 3 months after the preceding one. The hypobaric hypoxia stimulus was applied in a computer-controlled hypobaric chamber (CHEx-1; Moelco, Spain) for 3 h on 3 consecutive days, always from 5 to 8 a.m. (subjects having spent the previous week following the habitual diet and physical activity and with no detected illnesses or chronobiological changes); the simulated altitude was 5,000 m (400 mmHg = 535 hPa), reached in 10 min and returning to sea level pressure in 15 min.

Muscle electrostimulation was applied by means of a Winform Stimulation System (Model W5 multi frequency training, Winform S.r.l., Venice, Italy) according to a widely accepted procedure as described elsewhere [5]. Surface electrodes were fixed on both knee extensors and abdominal wall muscles. Stimulation was achieved at the maximal tolerated intensity (regulated individually by each experimental subject) during two periods of 25 min: one in the first-half period of hypobaric chamber stay (90 min) and the other in the second 90-min period of stay. The protocol of OME was the same as HME and also took place inside the hypobaric chamber. However, as the door was open, there was no hypoxic stimulus. Oxygen arterial saturation was measured at rest during each hypoxia exposure session by means of a pulsioxymeter (Onyx II 9550, Nonin Medical Inc., Plymouth, MN). The study was conducted according to the Helsinki Declaration, and the experimental protocol was approved by the institutional University of Barcelona Ethics Committee.

25.2.2 Blood Sampling, CD34⁺ Staining, and Flow Cytometry Assay

In order to detect possible individual oscillations, baseline blood samples were drawn on each of the 3 days prior to the first experiment (OH). Subsequently, blood samples were always obtained just before each of the experimental sets (OH, HME, and OME) and 24, 48 h, 4 and 7 days later. In the third protocol (OME), an additional sample was taken 10 days after the end of muscular electrostimulation. All samples were obtained between 8:15 and 8:30 a.m. following the same extraction methodology as detailed below. Samples were preserved, without any previous processing, at a temperature between 4°C and 6°C until transfer to the hematology laboratory. There, they were processed according to a blinded design (the technicians involved had no knowledge of either the experimental subject or the protocol).

Peripheral blood samples were collected by puncture of an antecubital vein and placed in tubes treated with 0.34 M dipotassium ethylenediaminetetraacetic acid anticoagulant. All samples were stored at 4°C and processed within 24 h of arrival at the laboratory. Blood cell count was assessed by use of an automatic cell counter (Ac·T-diff; Beckman Coulter, Miami, FL). Samples were incubated for cytometric absolute count with antihuman fluorescein isothiocyanate (FITC)-conjugated CD45 monoclonal antibody (Beckman Coulter, clone J.33) and antihuman phycoerythrin (PE)-conjugated anti-CD34 (clone 8G12, Becton Dickinson) in PBS containing 1% albumin and 0.1% sodium azide for 15 min at room temperature. Red blood cells were lysed with 1 mL of quick lysis solution (CYT-QL-1, Cytognos) for 15 min at room temperature. Samples were incubated in the dark and analyzed immediately. To ensure accuracy, reverse pipetting was used to dispense the volumes.

A single-platform protocol with Perfect-Count Microspheres CYT-PCM-50 (Cytognos, Salamanca, Spain) was used according to the manufacturer's instructions. The Perfect-Count Microspheres system contains two different fluorospheres in a known proportion (A and B beads), thus assuring the accuracy of the assay by verifying the proportion of both types of beads. Known volumes (25 μL) of Perfect-Count Microspheres were added to the same known volume (25 μL) of stained blood in a lyse/no-wash technique, and the beads were counted along with the cells. Cell viability was measured by staining the samples with the vital dye 7-aminoactinomycin D (7-AAD), as proposed by the ISHAGE guidelines [21]. Samples were analyzed on a FACScan/Calibur flow cytometer (BD Biosciences) with a 488-nm argon laser and Cell Quest 3.1 software (BD Biosciences). The instrument was aligned and calibrated daily using a three-color mixture of Calibrite™ beads (BD Biosciences) with FACSComp software (BD Biosciences). The gating strategy also followed ISHAGE guidelines [21].

25.3 Additive Effects of Intermittent Hypobaric Hypoxia Exposure and Surface Muscle Electrostimulation on Circulating CD34⁺ Cells

The main result of the present study is the synergic capacity of a short-term IH stimulus plus surface-electrode muscle electrostimulation to increase the circulating concentrations of hematopoietic CD34⁺ stem cells in a group of four healthy men aged around 50 years of age. Only the HME experimental data set showed a clear increase for all the subjects (about threefold) in the percentage of circulating CD34⁺ cells. Moreover, the number of circulating CD34⁺ cells increased in this experiment from a median value of 0.95 cells·μL^{-1} (range: 0.5–2.1) to a median level of 6.65 cells·μL^{-1} (range: 3.7–10.7); this increase being highly significant ($p = 0.009$) (Fig. 25.1).

This increase can be considered as substantial, because it is generally accepted that a concentration of 7 cells/μL is equivalent to approximately 5×10^5 cells·kg^{-1} in an adult subject. This concentration can be assumed to be useful for harvesting purposes and corresponds to a considerable fraction of the increase in CD34⁺ cells obtained after a standard 5-day treatment involving 2-day doses of granulocyte colony-stimulating factor (G-CSF). It also seems that the increases in CD34⁺ produced by G-CSF have a nonprogressive tendency, as reported in a study of patients with myocardial infarction, in whom circulating CD34⁺ levels began to decrease the day after the fourth consecutive dose of G-CSF, reaching the previous concentrations between days 6 and 10 after the end of G-CSF treatment [48]. In the present study, CD34⁺ levels appear to continue increasing 7 days after the last hypoxia session, and thus, it is not clear whether a plateau or maximum value was reached. It should also be taken into account that G-CSF shows some pro-thrombotic effects [14, 18]. Other lines of hematological studies can be of interest, for instance, the most important chemokine involved in endothelial progenitor cells mobilization is thought to be stromal-derived factor 1 (SDF1), and CXC receptor 4 (CXCR4) is the predominant receptor for SDF1 and is widely expressed by many tissues including hematopoietic cells and endothelial cells. The precise mechanism of action of CXCR4 has yet to be elucidated, although it may be implicated in mobilization from different niches [47]. CXCR4 enhances engraftment of muscle progenitor cells in mice, suggesting a possible role in the treatment of some muscular dystrophies [32].

No other studied leukocyte parameter showed changes in this experimental block. Furthermore, neither OH nor OME experimental data showed statistically significant changes across the study for general leukocyte parameters or circulating CD34⁺ cells. The lack of response in the OME experiment does not seem attributable to the age of the participants, since a clear HSC response to physical exercise was detected in a group of 63-year-old men [19]. However, there are two

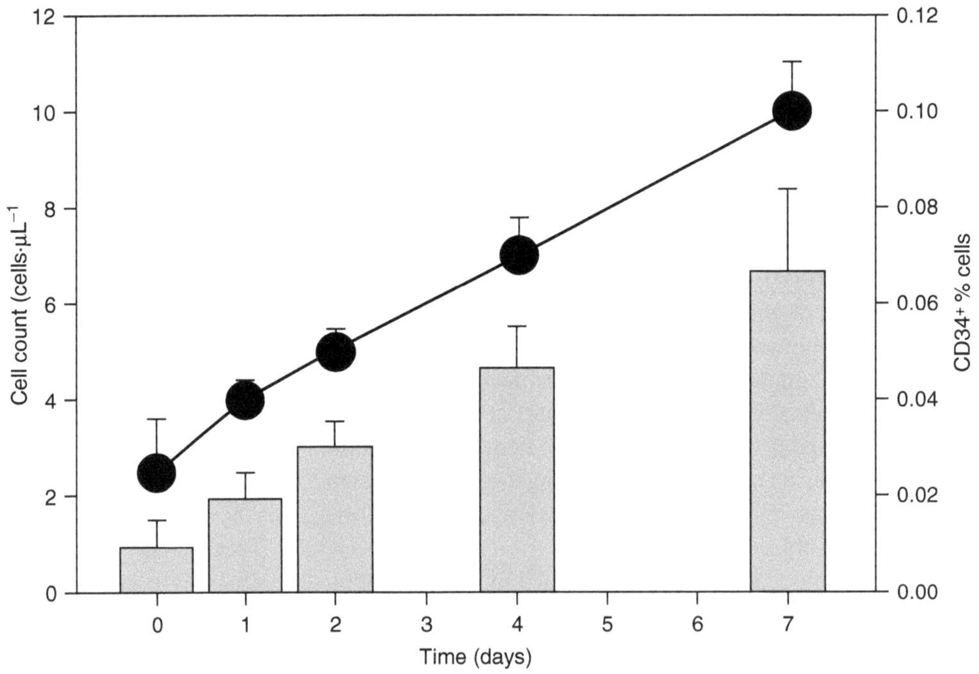

Fig. 25.1 CD34⁺ cells after hypobaric hypoxia and muscle electrostimulation. Time course of the CD34⁺ cell count (*left axis*; *bars*) and percentage (*right axis*; *circles*) after a program of 3 consecutive days of daily hypobaric hypoxia sessions combined with surface muscle electrostimulation during hypobaric exposure (HME experimental set). Category medians and positive standard errors are shown for the two variables. A statistically significant increase for CD34⁺ concentration (cells·µL⁻¹) was found ($p=0.009$)

alternative explanations for these findings. First, there was a relatively short duration of the hypoxic stimulus (a total of 9 h), whereas positive neurogenesis in rats was demonstrated after applying a hypoxic stimulus of 4 h/day over 2 weeks [53], while other studies detected a positive SC response to physical exercise after about 3 months of routine physical activity [19, 44]. Myocardial infarction was enough to increase the number of CD34⁺ cells after 7 days [42], and a single bout of intense exercise increases HSC 24–48 h later [1, 24]. Second, the low intensity of the stimulus in our study (used in order to be applied and tolerable to a large majority of healthy people) compared with some in vitro studies, in which more severe hypoxic atmospheres were used [17, 34]. Obviously, a higher number of repeated hypoxia sessions could be applied; however, it does not seem reasonable to use much more intense sessions (higher simulated altitude), as these might not be so well tolerated by some patients. On the other hand, longer hypoxic sessions could have a greater interference on daily activities and make the protocol much more difficult to comply.

It is also worth noting some of the advantages of muscular electrostimulation over exercise during hypoxia exposure: (a) it is easy to measure and reproduce; (b) it can be applied in a hypoxic atmosphere (hypobaric chamber or breathing a hypoxic mixture); and (c) it can be applied to most humans, even those with mild or severe physical limitations for standard exercise. It is not clear from the present study whether muscular electrostimulation should necessarily be applied simultaneously during hypoxia exposure.

The major limitations of the present study are the short total duration of the hypoxic stimulus in OH (which was sufficient in HME) and the small sample size. However, given the clarity of the data obtained, it does not seem likely that a larger sample size would produce different results. The lack of a more complete hematologic study means we cannot rule out the possibility that the CD34⁺ increase is caused by a decrease in "homing" mechanisms in possible target tissues, although this does not seem a likely phenomenon in this case.

The optimal stimulation timing in order to produce a stable increase in CD34⁺ cells with this procedure remains to be established, although the apparent maintained effect observed (CD34⁺ increasing 7 days after the stimulus) suggests that some repeated "doses" might alone be enough.

Further studies are required to address several questions derived from our current research: (a) elucidating the possibility that the OH or OME stimulus applied via more persistent schedules or by other means might also induce a measurable increase in HSC. A recent study [39] has found consistent results with a normobaric hypoxia exposure program that was able to enhance innate immunity by mobilizing HSC, activating neutrophils, and increasing circulating complement and immunoglobulins; (b) evaluating the potential repercussions of the CD34⁺ increases on different pathologies: it might be possible to increase HSC homing in injured tissues because after the release of HSCs from bone marrow, cells home to ischemic or damaged regions via alterations of the affected tissue [50]; (c) determining the most efficient protocols to induce an optimal and maintained increase in HSC; and (d) meeting the need for a more exhaustive study of the possible subclasses of HSC released under HME conditions.

Conclusions

A simple protocol stimulating healthy humans with hypoxia plus muscle electrostimulation can quickly induce a notable increase in blood HSC. Muscle electrostimulation can be a useful tool for patients with a wide variety of conditions limiting classical physical exercise. The significant differences obtained when combining hypoxic stimulus and muscle contraction, over such a short period of time, coupled with the ease of application of these two combined stimuli, make this method an interesting tool to increase peripheral HSC concentration. This can be a cheaper, noninvasive alternative to G-CSF treatment in blood banks and hemotherapy units for the improvement of HSC collection. A wide variety of different tools and programs of intermittent hypoxia (hypobaric or normobaric) exposure should be examined with a view to possible future application in the treatment of several pathologies, in order to evaluate their possible favorable effects and their persistence.

Acknowledgments The authors are grateful to Dr. Gregorio Martín-Henao and Ms. Carmen Azqueta from Unitat de Teràpia Cel·lular (Centre de Transfusió i Banc de Teixits) for their key contribution in HSC quantification. We also acknowledge Mr. Víctor Gómez for his kind support to our research group and for his critical participation in the installation of the hypobaric chamber and annexed facilities. We are also grateful to Mr. Juan A. Silva from Universidad de Antofagasta (Chile) by his collaboration in some data collection, and to Mr. Robin Rycroft (Language Advice Service, Universitat de Barcelona) for his useful help in editing the manuscript. Finally, we wish to express our gratitude and appreciation to Prof. Ramon Segura for his mentoring tasks of our research group and to Prof. Luis Palacios for his support and ideas and his pioneering impulse on hypobaric studies.

Competing Interests This study was performed without support from any public or private fund, agency, or company. The authors declare that they have no competing interests. This chapter is based on a previous study that was published in J Transl Med (2009) 7:91.

References

1. Adams V, Lenk K, Linke A, et al. Increase of circulating endothelial progenitor cells in patients with coronary artery disease after exercise-induced ischemia. Arterioscler Thromb Vasc Biol. 2004; 24:684–90.
2. Asahara T, Murohara T, Sullivan A, et al. Isolation of putative progenitor endothelial cells for angiogenesis. Science. 1997;275:964–7.
3. Assmus B, Schachinger V, Teupe C, et al. Transplantation of progenitor cells and regeneration enhancement in acute myocardial infarction (TOPCARE-AMI). Circulation. 2002;106:3009–17.
4. Bahlmann FH, de Groot K, Spandau J, et al. Erythropoietin regulates endothelial progenitor cells. Blood. 2004;103:921–6.
5. Bennie SD, Petrofsky JS, Nisperos J, et al. Toward the optimal waveform for electrical stimulation of human muscle. Eur J Appl Physiol. 2002;88:13–9.
6. Bonsignore MR, Morici G, Riccioni R, et al. Hemopoietic and angiogenetic progenitors in healthy athletes: different responses to endurance and maximal exercise. J Appl Physiol. 2010;109:60–7.
7. Brocherie F, Babault N, Cometti G, et al. Electrostimulation training effects on the physical performance of ice hockey players. Med Sci Sports Exerc. 2005;37:455–60.
8. Burtscher M, Pachinger O, Ehrenbourg I, et al. Intermittent hypoxia increases exercise tolerance in elderly men with and without coronary artery disease. Int J Cardiol. 2004;96:247–54.
9. Casas M, Casas H, Pagès T, et al. Intermittent hypobaric hypoxia induces altitude acclimation and improves the lactate threshold. Aviat Space Environ Med. 2000;71:125–30.
10. Cashen AF, Lazarus HM, Devine SM. Mobilizing stem cells from normal donors: is it possible to improve upon G-CSF? Bone Marrow Transplant. 2007;39:577–88.
11. Crameri RM, Weston A, Climstein M, et al. Effects of electrical stimulation-induced leg training on skeletal muscle adaptability in spinal cord injury. Scand J Med Sci Sports. 2002;12:316–22.
12. Esteva S, Panisello P, Torrella JR, et al. Blood rheology adjustments in rats after a program of intermittent exposure to hypobaric hypoxia. High Alt Med Biol. 2009;10:275–81.
13. Esteva S, Panisello P, Ramon Torrella J, et al. Enzyme activity and myoglobin concentration in rat myocardium and skeletal muscles after passive intermittent simulated altitude exposure. J Sports Sci. 2009;27:633–40.
14. Falanga A, Marchetti M, Evangelista V, et al. Neutrophil activation and hemostatic changes in healthy donors receiving granulocyte colony-stimulating factor. Blood. 1999;93:2506–14.
15. Ferrario M, Massa M, Rosti V, et al. Early haemoglobin-independent increase of plasma erythropoietin levels in patients with acute myocardial infarction. Eur Heart J. 2007;28:1805–13.
16. Flames N, Pla R, Gelman DM, et al. Delineation of multiple subpallial progenitor domains by the combinatorial expression of transcriptional codes. J Neurosci. 2007;27:9682–95.
17. Grayson W, Zhao F, Bunnell B, et al. Hypoxia enhances proliferation and tissue formation of human mesenchymal stem cells. Biochem Biophys Res Commun. 2007;358:948–53.
18. Gutierrez-Delgado F, Bensinger W. Safety of granulocyte colony-stimulating factor in normal donors. Curr Opin Hematol. 2001;8:155–60.
19. Hoetzer GL, Van Guilder GP, Irmiger HM, et al. Aging, exercise, and endothelial progenitor cell clonogenic and migratory capacity in men. J Appl Physiol. 2007;102:847–52.
20. Katayama K, Ishida K, Iwasaki K, et al. Effect of two durations of short-term intermittent hypoxia on ventilatory chemosensitivity in humans. Eur J Appl Physiol. 2009;105:815–21.
21. Keeney M, Chin-Yee I, Weir K, et al. Single platform flow cytometric absolute CD34+ cell counts based on the ISHAGE guidelines. International Society of Hematotherapy and Graft Engineering. Cytometry. 1998;34:61–70.
22. Kondo T, Hayashi M, Takeshita K, et al. Smoking cessation rapidly increases circulating progenitor cells in peripheral blood in chronic smokers. Arterioscler Thromb Vasc Biol. 2004;24:1442–7.
23. Koutedakis Y, Frischknecht R, Vrbova G, et al. Maximal voluntary quadriceps strength patterns in Olympic overtrained athletes. Med Sci Sports Exerc. 1995;27:566–72.
24. Laufs U, Urhausen A, Werner N, et al. Running exercise of different duration and intensity: effect on endothelial progenitor cells in healthy subjects. Eur J Cardiovasc Prev Rehabil. 2005;12:407–14.
25. Levine BD, Stray-Gundersen J. "Living high-training low": effect of moderate-altitude acclimatization with low-altitude training on performance. J Appl Physiol. 1997;83:102–12.
26. Levine BD. Intermittent hypoxic training: fact and fancy. High Alt Med Biol. 2002;3:177–93.
27. Meng X, Ichim T, Zhong J, et al. Endometrial regenerative cells: a novel stem cell population. J Transl Med. 2007;5:57.

28. Miller-Kasprzak E, Jagodzinski PP. Endothelial progenitor cells as a new agent contributing to vascular repair. Arch Immunol Ther Exp (Warsz). 2007;55:247–59.
29. Mobius-Winkler S, Hilberg T, Menzel K, et al. Time-dependent mobilization of circulating progenitor cells during strenuous exercise in healthy individuals. J Appl Physiol. 2009;107:1943–50.
30. Panisello P, Torrella JR, Esteva S, et al. Capillary supply, fibre types and fibre morphometry in rat tibialis anterior and diaphragm muscles after intermittent exposure to hypobaric hypoxia. Eur J Appl Physiol. 2008;103:203–13.
31. Panisello P, Esteva S, Torrella R, et al. Intermittent hypobaric hypoxia induces changes at a different extent in biochemical parameters depending on muscle activity degree. Comp Biochem Physiol A Mol Integr Physiol. 2007;146:S184.
32. Perez AL, Bachrach E, Illigens BM, et al. CXCR4 enhances engraftment of muscle progenitor cells. Muscle Nerve. 2009; 40:562–72.
33. Perin EC, Dohmann HF, Borojevic R, et al. Transendocardial, autologous bone marrow cell transplantation for severe, chronic ischemic heart failure. Circulation. 2003;107:2294–302.
34. Qiang X, Shaoxia W, Xijuan J, et al. Hypoxia-induced astrocytes promote the migration of neural progenitor cells via vascular endothelial factor, stem cell factor, stromal-derived factor-1α and monocyte chemoattractant protein-1 upregulation in vitro. Clin Exp Pharmacol Physiol. 2007;34:624–31.
35. Ricart A, Casas H, Casas M, et al. Acclimatization near home? Early respiratory changes after short-term intermittent exposure to simulated altitude. Wilderness Environ Med. 2000;11:84–8.
36. Roberts N, Xiao Q, Weir G, et al. Endothelial progenitor cells are mobilized after cardiac surgery. Ann Thorac Surg. 2007;83: 598–605.
37. Rodriguez FA, Ventura JL, Casas M, et al. Erythropoietin acute reaction and haematological adaptations to short, intermittent hypobaric hypoxia. Eur J Appl Physiol. 2000;82:170–7.
38. Rodriguez FA, Casas H, Casas M, et al. Intermittent hypobaric hypoxia stimulates erythropoiesis and improves aerobic capacity. Med Sci Sports Exerc. 1999;31:264–8.
39. Serebrovskaya TV, Nikolsky IS, Nikolska VV, et al. Intermittent hypoxia mobilizes hematopoietic progenitors and augments cellular and humoral elements of innate immunity in adult men. High Alt Med Biol. 2011;12:243–52.
40. Serebrovskaya TV. Intermittent hypoxia research in the former Soviet Union and the Commonwealth of independent states: history and review of the concept and selected applications. High Alt Med Biol. 2002;3:205–21.
41. Shatilo VB, Korkushko OV, Ischuk VA, et al. Effects of intermittent hypoxia training on exercise performance, hemodynamics, and ventilation in healthy senior men. High Alt Med Biol. 2008;9:43–52.
42. Shintani S, Murohara T, Ikeda H, et al. Mobilization of endothelial progenitor cells in patients with acute myocardial infarction. Circulation. 2001;103:2776–9.
43. Stamm C, Westphal B, Kleine HD, et al. Autologous bone-marrow stem-cell transplantation for myocardial regeneration. Lancet. 2003;361:45–6.
44. Steiner S, Niessner A, Ziegler S, et al. Endurance training increases the number of endothelial progenitor cells in patients with cardiovascular risk and coronary artery disease. Atherosclerosis. 2005; 181:305–10.
45. Theiss HD, David R, Engelmann MG, et al. Circulation of $CD34^+$ progenitor cell populations in patients with idiopathic dilated and ischaemic cardiomyopathy (DCM and ICM). Eur Heart J. 2007; 28:1258–64.
46. Thijssen DH, Vos JB, Verseyden C, et al. Haematopoietic stem cells and endothelial progenitor cells in healthy men: effect of aging and training. Aging Cell. 2006;5:495–503.
47. Tilling L, Chowienczyk P, Clapp B. Progenitors in motion: mechanisms of mobilization of endothelial progenitor cells. Br J Clin Pharmacol. 2009;68:484–92.
48. Valgimigli M, Rigolin GM, Cittanti C, et al. Use of granulocyte-colony stimulating factor during acute myocardial infarction to enhance bone marrow stem cell mobilization in humans: clinical and angiographic safety profile. Eur Heart J. 2005;26: 1838–45.
49. Valina C, Pinkernell K, Song Y, et al. Intracoronary administration of autologous adipose tissue-derived stem cells improves left ventricular function, perfusion, and remodelling after acute myocardial infarction. Eur Heart J. 2007;28:2667–77.
50. Wahl P, Brixius K, Bloch W. Exercise-induced stem cell activation and its implication for cardiovascular and skeletal muscle regeneration. Minim Invasive Ther Allied Technol. 2008;17:91–9.
51. Werner N, Kosiol S, Schiegl T, et al. Circulating endothelial progenitor cells and cardiovascular outcomes. N Engl J Med. 2005;353:999–1007.
52. Westenbrink BD, Lipsic E, van der Meer P, et al. Erythropoietin improves cardiac function through endothelial progenitor cell and vascular endothelial growth factor mediated neovascularization. Eur Heart J. 2007;28:2018–27.
53. Zhu L, Zhao T, Li H, et al. Neurogenesis in the adult rat brain after intermittent hypoxia. Brain Res. 2005;1055:1–6.

Index

L. Xi, T.V. Serebrovskaya (eds.), *Intermittent Hypoxia and Human Diseases*,
DOI 10.1007/978-1-4471-2906-6, © Springer-Verlag London 2012

I

MIX
Papier aus verantwortungsvollen Quellen
Paper from responsible sources
FSC® C105338

If you have any concerns about our products,
you can contact us on
ProductSafety@springernature.com

In case Publisher is established outside the EU,
the EU authorized representative is:
Springer Nature Customer Service Center GmbH
Europaplatz 3, 69115 Heidelberg, Germany

Printed by Libri Plureos GmbH
in Hamburg, Germany